Mandatory staffing

Entry into practice

Workplace violence

# PROFESSIONAL ISSUES IN NURSING

## CHALLENGES & OPPORTUNITIES

**Carol J. Huston,** RN, MSN, MPA, DPA, FAAN
*Director, School of Nursing*
California State University, Chico
Chico, California

Wolters Kluwer | Lippincott Williams & Wilkins
Health

Philadelphia · Baltimore · New York · London
Buenos Aires · Hong Kong · Sydney · Tokyo

*Acquisitions Editor:* Christina C. Burns
*Product Manager:* Paula C. Williams
*Vendor Manager:* Bridgett Dougherty
*Manufacturing Coordinator:* Karin Duffield
*Design Coordinator:* Holly McLaughlin
*Production Services:* S4Carlisle Publishing Services

Copyright © 2014 Lippincott Williams & Wilkins, a Wolters Kluwer business

351 West Camden Street       Two Commerce Square
Baltimore, MD 21201          2001 Market Street
                             Philadelphia, PA 19106

Printed in China

9 8 7 6 5 4 3 2

**Library of Congress Cataloging-in-Publication Data**
Huston, Carol Jorgensen.
    Professional issues in nursing : challenges & opportunities / Carol J. Huston. — 3rd ed.
        p. ; cm.
    Includes bibliographical references.
    ISBN 978-1-4511-2833-8
    I. Title.
    [DNLM: 1.   Nursing—trends—United States. 2.   Ethics, Nursing—United States. 3.   Nurse's Role—United
States. 4.   Nursing—manpower—United States. 5.   Professional Competence—United States.   WY 16]

    610.73—dc23
                                                                                    2012038966

CCS1213

I dedicate this book in memory of my father, Leo N. Jorgensen.
You always believed in me and supported me.
Thank you for being an amazing father and role model.

Carol Jorgensen Huston

# CONTRIBUTORS

**Marjorie Beyers,** RN, PhD, FAAN
*Consultant*
Patient Care Services
Barrington, Illinois
(CHAPTER 24)

**Rebekah Damazo,** RN, PNP, MSN
*Rural Northern California Clinical*
   *Simulation Center Project*
   *Coordinator*
*Certified Pediatric Nurse*
*Practitioner*
*Professor*
School of Nursing
California State University, Chico
Chico, California
(CHAPTER 4)

**Lynn Gallagher-Ford**, PhD, RN,
   NE-BC
*Director*
Center for Transdisciplinary
Evidence-based Practice
College of Nursing
The Ohio State University
Columbus, Ohio

**Sherry D. Fox,** RN, PhD
*Emerita Professor*
School of Nursing
California State University
Chico, California
(CHAPTER 4)

**Charmaine Hockley,** PhD, LLB,
   GDLP, RN, FACON, JP.
Charmaine Hockley & Associates
*Director*
*Workplace Relationships Consultant*
PO Box 741
Strathalbyn, South Australia 5255
AUSTRALIA
(CHAPTER 13)

**Deloras Jones,** RN, MS
*Executive Director*
California Institute for Nursing &
Health Care
Oakland, California
(CHAPTER 10)

**Jennifer Lillibridge,** PhD, RN
*Professor*
California State University, Chico
School of Nursing
Chico, California
(CHAPTER 17)

**Jeanne Madison,** PhD, RN
*Retired*
University of New England
Armidale, Australia
(CHAPTER 8)

**Kathy Malloch,** PhD, MBA, RN,
   FAAN
*President*
KMLS, LLC
*Associate Professor*
ASU College of Nursing and
Health Innovation
Phoenix, Arizona
*Clinical Consultant*
API Healthcare Inc.
Hartford, Wisconsin
(CHAPTER 3)

**Bernadette M. Melnyk,** PhD, RN,
   CPNP/PMHNP, FNAP, FAAN
*Dean*
College of Nursing
Ohio State University
Columbus, Ohio
(CHAPTER 3)

**Donna M. Nickitas,** PhD, RN,
   NEA-BC, CNE
*Professor*
Hunter College, City University of
New York Hunter-Bellevue School
of Nursing
New York, New York
(CHAPTER 23)

**Suzanne S. Prevost,** PhD, RN
*Associate Dean*
Practice and Community Engagement
College of Nursing
University of Kentucky
(CHAPTER 2)

**Margaret J. Rowberg,** DNP, APN
*Certified Adult Nurse Practitioner*
*Professor*
School of Nursing
California State University, Chico
Chico, California
(CHAPTER 22)

**Nikki West,** MPH
*Project Manager*
California Institute for Nursing &
Health Care
Oakland, California
(CHAPTER 10)

# REVIEWERS

**Lynne M. Connelly,** PhD
*Director*
Department of Nursing
Benedictine College
Atchison, Kansas

**Karla Haug,** MSN, BSN
*Assistant Professor*
North Dakota State University
Fargo, North Dakota

**Juanita Hickman,** PhD
*Associate Dean*
Cochran School of Nursing
Yonkers, New York

**Monique Mallet-Boucher,** MEd,
  MN, PhD (c)
*Senior Teach Associate*
University of New Brunswick
New Brunswick, Canada

**Jodi Orm,** MSN, CNE
*Assistant Professor*
Lake Superior State University
Sault Ste. Marie, Michigan

**Dianna Rivers,** DrPH,
  MPH/N, BSN
*Professor of Nursing*
Lamar University
Beaumont, Texas

**Karen Zapko,** MSN, PhD (c)
*Assistant Professor*
Kent State University

**Jane Leach,** PhD, RNC
*Assistant Professor*
Midwestern State University
Wichita Falls, Texas

**Ruth Schaffler,** PhD, ARNP
*Associate Professor*
Pacific Lutheran University
Parkland, Washington

**Jack Rydell,** RN, MS
*Assistant Professor*
Concordia College
Moorhead, Minnesota

**Bonnie Fuller,** PhD(c), MSN,
  RN, CNE
*Clinical Assistant Professor*
Towson University
Towson, Maryland

# PREFACE

As a nursing educator for more than 30 years, I have taught many courses dealing with the significant issues which impact the nursing profession. I often felt frustrated that textbooks that were supposed to be devoted to professional issues in the field instead deviated significantly into other areas including nursing research and theory. In addition, while many of the existing professional issues books dealt with the enduring issues of the profession, it was difficult to find a book for my students that incorporated those with the "hot topics" of the time.

The first and second editions of *Professional Issues in Nursing: Challenges & Opportunities* were efforts to address both of these needs. The third edition maintains this precedent with content updates as well as the addition of chapters on the need to develop effective leaders to meet 21st-century health care challenges for nursing as well as the use of residencies for new graduate nurses as a transition to practice. The implications of health care reform and the Institute of Medicine (IOM) recommendations noted in *The Future of Nursing: Leading Change, Advancing Health* have influenced this edition greatly.

This book continues, however, to be first and foremost a professional issues book. While an effort has been made to integrate research and theory into chapters where it seemed appropriate, these topics in and of themselves are too broad to be fully addressed in a professional issues book. This book is also directed at what I and my expert nursing colleagues have identified as both enduring professional issues and the most pressing contemporary issues facing the profession. It is my hope, then, that this book fills an unmet need in the current professional issues text market. It has an undiluted focus on professional issues in nursing and includes many timely issues not addressed in other professional issues texts. The book is edited with the primary author contributing 14 chapters and guest contributors with expertise in the specific subject material, contributing the remaining 10 chapters.

This book has been designed for use at both the baccalaureate and graduate level. It is envisioned that this book will be used as a primary textbook or as a supplement for a typical two- to three-unit professional issues course. It would also be appropriate for most RN–BSN bridge courses and may be considered by some faculty as a supplemental reader to a leadership/management course that includes professional issues.

The book can be used in both the traditional classroom and in online courses because the discussion question format works well for both small and large groups onsite as well as in bulletin board and chat room venues.

## ORGANIZATION AND FEATURES

The book is divided into five units, representing contemporary and enduring issues in professional nursing. The five sections include, Furthering the Profession, Workforce Issues, Workplace Issues, Legal and Ethical Issues, and Professional Power. Each unit has four to six chapters.

## Features

Each chapter begins with **Learning Objectives** and an overview of the professional issue being discussed. Multiple perspectives on each issue are then identified in an effort to reflect the diversity of thought found in the literature as well as espoused by experts in the field and varied professional nursing and health care organizations. **Discussion Points** encourage readers to pause and reflect on specific questions (individually or in groups), and **Consider This** features encourage active learning, critical thinking, and values clarification by the users. In addition, at least one research study is profiled in every chapter in **Research Study Fuels the Controversy** an effort to promote evidence-based analysis of the issue. Each chapter concludes with **Conclusions** about the issues discussed, questions **For Additional Discussion**, a comprehensive and current reference list, and an expansive bibliography of resources for further exploration (electronic links, news media, and print resources). Each chapter also includes multiple displays, boxes, and tables to help the user visualize important concepts.

## NEW TO THIS EDITION

- Chapters on developing effective leaders to meet 21st-century health care challenges as well as the use of residencies for new graduate nurses as a transition to practice have been added, while a chapter on blending the new essentials of baccalaureate education and distance learning education was deleted.

- New or updated content has been added throughout the book to reflect cutting-edge trends in health care including an ever-increasing demand for quality and safety in the workplace for patients as well as workers; the impact of health care reform; the IOM recommendations put forth in *The Future of Nursing: Leading Change, Advancing Health;* workforce projections and changing population demographics; and the challenges and opportunities which accompany providing nursing care in an increasingly global, rapidly changing, technology-driven world.

## TEACHING/LEARNING RESOURCES

*Professional Issues in Nursing: Challenges and Opportunities,* Third Edition, includes additional resources for both instructors and students that are available on the book's companion website at http://thePoint.lww.com/Huston3e.

### Instructor Resources

Approved adopting instructors will be given access to the following additional resources:

- Test Generator containing NCLEX-style questions
- PowerPoint Presentations
- Journal Articles
- Answers to Journal Articles Critical Thinking Questions
- Lab Activities with Answers
- Teaching/Learning Activities

### Student Resources

Students who have purchased *Professional Issues in Nursing: Challenges and Opportunities,* Third Edition, have access to the following additional resources:

- Journal Articles
- Journal Articles Critical Thinking Questions
- Spanish—English Audio Glossary
- Learning Objectives

In addition, purchasers of the text can access the searchable full text online by going to the *Professional Issues in Nursing: Challenges and Opportunities,* Third Edition, website at http://thePoint.lww.com/Huston3e. See inside the front cover of this text for more details, including the passcode you will need to gain access to the website.

*Carol J. Huston, RN, MSN, MPA, DPA, FAAN*

# CONTENTS

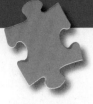

## V. PROFESSIONAL POWER

# Unit 1

# Furthering the Profession

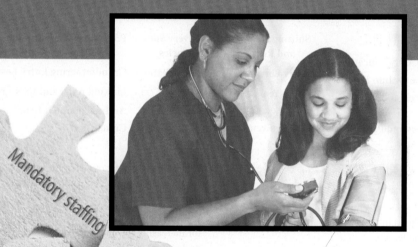

Mandatory staffing

Workplace violence

Entry into practice

Chapter **1**

# Entry Into Practice
## *The Debate Rages On*

Carol J. Huston

## ADDITIONAL RESOURCES

Visit thePoint for additional helpful resources
- eBook
- Journal Articles
- WebLinks

## CHAPTER OUTLINE

## LEARNING OBJECTIVES

*The learner will be able to:*

1. Differentiate between technical and professional nurses as outlined in Esther Lucille Brown's classic *Nursing for the Future.*

2. Identify what if any progress has been made on increasing the educational entry level for professional registered nursing since publication of the 1965 position paper of the American Nurses Association on entry into practice.

3. Identify similarities and differences between contemporary associate and baccalaureate degree nursing programs.

4. Describe basic components of associate degree educational programs as outlined by Mildred Montag and compare those with typical associate degree programs in the 21st century.

5. Analyze how having one NCLEX for entry into practice, regardless of educational entry level, impacts the entry-into-practice dilemma.

6. Identify key driving and restraining forces for increasing the educational entry level for professional nursing.

7. Analyze the potential impacts of raising the educational entry level on the current nursing shortage, workforce diversity, and intraprofession conflict.

8. Examine current evidence-based research that explores the impact of registered nurse educational level on patient outcomes.

9. Explore how shifting health care delivery sites and increasing registered nursing competency requirements are impacting employer preferences for hiring a more educated nursing workforce.

10. Compare the nursing profession's educational entry standards with that of the other health care professions.

11. Identify positions taken by specific professional organizations, certifying bodies and employers

regarding the appropriate educational level for entry into practice for professional nursing.

12. Explore personal values, beliefs, and feelings regarding whether the educational entry level in nursing should be increased to a baccalaureate or higher degree.

Few issues have been as long-standing or as contentious in nursing as the entry-into-practice debate. Taylor (2008) agrees, suggesting that "the issues surrounding entry into practice have been a rock in the shoe of nursing for many years" (p. 611). Although the entry-into-practice debate dates back to the 1940s with the publication of Esther Lucille Brown's classic *Nursing for the Future*, the debate came to the forefront with a 1965 position paper by the American Nurses Association (ANA, 1965a, 1965b). This position paper suggested an orderly transition from hospital-based diploma nursing preparation to nursing education in colleges or universities based on the following premises:

- The education of all those who are licensed to practice nursing should take place in institutions of higher education.

- Minimum preparation for beginning professional nursing practice should be baccalaureate education in nursing.

- Minimum preparation for beginning technical practice should be associate education in nursing.

- Education for assistants in the health care occupations should be short, intensive, preservice programs in vocational education institutions rather than on-the-job training programs.

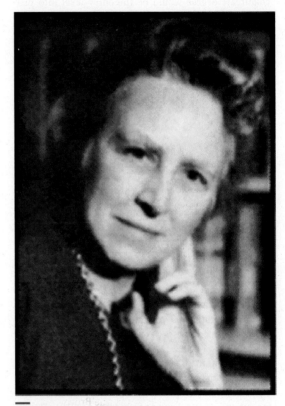

**Figure 1.1** Mildred Montag.

In essence, two levels of preparation were suggested for registered nurses (RNs): *technical* and *professional*. Persons interested in technical practice would enroll in junior or community colleges and earn associate degrees in 2-year programs. Those interested in professional nursing would enroll in 4-year programs in colleges or universities. Hospital-based diploma programs were to be phased out.

The curriculums for the two programs were to be very different, as were each program's foci. The 2-year technical degree was to result in an associate degree in nursing (ADN). This degree, as proposed by Mildred Montag (Fig. 1.1) in her dissertation in 1952, with direction and support from R. Louise McManus, would prepare a beginning, technical

practitioner who would provide care in acute care settings, under the supervision of a professional nurse.

In a typical associate degree program, approximately half of the credits would be fulfilled by general education courses such as English, anatomy, physiology, speech, psychology, and sociology and the other half were fulfilled by nursing courses. The 4-year degree would result in a bachelor of science in nursing (BSN) and would encompass coursework taught in ADN programs as well as more in-depth treatment of the physical and social sciences, nursing research, public and community health, nursing management, and the humanities. The additional course work in the BSN was intended to enhance the students' professional development, prepare them for a broader scope of practice, and provide a better understanding of the cultural, political, economic, and social issues affecting patients and health care delivery.

The ANA 1965 position statement was reaffirmed by a resolution at the ANA House of Delegates in 1978, which set forth the requirement that the baccalaureate degree would be the entry level into professional nursing practice by 1985. Associate degree and diploma programs responded strongly to what they viewed as inflammatory terminology and clearly stated that not being considered "professional" was unacceptable. In the end, both ADN and diploma programs refused to compromise title or licensure. Dissension ensued both within and among nursing groups, but little movement occurred to make the position statement a reality.

> CONSIDER THIS  Titling (professional vs. technical) was and will be an important consideration before consensus can be reached on the entry-into-practice debate.

Finally in 2008, 30 years later, the ANA House of Delegates stepped forth once again to pass a resolution supporting initiatives to require diploma and associate degree educated nurses to obtain a BSN within 10 years of license (Starr & Edwards, 2010). Requiring a return to school within 10 years after graduation supports the view that nursing is constantly changing and that education and knowledge are needed to appropriately care for patients today (Lane & Kohlenberg, 2010). The responsibility for mandating and implementing this new resolution was passed on to individual states.

Just one state, however, North Dakota, became successful in changing the nurse practice act so that baccalaureate education was necessary for RN licensure. For 15 years, it was the only state to recognize baccalaureate education as the minimal education for profesional nursing, despite challenges from opposing groups. Smith (2010) suggests this occurred because the public perceived a true sense of unity and dedication to the cause and the interest groups representing the health care industry were no match for the positive public opinion generated by the unity within the nursing community. Unfortunately, however, North Dakota repealed this act in 2003, bowing to pressure from nurses and some health care organizations, to once again allowing nonbaccalaureate entry into practice.

Other states, however, continue to consider increasing educational entry levels. California, for example, requires a BSN for certification as a public health nurse in that state, and multiple states require a BSN to be a school nurse because that is considered to be a part of public health nursing. In addition, state nursing associations or other nursing coalitions in California, New York, Rhode Island, and New Jersey have, over the past few years, called for initiatives to establish the BSN as the entry level for nursing in their respective state. These initiatives have either stalled or met such resistance that they have been discarded. In addition, Boyd (2011) notes that as many as 18 states are currently preparing some type of initiative requiring newly graduated RNs to obtain a BSN within a certain time frame in order to maintain their licensure.

The end result is that almost 60 years after the initial ANA resolution, entry into practice at the baccalaureate level has not been accomplished. Even the strongest supporters of the BSN for entry into practice cannot deny that despite almost six decades of efforts, RN entry at the baccalaureate level continues to be an elusive goal.

## PROLIFERATION OF ADN EDUCATION

It is doubtful that Mildred Montag had any idea in 1952 that ADN programs would someday become the predominant entry level for nursing practice or that this education model would proliferate like it did in the 1960s—just one decade after she completed her doctoral work. While the overwhelming majority of nurses in the early 1960s were educated in diploma schools of nursing, enrollment in baccalaureate programs was increasing and associate degree programs were just beginning. By the year 2000, diploma education had virtually disappeared, and although BSN education had increased significantly, it was ADN education which represented nearly two thirds of all nursing school graduates.

Indeed, ADN education continues to be the primary model for initial nursing education in the United States today. As of 2009, 59% of nurses initially graduate from associate degree programs, followed by baccalaureate programs (37%), and then diploma programs (4%) (Johnston, 2009).

Yet enrollment in baccalaureate nursing programs is also on the rise, increasing by 6.1% from 2009 to 2010, marking the 10th consecutive year of enrollment growth

(The American Nurse, 2011). The American Association of Colleges of Nursing (AACN, 2011a) states that as of 2008, 50.0% of the RN workforce holds a baccalaureate or graduate degree whereas 36.1% earned an associate degree and 13.9% a diploma in nursing. The greatest increase appears to be in graduate degree program enrollment with nursing schools with master's programs reporting a 9.6% increase in enrollment (409 schools reporting) and a 10.5% increase in graduations (380 schools reporting; AACN, 2009).

## LICENSURE AND ENTRY INTO PRACTICE

Critics of BSN as a requirement for entry into practice argue that there is no need to raise entry levels because passing rates for the National Council Licensure Examination (NCLEX) show no significant differences between ADN, diploma, and BSN graduates (Table 1.1). Although some might argue that this suggests similar competencies across the educational spectrum, the more common precept is that the NCLEX is a test that measures minimum technical competencies for safe entry into basic nursing practice and, as such, may not measure performance over time or test for all of the knowledge and skills developed through a BSN program. One must also ask why the nursing profession has not differentiated RN licensure testing based on educational preparation for RNs, just as has been done for practical nurses, RNs, and advanced practice nurses.

> ### DISCUSSION POINT
>
> Should separate licensing examinations be developed for ADN-, diploma-, and BSN-educated nurses?

Complicating the picture is that both ADN and BSN schools preparing graduates for RN licensure meet similar criteria for state board approval and have roughly the same number of nursing coursework units. All of these factors contribute to confusion about differentiations between ADN- and BSN-prepared nurses and result in an inability to move forward on implementing the BSN as the entry level for professional nursing.

> CONSIDER THIS   Critics of BSN entry into practice argue that ADN-, diploma-, and BSN-educated nurses all take the same licensing examination and therefore have earned the title of RN. In addition, nurses prepared at all three levels have successfully worked side by side, under the same scope of practice, for more than 50 years.

Research also suggests that there are differences in the demographics of BSN and ADN graduates. Sexton, Hunt, Cox, Teasley, and Carroll's (2008) study of more than 5,000 nurses found that the BSN nurses in their convenience sampling were younger than the ADN-educated nurses, with 28% of the baccalaureate-educated nurses being born in or after 1980 as compared to 13% of the associate degree nurses. It is also generally believed that ADN graduates represent greater diversity in race, gender, age, and educational experiences than BSN-prepared nurses. Critics of the BSN requirement for entry into professional nursing suggest that greater diversity is needed in nursing, and this may be lost if entry levels are raised.

In addition, many employers state they are unable to differentiate roles for nurses based on education because both ADN- and BSN-prepared nurses hold the same license. Ironically, state boards of nursing have asserted their inability to develop a different licensure system given the fact that employers have not developed different roles.

Furthermore, many employers provide no incentives for BSN education in terms of pay, recognition, or career mobility and are afraid to do so, fearing they may be unable

**TABLE 1.1   2010 NCLEX-RN Passage Rate per Educational Program Type**

| Program Type | Number of Graduates | NCLEX-RN Passage Rate |
|---|---|---|
| Diploma | 3,753 | 89.66% |
| Associate degree | 81,618 | 86.46% |
| Baccalaureate degree | 55,414 | 88.69% |

*Source:* National Council of State Boards of Nursing. (2011). *NCLEX examiniation pass rates*. Retrieved February 5, 2011, from https://www.ncsbn.org/Table_of_Pass_Rates_2010.pdf

to fill vacant nursing positions. The starting rate of pay for ADN- and BSN-prepared nurses historically has not been significantly different, although this appears to be changing.

Finally, some empassioned supporters of maintaining ADN education as the entry level for nursing practice argue that associate degrees allow students to graduate in a shorter amount of time so that they can support their family and that the cost of baccalaureate education would be cost or time prohibitive to many working students with families (Moltz, 2010).

## EDUCATIONAL LEVELS
## AND PATIENT OUTCOMES

Perhaps the most common argument against raising the entry level in nursing is an emotional one, with ADN-prepared nurses arguing that "caring does not require a baccalaureate degree." Many ADN-educated nurses argue passionately that patients do not know or care what educational degree is held by their nurse as long as they receive high-quality care by the nurse at their bedside. ADN nurses also frequently claim that BSN-prepared nurses are too theoretically oriented and thus are not in touch with real practice. In addition, many ADN nurses suggest baccalaureate-prepared nurses are deficient in basic skills mastery and conclude that care provided by ADN nurses is at least as good as, if not better than, that provided by their BSN counterparts. This was supported in research completed by Rosenfeld, Chaya, Lewis-Holman, and Davin (2010), which suggested that the performance of ADN and BSN nursing graduates, working as interns

with the Visiting Nurse Service of New York, was comparable (see Research Study Fuels the Controversy 1.1).

---

CONSIDER THIS   Most ADN-prepared nurses argue that significant differences exist between their practice and that of a licensed vocational/practical nurse (LVN/LPN), despite there typically being only 12 months difference in length of educational preparation. Yet many ADN-educated nurses argue that the additional education that BSN-educated nurses have makes little difference in their practice over that of their ADN counterparts. How can this argument be justified?

---

An increasing number of studies, however, report differences between the performance levels of ADN- and BSN-prepared nurses. In a landmark 2003 study, Linda Aiken and her colleagues at the University of Pennsylvania identified a clear link between higher levels of nursing education and better patient outcomes (AACN, 2011b). This study found that surgical patients have a 'substantial survival advantage' if treated in hospitals with higher proportions of nurses educated at the baccalaureate or higher degree level and that a 10% increase in the proportion of nurses holding BSN degrees decreased the risk of patient death and failure to rescue by 5% (AACN, 2011b).

Research by Aiken and colleagues also showed that hospitals with better care environments, the best nurse staffing levels, and the most highly educated nurses had the lowest surgical mortality rates. In fact, the researchers found

## RESEARCH STUDY FUELS THE CONTROVERSY 1.1

### COMPARING BSN AND ADN GRADUATES IN AN INTERNSHIP

This quasi-experimental study compared ADN and BSN nursing graduates, working as interns with the Visiting Nurse Service of New York, in terms of their retention in the internship, clinical thinking, assessment skills, productivity, and intention to remain in nursing. Data were collected at pre- and postintervention intervals.

Rosenfeld, P., Chaya, J., Lewis-Holman, S., & Davin, D. (2010). Can an ADN internship program prepare new RNs for careers in home health care nursing? Findings from an evaluation study at visiting nurse service of New York. *Home Health Care Management & Practice, 22*(4), 254–261.

### STUDY FINDINGS

Findings revealed few significant differences between the ADN and BSN interns, suggesting that with competitive recruitment, appropriate support, and supplementary training, ADN interns can perform on par with their BSN counterparts. The small number of participants in the internship programs was identified as a significant limitation to the study findings.

## RESEARCH STUDY FUELS THE CONTROVERSY 1.2

### EFFECT OF EDUCATION ON PATIENT OUTCOMES

Data from 10,184 nurses and 232,342 surgical patients in 168 Pennsylvania provided stinging evidence that educational entry level makes a difference in patient outcomes.

Aiken, L., Clarke, S. P., Sloane, D. M., Lake, E. T., & Cheney, T. (2008). Effects of hospital care environment on patient mortality and nurse outcomes. *Journal of Nursing Administration, 38*(5), 223–229.

### STUDY FINDINGS

This study found that patients experienced significantly lower mortality and failure to rescue rates in hospitals where more highly educated nurses were providing direct patient care. Nurses reported more positive job experiences and fewer concerns with care quality, and patients had significantly lower risks of death and failure to rescue in hospitals with better care environments.

---

that every 10% increase in the proportion of BSN nurses on the hospital staff was associated with a 4% decrease in the risk of death (Aiken, Clarke, Sloane, Lake, & Cheney, 2008; see Research Study Fuels the Controversy 1.2).

As more outcome research becomes available suggesting an empirical link between educational entry level of nurses and patient outcomes, nursing leaders, professional associations, and employers are increasingly speaking out on the need to raise the profession's entry level as a means of improving quality patient care and patient safety. Lane and Kohlenberg (2010, p. 220), concur, arguing that the role of the nurse is changing with the transformation of health care, yet despite the benefits of better patient outcomes and the potential to expand the discipline of nursing, the typical level of education for nurses remains the same.

Patricia Benner, director of a recent landmark Carnegie study on nursing, professor emerita at the University of California at San Francisco School of Nursing, and a former graduate of an ADN program, concurs, asserting that "I'm not against community college nursing programs, and this is not a diatribe against community colleges. But something is out of whack when students get a degree that doesn't allow them to go on to advanced practice. It's just not adequate to meet current demands" (Moltz, 2010, para. 6).

Ward-Smith (2011) agrees, suggesting that as frontline providers, nurses are critical to changing the health care environment but questions how a nurse educated at the ADN or diploma level can be expected to be capable of providing the same level of care as a nurse with a BSN. She points out that the October 2010 Institute of Medicine (IOM) report, *The Future of Nursing* (IOM, 2010), suggests that RNs are expected to coordinate care with other health care professionals, such as pharmacists and physical, occupation, and speech therapists, most of whom have master's or doctoral degrees. She argues that such a situation appears to set the ADN or diploma-educated nurse up to fail, since it seems unlikely that these skills can be taught in a 2 or 3-year educational process.

## EMPLOYERS' VIEWS AND PREFERENCES

Nursing employers are divided on the issue of entry into practice. The academic requirements of associate degree, diploma, and baccalaureate programs vary widely, yet health care settings that employ nursing graduates often make no distinction in the scope of practice among nurses who have different levels of preparation.

Employers, however, appear to be increasingly aware of purported differences between BSN and ADN graduates, and this is increasingly being reflected in their hiring preferences. In addition, some employers are now giving preference for clinical placements to students in baccalaureate and higher degree programs over those enrolled in associate degree programs.

Nickitas (2010) makes an empassioned plea to nurse executives, nurse managers, and nurse academics to strongly encourage RNs to advance their careers. She suggests that entry-level employers have an obligation to make a clear case for educational advancement to the baccalaureate degree and then for the graduate degree. Indeed, many more position descriptions for nursing managers and administrators now require or at least prefer a BSN degree. In addition, magnet hospitals are required to have a higher percentage of nurses educated at the baccalaureate level.

**DISCUSSION POINT**

If indeed employers prefer hiring BSN-prepared RNs, why don't more employers offer pay differentials for nurses with BSN degrees?

The Veterans Administration (VA), with its 35,000 nurses on staff, is leading the nation in raising the bar for a higher educational entry hire level in nursing. The VA established the BSN as the minimum education level for new hires and required all nonentry-level nurses have at least a BSN by 2005. A 2009 VA description of hiring programs and incentives suggests that VA nurses who want to advance beyond Nurse Level 1 must earn a BSN degree (U.S. Department of Veterans Affairs, 2009). As the nation's largest employer of RNs, the VA committed US$50 million over a 5-year period to help VA nurses obtain baccalaureate or higher nursing degrees (AACN, 2011b). In addition, the U.S. Army, Navy, and Air Force require the baccalaureate degree for active duty as an RN, and the U.S. Public Health Service requires the baccalaureate degree in nursing for a nurse to be a commissioned officer (Johnston, 2009).

## SHIFTING HEALTH CARE DELIVERY SITES AND REQUIRED COMPETENCIES

Although hospitals continue to be the main site of employment for nurses, there is an ongoing shift in health care from acute-care settings to the community and integrated health care settings. This shift will clearly require more highly educated nurses who can function autonomously as care givers, leaders, managers, and change agents. These are all skills which are emphasized in a baccaluareate nursing curriculum.

CONSIDER THIS    Baccalaureate and graduate-level skills in research, leadership, management, and community health are increasingly needed in nursing as health care extends beyond the acute care hospital.

Ellenbecker (2010) concurs, arguing that we are not preparing nurses with the right skills to fully participate in a reformed health care system or for the workforce of the future. "Today's environment of expanding knowledge, the call for interdisciplinary healthcare delivery teams, and evidence of the relationship between nurse education and improved patient outcomes strongly indicate the need for nurses prepared at the baccalaureate level. Requiring a baccalaureate degree for entry into nursing practice, and as the initial degree of nursing education would prepare nurses earlier for graduate education and the much needed roles of educator, researcher and advanced practice nurse" (Ellenbecker, 2010).

In May 2010, the Tri-Council for Nursing, a coalition of four steering organizations for the nursing profession (AACN, ANA, the American Organization of Nurse Executives [AONE], and the National League for Nursing [NLN]), issued a consensus statement calling for all RNs to advance their education in the interest of enhancing quality and safety across health care settings. The statement suggested that a more highly educated nursing workforce will be critical to meeting the nation's nursing needs and delivering safe, effective patient care and that failure to do so will place the nation's health at further risk (AACN, 2012).

The recommendations of the IOM (2010) report, *The Future of Nursing*, were even stronger. This landmark report called for increasing the number of baccalaureate-prepared nurses in the workforce from 50% to 80% over the next 10 years and doubling the population of nurses with doctorates to meet the demands of an evolving health care system and changing patient needs.

In addition, in December 2009, Patricia Benner and her team at the Carnegie Foundation for the Advancement of Teaching released a new study titled *Educating Nurses: A Call for Radical Transformation*, which recommended preparing all entry-level RNs at the baccalaureate level and requiring all RNs to earn a master's degree within 10 years of initial licensure (Benner, Sutphen, Leonard, & Day, 2010). The authors found that many of today's new nurses are "undereducated" to meet practice demands across settings. Their strong support for high-quality baccalaureate degree programs as the appropriate pathway for RNs entering the profession is consistent with the views of many leading nursing organizations, including AACN (AACN, 2011b).

Similarly, the National Advisory Council on Nurse Education and Practice (NACNEP) suggests that nursing's role for the future calls for RNs to manage care along a continuum, to work as peers in interdisciplinary teams, and to integrate clinical expertise with knowledge of community resources. This increased complexity of scope of practice will require the capacity to adapt to change; critical thinking and problem-solving skills; a social foundation in a broad range of basic sciences; knowledge of behavioral, social, and management sciences; and the ability to analyze and communicate data

(AACN, 2011b). All these are integral components of BSN education. As a result, NACNEP has recommended to Congress that at least two thirds of the nurse workforce hold baccalaureate or higher degrees in nursing by 2010 (AACN, 2011a).

The Council on Physician and Nurse Supply also released a statement in 2007 calling for a national effort to substantially expand baccalaureate nursing programs, citing the growing body of evidence that nursing education impacts both the quality and safety of patient care. Consequently, the group is calling on policy makers to shift federal funding priorities in favor of supporting more baccalaureate-level nursing programs (AACN, 2011b). Some nurse leaders have even suggested that a BSN degree may not be an adequate preparation for these expanded roles and that, instead, master's or doctoral degrees should be required for entry into practice for registered nursing.

> ### DISCUSSION POINT
>
> Would raising the entry level to the master's or doctoral degree eliminate the tension between supporters of ADN and BSN as entry levels into nursing, since both educational preparations would be considered inadequate? Is a graduate degree currently feasible as the entry level for professional nursing? If not, what would it take to make it happen?

## ENTRY LEVEL AND PROFESSIONAL STATUS

Nurses, consumers, and allied health care professionals are currently questioning why the entry level into professional nursing is so much lower than other health care professions. Does nursing require less skill? Is the knowledge base needed to provide nursing care skill based instead of knowledge based? Should nursing be reclassified as a vocational trade and not a profession? The answer to these questions, of course, is no. Yet clearly, nurses have resisted the normal course of occupational development that other health care professions have pursued. As a result, nurses are now the least educated of the health care professionals, with most health care professions now requiring graduate degrees for entry. Indeed, one must question whether nursing is at risk for losing its designation as a profession because of its failure to maintain educational equity.

The primary identity of any professional group is based on the established education entry level. Attorneys, physicians, social workers, engineers, clergy, and physical therapists, to list a few examples, have in common an essential education at the bachelor's level. Nursing is unique among the health care professions in having multiple educational pathways lead to the same entry level license to practice. In fact, advanced degrees are required in many professions for entry positions at the professional level. Only nursing continues the hypocrisy of pretending that education is unimportant and does not make a difference. Only nursing allows individuals with no college course work, or with limited college study that lacks a well-rounded global college education, to lay claim to the same licensure and identity as that held by nurses having a baccalaureate education.

Indeed, the educational gap between nursing and other health professions continues to grow (Table 1.2). Disciplines such as occupational therapy, physical therapy, speech therapy, and social work all require master's or doctoral degrees. Pharmacy has also raised its educational standards to that of a doctoral degree.

| TABLE 1.2 Entry Level Degrees for the Health Professions | |
| --- | --- |
| **Health Profession** | **Entry-Level Degree** |
| Medicine | Doctorate |
| Pharmacy | Doctorate |
| Social work | Master's |
| Speech pathology | Master's |
| Physical therapy | Master's transitioning to doctorate |
| Occupational therapy | Master's |
| Nursing | Associate |

CONSIDER THIS  Unlike the other health care professions which now require master's and doctoral degrees, nursing continues to put forth an argument that educational degree does not matter or that requiring a BSN for entry into practice is elitist.

## DISCUSSION POINT

Is nursing in danger of losing its designation as a "profession" if it fails to maintain educational entry levels comparable to those of the other health professions?

## DISCUSSION POINT

Should licensure be equated with professional status?

Failure to maintain educational parity with other health care professions also contributes to nursing being viewed as a "second-class citizen" in the health care arena. It is difficult to justify the profession's argument that nursing should be an equal partner in health care decision making when other professions are so much better educated, suggesting that nurses are either under-educated for the roles they assume or that the nursing role lacks complexity.

CONSIDER THIS  Nursing is the only health care "profession" that does not require at least a bachelor's or higher degree for entry into practice.

## THE 2-YEAR ADN PROGRAM?

Many ADN-prepared nurses also express frustration when discussing the need to raise the entry level in professional nursing because they feel the ADN degree does not appropriately represent the scope of their education or the time they had to put in to earn what is typically considered to be a 2-year degree. ADN nurses argue that the "2-year" ADN program is a myth. Many ADN students follow nontraditional education paths, and almost all ADN programs currently require 3 or more years of education, not 2, with a minimum of 12 to 24 months of prerequisites and a full 2 years of nursing education. Most associate's degrees require approximately 60 semester units or 90 quarter units of coursework although there is a great deal of variance with some programs now requiring more than 70 semester units and over 100 quarter units.

CONSIDER THIS  The 2-year ADN program is a myth.

Indeed, it is almost impossible to graduate from an ADN program in less than 3 years and often 4 or more years are required to complete the general education, prerequisite, and nursing requirements. Given that most BSN programs require approximately 120 semester units for graduation, the question must be asked whether requiring so many units at the associate degree level, without granting the upper division credit that could lead to a BSN degree, is an injustice to ADN graduates. Patricia Benner goes so far as to suggest that "if the baccalaureate were made the minimum requirement for entrance into the field, then community college programs would at least have to be more honest about how much time it takes students to get through their programs and how much opportunity cost is there for them" (Moltz, 2010, para. 4).

This addition of units and extension of educational time in ADN programs has generally been attributed to the need to respond to a changing job market; that is, the need to prepare ADNs to work in more diverse environments (nonhospital) and to increasingly assume positions requiring management skills. While Montag clearly intended a differentiation between level of education and level of practice between ADN- and BSN-prepared nurses, many ADN programs have added leadership, management, research, and home health and community health courses to their curriculums in the past two decades.

One must ask then what part of the associate degree curriculum should be cut to add these new experiences. What should the balance be between community and acute-care experiences in ADN programs? How much management content do ADN nurses need and what roles will they be expected to assume? If no content is deleted from the ADN programs to accommodate the new content, how can ADN education reasonably be completed within a 2-year framework?

Montag expressed concern that when ADN programs add content inappropriate for technical practice, appropriate content may have to be deleted to maintain the estimated time for completion. The question that follows then is, If ADN education now incorporates much of what was meant to be BSN content, and if the time needed to complete this education is near that of a bachelor's degree, why are ADN graduates being given associate degrees, which reflect expertise in technical practice, rather than BSN degrees, which reflect achievement of these higher-level competencies?

## SHORTAGES AND ENTRY-LEVEL REQUIREMENTS

Whenever there are shortages, legislators and workforce experts suggest a need to reexamine or reduce educational requirements. Indeed, Montag's original project to create ADN education was directed at reducing the workforce shortage of nurses that existed at that time, by reducing the length of the education process to 2 years. Clearly, the immediate short-term threat of raising the entry level to the bachelor's degree may be to exacerbate predicted nursing shortages. In the long run, however, raising the entry level may elevate the public image of nursing and increase recruitment to the field since the best and the brightest may seek professions with greater academic prestige.

In addition, raising the entry level may impact retention rates in nursing. Research suggests that nurses who have a BSN are more likely to report higher job satisfaction scores in relation to opportunities for growth and remain in practice longer (Starr & Edwards, 2010).

Having more BSN nurses may actually then stabilize the nursing workforce as a result of their higher levels of job satisfaction, a key to nurse retention.

> CONSIDER THIS   The impact of raising the entry level in nursing to the baccalaureate level on the current nursing shortage is not known.

The other reality is that a chronic shortage of nursing personnel has persisted despite the proliferation of ADN programs. This negates the argument that the current nursing shortage should be used as an excuse for postponing action to raise educational standards. A nursing shortage existed at the time of the 1965 ANA proposal and has occurred intermittently since that time. Clearly, nursing has been swept along by a host of social, economic, and educational circumstances that have little to do with nursing or the clients we serve. Perhaps, then, the decision to raise the entry-to-practice level in nursing should be made because it is the right and necessary thing to do and not as a result of the influence of external communities of interest.

Taylor (2008) agrees, going so far as to suggest that as a result of research that clearly shows a link between nurse's educational entry level and patient outcomes, "employers who hire nurses with less than a bachelor's degree are doing their patients a disservice" (p. 4). He goes on to say that "the nursing shortage should not be an excuse to push for the continuance of associate degree programs only to graduate more nurses to fill the ever-increasing number of positions nationwide."

> CONSIDER THIS   Nurses, professional health care and nursing organizations, credentialing programs, and employers are divided on the entry-into-practice issue.

Debate over entry into practice is as varied among professional health care and nursing organizations, credentialing programs, and employers as it is among individual nurses. Getting support for the BSN as the entry-level requirement for nursing will be difficult because the overwhelming majority of nurses are currently ADN prepared and there are inadequate workplace incentives to increase entry requirements to the BSN degree.

## PROFESSIONAL ORGANIZATIONS, UNIONS, AND ADVISORY BODIES SPEAK OUT

Not surprisingly, a 2006 position statement issued by the NOADN (2011a) on entry into practice reaffirms the role and value of associate degree nursing education and practice. The position statement suggests that graduates of ADN programs are professional nurses who are essential members of the interdisciplinary health care team, that these nurses are prepared to function in diverse health care settings, and that associate degree education provides a dynamic pathway for entry into professional RN practice. A follow-up position statement issued by the NOADN in 2008 goes on to say that a BSN should not be required for continued practice beyond initial licensure as an RN and that the choice to pursue further education should remain the choice of each ADN graduate based on his or her personal preferences and professional career goals (NOADN, 2008, 2011b).

Similarly, the position of the NLN, the national voice for nurse educators in all types of nursing education programs, has historically been that the nursing profession should have multiple entry points (NLN, 2007). As such, the NLN suggests that instead of investing energy debating entry into the profession, the focus should turn toward opportunities for lifelong learning and progression for those who enter the nursing profession through diploma and associate degree programs.

In addition, the Nurse Alliance of the Service Employees International Union (SEIU) Healthcare, an organization of 85,000 RNs, has firmly rejected any bill that would limit entry into or maintenance of practice to the BSN, arguing this would only exacerbate the current nursing shortage (SEIU, 2008). Instead, they argue that more resources must be made available to support nursing education at all levels, to give academic credit for work experience, to provide workplace support for nurses who wish to return to school, and to develop more online and hybrid programs for nurses who cannot attend traditional on-site classes to advance their education.

An increasing number of professional nursing organizations, however, are now supporting the BSN requirement for entry into professional nursing. The ANA, however, is no longer the standard bearer in this effort. Instead, organizations such as the AACN, the National Association of Neonatal Nurses (NANN), the American Nephrology Nurses' Association (ANNA), the Association of Operating Room Nurses (AORN), and the AONE have published position statements supporting BSN entry.

For example, the AACN suggests that the primary pathway for entry into professional-level nursing, as compared to technical-level practice, is a 4-year bachelor of science degree in nursing (BSN). NANN issued its position statement in 2009, arguing that "the increasing acuity of patients and their more complex needs for care in community and home settings demand a higher level of educational preparation for nurses than was necessary in the past" (NANN, 2009, para. 1).

AORN has also supported the baccalaureate degree for entry into nursing since 1979. AORN's current position statement on entry into practice reaffirms its belief that there should be one level for entry into nursing practice and that the minimal preparation for future entry into the practice of nursing should be the baccalaureate degree (AORN, 2011). In 2004, the AONE also published guiding principles suggesting that "the educational preparation of the nurse of the future should be at the baccalaureate level."

The National Advisory Council on Nurse Education and Practice, which advises the Secretary of the U.S. Department of Health and Human Services and the U.S. Congress on policy issues related to nurse workforce supply, education, and practice improvement, also urged in 2007 that a minimum of two thirds of working nurses hold baccalaureate or higher degrees in nursing by 2010 (AACN, 2012). Yet federal and state regulation of entry into practice has, for the most part, not occurred.

## GRANDFATHERING ENTRY LEVELS

Traditionally, when a state licensure law is enacted, or when a current law is repealed and a new law enacted, a process called "grandfathering" occurs. Grandfathering allows individuals to continue to practice his or her profession or occupation despite new qualifications having been enacted into law. Should the entry-level requirement for nursing be raised to a bachelor's or higher degree, debate will undoubtedly occur as to how and when grandfathering should be applied.

> **CONSIDER THIS**  "Grandfathering" current ADN nurses as professional nurses would smooth political tensions between current educational entry levels but threatens the essence of the goal.

Several professional organizations have actively advocated that all RNs should be grandfathered if the entry level is raised. Other professional organizations have argued that it should not occur at all. Still others believe that grandfathering should be conditional. For example, all RNs licensed at the time of the law would be allowed to retain their current title for a certain time, but would be required to return to school to increase their educational preparation if it did not meet the new entry level.

## LINKING ADN AND BSN PROGRAMS

Returning to school, unfortunately, is not part of the career path for most nurses, which makes the entry level even more important. Starr and Edwards (2010) suggest that many nurses who have been out of school for some time relate they are intimidated by the thought of going back to school, fearing they will be unsuccessful in the academic setting.

McGrath (2008) suggests that many nonbaccalaureate RNs do not even consider returning to school. They question why anyone would want to do that, what it would get them, what impact it would have on their family, and what resources would be needed to do so. In addition, she notes that while employers prefer baccalaureate-educated nurses, they may overtly or covertly discourage the RNs from returning to school for fear they might "lose their best staff nurses" to other institutions or other areas of nursing (p. 88).

McGrath (2008) goes on to say that cost is frequently perceived as the chief obstacle to obtaining advanced education. Given that many practicing nurses are in their 40s, there are appropriate concerns regarding the cost–benefit of returning to school. In addition, younger nurses considering a return to school are often advised to get more clinical experience in a specialty area first. This kind of thinking is unique to nursing as most professions encourage more education as soon as possible for their best and brightest.

These same concerns were cited by Megginson (2008), who found that approximately 70% of practicing RNs in the United States are educated at the associate degree or diploma level and only 15% ever move on to achieve a higher degree. Using phenomenological inquiry via focus group interviews, Megginson found that barriers for return to school included (1) time; (2) fear; (3) lack of recognition for past educational and life accomplishments; (4) equal treatment of BSN, ASN, and diploma RNs; and (5) negative ASN or diploma school experience. Incentives to return to school for RNs included (1) being at the right time in life, (2) working with options, (3) achieving a personal goal, (4) being provided with a credible professional identity, (5) encouragement from contemporaries, and (6) user-friendly RN-to-BSN programs.

Currently, more than 630 RN-to-BSN programs nationally build on the education provided in diploma and ADN programs, including more than 390 programs that are offered at least partially online (AACN, 2011a). In addition, 160 RN-to-master's degree programs are available which cover the baccalaureate content missing in the other entry-level programs as well as graduate-level course work (AACN, 2011a).

In addition, statewide articulation agreements exist in many states, including Florida, California, Connecticut, Arkansas, Texas, Iowa, Maryland, South Carolina, Idaho, Alabama, and Nevada, to facilitate credit transfer from community colleges to universities with BSN programs.

Unfortunately, however, sometimes there is little integration, standardization, or cooperation between

> **CONSIDER THIS** A broad new system, composed of direct transfer, linkage, and partnership programs, is needed between community college and baccalaureate institutions to ensure a smooth transition from ADN to BSN as the entry-level requirement for professional nursing practice. This transition will be costly.

public systems of education. Such integration, standardization, and cooperation will be essential for transition to BSN entry levels. This is why one of the key recommendations in *The Future of Nursing* was that all nursing schools should offer defined academic pathways that promote seamless access for nurses to higher levels of education (IOM, 2010). Transition programs or services for non-baccalaureate-prepared nurses must be designed, which facilitate entry into baccalaureate and advanced education and practice programs. In addition, funding must continue to be increased for colleges and universities sponsoring baccalaureate and advanced practice nursing education programs.

Clearly, barriers for educational reentry must be removed if the educational entry level in nursing is to be raised to a bachelor's or higher degree. Alternative pathways for RN education must be developed to create opportunities for learners who might not otherwise be able to pursue additional nursing education.

Finally, raising the entry level in professional nursing practice will be costly. University education simply costs more than education at community colleges and significant increases in federal and state funding for baccalaureate and graduate nursing education will need to occur. Given the significant budget deficit currently faced by almost all states, the likelihood of funding increases for nursing education is directly related to the public and legislative understanding of the complexity of roles nurses assume each and every day and the educational level they perceive is needed to accomplish these tasks.

## AN INTERNATIONAL ISSUE

The entry-into-practice debate in nursing is not limited to the United States, although several countries have already established the baccalaureate degree as the minimum entry level and grandfathered all those with a license before that date. For example, since 1982, all provincial and territorial nurses associations in Canada have advocated the baccalaureate degree as the education entry-to-practice standard and most provincial and territorial regulatory bodies have achieved this goal. The Canadian Nurses Association (CNA) and the Canadian Association of Schools of Nursing (CASN) reaffirmed this goal in a joint statement released in 2004.

Similarly, Australia moved toward the adoption of a BSN for entry into nursing during the 1980s, initially encountering resistance by both physicians and by nurses themselves, who viewed university education would minimize needed hands-on training. Registered nursing as a university degree, however, was mandated in the 1990s. *Enrolled nurses* (scope of practice similar to LPNs/LVNs in the US) continue to be educated in diploma programs and work under the supervision of the RN.

Similarly, in South Africa, nurses who complete a 2-year course of study are called *enrolled nurses* or *staff nurses*, whereas those who complete 4 years of study attain *professional nurse* or *sister* status. Enrolled nurses can later complete a 2-year bridging program and become *registered general nurses* (The high-tech end of training. (2007/2008). *Nursing Update*, 31(11), 42–43).

Wales, Scotland, and Northern Ireland also offer only one entry point for nursing entry and that is a 3-year university degree. Other one entry-point countries include Italy, Norway, and Spain (3-year university degree); Ireland (4-year university degree); and Denmark (3.5-year degree at nursing school in university college sector). Many countries, such as Sweden, Portugal, Brazil, Iceland, Korea, Greece, and the Philippines already require a 4-year undergraduate degree to practice nursing (Boyd, 2011). England is currently considering a move to degree-only nursing across the United Kingdom, although the overwhelming majority of nurses are supporting a resolution to investigate how appropriate nursing experience might be recognized and accredited (Kendall-Raynor & Harrison, 2011).

> CONSIDER THIS   A growing list of countries, states, and provinces now require baccalaureate education in nursing.

Yet conflict continues even in countries who have adopted or are moving toward the BSN entry level. Parker, Keleher, Francis, and Abdulwadud (2009) suggest that Australia continues to recognize both registered

(BSN) and enrolled (ADN) nurses as qualified and appropriately educated to provide nursing services to the Australian community. This is reflected in a position statement published by the Royal College of Nursing Australia (2008). Similarly, Rheaume, Dykeman, Davidson, and Ericson (2007) contend that the adoption of the baccalaureate degree in New Brunswick, Canada, in 1993 as basic preparation for entry into nursing has further complicated the lives of nurses, since baccalaureate-educated nurses provide less direct care to patients and instead take on more administrative roles. As a result, strain has developed between older and younger nurses, accentuating differences in working knowledge and work ethic. In addition, many of these nurses felt inadequately prepared to handle the increased emphasis on coordination activities as part of their BSN leader role.

## CONCLUSIONS

The entry-into-practice debate in the United States continues to be one of the oldest and hottest professional issues nurses face as we enter the second decade of the 21st century. It appears that little progress has been made since 1965 in creating a consensus to raise the entry level into professional nursing practice, although experts do not agree even on that issue. Donley and Flaherty (2008) suggest that if the 1965 ANA statement is viewed as "a call to close hospital schools of nursing and move nursing education inside the walls of universities or colleges" (p. 22), then it was successful. If, however, the position is viewed as "a mandate for a more educated nurse force to provide better patient care, the goal has not been achieved" (p. 22).

Achieving the BSN as the entry degree for professional nursing practice will take the best thinking of our nursing leaders. It will also require courage, as well as a respect for persons not seen in the entry debate, and collaboration of the highest order. It will also require nurses to depersonalize the issue and look at what is best for both the clients they serve and the profession, rather than for them individually.

Even the most patient planned-change advocate would agree that almost 50 years is a long time for implementation of a position. Clearly, the driving forces for such a change have not yet overcome the restraining forces, although movement is apparent. The question seems to come down to whether the nursing profession wants to spend another 50 years debating the issue or whether it wants to proactively take the steps necessary to make the goal a reality.

## FOR ADDITIONAL DISCUSSION

1. What are the greatest driving and restraining forces for increasing entry into practice to a bachelor's or higher level?

2. Are the terms *professional* and *technical* unnecessarily inflammatory in the entry-into-practice debate? Why do these terms elicit such a "personal" response?

3. Is calling the associate degree in nursing a 2-year vocational degree an injustice to its graduates?

4. What is the legitimacy of requiring so many units at the community college level for an ADN degree? Should the current movement by community colleges to award baccalaureate degrees in nursing be encouraged?

5. How does the complexity of nursing roles and responsibilities compare to that of other health professions with higher entry levels?

6. What is the likelihood that nurses and the organizations that represent them will be able to achieve consensus on the entry-into-practice issue?

7. If the entry level is raised, should grandfathering be used? If so, should this grandfathering be conditional?

8. Is the goal of BSN entry a realistic one by 2015? If not, when?

## REFERENCES

Aiken, L., Clarke, S. P., Sloane, D. M., Lake, E. T., & Cheney, T. (2008). Effects of hospital care environment on patient mortality and nurse outcomes. *Journal of Nursing Administration, 38*(5), 223–229.

American Association of Colleges of Nursing. (2009, December 2). Student enrollment expands at U.S. nursing colleges and universities for the 9th year despite financial challenges and capacity restraints. Retrieved February 6, 2011, from http://www.aacn.nche.edu/Media/NewsReleases/2009/StudentEnrollment.html

American Association of Colleges of Nursing. (2011a). *Fact sheet: Creating a more highly qualified nursing workforce.* Retrieved June 16, 2011, from http://www.aacn.nche.edu/Media/FactSheets/NursingWrkf.htm

American Association of Colleges of Nursing. (2011b). *Fact sheet: The impact of education on nursing practice.* Retrieved June 16, 2011, from http://www.aacn.nche.edu/Media/FactSheets/ImpactEdNP.htm

Association of Operating Room Nurses. (2011). *AORN position statement on entry into practice.* Retrieved June 16, 2011, from http://www.aorn.org/PracticeResources/AORNPositionStatements/Position_EntryIntoPractice/

The American Nurse. (2011, February 11). *Bachelor's program enrollment expands.* Retrieved June 16, 2011, from http://www.theamericannurse.org/index.php/2011/02/page/2/

American Nurses Association. (1965a). *A position paper.* New York, NY: Author.

American Nurses Association. (1965b). *Educational preparation for nurse practitioners and assistants to nurses: A position paper.* New York, NY: Author.

Benner, P., Sutphen, M., Leonard, V., & Day, L. (2010). *Educating nurses: A call for radical transformation* (The Carnegie Foundation for the Advancement of Teaching. Preparation for the professions). San Francisco, CA: Jossey-Bass.

Boyd, T. (2011). It's academic. *NurseWeek, 24*(3), 30–31.

Donley, S. R., & Flaherty, M. J. (2008, April 30). *Entry into practice: Revisiting the American Nurses Association's first position on education for nurses. A comparative analysis of the first and second position statements on the education of nurses.* Retrieved May 20, 2008, from http://www.nursingworld.org/mods/mod524/entry2.pdf

Ellenbecker, C. (2010). Preparing the nursing workforce of the future. *Policy, Politics & Nursing Practice, 11*(2), 115–125.

Institute of Medicine. (2010, October). *The future of nursing: Leading change, advancing health.* Retrieved June 16, 2011, from http://thefutureofnursing.org/IOM-Report

Johnston, K. A. (2009, April). The importance of a baccalaureate degree in nursing education. *Peoriamagazines.com*. Retrieved February 6, 2011, from http://www.peoriamagazines.com/ibi/2009/apr/importance-baccalaureate-degree-nursing-education

Kendall-Raynor, P., & Harrison, S. (2011). Experience needs recognition as profession moves to degree entry. *Nursing Standard, 25*(34), 10.

Lane, S., & Kohlenberg, E. (2010). The future of baccalaureate degrees for nurses. *Nursing Forum, 45*(4), 218–227.

McGrath, J. (2008). Why would I want to do that? Motivating staff nruses to consider BSN education. *Journal of Perinatal and Neonatal Nursing, 22*(2), 880–890.

Megginson, L. (2008). RN-BSN education: 21st century barriers and incentives. *Journal of Nursing Management, 16*(1), 47–55.

Moltz, D. (2010, January 7). *Nursing tug of war*. Retrieved June 16, 2011, from http://www.insidehighered.com/news/2010/01/07/nursing

National Association of Neonatal Nurses. (2009). *Educational preparation for nursing practice roles* (Position statement No. 3048, NANN Board of Directors). Retrieved February 6, 2011, from http://www.nann.org/pdf/09educational_prep.pdf

National Council of State Boards of Nursing. (2011). *NCLEX examiniation pass rates*. Retrieved February 5, 2011, from https://www.ncsbn.org/Table_of_Pass_Rates_2010.pdf

National League for Nursing. (2007, September). *Reflection and dialogue: Academic/professional progression in nursing*. Retrieved May 22, 2008, from http://www.nln.org/aboutnln/reflection_dialogue/refl_dial_2.htm

National Organization for Associate Degree Nursing. (2008). *Nursing facts*. Retrieved May 22, 2008, from https://www.noadn.org/resources/nursing-facts.html

National Organization for Associate Degree Nursing. (2011a). *Position statement of associate degree nursing*. Retrieved February 6, 2011, from https://www.noadn.org/component/option,com_docman/Itemid,250/task,cat_view/gid,87/

National Organization for Associate Degree Nursing. (2011b). *Position on the requirement of bachelor's degree in nursing (BSN) for continued practice*. Retrieved February 6, 2011, from https://www.noadn.org/component/option,com_docman/Itemid,250/task,cat_view/gid,87/

Nickitas, D. (2010). Getting RN entry-level employment right: What are we waiting for? *Nursing Economics, 28*(4), 225.

Parker, R. M., Keleher, H. M., Francis, K., & Abdulwadud, O. (2009). Practice nursing in Australia: A review of education and career pathways. *BMC Nursing, 8*(5). Retrieved July 18, 2012, from http://www.biomedcentral.com/1472-6955/8/5

Rheaume, A., Dykeman, M., Davidson, P., & Ericson, P. (2007). The impact of health care restructuring and baccalaureate entry to practice on nurses in New Brunswick. *Policy, Politics, & Nursing Practice, 8*(2), 130–139.

Rosenfeld, P., Chaya, J., Lewis-Holman, S., & Davin, D. (2010). Can an ADN internship program prepare new RNs for careers in home health care nursing? Findings from an evaluation study at visiting nurse service of New York. *Home Health Care Management & Practice, 22*(4), 254–261.

Royal College of Nursing Australia. (2008). *Position statements, guidelines, and communiques: Enrolled nurse (EN)*. Retrieved April 23, 2012, from http://www.rcna.org.au/WCM/RCNA/Policy/Position_statements/rcna/policy/position_statements_guidelines_and_communiques.aspx?hkey=5700bcdc-a03b-48e2-bd2c-a33128628d2d

Service Employees International Union. (2008). *Position statement on BSN requirement for RN practice*. Retrieved June 29, 2008, from http://www.seiu.org/health/nurses/bsn_requirement.cfm

Sexton, K. A., Hunt, C. E., Cox, K. S., Teasley, S. L., & Carroll, C. A. (2008). Differentiating the workplace needs of nurses by academic preparation and years in nursing. *Journal of Professional Nursing, 24*(2), 105–108.

Smith, T. (2010). A policy perspective on the entry into practice issue. *Online Journal of Issues in Nursing, 15*(1), 2.

Starr, S., & Edwards, L. (2010). Why should I get a BSN? *Tar Heel Nurse, 72*(3), 10–12.

Taylor, D. L. (2008, March). Should the entry into nursing practice be the baccalaureate degree? *AORN Journal, 87*(3), 611–614, 616, 619–620.

U.S. Department of Veterans Affairs. (2009, November 9). *Hiring programs and incentives*. Retrieved June 16, 2011, from http://www.va.gov/jobs/hiring_programs.asp#3

Ward-Smith, P. (2011). Everything old is new again. *Urologic Nursing, 31*(1), 9–10.

## BIBLIOGRAPHY

American Association of Colleges of Nursing. (2010, Spring). Amid calls for more highly educated nurses, new AACN data show impressive growth in doctoral nursing programs: final data from AACN's 2009 survey indicate ninth year of enrollment and admissions increases in entry-level baccalaureate nursing programs. *Dakota Nurse Connection, 8*(2), 22–24.

American Association of Colleges of Nursing (April 2, 2012). The impact of education on nursing practice. Available at: http://www.aacn.nche.edu/media-relations/fact-sheets/impact-of-education. Retrieved Sept. 11, 2012.

Boyd, T. (2010). A matter of degree: Hospitals begin to require BSNs, aren't waiting on BSN in 10 legislation: Part 3. *Nursing Spectrum—New York & New Jersey Edition, 22*(20), 22–23.

BSN requirement not a welcome change . . . "A matter of degree: Hospitals begin to require BSNs, aren't waiting on BSN in 10 legislation." (2011). *Nursing Spectrum—New England Edition, 15*(2), 8.

Chappy, S., Jambunathan, J., & Marnocha, S. (2010). Evidence-based curricular strategies to enhance BSN graduates' transition into practice. *Nurse Educator, 35*(1), 20–24.

Holmes, A. M. (2011). Transforming education. *Nursing Management, 42*(4), 34–38.

Johnson, D. (2009). Article about clarifies ADN-to-MSN programs . . . "Skipping the BSN." *NurseWeek (California/Mountain West), 22*(11), 12.

Klich-Heartt, E. (2010). Special needs of entry-level master's-prepared nurses from accelerated programs. *Nurse Leader, 8*(5), 52–54.

Lampe, S., & Schofield, L. N. (2011). The BSN requirement . . . "A failure to rescue ourselves," Viewpoint, November 2010. *American Journal of Nursing, 111*(2), 12–13.

Matthias, A. (2010). The intersection of the history of associate degree nursing and "BSN in 10": Three visible paths. *Teaching & Learning in Nursing, 5*(1), 39–43.

Mooneyham, J., Goss, T., Burwell, L., Kostmayer, J., & Humphrey, S. (2011). Employment incentives for new grads. *Nursing Management, 42*(3), 39–44.

Muma, R. D., Smith, B. S., Anderson, N., Richardson, M., Selzer, E., & White, R. (2011). Perceptions of U.S. physicians regarding the entry-level doctoral degree in physician assistant education. *Journal of Allied Health, 40*(1), 25–30.

Praeger, S. (2010). Developing competencies for entry into practice. *NASN School Nurse, 25*(3), 106.

Rizzuto, C., & Prada, J. (2010). Readers encourage nurse to pursue BSN. *Nursing Spectrum—New York & New Jersey Edition, 22*(18), 14–15.

Shipman, D., & Hooten, J. (2010). Employers prefer BSN nurses: But where's the financial compensation? *Nurse Education Today, 30*(2), 105–106.

Shipman, D., Roa, M., & Hooten, J. (2011). Healthcare organizations benefit by promoting BSN education. *Nurse Education Today, 31*(4), 309–310.

Simon, E., & Augustus, L. (2009). Comparative analysis of NLN NCLEX-RN readiness exam performance: BSN versus ADN. *Journal of Research in Nursing, 14*(5), 451–462.

Starr, S. (2010). Associate degree nursing: Entry into practice—Link to the future. *Teaching & Learning in Nursing, 5*(3), 129–134.

Student applauds system's aggressive BSN policy . . . Oct. 11 . . . "A matter of degree." (2010, November 22). *Nursing Spectrum—New York & New Jersey Edition, 22*(23), 10–11.

Thomas, C. M., Ryan, M. E., & Hodson-Carlton, K. E. (2011). Recruitment & retention report. What are your perceptions of new RN competency levels? *Nursing Management, 42*(12), 15–18.

Woo, A., & Dragan, M. (2012). Ensuring validity of NCLEX with differential item functioning analysis. *Journal of Nursing Regulation, 2*(4), 29–31.

# Chapter 2

# Evidence-Based Practice

Suzanne S. Prevost

## ADDITIONAL RESOURCES

Visit the Point for additional helpful resources
- eBook
- Journal Articles
- WebLinks

## CHAPTER OUTLINE

## LEARNING OBJECTIVES

*The learner will be able to:*

1. Differentiate between evidence-based practice and best practices.

2. Explain why the identification and implementation of evidence-based practice is important both for assuring quality of care and in advancing the development of nursing science.

3. Identify personal, professional, and administrative strategies, as well as support systems, that promote the identification and implementation of evidence-based practice.

4. Describe the types of knowledge and education that nurses need to prepare them for conducting research and leading best practice initiatives.

5. Recognize the need to ask critical questions in the spirit of looking for opportunities to improve nursing practice and patient outcomes.

6. Delineate research and nonresearch sources of evidence for answering clinical questions.

7. Describe and compare practices that have evolved in the workplace as a result of tradition-based and research-based inquiry.

8. Compare the efficacy of randomized, controlled trials, integrative reviews, or meta-analyses, with practice-based evidence for continuous process improvement (PBE-CPI) to answer clinical research questions.

9. Specify institutions, units, teams, or individuals in the community that could be considered regional or national benchmark leaders in the provision of a specialized type of medical or nursing care.

10. Explore reasons for the disconnect that often exists between nurse researchers and educators studying evidence-based practice and nurses who seek to implement research into their practice.

Nurses and other health care providers constantly strive to provide the best care for their patients. As new medications and health care innovations emerge, determining the best options can be challenging. This process has become more difficult in recent years as health care administrators, insurance companies and other payers, accrediting agencies, and consumers demand the latest and greatest health care interventions. Nurses and physicians are expected to select health care interventions that are supported by research and other credible forms of evidence. They may also be expected to provide evidence to demonstrate that the care they deliver is not only clinically effective but also cost-effective, and satisfying, to patients. In light of these challenges, the term *evidence-based practice* has emerged as a descriptor of the preferred approach to health care delivery.

This chapter begins by defining the concept of evidence-based practice. Examples of when and where nurses are using evidence-based practice are provided, as are strategies for determining and applying these practices. In addition, the *who* of evidence-based practice is addressed regarding how nurses in various roles can support this approach to care. Finally, future implications are discussed.

## WHAT IS EVIDENCE-BASED PRACTICE?

The term evidence-based practice is being used with increasing frequency among health care providers. Evidence-based practice has a variety of definitions and interpretations. The term evidence-based practice evolved in the mid-1990s when discussions of evidence-based medicine were expanded to apply to an interdisciplinary audience, which included nurses. David Sackett, one of the leaders of the movement, defined evidence-based medicine as "the conscientious and judicious use of current best evidence from clinical care research in the management of individual patients" (Sackett, Rosenberg, Gray, Haynes, & Richardson, 1996, p. 71). The Honor Society of Nursing, Sigma Theta Tau International (STTI) expanded this definition to address a broad nursing context with the following definition of evidence-based nursing practice: "An integration of the best evidence available, nursing expertise, and the values and preferences of the individuals, families and communities who are served" (STTI, 2005, p. 1).

Historically, various industries, in health care and beyond, have used the term *best practice* to describe the strategies or methods that work most efficiently or achieve the best results. This concept is often associated with the process of *benchmarking*, which involves identifying the most successful companies or institutions in a particular sector of an industry, examining their methods of doing business, using their approach as the goal or gold standard, and then replicating and refining their methods. Today, benchmarking data is one of the less scientific forms of evidence that is used, along with the results of formal research studies, to identify evidence-based nursing practices.

> CONSIDER THIS  Today, most nurse experts agree that the best practices in nursing care are also evidence-based practices.

Although this process of identifying the best evidence-based practices has become more scientific, the ultimate goal remains to provide optimal patient care, with the goal of enhancing nursing practice and, in turn, improving patient or system outcomes.

> ### DISCUSSION POINT
>
> Are there any situations in which an evidence-based practice might not be considered the best practice?

## WHY, WHEN, AND WHERE IS EVIDENCE-BASED PRACTICE USED?

Each week, new developments and innovations occur and are reported in health care—not only in research findings but also in the public media. Contemporary health care consumers are knowledgeable and demanding. They expect the most current, effective, and efficient interventions.

## Why Is Evidence-Based Practice Important?

In their quest to provide the highest quality care for their patients, nurses are challenged to stay abreast of new developments in health care, even within the limits of their areas of specialization. Simultaneous with the growth of health care knowledge, health care costs have increased and patient satisfaction has taken on greater importance. Administrators expect health care providers to satisfy their customers and to do it in the most clinically effective and cost-effective manner.

Control of health care costs was one of the early drivers of the evidence-based practice movement. As contracted and discounted reimbursement systems decreased revenue to hospitals and providers, it became increasingly apparent that some providers were capable of providing high-quality care in a more efficient and cost-effective manner than their peers. The practices of these industry leaders were quickly identified and emulated. Within the current litigious and cost-conscious health care environment, there remains a sense of urgency to select and implement the most effective and efficient interventions as quickly as possible.

Nurses are increasingly accepted as essential members, and often as leaders, of the interdisciplinary health care teams. To effectively participate and lead a health care team, nurses must have knowledge of the most effective and reliable evidence-based approaches to care, and as nurses increase their expertise in critiquing research, they are expected to apply the evidence of their findings to select optimal interventions for their patients.

The processes and tools of evidence-based practice can help nurses respond to these challenges. This approach to care is based on the latest research and other forms of evidence, as well as clinical expertise and patient preferences. All of these factors contribute to providing quality care that is clinically effective, cost-effective, and satisfying to health care consumers.

---

### DISCUSSION POINT

What type of knowledge and education do nurses need to prepare them for leading evidence-based practice initiatives as described?

---

## When and Where Is Evidence-Based Practice Used?

In recent years, the implementation of evidence-based practice has been identified as a priority across nearly every nursing specialty. Over the past decade, STTI, the International Honor Society for Nurses, has consistently received feedback from their membership surveys asking for support systems and resources to help nurses implement evidence-based practice. This feedback has been consistent across nursing specialties and across nursing roles and positions. Initiatives to help nurses understand and implement evidence-based practice have become a priority since that time. A review of recent literature yields case studies and recommendations for evidence-based practice implementation across several nursing specialties. These are shown in Table 2.1.

In addition to the universal application across nursing specialties, the concept of evidence-based practice is also valued across nursing roles and responsibilities. Sandstroma and colleagues discussed the importance of preparing nurse leaders and administrators to promote evidence-based practice (Sandstroma, Borglin, Nilsson, & Willman, 2011). Clinical nurse specialists are frequently called on to serve as leaders of evidence-based practice initiatives (Muller, McCauley, Harrington, Jablonski, & Strauss, 2011). Nursing professors are challenged to incorporate evidence-based practice into nursing curricula (Oh et al., 2010). Last but not least, staff nurses are frequently being expected to participate in, or lead, evidence-based practice initiatives (Grant, Hanson, Johnson, Idell, & Rutledge, 2011).

## Evidence-Based Practice Around the World

A commitment to evidence-based practice is not limited to the United States. A few countries—in particular, Australia, Canada, and the United Kingdom—adopted this approach to care several years before it became popular in the United States. The Joanna Briggs Institute, which started at the University of Adelaide, Australia, in 1996, now has over 70 centers collaborating to provide evidence-based resources to health care providers around the world. The Registered Nurses Association of Ontario has been developing and distributing evidence-based nursing practice guidelines for more than a decade. Nursing Knowledge International (NKI), a subsidiary of STTI, also serves as an international clearinghouse and facilitator to promote international nursing communication, collaboration, and sharing of resources in support of evidence-based practice.

| TABLE 2.1 | Evidence-Based Practice Across Nursing Specialties | | |
|---|---|---|---|
| **Area of Specialization** | **Author and Year** | **Title or Theme** | **Type of Report** |
| Administration | Everett and Sitterding (2011) | Promoting EBP | Nursing leadership competencies for EBP |
| Critical care | Ban (2011) | Using EBP to reduce ventilator-associated pneumonia | Report of a research study |
| Emergency | Kleiber, Jennissen, McCarthy, and Ansley (2011) | EBP for pediatric pain management in emergency departments | Report of a survey of ED nurses and MDs |
| Gerontology | Wilson, Ratajewicz, Els, and Asirifi (2011) | Using EBP to prevent elder abuse | Case studies and recommendations for practice |
| Medical-surgical | Deitrick, Baker, Paxton, Flores, and Swavely (2011) | Hourly rounding | Describes challenges associated with implementing an EBP rounding procedure |
| Mental health | Beebe, Adams, and El-Mallakh (2011) | Putting the "evidence" in EBP | Recommendations to promote EBP in psychiatric settings |
| Oncology | Alexander and Allen (2011) | EBP for fluid balance in oncology patients | Describes the EBP and the process for implementing it |
| Pediatrics | Randhawa, Roberts-Turner, Woronick, and DuVal (2011) | Reducing pediatric cardiopulmonary arrests | Describes an evidence-based tool and the process for implementation |
| Women's health | Kulie et al. (2011) | Obesity and women's health | Reviews the evidence linking obesity to other negative health outcomes in women |

*Note:* EBP = evidence-based practice.

CONSIDER THIS In the past decade, the concept of evidence-based practice has evolved and been embraced by nurses in nearly every clinical specialty, across a variety of roles and positions, and in locations around the globe.

## How Do Nurses Determine Evidence-Based Practices?

Evidence-based practice begins with questions that arise in practice settings. Nurses must be empowered to ask critical questions in the spirit of looking for opportunities to improve nursing practice and patient outcomes. In any specialty or role, nurses can regard their work as a continuous series of questions and decisions.

In a given day, a staff nurse may be called to ask and answer questions, such as "Should I give the analgesic only when the patient requests it, or should I encourage him to take it every 4 hours? Will aggressive ambulation expedite this patient's recovery, or will it consume too much energy? Will open family visitation help the patient feel supported, or will it interrupt her rest?"

A nurse manager or administrator might ask, "Who is the most qualified care provider for our sickest patient today? What is the optimal nurse-to-patient ratio for a specific unit? Do complication rates and sentinel events increase with less-educated staff? Do longer shifts result in greater staff fatigue and medication errors? Will higher quality and more expensive mattresses decrease the incidence of pressure ulcers? What benefits promote nurse retention? How does the use of supplemental (or agency) staffing affect the morale of existing staff? Can this population be treated on an outpatient, rather than an inpatient, basis? What is the optimal length of time for a comprehensive home care assessment? How many patients can a nurse practitioner see in 8 hours?"

Likewise, a nurse educator may ask, "Is it more effective to teach a procedure in the laboratory or on an actual patient? What are the most efficient methods of documenting continued competency? Do web-based students perform as well on standardized tests as students in traditional classrooms?"

Each type of question can lead to important decisions that affect outcomes, such as patient recovery, organizational effectiveness, and nursing competency. The best answers and consequently the best decisions come from informed, evidence-based analysis of each situation. See Box 2.1 for a list of questions to assist the nurse in the process of evidence-based decision making for various nursing scenarios.

## FINDING EVIDENCE TO ANSWER NURSING QUESTIONS

Nurses rely on various sources to answer clinical questions such as those cited previously. A practicing staff nurse might consult a nurse with more experience, more education, or a higher level of authority to get help in answering such questions. Institutional standards or policy and procedure manuals are also a common reference source for nurses in practice. Nursing coworkers or other health care providers, such as physicians, pharmacists, or therapists, might also be consulted. Although all of these approaches are extremely common, they are more likely to yield clinical answers that are *tradition based* rather than *evidence based*.

If evidence-based practice is truly based on best evidence, nursing expertise, and the values and preferences of patients, then local expertise and tradition is not sufficient. However, the optimal source of best evidence is often a matter of controversy.

---

### DISCUSSION POINT

In your preferred area of nursing specialization, what are some key questions and decisions that nurses address on a daily basis?

---

### DISCUSSION POINT

What are the best sources of evidence for answering clinical questions?

---

### BOX 2.1   KEY QUESTIONS TO ASK WHEN CONSIDERING EVIDENCE-BASED PRACTICES

- Why have we always done "it" this way?
- Do we have evidence-based rationale? Or, is this practice merely based on tradition?
- Is there a better (more effective, faster, safer, less expensive, more comfortable) method?
- What approach does the patient (or the target group) prefer?
- What do experts in this specialty recommend?
- What methods are used by leading, or benchmark, organizations?
- Do the findings of recent research suggest an alternative method?
- Is there a review of the research on this topic?
- Are there nationally recognized standards of care, practice guidelines, or protocols that apply?
- Are organizational barriers inhibiting the application of evidence-based practice in this situation?

Research is generally considered a more reliable source of evidence than traditions or the clinical expertise of individuals. However, many experts argue that some types of research are better, or stronger, forms of evidence than others. In medicine and pharmacology, the *randomized, controlled trial* (RCT) has been considered the gold standard of clinical evidence. RCTs yield the strongest statistical evidence regarding the effectiveness of an intervention in comparison to another intervention or placebo. For many clinical questions in medicine and pharmacy, there may be multiple RCTs in the literature addressing a single question, such as the effectiveness of a particular drug. In such situations, an even stronger form of evidence is an *integrative review or meta-analysis* wherein the results of several similar research studies are combined or synthesized to provide the most comprehensive answer to the question.

In nursing literature, RCTs, meta-analyses, and integrative reviews are significantly less common than in medical or pharmaceutical literature. For many clinical questions in nursing, RCTs may not exist, or they may not even be appropriate. For example, if a nurse is considering how best to prepare a patient for endotracheal suctioning, it would be helpful to inform the patient what suctioning feels like. This type of question does not lend itself to an RCT, but rather to descriptive or qualitative research. In general, qualitative, descriptive, or quasi-experimental studies are much more common methods of inquiry in nursing research than RCTs or meta-analyses. Furthermore, the body of nursing research overall is newer and less developed than that of some other health disciplines. Thus, for many clinical nursing questions, research studies may not exist.

Recently, a new research method has evolved that provides excellent support for evidence-based practice. Fittingly, this research method is referred to as *practice-based evidence for continuous process improvement* (PBE-CPI). PBE-CPI incorporates the variation from routine clinical practice to determine what works best, for which patients, under what circumstances, and at what cost. It uses the knowledge of frontline caregivers, who help to develop the research questions and define variables (Horn & Gassaway, 2010). This method can provide a more comprehensive picture than a randomized, controlled study that only examines one intervention with a very limited population under strictly controlled, laboratory-like circumstances. Although research results are usually considered the optimal form of evidence, many other data sources have been used to support the identification of optimal interventions for nursing and other health care disciplines. Some of the additional sources are as follows:

- Benchmarking data
- Clinical expertise
- Cost-effectiveness analyses
- Infection-control data
- Medical record review data
- National standards of care
- Pathophysiologic data
- Quality improvement data
- Patient and family preferences

Another dilemma for the practicing nurse is the time, access, and expertise needed to search and analyze the research literature to answer clinical questions. In the midst of the current nursing shortage, few practicing nurses have the luxury of leaving their patients to conduct a literature search. Many staff nurses practicing in clinical settings have less than a baccalaureate degree; therefore, they likely have not been exposed to a formal research course. Findings from research studies are typically very technical, difficult to understand, and even more difficult to translate into applications. Searching, finding, critiquing, and summarizing research findings for applications in practice are high-level skills that require substantial education and practice.

### DISCUSSION POINT

If a practicing nurse has no formal education or experience related to research, what strategies should she or he use to find evidence that answers clinical questions and supports evidence-based practice?

## SUPPORTING EVIDENCE-BASED PRACTICE

In light of the challenges of providing or implementing evidence-based practice, nurses must consider some alternative support mechanisms when searching for the best evidence to support their practice. Recommended mechanisms of support are summarized in Box 2.2.

### Garner Administrative Support

The first strategy is to garner administrative support. The implementation of evidence-based practice should not be an individual, staff nurse–level pursuit. Administrative support is needed to access the resources, provide the support

## BOX 2.2    MECHANISMS TO PROMOTE EVIDENCE-BASED PRACTICE

- Garner administrative support.
- Collaborate with a research mentor.
- Seek assistance from professional librarians.
- Search for sources that have already reviewed or summarized the research.
- Access resources from professional organizations.
- Benchmark with high-performing teams, units, or institutions.

## BOX 2.3    STRATEGIES FOR THE NEW NURSE TO PROMOTE EVIDENCE-BASED PRACTICE

- Keep abreast of the evidence—subscribe to professional journals and read widely.
- Use and encourage use of multiple sources of evidence.
- Find established sources of evidence in your specialty; do not reinvent the wheel.
- Implement and evaluate nationally sanctioned clinical practice guidelines.
- Question and challenge nursing traditions, and promote a spirit of risk taking.
- Dispel myths and traditions not supported by evidence.
- Collaborate with other nurses locally and globally.
- Interact with other disciplines to bring nursing evidence to the table.

personnel, and sanction the necessary changes in policies, procedures, and practices. Recently, nursing administrators have had increased incentives to support evidence-based practice because this approach to care has become recognized as the standard expectation of organizations, such as the Joint Commission, which accredits hospitals and other health care institutions. Evidence-based practice is also one of the expectations associated with the highly regarded Magnet Hospital Recognition program. Most nursing administrators who want their institutions to be recognized for providing high-quality care will understand the value of evidence-based practice and therefore should be willing to provide resources to support it.

## Collaborate With a Research Mentor

One way nurse administrators can support the use of evidence-based practice is through the provision of nurse experts who can function as research mentors. Advanced practice nurses, nurse researchers, and nursing faculty are examples of nurses who may provide consultation and collaboration to support the process of searching, reviewing, and critiquing research literature and databases to answer clinical questions and identify best practices. Most staff nurses do not have the educational background, research expertise, or time to effectively review and critique extensive research literature in search of the evidence to support evidence-based practice. Research mentors can assist with these processes, whereas staff nurses can often provide the best insight on clinical needs and patient preferences. Box 2.3 includes a list of strategies for the new graduate nurse to promote evidence-based practice.

## Seek Assistance From Professional Librarians

Another valuable type of support that is available in academic medical centers, and in some smaller institutions, is consultation from medical librarians. A skilled librarian can save nurses a tremendous amount of time by providing guidance in the most comprehensive and efficient approaches to search the health care literature to find research studies and other resources to support the implementation of evidence-based practice.

## Search Already Reviewed or Summarized Research

A strategy nurses can use to expedite the search for evidence-based practice is to specifically seek references that have already been reviewed or summarized in the research literature. For example, some journals, such as *Evidence-Based Nursing* and *WorldViews on Evidence-Based Nursing*, specifically focus on providing summaries, critiques, and practice implications of existing nursing research studies. For example, the 2011 issues of *WorldViews on Evidence-Based Nursing* included reviews and summaries on the following topics:

- Cancer-related fatigue
- Cultural sensitivity in advanced directives
- Nursing interventions for sleep promotion
- Management of aggressive patients
- Weaning from mechanical ventilation

When conducting a literature search, use of keywords, such as "research review" or "meta-analysis," can assist the nurse in identifying research review articles that have been published on the topic of interest.

The *Cochrane Collaboration* is a large international organization composed of several interdisciplinary teams of research scholars that are continuously conducting reviews of research on a wide variety of clinical topics. The Cochrane Collaboration promotes the use of evidence-based practice around the world. The Cochrane reviews tend to focus heavily on evaluating the effectiveness of medical interventions, for example, comparing the effects of different medications for specific conditions. Therefore, many of the Cochrane review summaries are more useful for primary care providers, such as physicians and nurse practitioners, than for staff nurse clinicians. Some of the Cochrane projects of interest to nurses in direct care positions include their reviews of products designed to prevent pressure ulcers, nursing interventions for smoking cessation, interventions to help patients follow their medication regimens, and interventions to promote collaboration between nurses and physicians.

The Agency for Healthcare Research and Quality (AHRQ) is also a good resource for identifying research reviews and summaries that have been compiled by national panels of experts. One particularly helpful AHRQ resource is the *National Guideline Clearinghouse* (NGC), a link to which can be found on thePoint and is also available at www.guidelines.gov. The mission of the NGC is to "provide physicians and other healthcare providers . . . an accessible mechanism for obtaining objective, detailed information on clinical practice guidelines and to further their dissemination, implementation and use" (AHRQ, 2011, para. 2).

All of the practice guidelines available through this site are developed through systematic searches and reviews of research literature and scientific evidence by a professional organization, health care specialty association, or government agency. Nursing organizations that have contributed guidelines to the NGC include the American Association of Neuroscience Nurses; Association of Women's Health, Obstetric, and Neonatal Nursing; Emergency Nurses Association; the Oncology Nursing Society; and the Registered Nurses Association

of Ontario. Each guideline includes an abstract summary and a list of recommended practices, strategies, or interventions for a specific clinical condition. The NGC contains more than 2,500 unique practice guidelines.

## Access Resources From Professional Organizations

Professional nursing organizations can also provide a wealth of resources to support evidence-based practice. For example, the American Association of Critical Care Nurses has published several *Practice Alerts* that are relevant to nursing care in critical care units. These documents are based on extensive literature reviews conducted by national panels of nurse researchers and advanced practice nurses. They provide concise recommendations focused on areas where current common practices should change on the basis of the latest research. Some of the topics covered in the *Practice Alerts* include delirium assessment and management, prevention of ventilator-associated pneumonia, pulmonary artery pressure monitoring, and family presence during resuscitation.

The Association of Women's Health, Obstetric, and Neonatal Nursing (AWHONN) also provides several resources to support evidence-based practice. The AWHONN Research-Based Practice Projects are designed to "translate research into nursing practice, ultimately advancing evidence-based clinical practice" (AWHONN, 2011, para. 1). Through this program, several nationwide, multiyear projects have been completed. Topics addressed through this mechanism have included management of women in second-stage labor, urinary continence for women, neonatal skin care, and cyclic pelvic pain and discomfort management.

AWHONN also sponsored an Evidence-Based Clinical Practice Guideline Program. Each of their guidelines includes clinical practice recommendations, referenced rationale statements, quality of evidence ratings for each statement, background information describing the scope of the clinical issue, and a quick care reference guide for clinicians. Cardiovascular health for women and perimenstrual pain and discomfort are two of the guideline topics produced through this program (AWHONN, 2011).

The American Association of Operating Room Nurses (AORN), the Oncology Nursing Society (ONS), and STTI also provide Web-based resources to facilitate implementation of evidence-based practice. AORN has published *Evidence-Based Guidelines for Safe Operating Room Practices,* the ONS provides an *Evidence-Based Practice*

*Resource Area,* and STTI publishes Web-based continuing education programs and several supportive publications, including *Worldviews on Evidence-Based Nursing.*

**DISCUSSION POINT**

What institutions, units, teams, or individuals can you identify in your region that would be considered regional or national benchmark leaders in the provision of a specialized type of medical or nursing care?

## Benchmark With High-Performing Teams, Units, or Institutions

Finally, nurses can use benchmarking strategies to poll nurse experts from high-performing teams, units, or institutions to learn more about their practices for specific clinical problems or patient populations. Leaders of professional nursing organizations, such as STTI or the National Association of Clinical Nurse Specialists, can help nurses locate and contact established nurse experts in various areas of specialization. Accrediting organizations, such as the Joint Commission, can assist in identifying institutions that are known as national leaders in providing specific types of care. The University of Iowa, Arizona State University, and McMaster University of Ontario are three North American institutions that have established reputations as leaders in evidence-based nursing practice.

**DISCUSSION POINT**

When the investigation reveals a need for an evidence-based change in practice, what strategies are useful for implementing change?

## CHALLENGES AND OPPORTUNITIES: STRATEGIES FOR CHANGING PRACTICE

Nurses use several mechanisms for incorporating new research into current practice in the pursuit of promoting evidence-based practice. Perhaps the most common mechanism is through the development and refinement of research-based policies and procedures. Fortunately, the JCAHO has mandated that health care institutions must implement formal processes for reviewing the latest research and assuring that institutional policies and procedures are consistently revised in keeping with current research findings.

Protocols, algorithms, decision trees, standards of care, critical pathways, care maps, and institutional clinical practice guidelines are additional mechanisms used to incorporate new evidence into clinical practice. Each of these formats is used by health care teams to guide clinical decision making and clinical interventions. Although nurses often take the lead in developing or revising these devices, participation and buy-in from the interdisciplinary health care team are essential to achieve successful implementation and consistent changes in practice.

In addition to consensus from the interdisciplinary team, support from patients and their families is important. This element of the evidence-based practice process is frequently overlooked or not thoroughly considered. As previously mentioned, evidence-based nursing practice involves "an integration of the best evidence available, nursing expertise, and the values and preferences of the individuals, families and communities who are served" (STTI, 2005, p. 1).

If the review of evidence leads the health care team to recommend an intervention that is inconsistent with the patient or family's values and preferences (such as a specific dietary modification or transfusion of blood products), the recommendation may lead to poor adherence or total disregard by the patient, not to mention a loss of the patient's trust and confidence in the health care team.

**DISCUSSION POINT**

Can you think of situations in which the latest research may be inconsistent with the values of an individual or group of patients?

## Challenges to Implementing Evidence-Based Practice

Although evidence-based practice is being discussed and pursued by nurses around the world, several obstacles continue to inhibit the movement. Funk, Champagne, Wiese, and Tornquist (1991) originally studied this problem, and Retsas (2000) used a modification of their survey to poll 400 Australian nurses. He identified several barriers that he grouped into four main factors: accessibility of research findings, anticipated outcomes of using research, support from others, and lack of organizational

## RESEARCH STUDY FUELS THE CONTROVERSY

**EVIDENCE-BASED PRACTICE BARRIERS AND FACILITATORS FROM A CONTINUOUS QUALITY IMPROVEMENT PERSPECTIVE: AN INTEGRATIVE REVIEW**

In 2011, these authors synthesized the results of 23 different research studies that were conducted in the United States and Canada between 2004 and 2009. The collection included descriptive research projects that addressed the question: What are the barriers to evidence-based nursing practice in the workplace? They also included interventional studies that described strategies or solutions to increase evidence-based practice utilization. Nurses were participants or respondents in all of the research studies.

Solomons, N. M., & Spross, J. A. (2011). Evidence-based practice barriers and facilitators from a continuous quality improvement perspective: An integrative review. *Journal of Nursing Management, 19*(1), 109–120.

### STUDY FINDINGS

The most common barriers identified across these studies were lack of time or ability to effectively review the research literature and lack of authority to make changes to practice. Other barriers included difficulty accessing research articles, information overload, insufficient resources, a preference for knowledge received through coworkers and practice experience—rather than through journal articles—and a lack of interest or value for research. Strategies that were found to increase evidence-based practice by nurses in these settings were the presence of "EBP Champions," especially if the chief nursing officer was a supporter of evidence-based practice; open access to the Internet and electronic literature databases; pursuit of Magnet hospital status; continuing education programs to explain the process; and the presence and use of nurse mentors.

---

support, which was perceived to be the most significant limitation. In recent years, other researchers have investigated the same questions with similar results.

In 2011, Solomons and Spross published an integrative review of several studies about the barriers and facilitators to evidence-based practice (see Research Study Fuels the Controversy for a summary of their findings).

### DISCUSSION POINT

What obstacles would limit your involvement in the process of pursuing evidence-based practice?

---

## CONCLUSIONS

Many nurses are experiencing success in promoting evidence-based practice. Organizations such as the AHRQ and the Cochrane Collaboration provide support to help clinicians overcome some of the barriers, such as the difficulties in obtaining and understanding research reports, and the lack of time to synthesize research findings into recommended practices. The many agencies that support teams of research experts to collect, critique, and summarize the research and other forms of evidence pave the way for frontline clinicians to find and adopt evidence-based practices.

Yet challenges continue. Too few nurses understand what evidence-based practice is all about. Organizational cultures may not support the nurse who seeks out and uses research to change long-standing practices rooted in tradition rather than science. In addition, a stronger connection needs to be established between researchers and academicians who study evidence-based nursing practice and staff nurses who must translate those findings into the art of nursing practice. Nursing cannot afford to value the art of nursing over the science. Both are critical to making sure that patients receive the highest quality of care possible.

## FOR ADDITIONAL DISCUSSION

**1.** Can decision support tools such as algorithms, decision trees, clinical pathways, and standardized clinical guidelines ever replace clinical judgment?

**2.** Why does at least some level of disconnect exist between nurse researchers or faculty studying evidence-based practice and the nurses who seek to implement such research into their practice? Is the problem a lack of communication?

**3.** Do most nurses have access to evidence-based nursing research findings?

**4.** Are evidence-based practice findings consistent over time? Can you identify an evidence-based practice that was later found to be ineffective or inappropriate?

**5.** Should evidence-based practices be institution specific, or should they be more generalizable across different settings?

**6.** Is evidence-based nursing research grounded more in quantitative or qualitative research? Are both needed?

**7.** What can be done to increase the research knowledge base of practicing registered nurses (RNs), given that a significant portion of those nurses have been educated at the associate-degree level?

## REFERENCES

Agency for Healthcare Research and Quality. (2011). *National Guideline Clearinghouse*. Retrieved January 3, 2012, from http://www.guideline.gov/about/index.aspx

Alexander, L., & Allen, D. (2011). Establishing an evidence-based inpatient medical oncology fluid balance measurement policy. *Clinical Journal of Oncology Nursing, 15*(1), 23–25.

Association of Women's Health, Obstetric and Neonatal Nursing. (2011). *Research-based practice projects*. Retrieved January 2, 2012, from http://www.awhonn.org/awhonn/content.do?name=03_JournalsPubsResearch%2F3G_ResearchBasedPracticeProjects.htm

Ban, K. O. (2011). The effectiveness of an evidence-based nursing care program to reduce ventilator-associated pneumonia in a Korean ICU. *Intensive and Critical Care Nursing, 27*(4), 226–232.

Beebe, L., Adams, S., & El-Mallakh, P. (2011). Putting the "evidence" in evidence-based practice: Meeting research challenges in community psychiatric settings. *Issues in Mental Health Nursing, 32*(8), 537–543.

Deitrick, L. M., Baker, K., Paxton, H., Flores, M., & Swavely, D. (2011). Hourly rounding: Challenges with implementation of an evidence-based process. *Journal of Nursing Care Quality, 27*(1), 13–19.

Everett, L. Q., & Sitterding, M. C. (2011). Transformational leadership required to design and sustain evidence-based practice: A system exemplar. *Western Journal of Nursing Research, 33*(3), 398–426.

Funk, S. G., Champagne, M. T., Wiese, R. A., & Tornquist, E. M. (1991). Barriers to using research findings in practice: The clinician's perspective. *Applied Nursing Research, 4*(2), 90–95.

Grant, M., Hanson, J., Johnson, S., Idell, C., & Rutledge, D. N. (2011). Evidence-based practice for staff nurses. *Journal of Continuing Education in Nursing, 8*, 1–8.

Horn, S. D., & Gassaway, J. (2010). Practice based evidence: Incorporating clinical heterogeneity and patient-reported outcomes for comparative effectiveness research. *Medical Care, 48*(6 Suppl.), S17–S22.

Kleiber, C., Jennissen, C., McCarthy, A. M., & Ansley, T. (2011). Evidence-based pediatric pain management in emergency departments of a rural state. *Journal of Pain, 12*(8), 900–910.

Kulie, T., Slattengren, A., Redmer, J., Counts, H., Eglash, A., & Schrager, S. (2011). Obesity and women's health: An evidence-based review. *Journal of the American Board of Family Medicine, 24*(1), 75–85.

Muller, A., McCauley, K., Harrington, P., Jablonski, J., & Strauss, R. (2011). Evidence-based practice implementation strategy: The central role of the clinical nurse specialist. *Nursing Administration Quarterly, 35*(2), 140–151.

## REFERENCES *(continued)*

Oh, E. G., Kim, S., Kim, S. S., Cho, E. Y., Yoo, J. S., Kim, H. S., . . . Lee, H. (2010). Integrating evidence-based practice into RN-to-BSN clinical nursing education. *Journal of Nursing Education, 49*(7), 387–392.

Randhawa, S., Roberts-Turner, R., Woronick, K., & DuVal, J. (2011). Implementing and sustaining evidence-based nursing practice to reduce pediatric cardiopulmonary arrest. *Western Journal of Nursing Research, 33*(3), 443–456.

Retsas, A. (2000). Barriers to using research evidence in nursing practice. *Journal of Advanced Nursing, 31*(3), 599–606.

Sackett, D. L., Rosenberg, W. M., Gray, J. A., Haynes, R. B., & Richardson, W. S. (1996). Evidence based medicine: What it is and what it isn't. *British Medical Journal, 312*(7023), 71–72.

Sandstroma, B., Borglin, G., Nilsson, R., & Willman, A. (2011). Promoting the implementation of evidence-based practice: A literature review focusing on the role of nursing leadership. *Worldviews on Evidence-Based Nursing, 8*(4), 212–223.

Solomons, N. M., & Spross, J. A. (2011). Evidence-based practice barriers and facilitators from a continuous quality improvement perspective: An integrative review. *Journal of Nursing Management, 19*(1), 109–120.

Sigma Theta Tau International. (2005). *Evidence-based nursing position statement.* Retrieved December 31, 2011, from http://www.nursingsociety.org/aboutus/PositionPapers/Pages/EBNposition-paper.aspx

Wilson, D. M., Ratajewicz, S. E., Els, C., & Asirifi, M. A. (2011). Evidence-based approaches to remedy and also to prevent abuse of community-dwelling older persons. *Nursing Research and Practice, 2011*, 861484 (Epub).

## BIBLIOGRAPHY

Blazeck, A., Klem, M. L., & Miller, T. H. (2011). Building evidence-based practice into the foundations of practice. *Nurse Educator, 36*(3), 124–127.

Case, R., Haynes, D., Holaday, B., & Parker, V. G. (2010). Evidence-based nursing: the role of the advanced practice registered nurse in the management of heart failure patients in the outpatient setting. *Dimensions of Critical Care Nursing, 29*(2), 57–62; quiz 63–54.

Christian, B. J. (2011). Translational research: Creating excellent evidence-based pediatric nursing practice. *Journal of Peditric Nursing, 26*(6), 597–598.

Cronje, R. J., & Moch, S. D. (2010). Part III: Reenvisioning undergraduate nursing students as opinion leaders to diffuse evidence-based practice in clinical settings. *Journal of Professional Nursing, 26*(1), 23–28.

Dogherty, E. J., Harrison, M. B., & Graham, I. D. (2010). Facilitation as a role and process in achieving evidence-based practice in nursing: A focused review of concept and meaning. *Worldviews on Evidence-Based Nursing, 7*(2), 76–89.

Fineout-Overholt, E., Gallagher-Ford, L., Mazurek Melnyk, B., & Stillwell, S. B. (2011). Evidence-based practice, step by step: Evaluating and disseminating the impact of an evidence-based intervention: Show and tell. *American Journal of Nursing, 111*(7), 56–59.

Frace, M. (2010). Evidence-based nursing at the bedside: Are you walking the walk? *Medsurg Nursing, 19*(2), 77, 120.

Lehna, C., Love, P., Holt, S., Stokley, B., Vissman, A., Kupiec, T., . . . Dunlap, K. (2010). Nursing students apply evidence-based research principles in primary burn prevention projects. *Journal of Pediatric Nursing, 25*(6), 477–481.

Melnyk, B., & Fineout-Overholt, E. (Eds.). (2010). *Evidence-based practice in nursing & healthcare: A guide to best practice* (2nd ed.). Philadelphia, PA: Lippincott Williams & Wilkins.

Patrician, P. A., Loan, L., McCarthy, M., Brosch, L. R., & Davey, K. S. (2010). Towards evidence-based management: Creating an informative database of nursing-sensitive indicators. *Journal of Nursing Scholarship, 42*(4), 358–366.

Staffileno, B. A., & Carlson, E. (2010). Providing direct care nurses research and evidence-based practice information: An essential component of nursing leadership. *Journal of Nursing Management, 18*(1), 84–89.

# Chapter 3

# Developing Effective Leaders to Meet 21st Century Health Care Challenges

Bernadette M. Melnyk, Kathy Malloch, and Lynn Gallagher-Ford

## ADDITIONAL RESOURCES

Visit thePoint for additional helpful resources

- eBook
- Journal Articles
- WebLinks

## CHAPTER OUTLINE

## LEARNING OBJECTIVES

*The learner will be able to:*

1. Describe factors that are driving the need for innovative and transformational leaders in health care for the 21st century.

2. List five health care leadership challenges of the 21st century.

3. Delineate three effective strategies to promote and sustain an evidence-based practice organizational culture.

4. Explain why effective leaders in the 21st century must engage in mentoring of young leaders and succession planning today.

5. Describe the characteristics required of leaders in order to effectively promote innovation and change.

6. Discuss the importance of teamwork, effective communication, and transdisciplinary/de-siloed work as they relate to health care outcomes.

7. List 13 essential characteristics of effective leaders.

8. Recognize the areas of change that have occurred as a result of the "electronic world."

9. Discuss the strengths and weaknesses of three leaderships models: transactional, transformational, and complexity.

10. Distinguish the unique leadership components required in the complexity leadership model.

## TODAY'S HEALTH CARE: IN CRITICAL CONDITION

The American health care system is in critical condition, with a tripling of costs over the past two decades, poor-quality services, wasteful spending, and rise in medical errors (Hader, 2010). Half of the hospitals in the United States are functioning in deficit, and there are up to 200,000 unintended patient deaths every year (American Hospital Association, 2007). Furthermore, we are living in an era in which patients receive only approximately 55% of the care they should receive when they enter the health care system (Resar, 2006). The health care system is also facing the most severe shortage of health professionals, including physicians and nurses, it has ever encountered. The changing nature of morbidities in the United States (e.g., a high prevalence of overweight/obesity, chronic diseases, and mental health disorders), the current condition of the health care system, and the severe shortage of health care professionals call for transformational and innovative leaders who will develop new models of transdisciplinary care and interprofessional education that will lead to the highest quality of evidence-based care and patient outcomes and, at the same time, decrease health care costs (i.e., high-value health care) as well as limit the number of errors to attain high reliability (Melnyk, 2012).

This chapter presents nine critical leadership challenges for nurse leaders in the 21st century as well as 13 competencies needed to overcome these challenges. The chapter concludes with a discussion of leadership models for the 21st century and suggests that the complexity leadership model offers a new perspective for leadership and potential to support improved organizational performance.

## Twenty-First-Century Leadership Challenges

The foregoing health care issues provide challenges or "character-builders" specific to nurse leaders in the 21st century. These challenges are listed in Box 3.1. Each individual nurse leader will have the opportunity to leverage the challenges of these times or be overwhelmed by them. Old models of autocratic, hierarchical leadership will not be adequate to handle the fast-paced, complex health care environment of the future. Leaders of today and in the future need to be innovative, creative, flexible, engaging, courageous, relationship-based, and dynamic.

Leadership is not a "solo act"; it is imbedded in relationships, effective communication, shared ownership,

### BOX 3.1    NINE 21ST CENTURY LEADERSHIP CHALLENGES

- Meeting expectations for increased productivity within budgetary constraints
- Advancing evidence-based practice
- Planning for succession and mentoring young nurse leaders
- Facilitating and enhancing teamwork and effective communication
- Embracing and supporting transdisciplinary health care
- Positioning nursing to influence decision making in organizational and health policy
- Promoting workplace wellness
- Striking a balance between technology and interpersonal relationships to deliver best care
- Creating cultures of innovation and change

and coaching and motivating others. Leadership must move from an autocratic, transactional model to innovative complexity leadership. Leaders who are steeped in traditional leadership styles and unwilling to grow and change their own practices will be particularly challenged by the dynamics of the health care environment that lies ahead. Leaders who are proactive and embrace new approaches, who are better suited for chaotic times, will be in the best position for dealing with the following challenges.

### Meeting Expectations for Increased Productivity Within Rigorous Budgetary Constraints

Even in an era of major federal, state, and organizational budget reductions, leaders are expected to be highly productive with a scarcity of resources and financial constraints. In the theater of nursing, what exactly does "productive" encompass? Productivity includes both resource stewardship and delivery of the nursing "product" of safe, quality care. A major challenge for nurse leaders is to advocate for, attain, and maintain balance between these two key factors of nursing productivity.

Nurse leaders need to use strategies where "caring management and financial constraints can coexist while promoting quality patient care" (Cara, Nyberg, & Brousseau, 2011).

Nurse leaders also need to understand and clearly articulate the inextricable connectedness of nurse engagement, productivity, and retention with the production of caring and quality outcomes, which ultimately drive satisfaction and the financial well-being of the organization. Therefore, nurse leaders must be creative, innovative, entrepreneurial, and resourceful in garnering new resources and strategizing to maintain the core nursing value of caring to increase efficiency and to drive quality outcomes.

### Advancing Evidence-Based Practice When Care in Many Health Care Institutions Remains Steeped and Mired in Tradition

> CONSIDER THIS   A large number of medical errors occur because clinicians do not practice evidence-based health care.

The Institute of Medicine (IOM) named evidence-based practice (EBP) as a core competency for health care professionals (Greiner & Knebel, 2003). Shortly thereafter, the National Institutes of Health (NIH) Roadmap initiative prioritized the acceleration of the transfer of knowledge from research into practice (Zerhouni, 2005). Furthermore, studies have supported that evidence-based practice (EBP) enhances quality of care, improves patient outcomes, and decreases health care costs. Yet in spite of all of this, EBP is not the standard of practice in most health care organizations throughout the country (Melnyk & Fineout-Overholt, 2011).

Therefore, leaders must have the knowledge and skills to create cultures of EBP that ignite a spirit of inquiry throughout the organization and cultivate an environment where outcomes management flourishes. Unfortunately, although leaders report that they believe in the value of EBP, their own implementation of it is low (Sredl et al., 2010). It will be critical for nurse leaders to integrate evidence into their individual professional practices to deliver best leadership practice, as well as to serve as EBP role models, which will influence their staff's EBP beliefs and implementation of evidence-based care.

> **DISCUSSION POINT**
>
> As a new nurse executive, you are faced with an organization of nurses who in large part do not believe in or have the skills to deliver evidence-based care. What strategies would you embark upon early in your new role to begin to change that paradigm?

### Planning for Leadership Succession and Mentoring Young Nurse Leaders

Continuity is a vital aspect of effective organizations; it is critical to strategic and operational goals. Disruption in an organization's continuity can have dire consequences. Disruption is particularly challenging in health care organizations because of the potential damage to confidence from the community and employees, the cost of unfinished business and negative impact on financing, and the harm to the organization's image and history (Witt/Kieffer, 2004). Succession planning is the cure for this condition as the process is intended to create an internal leadership pipeline that delivers internal candidates to be promoted. These internal candidates require less time and effort to be oriented and are more likely to be successful in their new position. This, in turn, allows organizations to accomplish at least two major goals during times of transition and turnover: (1) effective resource stewardship and (2) ongoing focus on accomplishing their strategic mission.

Succession planning also can be a very positive experience for the "up and coming" leaders in the organization. As individuals in the organization are given expanded opportunities, planned support, intentional mentorship, and effective and meaningful rewards and recognition, they develop their leadership portfolio and are less likely to be a "flight risk" (Blouin & McDonagh, 2006) to the organization.

> CONSIDER THIS   Succession planning requires . . . planning! Have you thought about who will follow you and how you can influence their success?

One of the critical aspects of effective succession planning is mentoring. Studies have supported that nurses and physicians who have mentors tend to be more successful in and satisfied with their own careers

(Beecroft, Santner, Lacy, Kunzman, & Dorey, 2006; Sambunjak, Straus, & Marusic, 2006). Mentoring can run the gamut from informal "in the moment" coaching to formal, planned meetings. "Giving talented future leaders the time, energy, advice, and experiences to gain new competencies and learn how to begin to prepare for future roles and responsibilities becomes the 'gift' a current leader can bestow upon a future leader" (Blouin & McDonagh, 2006, p. 328). Evidence has supported that mentoring programs decrease nursing turnover rates (Zucker et al., 2006). Both mentors and mentees benefit from the process of mentoring as professional and personal growth occurs.

Yet, despite all of its associated positive benefits, there has not been enough mentoring and empowering of young nurse leaders by more seasoned leaders in the nursing profession (Huston, 2010). As a result, the profession is highly vulnerable as large numbers of established nurse leaders will be retiring in the next decade and the resulting talent gap may cause nursing to lose much of the ground gained in health care in recent years. Intentional as well as informal mentoring of young leaders and strategic succession planning is an imperative for current nurse leaders in order to sustain the positive changes and significant outcomes cultivated during their tenures.

### Facilitating and Enhancing Teamwork and Effective Communication

Communication has always been an important skill for all clinicians and teams with studies demonstrating the relationship between communication and patient safety. Effective communication among team members has been identified by the IOM as one of the markers of safe and highly reliable care (Kohn, Corrigan, & Donaldson, 2000).

Communication is not simply an exchange of information; it is a complex social process in which each party involved in the process brings history, assumptions, and expectations to the interaction (Lyndon, Zlatnik, & Wachter, 2011). "Effective (clinical) communication is clear, direct, explicit, and respectful" and "requires excellent listening skills, superb administrative support, and a collective commitment to move past traditional hierarchy and professional stereotyping" (p. 93). Communication, whether effective or ineffective, is jointly owned by all members of a team and each member is equally capable of engaging in good or bad communication tactics. Each member of the team enters the communication with different worldviews, values, fears, confidence level, and

assumed place within the hierarchy. Effective communication requires conscious effort, shared commitment, and hard work.

> CONSIDER THIS   Communication is a personal attribute and a learned skill. Do you have an understanding of your personal communication style? (How you communicate/how do you like to be communicated with?) There are many tools available that you can use to gain a better understanding of your style and how you interact with other individuals and teams and how you can modify your style to be more effective.

Leaders can significantly impact the success of teams and communication efforts in their organizations in a wide variety of ways. First, leaders must be effective communicators themselves and role model excellent communication skills in all settings. In addition, leaders are responsible to establish and uphold administrative structures to support and require effective teamwork and communication in their organizations. Finally, leaders must have the skills to effectively confront/manage conflicts that arise out of poor communications.

### Embracing and Supporting Transdisciplinary Health Care

The complexity and multidimensional nature of health care and health problems require a different approach than the traditional, segregated, discipline-siloed approach to patient care that has often been the standard in health care organizations for decades. Transdisciplinary care has received a great deal of attention lately and is emerging as an essential requirement for health care. This approach includes true interprofessional decision making and trust among a variety of health care providers (Légaré, Ratté, Gravel, & Graham, 2008). Transdisciplinary care assumes that merging the specialized knowledge from different health care disciplines together to act upon the same situation results in better and faster results for the recipient of that care (Vyt, 2008). Interprofessional collaboration, a key component of transdisciplinary care, has been demonstrated to improve patient care effectiveness for patients with chronic disease and a higher degree of work satisfaction in health care workers.

The challenge for leaders is to see the dynamics of health care through a contemporary lens, realize its complexities, and acknowledge that care must be evidence based and patient centered, both of which require a transdisciplinary, de-siloed approach. Leaders need to be well versed in tenets of this approach, able to model this approach in their leadership roles, and diligent in creating organizational settings and cultural milieus where this approach can thrive.

---

### DISCUSSION POINT

The physicians in your organization are reluctant to involve nurses in patient rounds. How would you deal with this situation?

---

### Positioning Nursing to Influence Decision Making in Organizational and Health Policy

Nurse leaders must not only be present in all health care and health policy venues but they must also be active contributors to key discussions and decision-making forums that influence the science and delivery of health care. They must also be proactive in assuring that nurses who are the best in representing certain topics are positioned at the right organizational and health policy tables. With an active presence at the "right tables," nurses are able to influence major decisions that positively influence health care quality, safety, and patient outcomes.

---

### DISCUSSION POINT

Nurses are the largest sector of health care professionals, yet nurses rarely participate in health care policy decisions. Why does this dilemma persist? What can nurses (individually and as a united group) do to change this?

---

### Promoting Workplace Wellness

Stress, burnout, and turnover continue to plague the nursing profession. This is particularly true for new graduates within the first year of employment (Cho, Laschinger, & Wong, 2006). Furthermore, although nurses are typically great caregivers of others, their own health and wellness often suffers. Wellness includes physical, emotional, mental health, and spiritual dimensions. Findings from a recent study by Laschinger, Grau, Finegan, and Wilk (2011) found that, in addition to workload and bullying, psychological capital (i.e., self-efficacy, optimism, hope, and resilience) was an important predictor of burnout in new nurses. In another recent study, depression was associated with prolonged absences from work (Franche et al., 2011). Therefore, promoting workplace wellness is critical, not only for the health of nurses directly but also to enhance productivity and decrease absences and high turnover rates, which are very costly to the health care system. Workplace wellness requires a culture of respect and support, including definitive programs that address workplace abuse from patients as well as coworkers (Franche et al., 2011).

---

### DISCUSSION POINT

How healthy is your workplace, physically and emotionally?
What single action could you take to make your workplace healthier? When can you initiate that action? How healthy are you? What are you doing to promote *your* physical and emotional well-being? What single action could you take to make yourself healthier? When can you initiate that action?

---

### Striking a Balance Between Technology and Interpersonal Relationships to Deliver Best Care

The impact of technology on health care in the past few decades has been startling, and this trend will surely continue into the future. The challenge for leaders as the next decades unfold will be in shifting from the current trend of technology driving our work to value-based health care quality and relationships as the drivers of our work, with technology supporting those drivers. Effective technology will need to be developed and designed with the "end users" (patients and providers) engaged, valued, and heard throughout the process.

Transformational and innovative leaders well versed in the concepts and language of technology development will be critical in forging the role and place of technology as an integrated component of health care in the future. They will need to understand and articulate the nonlinear and team-based nature of health care work, the innate complexity of the nature of life, and the essential requirement to deliver safe, timely, efficient, effective, equitable, patient-centered care through human interactions and relationships (Berwick, 2002).

### Creating Cultures of Innovation and Change

An innovation is more than an idea—it is an idea that comes to fruition and sustains. Although leaders may say that innovation is important, they often do not model it themselves or provide opportunities that foster innovation in others. In order for a change to be sustainable, it is not enough to simply create awareness about the change needed. In order to render a sustainable change, leaders must have the skills and capacity to manage the dynamics and processes associated with innovation as a lived experience (Porter-O'Grady & Malloch, 2010b).

In order to create a culture of innovation and change, leaders must acknowledge, embrace, and demonstrate engagement in innovation and change in their own leadership practices first. Only then are leaders able to help others to learn, embrace, and imbed the requirements of innovation and change into their individual practices. Creating a culture of innovation and change is not a passive process; it requires active participation, role-modeling, and mentorship by the leaders involved. Leaders of organizations who do not model innovation are a barrier in creating and sustaining an innovative environment where positive change and outcomes continually occur (Melnyk & Davidson, 2009).

CONSIDER THIS   Many people find change stressful. Many people inherently resist change. Embracing change/innovation is a challenge for many traditional managers and leaders.

## ESSENTIAL CHARACTERISTICS OF EFFECTIVE LEADERS

There are many characteristics that are essential for transformational and innovative leaders; 13 are detailed here (see Box 3.2). It is important to remember that titles do not make effective leaders; it is how individuals lead and their personal characteristics that earn them the respect of others in their organization. Informal leaders without titles who possess these characteristics are often far more respected than formal leaders with titles who do not possess these qualities.

### BOX 3.2   THIRTEEN CHARACTERISTICS OF TRANSFORMATIONAL AND INNOVATIVE LEADERS

- Vision and the ability to inspire a team vision/dream
- Passion for patient care and making a difference
- Transparency, honesty, integrity, and trust
- Effective communication skills
- The ability to lead/not micromanage
- Team, not "I," oriented
- Risk taking
- High level of execution
- Positive future orientation
- Innovative and entrepreneurial spirit
- Dedicated to coaching/mentoring
- Committed to motivating and empowering others to act/encouraging the heart
- Passion and persistence through the "character-building" experiences

### Vision and the Ability to Inspire a Team Vision/Dream

*Nothing happens unless first a dream.*

Carl Sandburg

There is nothing more important to achieving success than a potent dream/vision and an ability to inspire that vision in the team. The change efforts of many leaders fail because they focus too much on process and not enough on an exciting vision, although it does need to be recognized that vision without execution will also deter success. A motivational vision/dream will keep the energy of the leader and the team going when barriers, challenges, or fears are slowing or preventing outcomes from being achieved. Without an inspirational vision and a team who also buys into that vision, the likelihood of new initiatives being successfully attained is doubtful. In the health care environment of the future, characterized by constant change, switching directions, and continuous realignment of resources and priorities, the ability to set and achieve goals will be critical for a leader's success. Effective leaders in the 21st century will be those who can set a vision, guide others toward it, acknowledge progress along the way, and celebrate success relentlessly!

## Passion for Patient Care and Making a Difference

*The main thing is to keep the main thing the main thing.*

Stephen Covey

Historically, nurses have been perceived as *the* person on the health care team that "represents the patient" and "advocates for the patient." Placing the patient at the center of our work is not a stretch for nurses … it is part of nursing practice and it feels quite right to nurses. However, in the chaos and hustle-bustle of modern health care, it seems that this basic core value is lost at times. This simple idea must be reprioritized and be at the core of nursing, from the bedside to the nursing leadership suite. It must remain an integral part of not only what defines us as clinicians but also how it translates to the value we bring to patients as well as to the health care delivery milieu.

When patient care is the focus of the leader's efforts, all of the trials and tribulations of the day take on a new perspective. As long as the first question to be answered is "what is the best thing to do for this patient?" a plan can be constructed to get there. With the patient as the focus, it is possible to connect staff with their passion for serving others and define a shared commitment to a set of beliefs about the way patients will be cared for, how families will be treated, how leadership will support that vision, and how staff will help each other. As health care becomes more complex, consumers become more educated, and expectations continue to escalate, having a clear and simple focus that drives the work being done will help nurse leaders to be effective and valued.

## Transparency, Honesty, Integrity, and Trust

*Few things help an individual more than to place responsibility upon him and to let him know that you trust him.*

Booker T. Washington

Transparency, honesty, and integrity are all critical elements for establishing trust. Over the past several decades and across many disciplines, much has been written about the importance of trust. It is considered by many to be the foundation or the basic building block for healthy relationships and effective functional teams. Leaders who are wise know that trust is critical to their success and they work every day to attain and to sustain it. Trust is a "two-way street" and to reap the full benefits of trust, a leader must develop relationships where he/she is trusted by team members *and* where team members are trusted by him/her as well. When words and actions match, when one is perceived as authentic, and when humility and reflection are common actions … trust will flourish. The benefits and rewards of relationships forged from trust are immeasurable, and it is in every nurse leaders' best interest to cultivate this attribute.

---

### DISCUSSION POINT

As a nurse executive, you have a few nurse managers who hold things "tight to the vest" with their staff and are not transparent. As a result, there is pervasive mistrust among the staff. How would you handle the situation?

---

## Effective Communication Skills

Effective communication is critical to the safety of patients and the wellness of the workforce. By being effective communicators themselves and role modeling excellent communication skills at all times, leaders can significantly impact the success of teams and organizations. One of the earliest lessons presented in most nursing curriculums is to be attentive to verbal and nonverbal communication and to assess whether they are congruent in all interactions. This is a lesson that resonates whether one is taking care of a patient or presenting a strategic proposal at an executive board meeting. Words, tone, and nonverbal cues are all critically meaningful parts of communication. Effective leaders say what they mean, share as much information as they possibly can, and fully engage in their interpersonal interactions.

Within the scope of effective communication skills, the ability to listen cannot be emphasized enough. True listening to others is an incredibly powerful process. The effective listener not only obtains a tremendous amount of valuable information in the interaction but also begins, builds, or enhances their relationship with the other person.

However, it is not enough to simply have these skills and use them in the day-to-day operational context. Leaders must have the additional capacity and courage to use these skills effectively in the challenging times ahead in health care, to confront and manage the conflicts, dilemmas, and conundrums of the coming decades. Finally, in addition to being good communicators, leaders must fulfill their responsibility to establish and uphold administrative structures that assure effective teamwork and communication in their organizations.

## The Ability to Lead/Not Micromanage

*If you tell people where to go, but not how to get there, you'll be amazed at the results.*

General Patton

As a leader, it is critical to lead and sometimes to manage, but never micromanage. When you hire qualified people, you have to give them the freedom to carry out their jobs. Micromanagement is destructive at all levels and in every direction: vertical (manger/subordinate) as well as horizontal (peer/peer). When employees are micromanaged, they believe that their manager does not trust their work or judgment, which can often lead to employees' disengaging from their work and simply investing their time, but not their effort or creativity. The resulting dysfunctional work environment is characterized by employees feeling suffocated, which breeds contempt and distrust, both of which are extremely dangerous to teams, organizations, and leaders. This cycle is a leader's nightmare.

Effective leaders understand and recognize the differences between managing and leading, and they choose to lead whenever possible. Managing people is a skill, whereas leading people is an art and it is an investment. It requires commitment, relationships, emotional intelligence, critical thinking, finesse, and time. The rewards and joys of effective leading compared to the dangers and drain of micromanaging make the effort to lead worthwhile every time.

> CONSIDER THIS   Informal leaders without a title can be more effective than leaders with a formal title.

## Team, Not "I," Oriented

Teamwork is characterized by a set of interrelated activities accomplished by more than one person to achieve a common objective. Teamwork allows for engagement of many and the distribution of workload that enables each person to be more focused and efficient. Being on a team builds bonds among team members (being part of the team = being part of the solution), spawns creativity, and often generates a more robust outcome than could be achieved by a single individual. With all of this in mind, it would behoove any leaders to not squander the opportunity to work with and build effective teams.

Successful leaders understand the nature of teams and their role on a team. The effective leader, when working on a team, understands that the leader's goal is for the *team* to be successful. The effective leader knows that to be successful, each person must relinquish his or her own agenda for personal success and embrace the opportunity to share success with the team. The effective leader guides, motivates, listens to, critiques, and cheerleads the team, and in the end, earns the unique opportunity to celebrate successes as part of the team.

## Risk Taking

*Progress always involves risk; you can't steal second base and keep your foot on first.*

Frederick Wilcox

Many of the most successful people in life are the greatest risk takers. A definition of a risk taker is "a visionary change leader who can cope with the uncertainty that comes with change at the same time promoting innovation" (McGowan, 2007, p. 106). Risk taking is often related to "challenging the status quo," and it requires a rigorous spirit of inquiry and relentless curiosity about the possibilities.

Risk taking is a complex undertaking that includes weighing risks against rewards and moving into a process/project with a clear vision of the benefits overshadowing the doubts. At the same time, successful risk takers proactively recognize the vulnerabilities of moving forward and develop "back up" plans to address unexpected problems.

Leaders of the future will necessarily have to be comfortable with taking risks because the health care environment in the coming decades is bound to be chaotic, unpredictable, messy, and frenetic. Every day in health care will be peppered with opportunities to be risk aversive or risk engaging, and those leaders who embrace and leverage risk effectively will be the success stories looking at the others in their "rearview mirrors."

## High Level of Execution

*We are judged by what we finish, not by what we start.*

Unknown

Effective leaders understand that vision without execution will not lead to success, and so they begin their work with end point(s) in their mind and in their plan. They continuously think about outcomes, the bottom line, and/or the product to be delivered, but the critical difference of this attribute in great leaders is that they do this thinking/planning with finesse. They do not *only* focus on the outcome but also pay attention to the process and the people involved, but they never ever work without the end in mind.

## Positive Future Orientation

Transformational leaders aim high, have a positive future orientation, and "live comfortably in the gap between reality and the organization's vision" (Balik & Gilbert, 2010, p. 14). They are never satisfied, and they are energized by dissatisfaction as opposed to being distressed by it. They convey a positive spirit in their organization as they look to the challenges ahead of them as opportunities, not obstacles (2010). Leaders in the chaotic health care environment of the future who address their work with this type of spirit and energy will be more likely to survive and thrive. The key to this attribute is that every individual gets to choose how they will face their day, and those leaders who choose a positive future orientation in their work will be more effective and more likely to *have* a positive future.

## Innovative and Entrepreneurial Spirit

The current health care climate calls for leaders who are innovative and entrepreneurial. Resources are dwindling in most health care organizations, which require leaders to be more resourceful and creative in launching innovative and entrepreneurial initiatives that will lead to enhanced efficiency, revenue generation, and reduced costs. Leaders who create cultures of innovation and entrepreneurship will reap the benefits of an organization that thrives through uncertain times and budget constraints. According to Balik and Gilbert (2010), highly successful leaders in health care should "embrace a spirit of innovation, lead bold change, and find ways to lead from inside and outside health care—not only techniques, but changes in mind-set" and "learn to be prepared to lead an interdependent, agile organization with a non-hierarchical mentality that works as a team, with leaders defined by their actions, not by their title" (p. 256).

## Dedication to Coaching/Mentoring

Coaching and mentoring young leaders is an imperative for nurse leaders in order to sustain the positive changes and significant outcomes cultivated during their tenure.

The ability and desire to find and grow what is good in others is a hallmark of an effective leader. When you ask people . . . "have you ever been mentored by someone?" they are immediately able to tell you who their mentor was and what that mentor did for them that was so life changing. Mentoring is a deep and powerful experience that enriches both the mentee and the mentor. Effective leaders understand the potential power to help others grow and engage in mentoring relationships in order to build effective young leaders and, ultimately, better organizations.

### DISCUSSION POINT

What were the characteristics of individuals who have mentored you in your career? How did you *know* you were being mentored? Is there someone in your work environment who you could/should be mentoring now? What can you do to begin that process?

## Committed to Motivating and Empowering Others to Act/Encouraging the Heart

The ability to truly motivate and empower others is a skill that effective leaders must possess. People are keenly aware of imposters when it comes to motivation and empowerment. The wise and effective leader knows that this aspect of leadership should only be fulfilled with pure and real intention or the results will be disastrous. Strategies and approaches to connecting with others to motivate them, grow them, and empower them, such as Kouzes and Pozner's "encourage the heart," can serve leaders well in developing these attributes (Kouzes & Pozner, 2007). These authors stress that leaders must make sure that people must feel that what they do matters in their hearts. The practice of encouraging the heart is aligned with two commitments: (1) recognizing contributions by showing appreciation for individual excellence and (2) celebrating the values and victories by creating a spirit of community.

The sharing of stories can be an incredibly powerful tool for motivating and empowering others. Hearing about and relating to what others have lived, learned, or survived has served to help others for decades. Parents who have suffered the loss of a child who share their stories with other parents or with residents in training have demonstrated the power of storytelling. This type of exchange is emerging as a powerful tool for leaders to add to their toolkits (Melnyk & Fineout-Overholt, 2011).

## Passion and Persistence Through the "Character-Building" Experiences

*Many of life's failures are people who had not realized how close they were to success when they gave up.*

Thomas A. Edison

Passion is so critical, especially to avoid burnout and to keep you going when things get tough. Leaders need to know what their passion is and be able to access it and center on it when the environment intensifies. Persistence, described in the dictionary as an "enduring tenaciously," can be expressed quietly or loudly, but either way it is a key characteristic for effective health care. Persistence is deeply connected to passion in that what you are passionate about you are likely to be persistent about. Nurse leaders must learn the power of passion and persistence and leverage both wisely to attain vision and goals.

---

### DISCUSSION POINT

How many of these 13 essential characteristics have you mastered? Which of these characteristics do your coworkers, peers, direct reports, and supervisors attribute to you? What characteristics can you improve upon?

---

## MODELS OF LEADERSHIP FOR THE 21ST CENTURY

Over the last thirty years, different types and styles of leadership have been used by nurse leaders. Both transactional and transformational models are commonplace in varying degrees in health care organizations. In spite of many successes with these models, nurse leaders continue to struggle with patient quality, financial limitations, time management, knowledge access, information sharing, and effective communication. Not surprising, leaders are continually searching for the holy grail of leadership, that ultimate ideal model that effectively guides success in their respective organizations.

The work in today's health care organizations is increasingly complex and filled with digital tools and resources. Specifically, the digital world has changed when we work, where work takes place and the media for information transfer. The resulting changes in work processes; relationships between and among employees, patients, and the community; and the speed at which information is processed have challenged the best of traditional leadership models. Understanding the dynamics of these changes is the first step in determining the optimal leadership model.

Scharmer and Käufer (2000) identified four areas of change as a result of the electronic world: media, time, space, and structure. *Media* is the first and refers to the form in which information is documented, shared, and transmitted. In the information age, the Internet has revolutionized how information is transmitted. Flash drives and discs are the norm for data storage. The digitization of information has dramatically reduced the size and format of information. Less physical space is required for papers and files. In many cases, the information is virtual, requiring only electronic storage space. It is now possible for information to be sent to nearly anyone, at anytime, anywhere in the world. The majority of documents can be digitized and thus provide for increased consistency and quality of information. For leaders, the written or typed modality is no longer the most reliable; digitized documentation of information is now the more effective and efficient media for information.

With the nearly open access to the Internet, *time* for work is now wide open as well. The open access to individuals at any time of the day or night increases the emphasis on speed and efficiency. Lag times are decreased allowing for almost instantaneous responses and actions. Given the emphasis on speed and efficiency, this new reality of time as an open concept requires leaders think differently about when work is done. Furthermore, the new reality blurs the work–personal time boundaries creating more challenges. Leaders are now required to shift the emphasis on specific times for work based on a traditional five-day, eight-hour day in which an individual is present in the workplace to different models. Now, the leader is required to recognize and value work products wherever they are done rather than time present in the workplace. In health care, different models for work time necessarily exist for those providing patient care. The blurring of boundaries for work time necessarily creates two significant challenges—(a) being physically present when there is value in presence and (b) in assuring separation of work and personal time for healthy work–life balance.

As time and media conceptualizations have evolved, the *space* required for work also has changed. While single offices are still commonplace, the actual time spent by individuals in offices is decreasing. The portability of media and ready access to the Internet allows for work to be completed in many locations rather than in the traditional office. It is now possible to perform work wherever the information is accessible. Conference calls and electronic communication have decreased the need for physical gatherings. Individuals gathering at common physical sites are less and less the norm. The trend is to increase flexible spaces for individual and group meetings while decreasing individual office spaces.

The final major change is organizational *structure*. Given the new realities of information and communication exchange, the underlying structure for how work is organized is now open and free flowing. These changes impact organizational structure in numerous ways. The traditional levels of authority diagrams, communication pathways, and span of control are now secondary guides for the organization rather than the primary expectations for communication and permissions. In the digital age, any employee or patient or community members can now communicate with anyone in the organization using electronic mail. Documents or pictures can be shared with anyone in the organization at any time without seeking multiple layers of permissions. For these reasons, it is no wonder that leaders are struggling to be effective and efficient. The rules and principles under which transactional and transformational leadership emerged are quite different in the digital age as described by changes in media, time, space, and structure. In the next section, an overview of the strengths

and weaknesses of transactional and transformational leadership models followed by the emerging complexity leadership model are presented. Table 3.1 presents a comparison of the three model characteristics. This information is designed to assist leaders in understanding leadership models from a historical perspective and also to determine the role of leaders and leadership for the future.

*Transactional* or *instrumental* leadership is the most common and well-known leadership style used in health care. In this model, the focus is on task orientation, leader direction, follower participation with the expectation of rewards, threats, or disciplinary action from the leader (Bass & Bass, 2008; see Table 3.1). Research specific to transactional leadership supports the belief that personality traits are consistently correlated with the emergence and effectiveness of leaders. In a transactional model, leaders expect followers to support their goals; a job for the follower is exchanged for support of the leader's vision. In a transactional model, leaders have traditionally relied on traits believed to support and facilitate the role of the leader. Examples of trait theories which focus on the behaviors of the leader include the following:

- Great man theory: Throughout history, great men such as Abraham Lincoln, John Kennedy, and Bill Gates emerged as leaders.

## TABLE 3.1  Characteristics of Three Leadership Models

|  | **Transactional** | **Transformational** | **Complexity** |
|---|---|---|---|
| Focus | Planned work | Planned work | Emerging and transitional work |
| Locus of power | Individual leader-centric/position; formal | Individual leader-centric/position; formal | Team/group/relationship-centric network focus and informal |
| Work | Defined/prescribed; rule driven | Defined/prescribed; rule and principle driven | Emergent; principle driven |
| Communication direction | Top down; authoritarian | Top down; authoritarian | Multiple directions |
| Competencies | Plan, organize, direct, reward, punish | Plan, organize, direct, reward, punish, empower, collaborate | Facilitate, coach, collaborate |
| Organizational boundaries | Defined | Defined | Overlapping, informal |

- Biological-genetic theories: Some individuals were born to lead, a natural leader.

- Traits of individuals specific to qualities: Intelligence, scholarship, gender, dependability, situation, age, emotional competence, physique, fluency of speech, self-sufficiency, socioeconomic status, social activity, tact, popularity, and so on are common to leaders.

The limitations of transactional leadership include focus on a single individual as the source of knowledge and power; the role of the follower is to follow directions and support the vision of the leader. Creativity, self-actualization, and empowerment of followers are perceived as inappropriate in this model.

The second most common leadership model is *inspirational* or *transformational* and emphasizes the emotional and ideological appeals using exemplary behavior, confidence, symbolism, and intrinsic motivation (Bass & Bass, 2008). More recently, leaders have embraced the notion of transformational leadership, a style in which the leader forms relationships of mutual stimulation and elevation that converts followers into leaders (Bryman, Collinson, Grint, Jackson, & Uhl-Bien, 2011). In a transformational leadership model, the work of managing meaning, infusing ideological values, and co-creation of goals is recognized as processes of empowerment for both the leader and the follower. The exchange between the leader and the follower is elevated to include the value of personal growth for the follower.

Transformational leadership begins to engage followers to self-actualize and contribute to the organization and offers significant advantage over transactional leadership. The limitation of transformational leadership is the locus of power still remains with the leader; the leader is expected to begin the empowerment processes to engage employees rather than employees being expected to lead from their position in the organization. Formal leaders, those designated with an official leadership position, are the norm while informal leadership is not recognized.

In spite of the advancements in the transformational leadership model, the ability for the organization to optimize the knowledge and competencies of all members of the organization in a fluid and timely manner is still limited. Continuing to rely on bureaucratic, top-down processes is counterproductive in the presence of the critical dynamics of the digital media, time, space, and structure advancements. Considerations for the changes resulting from the digital advancements are needed to support the uncertain, emergent, and highly interconnected nature of the environment as well as the organizational culture.

Congruency between the leadership model, namely, how work occurs, and the underlying assumptions, values, and artifacts of the organization are positively correlated and impact organizational efficiency and effectiveness (Casida & Pinto-Zipp, 2008). Thus, a new leadership model must necessarily integrate the organization culture and local environment. Advancing our current leadership models to address the identified challenges of overwhelming work volumes, fewer financial resources, and increases in complexity of providing patient care will provide an improved framework for leaders. The *complexity leadership model* offers a new perspective for leadership and potential to support improved organizational performance.

Complexity leadership models are based on complexity leadership theory (CLT) and provide a new lens for leadership to increase effectiveness and efficiency (Uhl-Bien & Marion, 2008). This model recognizes health care organizations as networks of people, resources, knowledge, and other entities composed of overlapping, informal boundaries; leadership is both positional and informal, incorporating the full potential of human and social capital (Hanson & Ford, 2010, p. 6588).

The assumptions in a complexity leadership model are as follows:

- Positional and informal leaders fulfill diverse functions in the organization
  - Positional leaders carry authority focused on managing organizational dynamics and enabling informal initiatives rather than directing or mandating behaviors.
  - Informal leaders emerge based on relationships.

- Control is difficult if not impossible; uncertainty is the norm.

- System boundaries cannot be defined as all interactions are human and interconnected.

- Leadership is the accountability of every individual in the organization specific to the assigned role.

- Power does not rest solely with an individual(s); power is distributed among the members of the organization and is located within relationships.

- High degrees of individual interactions are the norm.

Within the CLT model, three types of leadership functions are identified; *administrative, adaptive,* and *enabling.* Interestingly, CLT embraces some aspects of transactional and transformational leadership. The CLT model provides a more robust and congruent model for leadership. The *administrative* leadership component is somewhat similar to the transactional model. This work is about coordinating and planning organizational activities with less hierarchy and formality and thereby sustaining the framework of the organization. The goal is minimize excessive control and bureaucracy and reinforce the adaptive work of others. The *adaptive* aspect of the model is about the emergence of optimal outcomes from interrelationships and interactions. Collaboration among individuals to produce collective best outcomes is the overall goal of the adaptive leadership role. Some similarities to the transformation model can be gleaned from the adaptive role. The *enabling* role is the new dimension and serves to foster and optimize adaptive work processes and mediate the tensions that occur between administrative and adaptive functions. Enabling leadership works to minimize bureaucratic controls, support the emergence of collective wisdom, and recognize the value of the multiple interactions of individuals as the way work occurs. This brief description of the CLT serves as the foundation for reframing the contemporary leadership model into a trimodal model to better meet the needs of today's challenges (Malloch, 2010).

The current work to meet the paradoxical nature of health care in which both stability and creativity are expected encompasses innovation and transition or transformation between operations and innovation. The organizational culture in a trimodal organization reinforces evidence-driven processes. It is also consistent with the work of innovation in which new ideas are encouraged, tested, validated, and implemented when evidence for improvement is available. The organizational culture also strongly supports the transition phase between innovation and operations. Oftentimes, new ideas are embraced and moved from innovation to operations without the necessary time to change to become embedded into the culture. Such changes are often discarded or at best modified. In the trimodal model, transition work is as important as operations and innovation work (Fig. 3.1).

The trimodal model reframes and identifies three vital work processes for leaders: operational stability, innovative leadership, and transformation from innovation to operations. These three categories are designed to manage the present, look to the future, and support the processes in between. A brief explanation of the three components excerpted from Porter-O'Grady and Malloch (2010a) follows.

Operations or the work of providing evidence-based patient care within a defined structure with supportive staff and resources comprises the majority of traditional health care work. This work is typically planned, funded, and evaluated within an operations model. Given the predictive nature of this work, it can be thought of as

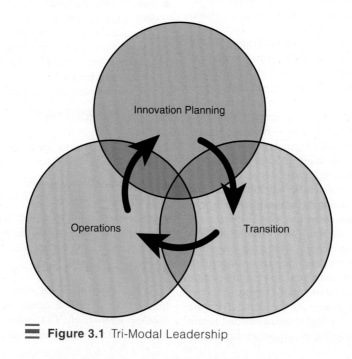

≡ **Figure 3.1** Tri-Modal Leadership

the technical work of an organization, provided by highly skilled professionals. Health care leaders balance and support multiple operational entities and initiatives, medical-surgical services, ambulatory services, pharmacy services, medical imaging, and others.

The new work, with greater variability and complexity, requires leaders to shift from an emphasis on operations to a model that values and integrates the work of change, innovation, and the transition between operations and innovation. It is unclear as to what the exact proportion of effort should be for each of these modes; however, it is clear that less time will be spent in operations, with increasing attention to innovation and transition to new levels of operational work.

Traditional operations change in several ways. The emphasis by operations on standardization shifts to one of accountability for work assignments and roles. There is a shift from an emphasis on rules to a focus on principles. Knowing that procedures will change, standardization and consistency must be continually challenged as new information and technologies are introduced. This approach recognizes the temporary nature of most work processes. The emphasis now shifts to the appropriateness of the work performed rather than the completion of checklists.

The second aspect of work in the trimodal model is innovation planning. In this model, innovation work is considered essential rather than optional. Innovation work includes those new ideas, challenges, and product consideration as the means to improve current work. Innovation planning focuses on the continual introduction, challenging, and evaluation of new ideas.

Challenging assumptions and asking what if this could happen are normative in innovation work. Innovation work considers any and all new technologies and processes as potential opportunities to advance and strengthen the work of the organization. The development of new approaches to health care that are safer, less invasive, and more cost-effective are the desired goals for this aspect of leadership. The tools of innovation provide structure and rigor for these processes to assure thorough consideration, testing, and pricing.

Numerous tools, spaces, and processes have been used to accomplish comprehensive evaluations. Many organizations have created physical space for this work; however, the emphasis is more on thinking differently, researching available technologies and the needs of clients. This thinking work does not require a specific physical space, but rather a physical or virtual space that supports creative, safe, and respectful dialog. Necessarily, the structure for this work is loose to allow for creativity and openness.

The work of innovation planning is not only about looking at new ideas and products but also includes improving or eliminating current ineffective or poorly functioning processes. Furthermore, when organizations are faced with fewer resources, negative outcomes, or shortages of workers, the innovation planning team can begin to assist with creative dialogue to seek greater efficiencies without compromising on quality.

The third aspect of the trimodal model is the transition work that is needed to sustain change and transform work processes. The significance and complexity of facilitating and assuring an effective transition between innovation and operations is too often overlooked or underestimated. Once new ideas are identified and determined to be suitable for future work, sustainable pathways to modify roles, competencies, infrastructure, technology, funding, and the cultural norms must also evolve. Changing the culture requires much more than a single educational program; it requires persistence and focus. When innovations are introduced into a traditional culture without adequate transition support and modification of the existing work, the innovations are most likely to be considered fads and dismissed quickly. New ideas are considered burdens rather than opportunities to remain competitive and achieve the highest quality outcomes. Participants are more likely to engage in new work at higher levels when they know the rationale for change, are able to test the knowledge in practice, and can support the ethical expectations for professional practice. Transition is about cultural transformation and requires time, reinforcement, and frequent course corrections to successfully embed new practices into the evolving culture.

The challenges in creating an organizational trimodal leadership model require both personal and organizational change. Knowledge of personal strengths and comfort with change and innovation are essential. Understanding one's approach to decision making, conflict-utilization style, comfort with change, uncertainty, errors, and challenging assumptions are essential for the innovation leader. In addition, basic knowledge of innovation principles, collaboration at the highest and most uncommon levels to foster diversity, and comfort with coaching other to fully engage in the work of the organization are selected competencies that all member of the organization are likely to pursue.

## CONCLUSIONS

In order to be successful, leaders must possess important characteristics to overcome the major challenges that plague health care in the 21st century. Major challenges facing today's leaders include dwindling resources, organizations and practices steeped in tradition, and intense pressures to achieve high-value, high-reliability organizations. Leaders must possess numerous essential characteristics, such as an ability to inspire a team vision, effective communication skills, integrity, and an ability to mentor and encourage their team to excel among others, in order to be effective. Although many leadership models exist, the complexity model combined with innovation leadership holds the most promise for best outcomes in dealing with 21st century leadership challenges.

## FOR ADDITIONAL DISCUSSION

1. How do traditional attributes associated with the nursing profession (caring, advocacy, service, etc.) promote effective leadership in the 21st century? How might these traditional attributes hinder effective leadership in the 21st century?

2. How could traditional nursing attributes be proactively and thoughtfully leveraged to influence health care decisions in the 21st century?

3. Are health care leaders "walking the talk"/role-modeling evidence-based practice by integrating evidence into their daily management decision making? How can this leadership paradigm shift be enhanced?

4. How could formal leadership training for nurse managers and leaders impact hospitals in terms of saving money related to recruitment, nursing satisfaction, nurse wellness, and retention?

5. Compare and contrast the three leadership models identified in Table 3.1. How does each model facilitate patient safety? Also, how can each model be a barrier to patient safety?

6. Is there a model of leadership that better supports leadership at the point of service? Why? Why not?

## REFERENCES

American Hospital Association. (2007). *TrendWatch Chartbook 2007: Trends affecting hospitals and health systems*. Retrieved from http://www.aha.org/aha/trendwatch/chartbook/2007/07chapter4.ppt#10

Balik, M. B., & Gilbert, J. A. (2010). *The heart of leadership: Inspiration and practical guidance for transforming your health care organization*. Chicago, IL: AHA Press.

Bass, B. M., & Bass, R. (2008). *Handbook of leadership: Theory, research, and management*. (4th ed.). New York, NY: Free Press.

Beecroft, P. C., Santner, S., Lacy, M. L., Kunzman, L., & Dorey, F. (2006). New graduate nurses' perceptions of mentoring: Six-year programme evaluation. *Journal of Advanced Nursing, 55*(6), 736–747.

Berwick, D. M. (2002). A user's manual for the IOM's "quality chasm" report. *Health Affairs, 21*(3), 80–90.

Blouin, A. S., & McDonagh, K. J. (2006). Leading tomorrow's healthcare organizations. *Journal of Nursing Administration, 36*(6), 325–330.

Bryman, A., Collinson, D., Grint, K., Jackson, B., & Uhl-Bien, M. (Eds.). (2011). *The SAGE handbook of leadership*. London, England: SAGE.

Cara, C. M., Nyberg, J. J., & Brousseau, S. (2011). Fostering the coexistence of caring philosophy and economics in today's health care system. *Nursing Administration Quarterly, 35*(1), 6–14.

Casida, J., & Pinto-Zipp, G. (2008). Leadership–organizational culture relationships in nursing units of acute care hospitals. *Nursing Economics, 26*(1), 7–15.

Cho, J., Laschinger, H. K. S., & Wong, C. (2006). Workplace empowerment, work engagement and organizational commitment of new graduate nurses. *Nursing Leadership, 19*(3), 43–60.

Franche, R. L., Murray, E., Ibrahim, S., Smith, P., Carnide, N., Cote, P., . . . Koehoorn, M. (2011). Examining the impact of worker and workplace factors on prolonged work absences among Canadian nurses. *Journal of Occupational and Environmental Medicine, 53*(8), 919–927.

Greiner, A. C., & Knebel, E., (Eds.). (2003). H*ealth professions education: A bridge to quality.* Washington, DC: The National Academies Press.

Hader, R. (2010). The evidence that isn't. *Nursing Management, 41*(9), 22–26. doi:10.1097/01. NUMA.0000387083.21113.09

Hanson, W. R., & Ford, R. (2010). Complexity leadership in healthcare: Leader network awareness. *Procedia Social and Behavioral Sciences, 2,* 6587–6596.

Huston, C. J. (2010). *Professional issues in nursing: Challenges & opportunities* (2nd ed.). Philadelphia, PA: Lippincott Williams & Wilkins.

Kohn, L. T., Corrigan, J. M., & Donaldson, M. (Eds.). (2000). *To err is human: Building a safer health system.* Washington, DC: Institute of Medicine.

Kouzes, J. M., & Posner, B. Z. (2007). *The leadership challenge* (4th ed.). San Francisco, CA: Jossey-Bass.

Laschinger, H. K. S., Grau, A. L., Finegan, J., & Wilk, P. (2011). Predictors of new graduate nurses' wellbeing: Testing the job demands-resources model. *Health Care Management Re*view, *37*(2), 175–186.

Légaré, F., Ratté, S., Gravel, K., & Graham, I. D. (2008). Barriers and facilitators to implementing shared decision-making in clinical practice: Update of a systematic review of health professionals' perceptions. *Patient Education and Counseling, 73*(3), 526–535.

Lyndon, A., Zlatnik, M., & Wachter, R. M. (2011). Effective physician–nurse communication: A patient safety essential for labor and delivery. *American Journal of Obstetrics & Gynecology, 205*(2), 91–96.

Malloch, K. (2010). Innovation leadership: New perspectives for new work. *Nursing Clinics of North America, 45*(1), 1–10.

McGowan, J. J. (2007). Swimming with the sharks: Perspectives on professional risk taking. *Journal of Medical Library Science, 95*(1), 104–113.

Melnyk, B. M. (2012). Achieving a high reliability organization through implementation of the ARCC Model for system-wide sustainability of evidence-based practice. *Nursing Administration Quarterly, 36*(2), 127–135.

Melnyk, B. M., & Fineout-Overholt, E. (2011). *Evidence-based practice in nursing & healthcare: A guide to best practice* (2nd ed.). Philadelphia, PA: Wolters Kluwer/ Lippincott, Williams & Wilkins.

Melnyk, B. M.,& Davidson, S. (2009). Creating a culture of innovation in nursing education through shared vision, leadership, interdisciplinary partnerships and positive deviance. *Nursing Administration Quarterly, 33*(4), 1–8.

Porter-O'Grady, T., & Malloch, K. (2010a). *Innovation leadership: Creating the landscape of health care.* Sudbury, MA: Jones and Bartlett.

Porter-O'Grady, T., & Malloch, K. (2010b), Innovation: Driving the green culture in healthcare. *Nursing Administration Quarterly, 34*(4), E1–E5.

Resar, R. K. (2006). Practical applications of reliability theory. Making noncatastrophic health care processes reliable: Learning to walk before running in creating high reliability organizations. *Health Services Research, 41*(4, Pt. 2), 1677–1689.

Sambunjak, D., Straus, S. E., & Marusic, A. (2006). Mentoring in academic medicine: A systematic review. *JAMA, 296*(9), 1103–1115.

Scharmer, C. O., & Käufer, K. (2000). *Universities as the birthplace for the entrepreneuring human being.* Retrieved August 14, 2011, from http://www. ottoscharmer.com/docs/articles/2000_Uni21us.pdf

Sredl, D., Melnyk, B. M., Hsueh, K.-H., Jenkins, R., Ding, C. D., & Durham, J. (2010). Health care in crisis: Can nurse executives' beliefs about and implementation of evidence-based practice be key solutions in health care reform? *Teaching and Learning in Nursing, 6,* 73–79.

Uhl-Bien, M., & Marion, R. (Eds.). (2008). *Complexity leadership, Part I: Conceptual foundations.* Charlotte, NC: Information Age.

Vyt, A. (2008). Interprofessional and transdisciplinary teamwork in healthcare. *Diabetes/Metabolism Research and Reviews, 24*(Suppl. 1), S106–S109.

Witt/Kieffer. (2004). *Putting succession planning in play: Identifying and developing the healthcare organization's successors.* Oak Brook, IL: Author.

Zerhouni, E. (2005). US biomedical research: Basic, translational, and clinical Sciences. *Journal of the American Medical Association, 294*(11), 1352–1358.

Zucker, B., Coss, C., Williams, D., Bloodworth, L., Lynn, M., Denker, A., & Gibbs, J. D. (2006). Nursing retention in the era of a nursing shortage. *Journal for Nurses in Staff Development, 22*(6), 302–306.

## BIBLIOGRAPHY

Anderson, B. J., Manno, M., O'Connor, P., & Gallagher, E. (2010). Listening to nursing leaders: Using national database of nursing quality indicators data to study excellence in nursing leadership. *Journal of Nursing Administration, 40*(4), 182–187.

Bradshaw, W. G. (2010). Importance of nursing leadership in advancing evidence-based nursing practice. *Neonatal Network: The Journal of Neonatal Nursing, 29*(2), 117–122.

Curtis, E. A., deVries, J., & Sheerin, F. K. (2011). Developing leadership in nursing: Exploring core factors. *British Journal of Nursing, 20*(5), 306–309.

Curtis, E. A., deVries, J., & Sheerin, F. K. (2011). Developing leadership in nursing: The impact of education and training. *British Journal of Nursing, 20*(6), 344–352.

Gordin, P. C., & Trey, B. (2011). Finding the leader within: Thoughts on leadership in nursing. *Journal of Perinatal & Neonatal Nursing, 25*(2), 115–118.

Jasper, M. (2011). Experiences of leadership in nursing management. *Journal of Nursing Management, 19*(4), 419–420.

Marshall, E. (2010). *Transformational leadership in nursing: From expert clinician to influential leader.* New York, NY: Springer.

Tomey, A. M. (2009). Nursing leadership and management effects work environments. *Journal of Nursing Management, 17*(1), 15–25.

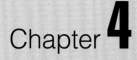

## Chapter 4

# Using Simulation to Teach Nurses

Sherry D. Fox and Rebekah Damazo

## ADDITIONAL RESOURCES

Visit thePoint for additional helpful resources
- eBook
- Journal Articles
- WebLinks

## CHAPTER OUTLINE

## LEARNING OBJECTIVES

*The learner will be able to:*

1. Describe the evolution of simulation technology used in teaching nurses from the late 1990s to the present.

2. Analyze the potential impact of simulation technology on nursing education's ability to produce graduates prepared for current workforce demands, despite inadequate numbers of nursing faculty and inadequate clinical placement sites for nursing students.

3. Explore how the use of simulation as an adjunct to clinical nursing education can mitigate or reduce provider errors and improve patient outcomes.

4. Identify how strategies such as debriefing and guided reflection can be used to stimulate collaborative dialogue and problem solving in simulated learning experiences.

5. Explore common challenges associated with using simulation to teach nurses, including cost, time constraints, a lack of realism, and educators who are unprepared for teaching with simulation.

6. Review and summarize the current literature regarding the effect of simulated learning on the achievement of desired learner outcomes.

7. Consider the strengths and limitations of high-fidelity patient simulators as a replacement for traditional acute care clinical experience in nursing education.

8. Explore the likelihood that certifying and licensing boards will look to simulation as one way to validate the initial and ongoing competency of health care professionals.

*continued*

9. Identify factors that should be considered and steps that should be taken before educational and health care facilities acquire simulation technology as a teaching tool.

10. Consider whether simulation could be used more effectively as a supplement to basic nursing education or ongoing continuing education of health care professionals.

Nurses the world over are familiar with the use of simulation for skills training. Most nursing students begin their exposure to clinical nursing cloistered in a skills lab, with static mannequins on which they practice positioning, turning, dressings, and inserting various tubes. The skill of injections is often practiced first on oranges, gel pads, or even classmates before the student approaches the real patient. Hypothetical patient interactions may be carried out in role-play.

Despite such rehearsals, the approach to the patient is often fraught with uncertainty, anxiety, and exposure to multiple contextual elements for which the skills lab has not prepared the student, and the practice of nursing turns out to be precisely *practice*. Many a wary patient has watched as a novice anxiously "practiced" some skill or assessment in the real world with varying degrees of success. The student is usually totally focused on the skill, barely able to interact with the patient or the environment. The pressure is compounded because hospitals are narrowing the ways in which students can participate in the health care setting. Some hospitals are severely limiting students' abilities to give medications or participate in procedures due to stringent oversight from accrediting bodies. Beyond the necessary psychomotor skills are the skills of clinical reasoning and decision making—picking up appropriate cues, making necessary assessments, and coming to appropriate conclusions about what the patient needs in a dynamic, fast-paced setting.

The skills needed to meet real-world demands cannot be easily rehearsed in traditional skills labs, with static mannequins such as the ubiquitous "Mrs. Chase." Nurse educators have tried to expand the scope of isolated skills lab practice by introducing computer vignettes, case studies, role playing, and other modalities, with positive results, but these teaching methods invariably lack many aspects of reality and interactivity for the student. Conversely, the real clinical setting lacks aspects of predictability and control in terms of the environment for learning. The instructor cannot ensure that each student attains the same, or even similar, experiences, resulting in highly variable learning outcomes.

These unmet needs were the impetus for the proliferation of high-fidelity patient simulators in the late 1990s and first decade of the 21st century. Technology innovations have provided new practice tools that include wireless, computer-driven mannequins with life-like features. Human patient simulation technology offers new possibilities for engaging student nurses in realistic patient scenarios with time to reflect and receive feedback to enhance learning. This chapter describes the emergence of sophisticated simulators as a tool for teaching nurses, provides the rationale for their use, and outlines the challenges inherent in determining how to incorporate simulation into nursing education. In addition, it presents preliminary outcomes of simulation use, as well as examples of emerging applications for staff training and competency assessment and regulatory trends. Components needed to develop a simulation center are summarized.

## THE EMERGENCE OF HIGH-FIDELITY PATIENT SIMULATORS

Within the last decade, the proliferation of high-fidelity patient simulators has set the stage for a revolution in how students are taught. Practicing nurses have also been affected as employers seek to quantify competency (Decker, Utterback, Thomas, Mitchell, & Sportsman, 2011). Patient simulators are full-sized, computerized mannequins that can be programmed to respond in realistic ways. They can provide dynamic assessment data in real time, display programmed signs and symptoms, and respond to nursing actions.

These sophisticated mannequins evolved from low-technology mannequins and task trainers (such as CPR mannequins and intravenous [IV] arms) as computer technology advanced. Human patient simulators are categorized as "high-fidelity" simulation, compared with the "lower fidelity" of task trainers (mannequins that have limited capabilities, designed for specific tasks, such as pelvic models and IV arms) and static mannequins such as the Mrs. Chase "dummy." Fidelity refers to the degree of realism.

In the 1980s, sophisticated simulators were in use for training anesthesiologists and military personnel (Hovancsek, 2007); nurse anesthetist programs also benefited. However, the costs for such early versions of patient simulators were prohibitive for most schools of nursing. As the industry has grown and the array of products has expanded, patient simulators are now within affordable ranges for many nursing schools and hospital systems and are poised to become an important technological adjunct for nursing education in the 21st century.

## CAPABILITIES OF PATIENT SIMULATORS

High-fidelity mannequins can be programmed to display selected signs and symptoms and to respond to the actions of the learner. The student can listen to preprogrammed heart, lung, and bowel sounds, can assess pulses at anatomically correct sites, can visualize respirations and pupil responses, and can observe displays of physiologic parameters such as the electrocardiogram (ECG), blood pressure, hemodynamic wave forms, pulse oximetry, and temperature on a simulated patient monitor. These parameters can all change in a preprogrammed pattern or under the control of a skilled operator. The simulators can be preprogrammed to speak or to respond through operator voices.

Three major companies produce a variety of simulators (infant, child, adult, birthing; Medical Education Technologies Incorporated CAE healthcare (formerly METI), Laerdal, and Gaumard), with more companies and products emerging rapidly. A range of sophisticated features is available, with the more complex models used for anesthesiology and military training.

Simulation is an educational strategy that allows realistic reproduction of aspects of real health care settings and patient events, which are designed by or under the control of the instructor. Students participate in the simulation scenario just as they would in the actual setting. Students interact with the mannequin, make physical assessments, monitor physiologic parameters, and observe the programmed trajectory of an episode. The student's interventions can affect the "patient's" course, for better or worse. All of the student's actions can be recorded for later reflection and debriefing and may be observed by peers to stimulate collaborative dialogue and problem solving. Possibly the most powerful component of simulations is the *debriefing*, which is a requisite at the completion of a scenario (Henneman, Cunningham, Roche, & Curnin, 2007). Debriefing, guided by a skilled educator, can produce insightful reflection on the events, help students to analyze and explain the reasoning behind actions, and facilitate the exploration of alternative approaches. Research indicates that debriefing is a key component in

the learning which occurs with simulation (Shinnick, Woo, Horwich, & Steadman, 2011a).

Decker (2007b) described the process of *guided reflection*, which she equated with the art of nursing. Decker hypothesized that "if simulated learning experiences are based on the principles of experiential learning, and guided reflection is embedded into the simulated learning experience, then the experience should promote the insight needed for the development of clinical judgment that promotes quality patient care" (p. 76). Research is needed to support this hypothesis, one of many challenges posed for nurse educators using simulation teaching strategies.

Rising to this challenge, Kuiper, Heinrich, Matthias, Graham, and Bell-Kotwall (2008) tested debriefing with a clinical reasoning model, comparing scores on a clinical reasoning tool for the same students in real clinical situations versus simulation. There was no significant difference between the clinical reasoning scores in the real and simulated experiences. The authors concluded that simulated experiences allow practice with clinical reasoning skills, promoting similar thinking as in authentic clinical experiences. Dreifuerst (2009) concurs, asserting that debriefing can be effective in helping students gain insight and clinical reasoning skills through reflection, thinking about their actions, and even beyond their actions. Shinnick et al. (2011a) determined through a two-group repeated measures design experiment that debriefing was a necessary component for knowledge acquisition after hands-on simulation.

> ### DISCUSSION POINT
>
> Following a critical patient incident, what type of discussion ensues in your clinical setting? Who provides input? What type of record is available to trace the actions that occurred (or were omitted)? (One example might be a debriefing session following a "code.")

There has been a surge in the sale and manufacture of new types of patient simulators and accompanying equipment, much of it fueled by the rapid adoption of simulators in nursing programs. A recent survey of 1,729 prelicensure RN programs in the United States explored the current use of simulators (Hayden, 2010). Eighty-seven percent of those who responded use simulation. The majority of programs use simulation in five or more clinical courses, with an evident trend of incorporating simulation throughout nursing curricula. Kardong-Edgren (2009) asserts, "In nursing education, simulation has become an essential instructional method" (p. e161). An international survey of simulation users (members of the International Nursing Association for Clinical Simulation and Learning [INASCL]) confirms that nursing educators worldwide are adopting simulation strategies (Gore, Van Gele, Ravert, & Mabire, 2012).

---

### DISCUSSION POINT

Think of a clinical occurrence in which you felt unprepared to handle the situation. What type of practice or rehearsal could have prepared you better?

---

## SIMULATION AND HEALTH CARE QUALITY

Nursing educators in academia, as well as in staff development, face challenges on many fronts in preparing and maintaining a well-educated, competent nursing workforce that is adequate in numbers and in appropriate skills to meet today's health care demands. Above all, the consumer of health care wants assurances that today's nurses are competent and that the care provided is safe and free from errors and omissions that can lead to prolonged illness or death.

The landmark Institute of Medicine (IOM) report *To Err Is Human* promoted simulation training as one way to prevent and mitigate errors (Kohn, Corrigan, & Donaldson, 2000). In simulation for modeling crisis management, "small groups that work together— whether in the operating room, intensive care unit, or emergency department—learn to respond to a crisis in an efficient, effective, and coordinated manner" (pp. 176–177). The report proposed the development of simulation technology, although it cautioned that simulation "that will allow full, interdisciplinary teams to practice interpersonal and technical skills in a nonjeopardy environment where they can receive meaningful feedback and reinforcement" (p. 177) would be a great challenge. Since this report, simulation technology and its implementation have made great strides in the area of simulation training for the professions and for interprofessional teams.

Simulation is poised to become an essential component of efforts to meet quality and safety initiatives. Medical errors continue to headline health care morbidity and mortality reports. The concern for patient safety has become a central theme for those who provide or receive care. Despite decades of research and scientific discovery, patients still experience harmful events with regrettable frequency (Freeth et al., 2009). Administrators are becoming more cognizant of the important role simulation could play in increasing the safety and quality of health care and the concomitant reduction in financial risk. Strouse (2010) advocates requiring staff to participate in multidisciplinary simulated learning experiences to reinforce principles of effective teamwork and communication.

Risk managers of health care systems are beginning to recognize the value of simulation training for containing the costs of legal suits. Harvard University Medical Center examined the high cost of malpractice for their anesthesiologists and pursued simulation as an anesthesia risk-control strategy. Because of success both in controlling costs and in malpractice litigation, the risk-control strategy was extended to obstetrical providers. The program was successful in developing, implementing, and evaluating an obstetric simulation-based team training course grounded in *crisis resource management* (CRM) principles. The results were highly satisfied participants who reported using the CRM principles in practice. Participants still valued their participation 1 year after completing the course, and, as an added benefit, received a 10% reduction in annual obstetrical malpractice premiums. This study supported the idea that simulation-based CRM training can serve as a strategy for mitigating adverse perinatal events and has the added benefit of reducing the cost of malpractice insurance (Gardner, Walzer, Simon, & Raemer, 2008).

Durham and Alden (2008), in a handbook for nurses produced by the federal Agency for Healthcare Research and Quality (AHRQ), proposed that the "use of simulation as a teaching strategy can contribute to patient safety and optimize outcomes of care, providing learners with opportunities to experience scenarios and intervene in clinical situations within a safe, supervised setting without posing a risk to a patient" (p. 1). Gantt and Webb-Corbett (2010) used simulation to integrate patient safety instruction into simulation experiences for undergraduate nursing students. Reducing medical errors is one area where the health care community can and should benefit from using simulation-based training to assure patient safety. However, it is important to note that simulation is only effective if it is designed and delivered appropriately.

---

CONSIDER THIS  The AHRQ supports simulation research through its patient safety program, funding 19 grant projects totaling US$5 million in 2006, to evaluate the role of simulation in improving the safety of health care. The agency asserted that simulation can provide safe learning environments to allow for testing new clinical processes and enhancing skills before bringing them to the patient (AHRQ, 2008). This agency continues to offer grant funding to support simulation research related to patient safety.

---

## New Graduate Nurse Readiness

Even with the best efforts of nursing academia to produce competent graduates, nursing educators know that a new graduate, at best, is a novice nurse, lacking confidence and competence in many areas. Lasater (2007b) reports there is a demand for nurses to enter professional practice with a "higher level of knowledge" in spite of the inconsistent practice that students receive. New nurses are often hired directly into settings demanding high-level competencies, without the luxury of practice experience in lower-acuity settings.

Practicing nurses must keep up with changes in technology and the effect on patient care, at the same time dealing with nursing staff shortages, rapid turnover, the use of traveling nurses, and the necessity for mentoring students and new nurses. Acuity levels in today's hospitals and other clinical settings do not allow for quiet reflection for decision making. The pace is fast, and the nurse who is not well practiced is at risk to make serious errors in omission and commission.

Del Bueno (2005), using a competency assessment tool, estimated that only 35% of new graduate registered nurses (RNs) meet expectations for entry-level clinical judgment. She attributed this deficiency to the tendency of nursing programs to focus on content rather than application. Students need consistent experience, in simulation and in real settings. A recent ranking of 36 new nurse graduate competencies by frontline nurse leaders in service settings (3,500 nurse managers, directors, educators, and charge nurses) revealed consistent agreements on new graduate deficiencies (Advisory Board Company, 2008). All six "Management of Responsibilities" competencies—appropriate follow-up, ability to take initiative, completion of tasks within the expected time frame, ability to track multiple responsibilities, ability to prioritize, and delegation of tasks—were in the lower one third of new-graduate proficiencies. Several critical thinking competencies (recognition of changes in patient status, interpretation of assessment data, and ability to anticipate risk) were also in the bottom one third of competencies. Only 10% to 19% of nurse leaders agreed that new graduates exhibited these competencies. Nursing educators, as well as nurses responsible for orienting new nurses, are faced with the challenge of developing the competency levels of new nurses.

Krautscheid, Orton, Chorpenning, and Ryerson (2011) explored anecdotal reports from clinical faculty and student nurses suggesting that students were not adequately prepared for safe entry into practice due to a lack of real-world medication administration scenarios. Researchers at the University of Portland in Portland, Oregon, found discrepancies in the way students were taught medication administration compared with current medication administration practice. Students wanted experience using relevant technology and tools needed for the hospital setting (Krautscheid et al., 2011). The practice of setting medications out on counters or in outdated medication carts did not prepare the student for the technology demands and distractions of a modern hospital.

Landmark research by Benner, Sutphen, Leonard, and Day (2010) summarizes the profound changes in 21st-century nursing and notes a significant gap between current practice and the education of nurses preparing them for practice. They call for radical changes in nursing education and the pedagogies involved. One recommendation for pedagogy change is keeping the student focused on the patient's experience, through unfolding cases, such as simulation scenarios; such teaching strategies will require resources to assist faculty to develop and implement effective clinical simulation exercises. Furthermore, they recommend the addition of competency assessments throughout the educational path, as well as with the NCLEX-RN examination, and again following a 1-year postlicensure residency, using simulation.

Fortunately, the "perfect storm" of health care chaos and increased demands on nursing educators is crossing paths with the recent revolution in high-technology patient simulators. Simultaneously, as production and market competition grow, these simulators are becoming priced at levels that make them more affordable. The planned integration of patient simulators in nursing, for academic education as well as for staff development, is one major avenue to producing higher levels of competency and safe practice for nursing.

## BENEFITS OF SIMULATION

Unlike real clinical practice, in which an instructor's vigilance is spread over many students and many patients, with simulation, the instructor can observe every step the student makes, allowing for many teachable moments and the possibility of coaching to correct fallacies of judgment and erroneous actions. In addition, simulations can expose students to rare events that they do not commonly see in the practice setting—events where competent performance is critical but rarely possible without practice opportunities.

Faculty can ensure that all students have exposure to specific critical learning experiences, providing more uniformity in student experience. Critical events that occur infrequently, such as cardiac arrest, can be practiced repeatedly in simulation, allowing for competent performance in the real setting. When life hangs in the balance, CPR must be initiated rapidly and correctly, yet CPR skills are usually practiced only briefly, every 2 years with CPR certification. Recent research by Leighton and Scholl (2009) revealed that nursing students could not successfully perform basic CPR steps just 22 weeks after their initial CPR certification. Moreover, the rapid assessment of patient deterioration and the advanced decision making needed to prevent the actual cardiac arrest are expert skills that need ongoing rehearsal and reinforcement, which students and novice nurses usually do not receive. On-the-job training is not the ideal place to develop such critical competencies.

Faculty who teach with simulation may choose not to rescue the "patient" by preventing student mistakes. Students may be allowed to experience the full consequences of their decisions, even to the point of the "death" of their "patients," which can profoundly affect the students' learning and retention of what they have learned.

The level of difficulty in simulation can be adapted for the student level. Simulators are differentiated according to the complexity needed for specific objectives. For example, anesthesiology training and advanced military training for casualty management involve highly complex simulators with advanced capabilities. However, the standard mannequins in use in most schools of nursing can be programmed for simple to advanced scenarios by manipulating one or more parameters to the level of difficulty. A novice student may have to respond to a simple declining blood pressure, whereas an advanced student may be dealing with a plummeting oxygen saturation, apparent respiratory distress, tachycardia, pharmacological effects, and distressed family members.

Beyond uses in teaching assessment and providing realistic skills practice, scenarios can be developed and validated to provide for the development of critical thinking and clinical decision making and can be used for competency evaluation (Decker, Sportsman, Puetz, & Billings, 2008). The ability for nurse educators to be able to observe a complete set of actions, question a student's line of thinking, and provide guidance when the student fails to notice or incorporate important cues is a powerful teaching adjunct, allowing for many more of the precious "teachable moments" valued by faculty.

Depending on how the learning environment is managed, students generally respond very positively to the learning opportunities in simulation, reporting increased self-confidence, competence, and lower anxiety levels (Hovancsek, 2007; Jeffries & Rizzolo, 2006; Yuan, Williams, & Fang, 2012). They also express value in learning from each other when a collaborative approach is used in which classmates observe and contribute to each other's scenarios (Lasater, 2007b).

Simulations can be designed for team practice, enhancing collaboration, and improving team communication skills. Simulations that provide for interdisciplinary training, including the full array of roles in a patient care scenario, are becoming an important part of staff development. Health care professionals are predominantly trained in their individual disciplines, yet they must be able to come together as teams, with little or no interdisciplinary training. Simulation can provide the common ground for health care teams to learn how to function as teams (Miller, Riley, Davis, & Hansen, 2008). Patient safety requires highly organized systems of care, yet the training of the individuals who comprise the teams has been neglected. The IOM report *To Err Is Human* emphasized the need for team training using simulation (Kohn et al., 2000).

Team STEPPS is a federally funded initiative by the AHRQ, designed to improve patient safety through effective teamwork. Institutions that are selected for participation receive standardized training materials and procedures. Simulation methods are offered as a powerful component of team training (Agency for Healthcare Research and Quality, n.d.).

## DISADVANTAGES OF SIMULATION

The use of patient simulators may not be a total panacea for educators. Initial costs for the acquisition of the simulators are prohibitive for many programs. New wireless high-fidelity simulators cost US$40,000 to US$90,000 and have an expected shelf life of around 3 years. More basic models are available but are rapidly being replaced with wireless models with improved reality features such as blinking eyes and the ability to measure values using real-world equipment. Models that sense and respond to medications and have other sophisticated features necessary for anesthesiology or military training can cost as much as US$250,000. Institutions must augment their traditional equipment budgets to accommodate this emerging technology. Beyond the initial investment in high-fidelity mannequins, ongoing considerations of space, technician support, and faculty training mandate continuing expenses.

The number of students who can work with the simulators at one time is limited, and students require intensive faculty involvement, which is often more time-consuming than regular clinical supervision for a group of students. Traditional student-to-faculty ratios may need to be evaluated as simulation users become more knowledgeable about the most effective use of simulation time schedules. Faculty may need to rethink the "8-hour" student shift and replace it with shorter, more frequent training days.

Students may feel put on the spot and experience anxiety, especially when being observed by faculty and peers. However, in her research analyzing the use of simulation to develop clinical judgment, Lasater (2007b) reported that, despite the fact students may report that simulations were "anxiety producing" or made them "feel like an idiot," the group participants consistently verbalized that they did learn through the scenarios. These findings corroborate other researchers who support the heightened learning achieved when students experience simulation (Beyea, von Reyn, & Slattery, 2007; Jarzemsky & McGrath, 2008; Jeffries & Rizzolo, 2006; Radhakrishnan, Roche, & Cunningham, 2007).

Another disadvantage is that students might not function as if the scenario was real, perceiving an artificiality to the setting (National Council of State Boards of Nursing [NCSBN], 2005). Most educators acknowledge where realism is lacking when discussing cases with students. It is important for the faculty designing the case scenario to understand the degree of realism required to accomplish the stated learning objectives. Although recognizing the promise of simulation, the NCSBN (2005) offered the caution that students "must practice in authentic situations." Although recognized as a complement to actual clinical practice, simulation should not replace it. Where simulation is done well, it provides experience and skill that will enhance practice. Finding the optimum balance, however, between clinical practice and simulation is not easy and will require ongoing research (see Research Study Fuels the Controversy 4.1).

## RESEARCH STUDY FUELS THE CONTROVERSY 4.1

### CAN SIMULATION DEVELOP NURSING EXPERTISE?

Day (2007) expressed concerns about the ability of nurses/students truly to develop expertise as described by Benner's model of "Novice to Expert" through simulation. Noting that expertise is developed within the complex context of practice settings, she asserted that the development of expertise in nursing requires experience and the "right kind of engagement with practice situations" (p. 507). She cautioned that simulations are removed from the context of the patient, requiring different assumptions and roles than those experienced by students in simulation. Acknowledging the promise of high-fidelity simulation, she expressed the belief that simulation will likely not speed the acquisition of skills for new graduates if clinical time with real patients is replaced.

In an alternative view, Beeman (2008) developed a tiered critical care education program based on Benner's model of "Novice to Expert." Simulations were developed to teach and assess levels of critical care expertise, from the advanced beginner to expert. Carefully designed scenarios for each level were used to foster clinical advancement and to provide for performance evaluation. The ultimate goal for this ambitious program was to demonstrate optimized patient outcomes and patient safety as a result of achieving clinical excellence (p. 50).

Both authors valued simulation, but Day saw the potential as much more limited than did Beeman. Beeman's approaches are used with practicing nurses, so the question of replacing clinical time is not an issue, as it might be with student

*continued*

nurses. However, Beeman evidenced confidence that the clinical reasoning needed to develop true expertise can be nurtured and evaluated through well-designed, complex scenarios with skilled faculty not necessarily requiring the context of the real patient encounter.

Day, L. (2007). Simulation and the teaching and learning of practice in critical care units. *American Journal of Critical Care, 16,* 504–507.

Beeman, L. (2008). Basing a clinician's career on simulation: Development of a critical care expert into a clinical simulation expert. In R. Kyle & W. Murray (Eds.), *Clinical simulation: Operations, engineering and management* (pp. 31–51). New York, NY: Elsevier.

---

### DISCUSSION POINT

1. Which position (Day or Beeman) do you find more compelling? (Consider the education of student nurses vs. ongoing proficiency development for practicing nurses.)
2. As a practicing nurse, would you consider ongoing training and evaluation with simulation as a requirement to advance your career as an opportunity or a threat?

Although it is important to note the cautionary views on simulation, it is noteworthy that those who are using and evaluating simulation are passionate champions of this rapidly advancing field. Today's simulation is not focused on isolated skill building. It builds on a skills foundation and requires students to acquire cognitive and affective skills and to develop clinical judgment (Lasater, 2007b). In many areas, students are required or encouraged to practice in a team of health professionals, building competencies essential for working within teams. One area of concern, however, relates to the student who becomes confident in simulation and may take on tasks beyond his or her level of expertise. It is essential that faculty provide simulations that are within the scope of practice geared to the student's level.

Perhaps the most significant barrier to the use of simulation is the need for well-trained faculty who can devise the best uses of simulation within specific curricula. All too often, expensive simulators are purchased but not effectively used, lacking a champion who can bring about the extensive curricular planning and faculty training needed. It is not uncommon for expensive mannequins to lie dormant in their shipping crates long after their arrival. Seasoned educators may find the technology interface daunting (Starkweather & Kardong-Edgren, 2008). Despite the availability of pre-developed scenarios for nursing education, nursing faculty will have their own priorities and will desire modifications that must be programmed into the computer. The availability of skilled technicians who can assist with the computer interface removes one of the major faculty hurdles but poses additional costs.

Effective simulations also require expert debriefing. Debriefing is a skilled function, bringing to bear the faculty member's clinical expertise, as well as his or her educational savvy. One approach to preparing faculty for the challenges is attendance at teaching conferences that focus on simulation; another approach is individual training sessions for groups of faculty. For example, California State University, Chico, integrates simulation training in the preparation of all nursing education master's students, preparing future educators with the skills needed to incorporate simulation into nursing education.

### SIMULATION FOR PRACTICE SETTINGS

Patient simulators are not and will not be relegated only to academic settings for the initial training of nursing students. Simulation has been used to test new procedures before bringing them to the patient bedside, as well as training individuals and teams for specific advanced skills for practicing nurses as well as for new nurse orientations.

Dartmouth-Hitchcock Medical Center initiated a nurse residency program using human patient simulation to address issues related to the orientation time required for new graduates to become competent and to feel confident (Beyea et al., 2007). A 12-week program was developed, with didactic courses, weekly simulation experiences, and clinical time with a preceptor. At the end of the residency, the nurses were evaluated with simulations designed to assess competence. The program resulted in a markedly reduced time for orientation, with the program participants able to take full patient assignments. Participants were better prepared for skills. The simulation experiences allowed early identification of areas in which participants needed remediation or more guidance. The residents improved in self-rated confidence, competence, and readiness for independent practice. An overwhelming majority of the participants were positive about the simulation experiences. Further outcomes from this continued project reinforced the value of the simulation-based residency program as a "powerful and effective strategy" (Beyea, Slattery, & von Reyn, 2010, p. e174). Recruitment and retention improved markedly. Nurse residents experienced significant improvement in perceived confidence, competence, and readiness for practice.

Similarly, Ackermann, Kenny, and Walker (2007) described the development of a simulator program to aid in the transition of new graduate nurses, promoting critical thinking, decision making, and clinical confidence. Stefanski and Rossler (2009) developed a critical care orientation program for new graduates, with similar positive outcomes in perceived confidence.

Morris et al. (2007) also incorporated the patient simulator as part of an overall critical care institute for orienting new graduates and inexperienced RNs into critical care units. The simulator facilitated the development of critical thinking skills and provided educators with ongoing assessment of the orientee's ability to apply knowledge.

Beeman (2008) described a tiered approach to nursing staff development, using simulation technology for three different levels of clinical expertise (based on Benner's model of Novice to Expert). An elaborate simulation center provides academic training, as well as staff development training, for medical residents, nurses, nurse technicians, respiratory therapists, pharmacists, and paramedics. Evaluation components are incorporated into the simulations and are used as part of performance evaluation for clinical advancement.

Kaddoura (2010) explored the use of simulation to develop critical thinking skills for graduates on critical care units. Participants reported that they were more confident in dealing with critical situations, and simulation helped to develop their critical thinking skills.

Anderson and Leflore (2008) described the benefits of simulation for operating room team training as a tool that can increase effective communication and overall team effectiveness. Wolf (2008) described the use of simulation to teach assessment and intervention skills for emergency nurses, using a "paradigm case" model described by Benner. Following 4 hours of classroom instruction, six nurses completed three to five simulation scenarios representing different diagnoses and indications for triage. The scenarios revealed gaps in the nurses' assessment and triage processes and indicated areas for refining training. All of the nurses felt that the combination of training methods was helpful and improved triage skills. Follow-up with chart reviews showed great improvement in triage accuracy, particularly for the least experienced nurses. Wolf concluded that simulation training can improve triage accuracy, leading to better patient care.

Yaeger and Arafeh (2008) described the value of simulation training for obstetric and neonatal care providers to obtain hands-on training of neonatal resuscitation. Studies have indicated that the ability to adequately perform neonatal resuscitation may not be achieved by traditional training methods. Simulation training is seen as an important enhancement to former models of neonatal resuscitation training.

Miller et al. (2008) described the use of "in situ" training in which human patient simulators are brought into the practice unit where the health care team normally functions to provide team training to enhance perinatal safety. This ambitious pilot study provided 35 simulations in six hospitals with more than 700 participants. Extensive debriefing following the simulations allowed participants to develop insight into communication lapses, team failures, and latent conditions. The authors emphasized the value of team versus individual training as a means to improve processes and safety.

In situ training has also been used for ambulatory care (Maynes, 2008) to provide emergency training to clinic staff. Maynes pointed out that in situ training allows staff to find and use equipment and supplies in their own units, often resulting in changes in the type of equipment as inadequacies became apparent during simulations. Similar results have been found in other in situ simulations, such as finding out that the anesthesiologist could not reach the crash cart in an operating room simulation or that emergency room staff could not locate an IV fluid warmer to deal with a near-infant drowning victim with hypothermia.

Acute care and ambulatory settings are finding patient simulators extremely valuable for ongoing staff development, as well as for interdisciplinary team training. Patient simulators are likely to be in every nurse's future to maintain practice competence and to develop new skills.

## RESEARCH ON SIMULATION OUTCOMES

Agencies that have instituted simulation training are usually very positive about their outcomes. However, research on simulation outcomes for nursing is in its infancy. Much of the literature is of a developmental nature, describing programs and processes but not evaluating outcomes. Is there evidence that these expensive programs lead to better learning than traditional teaching strategies? Schools of medicine, training in anesthesiology, and the military have been using sophisticated patient simulators for a long time and have performed studies on the effect on learning.

Issenberg, McGaghie, Petrusa, Gordon, and Scalese (2005) performed an extensive review of outcomes research on simulation in medical education conducted between the years 1969 and 2003. They focused on 109 studies that used a simulator as an educational assessment or intervention with quantitative measures, using experimental or quasi-experimental methodology. From this review they concluded, "While research in this field needs improvement in terms of rigor and quality, high-fidelity medical simulations are educationally effective and simulation-based education complements medical education in patient care settings" (p. 10). Their recommendations for effective learning with simulators are listed in Box 4.1. Although the research reviewed by Issenberg et al. was based on medical students, it is

reasonable to believe that these findings and recommendations apply to nursing education as well.

Scavone, Toledo, Higgins, Wojciechowski, and McCarthy (2010) evaluated 32 second-year anesthesiology residents who were randomly divided into two groups—half with simulation training and half without. In their study, they had residents who had completed their obstetric anesthesia rotation perform an emergency cesarean delivery. The students who underwent focused training on a patient simulator showed improved performance compared with similar trainees who did not have the simulation-based instruction.

A major study by Draycott et al. (2008) demonstrated the excellent potential for simulation training to affect health care outcomes. A retrospective, observational study compared the management and neonatal outcomes of births complicated by shoulder dystocia. All maternity staff was trained on birth training mannequins at a mandatory multiprofessional, 1-day training course at a British hospital. Birth records (15,908 births) for the 3 years before the training were compared with those (13,117 births) 3 years after the training. Clinical management improved after the training on several parameters. There was a significant reduction in neonatal injury. All of the outcomes could be attributed to several factors—the mandatory training of 100% of the staff, the teaching of simplified methods, and the use of a high-fidelity trainer. Further research would be needed to sort out the

---

### BOX 4.1   TIPS FOR EFFECTIVE TEACHING THROUGH SIMULATION

- Provide feedback during the learning experience with the simulator.
- Ensure that learners repetitively practice skills on the simulator.
- Integrate simulators into the overall curriculum.
- Ensure that learners practice with increasing levels of difficulty (if available).
- Adapt the simulator to complement multiple learning strategies.
- Ensure that the simulator provides for clinical variation.
- Ensure that learning on the simulator occurs in a controlled environment.
- Provide individualized (in addition to team) learning on the simulator.
- Clearly define outcomes and benchmarks for the learners to achieve by using the simulator.
- Ensure that the simulator is a valid learning tool.

*Source:* Issenberg, S., McGaghie, W., Petrusa, E., Gordon, D., & Scalese, R. (2005). Features and uses of high-fidelity medical simulations that lead to effective learning: A BEME systematic review. *Medical Teacher, 27*, 10–28.

contribution of each, but presumably the training's effectiveness was enhanced by the use of simulation practice.

## Nursing Student Perceptions of Simulation: Perceived Satisfaction, Decreased Anxiety, and Increased Confidence

Most of the studies performed in nursing have focused on how acceptable this mode of learning is to students and their satisfaction levels. In general, this mode of learning is very well received by students (Bantz, Dancer, Hodson-Carlton, & Van Hove, 2007; Jeffries, 2008; Robertson, 2006; Schoening, Sittner, & Todd, 2006).

Students who participated in a study by Kaddoura (2010) commented that they were able to sharpen their leadership skill, improve teamwork, and practice effective communication as part of the simulation experience. Students reported that they believe their real ICU patients were safer because they learned how to deal with similar situations in simulation.

Bremner, Aduddell, and Amason (2008) compared two groups of 1st-year nursing students to examine the effects of using the human patient simulator prior to the first clinical experience. One group ($n = 71$) worked with the simulator 1 week before the clinical experience; the other group ($n = 78$) experienced the traditional skills lab. The authors concluded that the intervention group experienced less anxiety and greater comfort in their first clinical experience. The simulator group believed that the experience gave them confidence in their assessment skills, helped to relieve stress on the first clinical day, and should be a component of the nursing curriculum.

Outcomes research on simulation extends beyond the United States; simulation is in use worldwide. Kiat, Mei, Nagammal, and Jonnie (2007) surveyed 260 second-year nursing students in Singapore 6 months after initiation of simulation in the curriculum. Each student experienced 20 hours in simulation training. The questionnaire asked about perceived benefits, the actual experience with the simulation, factors related to the effectiveness of the training, and whether they would choose to attend simulation training. Students were overwhelmingly positive about the experience, perceiving simulation as an enjoyable way to learn, which allows them to think on their feet, to identify areas for improvement, to make sure that mistakes, if they occur, do not cause harm, and to increase confidence. More than 95% of the students would choose to participate in more simulation training. The authors concluded that appropriately used simulation has the potential to revolutionize learning in nursing, bridging theory and practice.

## Learning Outcomes With Simulation

Perhaps most relevant to educators is the degree to which simulation experiences actually contribute to learning outcomes. Most of those who use simulation believe in the value of simulation for improving learning outcomes. The research literature is sparse in this area but is growing. However, research findings are not definitive. The majority of studies report qualitative data; many of those that have a quantitative focus use weak designs and small sample sizes, lack valid and reliable measurement tools, and present limited details on methodology (Lapkin, Levett-Jones, Bellchambers, & Fernandez, 2010; Shinnick, Woo, & Mentes, 2011b).

Several recent systematic reviews of research on simulation have attempted to determine the actual impact of simulation on outcomes (Cant & Cooper, 2009; Harder, 2010; Lapkin et al., 2010; Shinnick et al., 2011b). Harder (2010) examined 23 research studies applied to high-fidelity simulation published between 2003 and 2007. The majority reported an increase in students' clinical skills using simulation compared with other teaching methods. None found that clinical skills *decreased* in the simulation groups. Several reported increases in students' perceived self-confidence and competence. Although Harder concluded the evidence supports using simulation as a teaching tool, she found many gaps and limitations in simulation research. She notes the lack of formal evaluation tools designed to measure simulation outcomes as a serious limitation for simulation research.

Cant and Cooper (2009) performed a similar review, looking at studies using medium and/or high-fidelity mannequins. Twelve studies using experimental or quasi-experimental designs were reviewed. All 12 studies reported simulation was a valid teaching/learning strategy; six of the studies demonstrated statistically significant gains in knowledge, critical thinking, perceived clinical confidence, or satisfaction, compared with a control group. These reviewers noted the variability in designs and measurements and emphasized the need for a universal method to measure outcomes.

Lapkin et al. (2010) reviewed 8 studies that met inclusion criteria as experimental studies. Outcomes related to critical thinking, clinical skill performance, knowledge acquisition, self-reported confidence, and student satisfaction were examined. They found support for the use of human patient simulators to significantly improve knowledge acquisition, critical thinking, and the ability to identify deteriorating patients. The reviewers support the use of simulation as an active learning methodology, when implemented appropriately. At the same time, they note the need for better outcome measurement tools and more rigorous research methods.

Shinnick et al. (2011b) performed an extensive review of the literature, finding 8 quantitative studies with sample sizes greater than 20 that met inclusion criteria. They concluded that the literature shows that students like simulation and that self-efficacy improves with simulation. However, they found no evidence that simulation impacts students' ability to use critical thinking. They assert that, lacking solid research evidence, the efforts to integrate simulation into nursing education may be wasted. They recommend that studies need to be conducted with adequate sample sizes, using reliable and valid measurement tools for important learning outcomes (knowledge and skill acquisition and critical thinking) to establish definitive support for simulation in nursing education.

Recognizing the need for evaluation measurement tools, Lasater (2007a, 2007b) reported on students' experience with the development of clinical judgment through high-fidelity patient simulation. The first portion of the study (Lasater, 2007a) involved the development and pilot testing of a rubric to assess levels of performance in clinical judgment. The developed rubric provided clear expectations for student learning and a standard for providing feedback, serving as a guide for students' development of clinical judgment.

Kardong-Edgren, Adamson, and Fitzgerald (2010) reinforce the call for reliable and valid instruments to measure simulation learning outcomes. They surveyed available instruments and concluded that only four tools currently come close to addressing cognitive, psychomotor, and affective learning domains. They advocate reuse of existing tools, with emphasis on establishment of reliability and validity in multiple venues, to expand the science of simulation research. They suggest that further studies reporting only on self-report and satisfaction outcomes are not particularly useful at this point in simulation outcomes research (see Research Study Fuels the Controversy 4.2).

## RESEARCH STUDY FUELS THE CONTROVERSY 4.2

**SIMULATION MOST EFFECTIVE IN DEVELOPING HIGHER-LEVEL CRITICAL THINKING**

Johnson, Flagg, and Dremsa (2007) designed a prospective, randomized study to compare cognition and critical thinking outcomes using a patient simulator versus interactive CD-ROM in training for the care of combat casualties exposed to chemical agents. The study involved 99 volunteer health professionals from active duty or reserve military units. Following a carefully designed, valid, and reliable pretest on the care of casualties exposed to chemical agents, subjects were randomly assigned to a control group, a patient simulator group, or an interactive CD-ROM group. The two experimental groups completed instruction in the assigned modalities; the control group received no instruction. The patient simulator group interacted with three patient scenarios; the CD-ROM group was exposed to the same three scenarios, with the ability to make choices and receive computerized feedback on treatment choices. One month following the interventions, subjects were retested. The instrument contained items that measured lower-level cognition skills, as well as higher-level cognition and critical thinking skills.

Johnson, D., Flagg, A., & Dremsa, T. (2007). Effects of using a Human Patient Simulator (HPS™) versus a CD-ROM on cognition and critical thinking. *Medical Education Online, 13*(1). Retrieved July 29, 2008, from http://www.med-ed-online.org/pdf/T0000118.pdf

### STUDY FINDINGS

The baseline pretest showed no differences among groups on any of the cognitive levels. The posttest analyses showed no difference between the CD-ROM group and the patient simulator group on the lower-level cognitive skills. However, the simulator group had significantly higher scores on cognitive and critical thinking skills. The authors postulated that the teaching strategies used with the patient simulator provided the participants with the ability to see the actual effectiveness of interventions related to the use of atropine and fluid resuscitation in a simulated realistic situation. Because critical thinking is postulated to occur within the context of the situation, the authors concluded that the simulation training was the most effective in achieving higher-level critical thinking skills.

## REGULATORY TRENDS RECOGNIZE THE VALUE OF SIMULATIONS

Regulatory boards are challenged to describe continued competence for health professions. The NCSBN stated in 2005 that "it is time to address the challenge" of continued competency. Benner et al. (2010) assert that nursing licensure must be based on competency evaluation that extends far beyond the current multiple-choice NCLEX. They advocate a three-part performance assessment, beginning with the last year of nursing school, a second for licensure, and a third on completion of a 1-year postlicensure residency. Simulation would provide the method for these assessments.

The Accreditation Council for Graduate Medical Education (ACGME) and the American Board of Medical Specialties (ABMS) both have embraced simulation as one of a variety of tools that can assist in determining practitioner competency (Decker et al., 2011). The American Academy of Pediatrics (AAP) steering committee on Neonatal Resuscitation Programs (NRP) announced its commitment to base newborn resuscitation on the best evidence-based science available. With that in mind, AAP incorporates practice on an infant simulator as part of its Neonatal Resuscitation Program. This announcement prompted the Laerdal Corporation to collaborate with the AAP to develop an infant simulator specifically designed for NRP training (American Academy of Pediatrics, 2007).

As part of heightened emergency preparedness efforts, the U.S. Department of Health and Human Services (DHHS), together with the Joint Commission on the Accreditation of Healthcare Organizations and other agencies, is preparing to extend disaster training to the inpatient bedside environment. High-fidelity human patient simulators will be used for training in disaster and terrorism response and treatment, as well as in patient safety and other issues raised in the IOM report *To Err Is Human* (Ramirez, 2008).

## SIMULATION IN CONTINUING EDUCATION FOR NURSES

All licensed professions require ongoing education to maintain and expand the competency needed in a dynamic health care system. Yet traditional methods of continuing education are under scrutiny. An interdisciplinary conference on continuing education for the health professions acknowledged that professional continuing education is in disarray, with too little emphasis on improving clinical performance to provide high-quality care and the preponderance of continuing education offered in the form of lectures (Hager, Russell, & Fletcher, 2008). Freeth et al. (2009) describe the use of multidisciplinary obstetric-simulated emergency scenarios to promote patient safety with excellent results. Teamwork was an essential part of this training program, and upon reflection participants reported linking the training exercise with daily practice.

In addition, there is little evidence that lectures endured for continuing education requirements actually improve practice (see Chapter 19). Among many recommendations to improve the effectiveness of continuing education, the value of simulations was acknowledged: "Interactive scenarios and simulations are promising approaches to CE, particularly for skills development, whether the skill is a highly technical procedure, history taking or a physical examination technique" (Hager et al., 2008, p. 19).

National and international trends ensure that students, nurse educators, and practicing nurses will encounter high-fidelity human patient simulators in their career pathways. However, not every setting has embarked on the process of establishing such learning centers. The first step may be starting a center. Nurses in practice or in education settings may have to become the champions who instigate the establishment of simulation centers, as well as be involved in the initial planning stages.

## DEVELOPING A SIMULATION CENTER

Beginning on the pathway to developing a simulation center for an academic or service setting is a daunting task, with a steep learning curve. Despite the proliferation of such centers, many have been developed by serendipitous approaches rather than careful business plans. Few "how-to" resources were available for early adopters. More resources will be available for the next generation of centers, including work described by Seropian, Brown, Gavilanes, and Driggers (2004), Spunt (2007), and Kyle and Murray (2008). Most important, development of an effective simulation program requires much more than the purchase of a mannequin.

The American Hospital Association Committee on Health Professions (2007) delineated steps that should be taken before hospitals consider the acquisition of simulators. The first step should be an assessment of the simulators currently available within the institution and the region. Next, a clear purpose and specific objectives should be outlined to ensure regular use. Hospitals need to consider how the simulators will be used and by whom. Given the initial cost of developing a simulation center and maintaining it, a multiyear business plan is essential.

Human resources should also be assessed, such as potential champions, potential faculty, potential staffing, and the administrative structure for oversight. Space will need to be allocated in accordance with the types of trainings anticipated, with enough space to accommodate team trainings and observers. A budget plan that covers capital expenses, as well as maintenance, repair, and replacement is essential, including ongoing software upgrades. Plans for revenue generation should be considered. However, the committee cautioned that early centers have found that simulation is a "cost of doing business," not likely to bring a positive return on investment. Savings may result from risk reduction, but will be hard to quantify.

Given the high cost of simulation centers and the need to keep such centers fully functioning, partnerships in which several agencies collaborate and share financial sponsorship provide mutual benefits. Partnerships among academic centers and hospitals allow for ongoing maximal use of the center when the schools are out of session, as well as allow for expanded use covering more than one hospital shift (Metcalfe, Hall, & Carpenter, 2007). In addition to partnerships, use of nonfaculty nurses and retired nurses, either as volunteer or paid staff, can help to extend the faculty in labor-intensive simulations in a cost-effective manner (Foster, Sheriff, & Cheney, 2008).

Along with plans for developing the center, a plan for training of the faculty who will work with the students is essential. Teaching with simulation is not business as usual. Many faculty find the technology involved daunting. Even with skilled technicians to soften the technical interface, nursing faculty must deliberate on the best ways to integrate simulation into the curriculum. Clear learning outcomes must be delineated, along with specific objectives for each simulation. The degree of realism required to meet the learning objectives must be determined and incorporated. To achieve economical use of faculty and precious time with the simulators, faculty must develop strategies to engage groups of students so that more than one student can benefit from the learning in the scenario. The reflective learning that occurs after a scenario is completed requires skilled faculty (Bremner, Aduddell, Bennett, & VanGeest, 2006; Lasater, 2007a). Fortunately, many faculty are rising to the challenge. Most national nursing conferences now include sessions on the use of simulation, curriculum design, and ongoing research. Indeed, Decker (2007a) posed the question as to whether it is even ethical to train nurses without using simulation in an era in which these resources are readily available and when outcomes research suggests such positive outcomes (see Research Study Fuels the Controversy 4.3).

---

## RESEARCH STUDY FUELS THE CONTROVERSY 4.3

### IS IT ETHICAL TO TRAIN NURSES *WITHOUT* THE USE OF SIMULATION?

Given new simulation technology, which allows for much greater demonstration of competency before entering the real patient care setting, is it ethical to continue to educate students *without* simulation? Decker (2007a) discussed the educational ethics related to the use of patient simulators as a means to provide realistic training for students without endangering patients versus traditional clinical learning experiences in which patients are subjected to the ministrations of inexperienced students.

Decker, S. (2007). Simulations: Education and ethics. In P. Jeffries (Ed.), *Simulation in nursing education: From conceptualization to evaluation* (pp. 11–19). New York, NY: National League for Nursing.

---

### STUDY FINDINGS

Discussing ethical principles of justice, autonomy, beneficence, nonmaleficence, veracity, and compassion, Decker presented examples of how simulation training might lead to more ethical care for patients. For example, Decker asked, "Are nurse educators and other healthcare professionals demonstrating compassion when they allow students to perform procedures for the first time on clients instead of first providing students with simulated experiences?" (p. 16). Decker raised questions for nursing faculty to consider regarding their obligation to assure nursing student competencies prior to engaging in patient care, in light of the looming opportunities presented by patient simulators. She posed a need for a change in the culture of nursing education, related to use of simulation.

## CONCLUSIONS

The advance of technology in health care is relentless; simulation brings significant technological change to nursing education as well. Regardless of how nurses were initially educated, all nurses can anticipate exposure to simulation technology, whether as students or new graduates, in orienting to new roles or specialties, for demonstrating ongoing competency, and even for continuing education. Nurses in staff development or responsible for training nurses for specialty settings will need to consider simulation as a teaching and competency assessment strategy. In a profession that requires lifelong learning, the question of how best to learn new competencies is partially answered by the promise of simulation.

## FOR ADDITIONAL DISCUSSION

1. Consider your first skill applied to a real patient, such as giving an injection or starting an intravenous line. How confident were you of your skill? How anxious were you? How much of your anxiety was transmitted to the patient? Would simulation practice have improved your confidence and decreased your anxiety?

2. Reflect on a crisis situation in patient care that you had to solve quickly on your own. Would prior simulation practice have helped you in your ability to anticipate and critically analyze the situation? Why or why not?

3. Consider a clinical situation in which you experienced profound learning, something you will never forget. Is there a way to replicate that situation through simulation so that others could experience the same learning? Why or why not?

4. Simulation has been faulted for not being totally realistic. Which factors in patient care can readily be incorporated into simulation? Which cannot?

5. Consider the anxiety experienced by students in a simulation who are being observed by faculty and peers. In the clinical setting, is there more or less anxiety when you are uncertain of your actions and are being observed by patients, family, nurses, physicians, and others?

6. When a student approaches a patient procedure, is it ethical to ask for the patient's consent without fully disclosing the student's qualifications to perform the procedure?

7. In comparing traditional models of nursing education—skills labs followed by clinical practice—with simulation prior to clinical practice:

   a) Which model provides for greater patient safety?
   b) Which model provides for the greatest security for the patient?
   c) Which model provides for the greatest confidence building for students?

## REFERENCES

Ackermann, A., Kenny, G., & Walker, C. (2007). Simulator programs for new nurses' orientation: A retention strategy. *Journal for Nursing in Staff Development, 23*(3), 136–139.

Advisory Board Company. (2008). *Capturing the academic and industry perspectives.* Retrieved August 14, 2008, from http: www.advisoryboardcompany.com/offerings.html

Agency for Healthcare Research and Quality. (2008). *Improving patient safety through simulation research.* Retrieved August 30, 2008, from http://www.ahrq.gov/qual/simulproj.htm

Agency for Healthcare Research and Quality. (n.d.). *About Team STEPPS.* Retrieved April 27, 2011, from http://teamstepps.ahrq.gov/about-2cl_3.htm

American Academy of Pediatrics. (2007). NRP Celebrates 20th Anniversary. *NRP Instructor Update, 16*(2), 1–12.

American Hospital Association Committee on Health Professions. (2007). *Clinical simulators: Considerations for hospitals.* Retrieved July 27, 2008, from http://www.hret.org/hret/programs/content/simulatorsreport.pdf

Anderson, M., & Leflore, J. (2008). Playing it safe: Simulated team training in the OR. *AORN Journal, 87*(4), 772–779.

Bantz, D., Dancer, M., Hodson-Carlton, K., & Van Hove, S. (2007). A daylong clinical laboratory: From gaming to high-fidelity simulators. *Nurse Educator, 32*(6), 274–277.

Beeman, L. (2008). Basing a clinician's career on simulation: Development of a critical care expert into a clinical simulation expert. In R. Kyle & W. Murray (Eds.), *Clinical simulation: operations, engineering and management* (pp. 31–51). New York, NY: Elsevier.

Benner, P., Sutphen, M., Leonard, V., & Day, L. (2010). *Educating nurses: A call for radical transformation.* San Francisco, CA: Jossey-Bass.

Beyea, S. C., von Reyn, L., & Slattery, M. (2007). A nurse residency program for competency development using human patient simulation. *Journal for Nurses in Staff Development, 23*(7), 77–82.

Beyea, S., Slattery, M., & von Reyn, L. (2010). Outcomes of a simulation-based nurse residency program. *Clinical Simulation in Nursing, 6*(5), E169–E175.

Bremner, M., Aduddell, K., & Amason, J. (2008). Evidence-based practices related to the human patient simulator and first year baccalaureate nursing students' anxiety. *Online Journal of Nursing Informatics, 12*(1), 1–10.

Bremner, M., Aduddell, K., Bennett, D., & VanGeest, J. (2006). The use of human patient simulators: Best practices with novice nursing students. *Nurse Educator, 31*(4), 170–174.

Cant, R., & Cooper, S. (2009). Simulation-based learning in nurse education: Systematic review. *Journal of Advanced Nursing, 66*(1), 3–15.

Day, L. (2007). Simulation and the teaching and learning of practice in critical care units. *American Journal of Critical Care, 16*, 504–507.

Decker, S. (2007a). Simulations: Education and ethics. In P. Jeffries (Ed.), *Simulation in nursing education: from conceptualization to evaluation* (pp. 11–19). New York, NY: National League for Nursing.

Decker, S. (2007b). Integrating guided reflection into simulated learning. In P. Jeffries (Ed.), *Simulation in nursing education: From conceptualization to evaluation* (pp. 73–85). New York, NY: National League for Nursing.

Decker, S., Sportsman, S., Puetz, L., & Billings, L. (2008). The evolution of simulation and its contribution to competency. *Journal of Continuing Education in Nursing, 39*(2), 74–80.

Decker, S., Utterback, V., Thomas, M., Mitchell, M., & Sportsman, S. (2011). Assessing continued competency through simulation: A call to action. *Nursing Education Perspectives, 32*(2), 120–125.

Del Bueno, D. (2005). A crisis in critical thinking. *Nursing Education Perspectives, 26*, 278–282.

Draycott, T., Crofts, J., Ash, J., Wilson, L. V., Yard, E., Sibanda, T., & Whitelaw, A. (2008). Improving neonatal outcome through practical shoulder dystocia training. *Obstetrics & Gynecology, 112* (1), 1–7.

Dreifuerst, K. (2009). The essentials of debriefing in simulation learning: A concept analysis. *Nursing Education Perspectives, 30*(2), 109–114.

Durham, C., & Alden, K. (2008). Enhancing patient safety in nursing education through patient simulation. In R. G. Huges (Ed.), *Patient safety and quality: An evidence-based handbook for nurses* (AHRQ Publication No. 09-0043). Rockville, MD: Agency for Healthcare Research and Quality. Retrieved July 24, 2008, from http://www.ahrq.gov/qual/nurseshdbk/docs/durhamc_epsne.pdf

Foster, J., Sheriff, S., & Cheney, S. (2008). Using nonfaculty registered nurses to facilitate high-fidelity human patient simulation activities. *Nurse Educator, 33*(3), 137–141.

Freeth, D., Ayida, G., Berridge, E., Mackintosh, N., Norris, B., Sadler, C., & Strachan, A. (2009). Multidisciplinary obstetric simulated emergency scenarios (MOSES): Promoting patient safety in obstetrics with teamwork-focused interprofessional simulations. *Journal of Continuing Education in the Health Professions, 29*(2), 98–104.

Gantt, L., & Webb-Corbett, R. (2010). Using simulation to teach patient safety behaviors in undergraduate nursing education. *Journal of Nursing Education, 49* (1), 48–51.

Gardner, R., Walzer, T. B., Simon, R., & Raemer, D. B. (2008). Obstetric simulation as a risk control strategy: Course design and evaluation. *Journal of the Society for Simulation in Healthcare, 3*(2), 119–127.

Gore, R., Van Gele, P., Ravert, P., & Mabire, C. (2012). A 2010 Survey of the INACSL membership about simulation use. *Clinical Simulation in Nursing, 8*(4), e125–e133.

Hager, M., Russell, S., & Fletcher, S. (Eds.). (2008). *Continuing education in the health professions: Improving healthcare through lifelong learning.* New York, NY: Josiah Macy, Jr. Foundation.

Harder, N. (2010). Use of simulation in teaching and learning in health sciences: A systematic review. *Journal of Nursing Education, 49*(1), 23–28.

Hayden, J. (2010). Use of simulation in nursing education: National survey results. *Journal of Nursing Regulation, 1*(3), 52–57.

Henneman, E., Cunningham, H., Roche, J., & Curnin, M. (2007). Human patient simulation: Teaching students to provide safe care. *Nurse Educator, 32*(5), 212–217.

Hovancsek, M. (2007). Using simulation in nursing education. In P. Jeffries (Ed.), *Simulation in nursing education: from conceptualization to evaluation* (pp. 1–9). New York, NY: National League for Nursing.

Issenberg, S., McGaghie, W., Petrusa, E., Gordon, D., & Scalese, R. (2005). Features and uses of high-fidelity medical simulations that lead to effective learning: A BEME systematic review. *Medical Teacher, 27*, 10–28.

Jarzemsky, P., & McGrath, J. (2008). Look before you leap: Lessons learned when introducing clinical simulation. *Nurse Educator, 33*(2), 90–95.

Jeffries, P., & Rizzolo, M. (2006). Designing and implementing models for the innovative use of simulation to teach nursing care of ill adults and children: A national, multi-site, multi-method of study. In P. Jeffries (Ed.), *Simulation in nursing education: From conceptualization to evaluation* (pp. 147–159). New York, NY: National League for Nursing.

Jeffries, P. (2008). Designing simulations for nursing education. *Annual Review Nursing Education, 6*, 161–177.

Johnson, D., Flagg, A., & Dremsa, T. (2007). Effects of using a human patient simulator (HPS™) versus a CD-ROM on cognition and critical thinking. *Medical Education Online, 13*(1). Retrieved April 24, 2012, from http://med-ed-online.net/index.php/meo/article/view/4470/4650

Kardong-Edgren, S. (2009). A letter to nursing program administrators about simulation. *Clinical Simulation in Nursing, 5*, e161–e162.

Kaddoura, M. (2010). New graduate nurses' perceptions of the effects of clinical simulation on their critical thinking, learning, and confidence. *Journal of Continuing Education in Nursing, 41*(11), 506–515.

Kardong-Edgren, S., Adamson, K., & Fitzgerald, C. (2010). A review of currently published evaluation instruments for human patient simulation. *Clinical Simulation in Nursing, 6*, e25–e35.

Kiat, T., Mei, T., Nagammal, S., & Jonnie, A. (2007). A review of learners' experience with simulation based training in nursing. *Singapore Nursing Journal, 34*(4), 37–43.

Kohn, L., Corrigan, J., & Donaldson, M. (Eds.). (2000). *To err is human: Building a safer health system.* Washington, DC: National Academy Press.

Krautscheid, L., Orton, V., Chorpenning, L., & Ryerson, R. (2011). Student nurse perceptions of effective medication administration education. *International Journal of Nursing Education Scholarship, 8*(1), Article 7.

Kuiper, R., Heinrich, C., Matthias, A., Graham, M., & Bell-Kotwall, L. (2008). Debriefing with the OPT model of clinical reasoning during high fidelity patient simulation. *International Journal of Nursing Education Scholarship, 5*(1), Article 17. Retrieved December 30, 2008, from http://www.bepress.com/ijnes/vol5/iss1/art17

Kyle, R., & Murray, W. (Eds.). (2008). *Clinical simulation: Operations, engineering and management.* New York, NY: Elsevier.

Lapkin, S., Levett-Jones, T., Bellchambers, H., & Fernandez, H. (2010). Effectiveness of patient simulation manikins in teaching clinical reasoning skills to undergraduate nursing students: A systematic review. *Clinical Simulation in Nursing, 6*, e207–e222.

Lasater, K. (2007a). Clinical judgment development: Using simulation to create an assessment rubric. *Journal of Nursing Education, 46*, 496–503.

Lasater, K. (2007b). High-fidelity simulation and the development of clinical judgment: Students' experiences. *Journal of Nursing Education, 46*, 269–276.

Leighton, K., & Scholl, K. (2009). Simulated codes: Understanding the response of undergraduate nursing students. *Clinical Simulation in Nursing, 5*, 3187–3194. doi:10.1016/j.ecns.2009.05.058

Maynes, R. (2008). Human patient simulation in ambulatory care nursing. *AAACN Viewpoint, 30*(1), 11–14.

Metcalfe, S., Hall, V., & Carpenter, A. (2007). Promoting collaboration in nursing education: The development of a regional simulation laboratory. *Journal of Professional Nursing, 23*(3), 180–183.

Miller, K., Riley, W., Davis, S., & Hansen, H. (2008). In situ simulation. *Journal of Perinatal & Neonatal Nursing, 22*(2), 105–113.

Morris, L., Pfeifer, P., Catalano, R., Fortney, R., Hilton, E. L., McLaughlin, J., . . . Goldstein, L. (2007). Designing a comprehensive model for critical care orientation. *Critical Care Nurse, 27*(6), 37–61.

National Council of State Boards of Nursing. (2005). Clinical instruction in prelicensure nursing programs. Retrieved July 21, 2008, from http://www.ncsbn.org/Final_Clinical_Instr_Pre_Nsg_programs.pdf

Radhakrishnan, K., Roche, J., & Cunningham, H. (2007). Measuring clinical practice parameters with human patient simulation: A pilot study. *International Journal of Nursing Education Scholarship, 4*(1), Article 8. Retrieved December 30, 2008, from http://www.bepress.com/ijnes/vol4/iss1/art8/

Ramirez, M. (2008). Implications of NIMS integration plan for hospitals and healthcare. Retrieved August 2, 2008, from http://ezinearticles.com/?Implications-of-NIMS-Integration-Plan-For-Hospitals-and-Healthcare&id=672536

Robertson, B. (2006). An obstetric simulation experience in an undergraduate nursing curriculum. *Nurse Educator, 31*(2), 74–78.

Scavone, B., Toledo, P., Higgins, N., Wojciechowski, K., & McCarthy, R. (2010). A randomized controlled trial of the impact of simulation-based training on resident performance during a simulated obstetric anesthesia emergency. *Simulation in Healthcare, 5*(6), 320–324.

Schoening, A., Sittner, B., & Todd, M. (2006). Simulated clinical experience: Nursing students' perceptions and the educators' role. *Nurse Educator, 31*(6), 253–258.

Seropian, M., Brown, K., Gavilanes, J., & Driggers, B. (2004). An approach to simulation program development. *Journal of Nursing Education, 43*(4), 170–174.

Shinnick, M. A., Woo, M., Horwich, T. B., & Steadman, R. (2011a). Debriefing: The most important component in simulation? *Clinical Simulation in Nursing, 7*, e105–e111.

Shinnick, M., Woo, M., & Mentes, J. (2011b). Human patient simulation: State of the science in prelicensure nursing education. *Journal of Nursing Education, 50*(2), 65–72.

Spunt, D. (2007). Setting up a simulation laboratory. In P. Jeffries (Ed.), *Simulation in nursing education: From conceptualization to evaluation* (pp. 105–122). New York, NY: National League for Nursing.

Starkweather, R., & Kardong-Edgren, S. (2008). Diffusion of innovation: Embedding simulation into nursing curricula. *International Journal of Nursing Education Scholarship, 5*(1), Article 13. Retrieved December 30, 2008, from http://www.bepress.com/ijnes/vol5/iss1/art13/

Stefanski, R., & Rossler, K. (2009). Preparing the novice critical care nurse: A community-wide collaboration using the benefits of simulation. *Journal of Continuing Education in Nursing, 40*(10), 443–451.

Strouse, A. (2010). Multidisciplinary simulation centers: Promoting safe practice. *Clinical Simulation in Nursing, 6*(4), e139–e142.

Wolf, L. (2008). The use of human patient simulation in ED triage training can improve nursing confidence and patient outcomes. *Journal of Emergency Nursing, 34*(2), 169–171.

Yaeger, K., & Arafeh, J. (2008). Making the move: From traditional neonatal education to simulation-based training. *Journal of Perinatal & Neonatal Nursing, 22*(2), 154–158.

Yuan, H., Williams, B., & Fang, J. (2012). The contribution of high-fidelity simulation to nursing students' confidence and competence: A systematic review. *International Nursing Review, 59*, 26–33. doi:10.1111/j.1466-7657.2011.00964.x

## BIBLIOGRAPHY

Benner, P., Sutphen, M., Leonard, V., & Day, L. (2010). *Educating nurses: A call for radical transformation.* San Francisco, CA: Jossey-Bass.

DeBourgh, G., & Prion, S. (2011). Using simulation to teach prelicensure nursing students to minimize patient risk and harm. *Clinical Simulation in Nursing, 7*, e47–e56.

Hale, T., & Ahlschlager, P. (2010). *Simulation scenarios for nursing education.* Delmar, CA: Cengage Learning.

Hetzel Campbell, S., & Daley, K. (Eds.). (2009). *Simulation scenarios for nurse educators: Making it real.* New York, NY: Springer.

Howard, V., Englert, N., Kameg, K., & Perozzi, K. (2011). Integration of simulation across the undergraduate curriculum: Student and faculty perspectives. *Clinical Simulation in Nursing, 7*, e1–e20.

Kardong-Edgren, S. (2012). Why would simulation work? *Clinical Simulation in Nursing, 8*, e75–e76.

McGaghie, W., Issenberg, S. B., Petrusa, E., & Scalese, R. (2011). A critical review of simulation-based medical education research: 2003–2009. *Medical Education, 44*, 50–63.

Nehring, W., & Lashley, F. (2010). *High-fidelity patient simulation in nursing education.* Sudbury, MA: Jones & Bartlett.

Strouse, A. (2010). Multidisciplinary simulation centers: Promoting safe practice. *Clinical Simulation in Nursing, 6*, e139–e142.

Swanson, E., Nicholson, A., Boese, T., Cram, E., Stineman, A., & Tew, K. (2011). Comparison of selected teaching strategies incorporating simulation and student outcomes. *Clinical Simulation in Nursing, 7*, e81–e90.

Wilson, L., & Rockstraw, L. (Eds.). (2011). *Human simulation for nursing and health professions.* New York, NY: Springer.

# Unit 2

# Workforce Issues

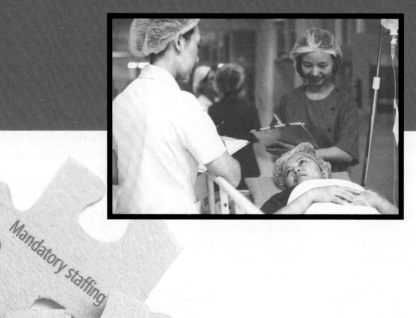

Mandatory staffing

Workplace violence

Entry into practice

# Chapter 5

# The Current Nursing Shortage
## Causes, Consequences, and Solutions

Carol J. Huston

## ADDITIONAL RESOURCES

Visit thePoint for additional helpful resources
- eBook
- Journal Articles
- WebLinks

## CHAPTER OUTLINE

## LEARNING OBJECTIVES

*The learner will be able to:*

1. Explore factors affecting the current supply of registered nurses (RNs) in the United States as well as the current and projected demand through 2020.

2. Compare regional differences in the supply and demand for RNs in the United States.

3. Discuss consequences of the current shortage on quality of health care, current working conditions for RNs, and RN retention rates.

4. Identify the relationship between the current nursing shortage and the state of the national economy.

5. Analyze the impact of salary as an incentive for resolving nursing shortages.

6. Address the educational challenges inherent in solving the nursing shortage given unfilled faculty positions, resignations, projected retirements, low faculty pay schedules, and the shortage of students being prepared for the faculty role.

7. Identify specific strategies being used to recruit and retain older nurses in the workforce.

8. Differentiate between and provide examples of both short-term and long-term solutions to nursing shortages.

9. Outline strategies directed at both supply and demand factors that have been proposed in an effort to reduce the current nursing shortage and analyze the efficacy of each.

10. Reflect upon his or her personal commitment to a career in professional nursing.

As government and private insurer reimbursement declined in the 1990s and managed care costs soared, many health care organizations, and hospitals in particular, began downsizing to achieve cost containment by eliminating registered nursing jobs or by replacing RNs with unlicensed assistive personnel. Even hospitals that did not downsize during this period often did little to recruit qualified RNs.

This downsizing and shortsightedness regarding recruitment and retention contributed to the beginning of an acute shortage of RNs in many health care settings by the late 1990s. Peter Buerhaus, an expert on health care workforce needs, suggested that the health care quality and safety movement also exacerbated the shortage in the late 1990s as research emerged to demonstrate the relationship between nurse staffing and patient outcomes and the public became aware of how important an adequately sized workforce was to patient safety (Roman, 2008).

Unlike earlier nursing shortages, which typically lasted only a few years, the current shortage has lasted longer and been more severe than any nursing shortage experienced thus far.

The nursing shortage is also widespread geographically (indeed, worldwide), with developed countries exacerbating the shortages in developing countries as a result of nurse migration (see Chapter 6). As of 2010, the overwhelming majority of states in the United States were reporting nursing shortages, ranging from a shortage of 200 nurses in Alabama to a shortage of 47,600 nurses in California (Trust for America's Health, 2011).

The shortage also exists in all practice settings, although the area of greatest demand has recently shifted from acute care hospitals to ambulatory care settings. Indeed, the U.S. Department of Labor (2010–2011) suggests that employment will grow only slowly in hospitals in the coming decade since the number of inpatients is expected to increase little, since patients are being discharged earlier, and since more procedures are being done on an outpatient basis. Rapid growth, however, is expected in hospital outpatient facilities, such as those providing same-day surgery, rehabilitation, and chemotherapy as well as in physicians' offices, and in outpatient care centers, such as freestanding ambulatory surgical and emergency centers.

In addition, the causes of the current shortage are numerous and multifaceted, which makes resolution even more difficult. How significant is the shortage? Projections made early in the 21st century suggested a national shortfall of at least 760,000 nurses by 2020. Recent estimates by Buerhaus and colleagues, however, cut that number in half as a result of recent increases

in nurse employment (Buerhaus, Auerbach, & Staiger, 2009b). Indeed, December 2010 data from the Health Resources and Services Administration (HRSA, 2010), demonstrated a 5.3% increase in the number of RNs in the United States (McNamara, 2010).

These increases in workforce data unfortunately reflect, at least in part, a large number of part-time nurses who have sought full-time employment during recent difficult economic times as well as nurses delaying or coming out of retirement for the same reason. Thus, the recent economic crisis has contributed to an obscurement of the current nursing shortage. Buerhaus et al. (2009b) concur, suggesting that significant nursing workforce shortages are still expected in the coming decade and caution that until nursing education capacity is increased, future imbalances in the nurse labor market will be unavoidable.

Indeed, Buerhaus, in an interview with *RN* editor Linda Roman (2008), stated

> We have reduced the magnitude of the future shortage hurricane from a Category Five, on a huge amount of steroids, down to a Category Three. But that can still kill you. It would cause unprecedented damage if it were to fully develop—It would shut down most of the system and cause care to be rationed.

In contrast, however, Tosto (2010), reporting on the job market in Minnesota for new nurses and the impact of the recession on the number of readily available RN positions, suggested that local schools were producing more nurses than the state needed to fill current vacancies. Indeed, Economic Modeling Specialists Inc. (EMSI), which consulted on this report, suggested that RNs were being overproduced in all states except Nevada and Alaska. A response by the Tri-Council for Nursing (AACN, 2010), however, questioned EMSI's data-collection procedures and how numbers were counted and encouraged nursing programs to work closely with their state workforce officials, boards of nursing, employers, and other stakeholders to determine workforce needs in terms of both absolute numbers and skill mix to meet population health care needs.

To more accurately assess the depth or significance of the current nursing shortage, data must be examined regarding both the demand for RNs and the supply. Assessing the demand for RNs is, in many ways, more complicated than assessing the supply. However, from an economic perspective, this shortage is being driven more by the supply side of the supply/demand equation than the demand side. This makes the problem even more difficult to solve because it will require more than the short-term, quick-fix solutions that have worked in the past.

CONSIDER THIS   This nursing shortage is not likely to be fixed by the same short-term, quick-fix solutions that worked in the past.

This chapter will explore the current nursing shortage, including the present and projected demand for RNs, as well as the supply. In addition, consequences of the shortage will be examined, together with strategies that have been proposed in an effort to confront what is likely one of the greatest current threats to quality health care.

## THE DEMAND

*Demand* is defined by the *Merriam Webster's Online Dictionary* (2011a) as the quantity of a commodity or service wanted at a specified price and time. In the case of nursing, demand would be the amount of a good or service (in this case, an RN) that consumers (in this case, an employer) would be willing to acquire at a given price. A shortage occurs when employers want more employees at the current market wages than they can get. Demand then is derived from the health status of a population and the use of health services.

The demand for professional nurses in both the short- and long-term future continues to increase. In fact, employment of RNs is expected to grow much faster than average for all occupations in the near future, despite significant job losses in 2011 in nearly all other major industries. Indeed, on April 1, 2011, the U.S. Bureau of Labor Statistics (BLS) reported that hospitals, long-term care facilities, and other ambulatory care settings added 37,000 new jobs in March 2011, the biggest monthly increase recorded by any employment sector (AACN, 2011a). In addition, the BLS has identified registered nursing as the top profession in terms of projected growth through 2018 (AACN, 2010).

## Causes of Increased Demand

There are multiple demand factors driving the current shortage, including a growing population, medical advances that increase the need for adequately educated nurses, and the increased acuity of hospitalized patients. Other factors driving demand are the technological advances in patient care and an increasing emphasis on health care prevention.

In addition, a growing elderly population with extended longevity and more chronic health conditions requires more nursing care. As life expectancy in the

United States increases, more nurses will be needed to assist the individuals who are surviving serious illnesses and living longer with chronic diseases. The AACN (2010) concurs, suggesting that as baby boomers enter their retirement years, their demand for care is escalating and health care reform will soon provide subsidies for more than 30 million citizens to more fully use the health care system. As a result, the demand for health care is expected to steadily increase in the next few decades and the numbers of nurses to care for these patients will lag behind.

## Geographical Maldistribution of Nurses

In addition, the nursing workforce is poorly distributed geographically across the United States with the greatest concentration of employed nurses being in New England and the lowest concentration in the Pacific region. The reality, however, is that virtually all states have been affected by the current shortage.

The situation in some states, however, is especially dire. For example, California, despite opening 35 additional nursing programs since 2005, still falls far short of the national average of 825 RNs employed per 100,000 population (Caine, 2011). With just 653 RNs employed per 100,000, the state's nursing shortage will climb to 80,000 by 2015 (Caine) and to 116,600 by 2020 (Winter, 2009).

The situation is similar in Texas. According to the Texas Organization of Nurse Executives (2010), demand for RNs in that state will exceed supply by 70,000 in the year 2020 as the state's rapidly growing population ages and requires more acute care, and as older nurse retire or reduce the hours they work. Alaska, however, has the largest nursing shortfall as a percentage of nursing positions left vacant with only 58% of nursing positions there being filled as of 2009 and only 40% expected to be filled as of 2015 (Winter, 2009).

## THE SUPPLY

*Supply* refers to the quantity of goods or services that are ready for use or purchase (*Merriam Webster's Online Dictionary*, 2011b). Currently, hospitals employ about 60% of working nurses. Eight percent of RNs hold jobs in physician offices, 5% in home health care services, 5% in nursing care facilities, and 3% in employment services. The remainder works mostly in government agencies, social assistance agencies, and educational services (U.S. Department of Labor, 2010–2011).

To evaluate the supply of RNs in the United States, it is necessary to look at both RNs who are currently working and those who are eligible to work, but do not. In addition, the current and potential student pool must be part of the supply discussion.

The United States currently has about 3 million RNs filling about 2.6 million jobs (U.S. Department of Labor, 2010–2011). Despite declining vacancy rates, particularly at hospitals, this does not appear to be enough to meet either short- or long-term needs in hospitals or other health care settings. According to a 2008 report released by the American Health Care Association, more than 19,400 RN vacancies exist in long-term care settings (AACN, 2011b). These vacancies, coupled with those in acute care hospitals translates into a national RN vacancy rate of 8.1% (AACN, 2011b). In addition, workforce analysts with the BLS project that more than 581,500 new RN positions will be created through 2018, increasing the size of the RN workforce by 22% (AACN, 2011b).

---

### DISCUSSION POINT

What factors cause turnover to be so high in long-term care facilities? Is the shortage of licensed health care professionals in long-term care more heavily influenced by supply or demand?

---

The bottom line is that the supply of RNs is expected to grow minimally in the coming decade, but large numbers of nurses are expected to retire. Indeed, Buerhaus suggested that the full effect of the shortage will not be felt until between 2015 and 2020, when demand for nurses is expected to grow well beyond the number of RNs available (Roman, 2008).

It must be noted, however, that despite evidence suggesting a significant current and projected nursing shortage, new nurse graduates in many parts of the country report having difficulty finding jobs, particularly in hospital settings. Wood (2011) notes that graduates who do find jobs often need to search harder and longer than in the past and may not get their first choice position.

In addition, Magnet hospitals prefer to hire baccalaureate graduates, making it more difficult for nurses educated in diploma or associate degree programs to find jobs. The 2010 IOM report, *The Future of Nursing,* recommends a rapid escalation of baccalaureate degree completion for RNs, and this too will further job-hunting challenges for newly graduated associate degree and diploma-educated nurses in the coming decade.

The current restricted job market for new graduate nurses, however, most likely reflects the current low vacancy rate in hospitals related to economy-induced delayed retirements and hiring freezes. In addition, "economic realities have forced healthcare systems to tighten budgetary belts, requiring their staff to handle more work rather than hire more staff and close services which are not profitable" (Metzger, 2010, p. 4). Wood goes so far then as to suggest that the current nursing shortage is really an "experienced nursing shortage," given the number of new graduates struggling to find work in the current job market.

## Enrollment in Nursing Schools

The number of students enrolled or projected to enroll in nursing programs is also an important factor in determining RN supply. Unfortunately, some schools of nursing have closed nursing programs due to funding cuts or to reduce program size. Still others have been forced to turn away potential students because of a lack of faculty. Despite this, enrollment in nursing schools has steadily increased every year for almost a decade (see Table 5.1). Unfortunately, however, these increases are not adequate to replace those nurses who will be lost to retirement in the coming decade.

In fact, the Council on Physician and Nurse Supply determined in 2008 that 30,000 additional nurses must be graduated annually to meet the nation's health care needs, an expansion of 30% over the number of annual nurse graduates that year (AACN, 2011b).

Unfortunately, enrollment increases are not possible without a significant boost in federal and state funding to prepare new faculty, enhance teaching resources, and upgrade nursing school infrastructure. More money is needed in the form of nursing scholarships and loans to encourage young people to enter nursing. In addition, individual nurses and professional organizations must support legislation to improve financial access to nursing education. The Tri-Council for Nursing (comprising the American Association of Colleges of Nursing, the American Nurses Association, the American Organization of Nurse Executives, and the National League for Nursing) has urged nurses to advocate for increased nursing education funding under Title VIII of the Public Health Service Act, as well as other publicly funded initiatives, so that there will be the necessary capacity and resources to educate future nurses.

There have been increases in federal money for nursing education over the last decade. The passage of legislation such as the 2002 Nurse Reinvestment Act encouraged more students to choose nursing as a career

**TABLE 5.1** Number of Candidates Taking the National Council Licensure Examination for Registered Nurses (NCLEX-RN): First-Time, U.S.-Educated Candidates Only

| Program | 2005 | 2006 | 2007 | 2008 | 2009 | 2010 |
|---|---|---|---|---|---|---|
| Diploma | 3,540 | 3,810 | 3,688 | 3,666 | 3,677 | 3,753 |
| Baccalaureate | 35,496 | 41,349 | 45,781 | 49,739 | 52,241 | 55,414 |
| Associate | 60,053 | 65,390 | 69,890 | 75,545 | 78,665 | 81,618 |
| Total | 99,187 | 110,713 | 119,579 | 129,121 | 134,708 | 140,889 |

*Source:* National Council State Boards of Nursing. (2011). *NCLEX examination pass rates.* Retrieved June 11, 2011, from https://www.ncsbn.org/1237.htm

and helped students financially to complete their education. It also encouraged graduate students to complete their studies and assume teaching positions in nursing schools. In addition, many states introduced or passed legislation designed to improve working conditions and attract more nurses.

In addition, some hospitals have joined forces with local schools of nursing to offer scholarships in exchange for a student's willingness to work in that institution after graduation. Hospitals are also lending master's and doctorally prepared advanced nurses such as nurse practitioners, clinical nurse specialists, and clinical nurse leaders to supplement faculty positions.

Private foundations have also stepped up to offer funding for nursing education. For example, in 2008, the Robert Wood Johnson Foundation (RWJF) joined with the American Association of Colleges of Nursing (AACN) to create the Robert Wood Johnson Foundation New Careers in Nursing (RWJF, 2010). Through grants to schools of nursing, the program funds up to 1,500 scholarships of US$10,000 each annually to schools that offer accelerated baccalaureate and master's nursing programs. Similarly, foundations set up by nursing organizations such as the Association of Perioperative Registered Nurses (AORN), the National Student Nurses' Association (NSNA), and the American Nurses Association (ANA) provide scholarships and financial assistance to students and RNs pursuing degrees in nursing.

Ironically, recruitment efforts into the nursing profession in the last decade have been very successful, and the problem is no longer a lack of nursing school applicants. Indeed, enrollment in nursing programs of education has increased steadily since 2001. The problem is that there are inadequate resources to provide nursing education to those interested in pursuing nursing as a career, including an insufficient number of clinical sites,

classroom space, nursing faculty, and clinical preceptors. As a result, qualified applicants are turned away, despite the current shortage of nurses. Indeed, the AACN (2011a) reported that 67,563 qualified applicants were turned away from baccalaureate nursing programs alone in 2010 and that number is likely higher in associate degree programs. In addition, 10,223 qualified applicants were turned away from master's programs, and 1,202 qualified applicants were turned away from doctoral programs (AACN, 2011a). The primary reason for not accepting all qualified students was a shortage of faculty.

Educational costs are also a deterrent to increasing nursing school enrollment. Nursing is often called an "expensive major" given relatively low faculty to student ratios in clinical courses and the need for financially strapped states to subsidize the cost of education at state universities.

> **DISCUSSION POINT**
>
> Should the increased cost of nursing education be passed on to students? Would students enrolled in public universities be willing to pay more for their education than students in other majors?

The greatest challenge, however, to increasing nursing school enrollment, is an inadequate number of nursing faculty to teach students interested in pursuing nursing as a career. By 2007, 71.4% of nursing schools cited faculty shortages as the major reason they had denied qualified students admission (AACN, 2011a). According to a Special Survey on Vacant Faculty Positions released by AACN in September 2010, a total of

880 faculty vacancies were identified in a survey of 556 nursing schools with baccalaureate and/or graduate programs across the country, creating a national nurse faculty vacancy rate of 6.9% (AACN, 2011a). Besides the vacancies, schools cited the need to create an additional 257 faculty positions to accommodate student demand. Most of the vacancies (90.6%) were faculty positions requiring or preferring a doctoral degree. The top reasons cited by schools having difficulty finding faculty were noncompetitive salaries compared with positions in the practice arena (30.2%) and a limited pool of doctorally prepared faculty (30.4%; AACN, 2011a).

Research conducted by the National League for Nursing (NLN) and the Carnegie Foundation Preparation for the Professions Program found an aging, overworked faculty earning far less than nurses entering clinical practice (NLN, 2010). In fact, this study reported that nurse faculty earned only 76% of the salary that faculty in other academic disciplines earned and that they earned far less than their RN counterparts in clinical practice.

*At the professor rank, nurse educators suffered the largest deficit with salaries averaging 45% lower than those of their non-nurse colleagues. Associate and assistant nursing professors were also at a disadvantage, earning 19 and 15% less than similarly ranked faculty in other fields. Those employed as nursing instructors experienced the only advantage, with salaries averaging 8% higher than those of non-nurses.* (National League for Nursing Releases Faculty Census Data, 2010, para. 2)

This lack of competitive pay for nurse educators is a significant obstacle to recruiting new nursing faculty.

Mary Ann Peters, the director of graduate nursing programs at La Salle University in Philadelphia, went so far as to suggest that nurse educators might be considered as candidates for the endangered species list (Issues in Nursing, 2008). She suggested that this is because there simply are not enough nurses with the educational credentials needed for the faculty role and because academic institutions do not provide a high-enough salary to draw new individuals to it. She concluded that the profession and society must develop a strategic plan and support it with adequate funding because excellent education is essential to the future of a vital evolving profession and superior patient care.

Increasing the number of nursing students in the pipeline as a strategy for addressing the current nursing shortage clearly depends on having enough qualified faculty to teach them. Clearly, the same energy that was directed at recruiting young people for nursing must now be directed at recruiting nursing faculty.

In response, programs have been created both to encourage nurses to consider careers in nursing education and to support them in that role. For example, the Division of Labor Workforce Investment Act has created a Faculty Loan Repayment Program, for nurses willing to serve in faculty roles after graduation. Furthermore, the NINR, the Agency for Health Care Research and Quality Department of Veterans Affairs, and other private foundations have funds available to enhance nursing education and faculty development (Williams, 2011).

In addition, AACN and the Johnson & Johnson Campaign for Nursing's Future announced the creation of a Minority Nurse Faculty Scholars program in 2008 (AACN, 2011a). This program seeks to address the nursing faculty shortage and diversity of the faculty population by providing financial support to graduate nursing students from minority backgrounds who agree to teach in a school of nursing after graduation.

To support the retention of new nursing faculty, the Elsevier Foundation awarded a grant to the Sigma Theta Tau International (STTI) Foundation for Nursing in 2009 to create a Nurse Faculty Mentored Leadership Development Program. Early career nurse educators with an advanced degree were selected to receive 18 months of leadership training designed to help them overcome the challenges of transitioning from nursing practice to faculty (Elsevier Foundation, 2011). "The program reflects the Elsevier Foundation's effort to alleviate the nurse faculty crisis by providing knowledge, skill development opportunities and support to retain new nurse educators who have transitioned into the role" (Elsevier Foundation, 2011, para. 5). Other long-term strategies for addressing the nursing faculty shortage are shown in Box 5.1.

---

CONSIDER THIS Unfilled faculty positions, resignations, and projected retirements continue to pose a threat to the nursing education workforce.

---

## Part-Time and Unemployed Nurses: An Untapped Pool?

Some experts have suggested that too much emphasis has been placed on recruiting young people to solve the nursing shortage and that supply could more easily be increased by bringing unemployed or part-time nurses

**BOX 5.1 LONG-TERM STRATEGIES FOR ADDRESSING THE NURSING FACULTY SHORTAGE**

**1.** Recruitment
- Provide a positive image/role model for advanced education in nursing education.
- Recruit young people from middle and high schools to become nursing faculty.
- Streamline the education track to higher academics.
- Provide financial support or tuition forgiveness in exchange for teaching service.
- Develop mentoring/support programs for new academics.

**2.** Retention
- Provide better salaries and benefits for nursing faculty.
- Create positive work environments and reasonable teaching assignments.
- Reward teaching excellence.
- Create faculty development and mentorship programs.

**3.** Collaboration
- Develop relationships with state legislators for support and funding.
- Partner with high schools, colleges, health care institutions, and governmental agencies to create support for higher education in nursing.

*Source:* Allen, L. (2008). The nursing shortage continues as faculty shortage grows. *Nursing Economics, 26*(1), 35–40.

back to nursing full-time. The reality, however, is that the percentage of RNs who are not employed in nursing has dropped significantly since 1977, from more than one in four RNs to one in six (Buerhaus et al., 2009b). In addition, the number of RNs working full-time increased from 68% in 1977 to just greater than 70% in 2004, and the number of hours during a given week worked by both full- and part-time RNs combined increased by approximately 6.5% between 1983 and 2006 (Buerhaus et al., 2009b). Thus, the pool of part-time and unemployed nurses has already been tapped.

In addition, the literature on reentry of RNs into the workplace is often pessimistic, suggesting that such programs take a great deal of effort for the results they provide. Yet Buerhaus et al. (2009b) suggest that the current shortage has been lessened, at least in part, by the reentry of older RNs into employment. This was especially true earlier in the past decade when the U.S. economy first began to stall. In fact, the "employment growth of older RNs (over the age of 50) has increased every year since 2000 for an astounding net gain of more than 257,000 full time equivalent (FTE) RNs" (Buerhaus et al., 2009b, p. 119). In contrast, the total net employment growth of RNs aged 21 to 34 was only roughly 36,000, which was effectively negated by a similar net

decrease in employment (roughly 40,000 FTE RNs) by RNs aged 35 to 59. Buerhaus et al. warned, however, that the increased demand by boomers and the aging workforce will make the reentry of older RNs only a brief reprieve in a shortage that is far from over.

## Using Foreign-Born Nurses to Relieve the Shortage

The shortage has also been alleviated at least in part by the importation of RNs from foreign markets. Buerhaus, Staiger, and Auerbach (2009a) suggested that the number of foreign-born RNs in the U.S. workforce between 1994 and 2001 averaged 6.0% each year. By 2002, it doubled to 12.5%. After a temporary decline in 2005, likely related to the expiration of work visas, the employment of foreign-born nurses surged forward again in 2006, outstripping the growth in employment among nurses born in the United States: "Overall, the rapid growth in employment of foreign-born RNs accounts for more than one-third (37%) of the total growth of total RN employment in the United States since 2002" (Buerhaus et al., 2009a, p. 118).

Widespread, transnational nursing migration is likely to continue for some time, given the success hospitals have had with foreign recruitment and the time required to strengthen the domestic nurse supply pipeline. Such practice, however, could potentially have negative implications in terms of the domestic job market and health care quality. In addition, using foreign-born labor has complex international implications, creating a drain on some countries' health care systems while shoring up the economies of countries that purposefully export their workers. Because the importation of nurses has such complex ramifications, a separate chapter is devoted to its discussion (see Chapter 6).

## ROOTS OF THE SHORTAGE

Many factors contribute to the current nursing shortage in acute care settings, including an aging workforce, high turnover due to worker dissatisfaction, inadequate long-term pay incentives, and an increasing recognition by nurses that they can make more money and act more autonomously as free agents than as full-time employees of a health care organization. These factors and others (Box 5.2) will be discussed in this section.

### Nursing as a "Graying" Population

Nursing is a graying population—even more so than the population at large. This means that the nursing workforce is retiring at a rate faster than it can be replaced. The national RN survey (2008 National Sample Survey of Registered Nurses), released in 2010, suggested that while 444,668 nurses received their license to practice from 2004 through 2008, the U.S. nursing workforce only grew by 153,806 RNs during this timeframe, indicative of the large-scale retirements, which the aging nursing profession has begun and will continue to experience (HRSA, 2010).

This same survey showed that the average age of the RN population in 2008 was 46, up from 45.2 in 2000. Given the demographics of the nursing workforce, this pattern is expected to continue over the next decade. Indeed, the average age of the working nurse has been increasing for some time, reflecting a two- to three-decade-long trend toward older students entering nursing education programs, as well as a general decline in interest in nursing as a career among younger people.

A 2007 study, however, first suggested that this trend might be reversing. Auerbach, Buerhaus, and Staiger (2007) found that although the number of people entering nursing in their early to mid-20s remains at its lowest point in 40 years, greater numbers of individuals in their late 20s and 30s are entering the field, which should serve to decrease the age of the average nurse. In addition, the study showed that people born in the 1970s are now almost as likely to become nurses as people born during the 1950s, when interest in nursing careers was at its height. The researchers suggested that this projected increase in nursing will mitigate the severity of the nursing shortage in 2020. Indeed, a 2010 study by HRSA

---

**BOX 5.2  CAUSES OF THE CURRENT NURSING SHORTAGE**

- Increasing elderly population (more individuals who are chronically ill)
- Increased acuity in acute care settings, requiring higher-level nursing skills
- Downsizing and restructuring of the late 1990s, which eliminated many RN positions
- A relatively healthy economy in the late 1990s and early 2000s, which encouraged some nurses to change from full-time employment to part-time or to quit
- Aging RN workforce
- Workplace dissatisfaction
- Women choosing fields other than nursing for a career
- Aging faculty for RN programs
- Inadequate nursing programs to accommodate interested applicants
- Low ceiling on wages for RNs without advanced degrees
- Future educator pool for RNs more limited than demand

found for the first time in 3 years that the youngest population of nurses was growing—an important move in replenishing the RN pool (McNamara, 2010).

Yet retirement projections for the profession continue to be grim. Hirschkorn, West, and Hill (2010) reported that 55% of nurses plan to retire between 2011 and 2020. Another survey, by AMN Healthcare, suggested that 35% of baby-boomer nurses said that they "plan to retire, change profession, work part-time, switch to a less demanding role, or work as travel nurses" in the next 1 to 3 years (Baby-Boomer Nurses Are on Their Way Out, 2008, para. 1). The most common reason given for their intent to change their current work situation was burnout and declining satisfaction with the work.

Although many nurses have temporarily delayed retirement due to the recession, a wave of retiring nurses is coming and this will result in an "intellectual drain of institutional and professional nursing knowledge" (Wood, 2011, para. 15). Letvak (2008) stated that we cannot afford to lose the experience of so many older nurses. He pointed out that older workers typically have higher job satisfaction and lower turnover. In addition, "they are more dedicated to their jobs, take pride in a job well done, have good listening skills, are not intimidated by difficult personalities, and demonstrate maturity" (p. 22).

---

### DISCUSSION POINT

What factors have led to the "graying" of the nursing workforce? Does there appear to be any short-term resolution of these factors?

---

### DISCUSSION POINT

Why is there so little discussion about the "expertise gap" that will occur as a result of impending nursing retirements?

---

## The Nursing Faculty Are Grayer Yet

To further confound the nursing shortage and efforts to address it, the average age of nursing faculty members continues to increase, narrowing the number of productive years nurse educators can teach. According to AACN's report *2010–2011 Salaries of Instructional and Administrative Nursing Faculty in Baccalaureate and Graduate Programs in Nursing,*

*the average ages of doctorally-prepared nurse faculty holding the ranks of professor, associate professor, and assistant professor were 60.5, 57.1, and 51.5 years, respectively. For master's degree-prepared nurse faculty, the average ages for professors, associate professors, and assistant professors were 57.7, 56.4, and 50.9 years, respectively.* (AACN, 2011a, para. 7)

Faculty census data collected by the NLN in 2010 also demonstrates an aging nursing faculty. The percentage of faculty ages 30 to 45 and ages 46 to 60 both dropped by 3% between 2006 and 2009, while the percentage of full-time educators above age 60 grew dramatically from only 9% in 2006 to nearly 16% in 2009 (PR WEB, 2010).

One must question where the faculty will come from to teach the new nurses needed to solve the current shortage. In addition, given the lag time required to educate master's- or doctorally prepared faculty, the faculty shortage may end up being the greatest obstacle to solving the current nursing shortage.

---

CONSIDER THIS   Even if enough students can be recruited to become nurses, there will likely not be enough faculty to teach them.

---

Fortunately, many foundations and funders have stepped forward to provide solutions. In June 2011, the American Association of Colleges of Nursing (AACN) and the Jonas Center for Nursing Excellence entered into a collaboration to increase the number of doctorally prepared faculty available to teach in nursing schools nationwide. This US$2.5-million initiative will be managed by AACN as part of the Jonas Center's larger effort to support 150 new doctoral students across all 50 states (AACN, 2011c). The program provides financial assistance, leadership development, and mentoring support to expand the pipeline of future nurse faculty into research-focused (PhD, DNS) and practice-focused (DNP) doctoral nursing programs.

## The Free Agent Nurse

An increase in the number of free agent nurses is another aspect that must be examined in assessing supply and demand factors of the current nursing shortage. Full-time employment of nurses is decreasing. Instead, nurses are increasingly assuming the role of *free agent*, a term more common to Generation X than their older counterparts, and this contributes to a shortage in acute care agencies. A free agent nurse is often an independent contractor who sells his or her services to an employer, with the condition that he or she maintains control over the number of hours they are willing to work and working conditions.

*Per-diem* and *traveling nurses* are two types of free agents. The relationship between the free agent and his or her employing organization is based on a free and open exchange, more of a partnership than an unequal dependency relationship. Typically, the free agent nurse makes a higher hourly wage than other full-time or part-time employees in a health care organization in exchange for not receiving health care and retirement benefits. Such nurses also have greater control over if and when they want to work.

Historically, health care organizations have sought to employ full-time workers (employees) so that they could better control the availability of needed human resources. However, the free agent model of nursing is gaining momentum in health care organizations as they recognize that they need to supplement their full-time employee pool with these skilled workers and that significant benefit costs can be saved from using free agent or temporary workers.

Critics of the increased use of free agent nurses, particularly traveling nurses, suggest that this practice may negatively affect the quality of care related to inconsistency of caretakers and a reduced ability to determine the competencies of the specific free agent nurse. More research is needed, however, on the effect of the free agent nurse on the current nursing shortage.

## Workplace Dissatisfaction

Perhaps one of the most significant yet least addressed factors leading to the current RN shortage is workplace dissatisfaction, resulting in high turnover levels and nurses leaving the profession. Long shifts, low autonomy, mandatory overtime, and being forced to work weekends, nights, and holidays prompts many nurses to look for other jobs.

A recent international study by Aiken et al. (2011) suggested that a third or more of hospital nurses, in a majority of countries studied, were dissatisfied with their jobs and experiencing burnout. Higher levels of dissatisfaction were associated with lower patient satisfaction with care and increased risks to patient safety and care quality.

*Hospitals with consistently better work environments had lower burnout, lower likelihoods of having nurses who were dissatisfied with their jobs and who thought that the quality of care on their unit was only fair or poor*

*and higher likelihoods of having nurses report that their patients were ready for discharge. This was true across virtually all of the countries despite different health-care systems and cultures.* (Aiken et al., 2011, p. 7)

Aiken et al. concluded that hospital leaders wanting to preserve their nursing workforce should work to improve staffing as well as nurse and physician relationships, involve nurses in hospital decision making, and give greater managerial support to those nurses who provide clinical care at the bedside. In doing so, the researchers concluded that substantial gains could be made in "stabilizing the global nurse workforce while also improving quality of hospital care throughout the world" (pp. 7–8).

Calarco's (2011) research findings were similar, suggesting that improved work environments result in both enhanced patient care delivery and nurse retention. Calarco's 5-year study found that nursing work satisfaction increases when nurses are engaged in work cultures that enhance communication and collaboration and which actively involve nurses in organizational and clinical decision making.

> CONSIDER THIS    The nursing shortage cannot be resolved until we address the underlying issues of worker dissatisfaction that caused it in the first place.

## Is Pay an Issue?

Salaries also provide mixed incentives for young people to become nurses and for nurse retention. The economy at the end of the 20th century was fairly strong, with low unemployment and rising consumer confidence. This resulted in some RNs, who were often the second breadwinner in the family unit, reducing their work hours or leaving the workplace entirely. Many of these same RNs, however, returned to work in the past decade as a result of declining stock market values, a rising recession, and lower levels of consumer confidence.

Wages for RNs have, however, increased with rising demand and progression of the shortage. The median annual wages of RNs as of May 2008 were US$62,450 (U.S. Department of Labor, 2010–2011). The middle 50% earned between US$51,640 and US$76,570, the lowest 10% earned less than US$43,410, and the highest 10% earned more than US$92,240.

Nursing salaries also vary by state and within states. For example, the average hourly wage for RNs in the state of California varies from US$24.04 to US$50.10 as compared to US$19.39 to US$31.05 in Ohio (Payscale, 2011a). Experienced nurses (more than 20 years), on average, earn significantly more than those with less than 1-year experience (up to US$42.52 per hour as compared to US$29.04; Payscale, 2011a).

---

### DISCUSSION POINT

Historically, nursing has been considered an altruistic profession. How critical do you think pay is as a motivator for people who want to become nurses today?

---

In contrast to the findings for staff nurses, salary is clearly a deterrent for nursing faculty: One reason that nursing faculty salaries are so poor comparatively is that nursing education has never had the same federal funding support as medical education. In addition, "not only are academic salaries lower than they are for clinical practice, and administrative positions of advanced practice nurses, but the cost of securing advanced academic degrees is costly" (Allen, 2008, p. 37). Indeed, many graduate students who may have become educators in the past are now opting instead for better-paying positions in clinical and private practice.

Average base salaries for nurse practitioners in 2011 ranged from US$59,150 to US$98,988 with bonuses and profit sharing adding up to US$20,000 additional wages annually (Payscale, 2011b). In contrast, the AACN (2011a) reported that full-time associate professor nurse faculty with a master's degree earned an annual average salary of US$66,588. Clearly, increasing faculty salaries and providing tuition support for graduate students considering a career as a nursing faculty will be an essential part of addressing the increasing faculty shortage. Feeg and Nickitas (2011) concur, suggesting that to get the right numbers of nurses with doctorates, competitive salary and benefit packages must be available so that highly qualified academic and clinical nurse faculty can be recruited and retained.

---

### DISCUSSION POINT

What incentives should be offered to nurses who earn a master's or doctoral degree to become nursing faculty members rather than advanced practice nurses engaged in clinical practice?

---

## Retention: An Undervalued Strategy

Some organizational turnover is normal and, in fact, desirable since it infuses the organization with fresh ideas. It also reduces the probability of *groupthink*, in which everyone shares similar thought processes, values, and goals (Marquis & Huston, 2012). However, excessive or unnecessary turnover reduces the ability of the organization to produce its end product. Thus, retention becomes a critical goal when work force shortages exist and the achievement of desired outcomes is critical to organizational success.

Unfortunately, many highly trained, employable nurses are *voluntarily* leaving the profession because they are dissatisfied with their work or the environment in which they work. This is especially true in long-term care settings where historical data suggests annual turnover rates between 55% and 75% for all health care workers including RNs (Mukamel et al., 2009). Annual turnover in acute care hospitals is currently approximately 15% (Alter Group, 2011).

High levels of turnover are disruptive to organizational functioning and threaten the quality of patient care. This was apparent in research done by Bae, Mark, and Fried (2010), which suggested that units with lower turnover levels had higher workgroup learning, workgroup cohesion, and relational satisfaction, leading to greater patient satisfaction and a reduction in severe medication errors (See Research Study Fuels the Controversy).

High turnover rates are also generally expensive. According to the American Organization of Nurse Executives (AONE), a conservative estimate of the price of hiring a new nurse totals US$10,000 in direct recruitment costs (recruiting a new nurse, hiring the optimal candidate, and training that individual) (Alter Group, 2011). These direct costs, however, represent only a small portion of the expense of hiring and training a nurse. "It is the hidden costs—such as signing bonuses and other incentives, lost productivity because of the vacant position, and the expenses associated with training—that drive up the price of replacing RNs" (Alter Group, 2011, para. 2).

According to AONE estimates, the actual cost to replace a medical/surgical nurse is US$42,000 and US$64,000 for a specialty nurse (Alter Group, 2011). Kaiser Permanente suggests the cost to replace a medical surgical nurse is US$47,403 and US$85,197 for a specialty nurse, so for a hypothetical 400-nurse hospital, the cost of replacing just 80 nurses annually could total US$4 million in direct and hidden costs (Alter Group, 2011).

Not all health care organizations, however, have high turnover rates. Research by Rondeau, Williams, and

## RESEARCH STUDY FUELS THE CONTROVERSY

### IMPACT OF NURSING UNIT TURNOVER ON WORKGROUP PROCESSES AND PATIENT OUTCOMES

The aim of this study was to examine how nursing unit turnover affects key workgroup processes and how these processes mediate the impact of nursing turnover on patient outcomes. This study used RN and patient data from 268 nursing units at 141 hospitals collected as part of the Outcomes Research in Nursing Administration (ORNA II) project. Nursing units provided monthly nursing unit turnover rates for 6 consecutive months, and RNs completed questionnaires measuring workgroup processes (group cohesion, relational coordination, and workgroup learning). Patient outcome measures included unit-level average length of patient stay, patient falls, medication errors, and patient satisfaction scores.

Bae, S., Mark, B., & Fried, B. (2010). Impact of nursing unit turnover on patient outcomes in hospitals. *Journal of Nursing Scholarship*, 42(1), 40–49.

### STUDY FINDINGS

The researchers found that nursing units with moderate levels of turnover were likely to have lower levels of workgroup learning compared to those with no turnover ($p < 0.01$). Surprisingly, nursing units with low levels of turnover were likely to have fewer patient falls than nursing units with no turnover ($p < 0.05$). In addition, workgroup cohesion and relational coordination had a positive impact on patient satisfaction ($p < 0.01$), and increased workgroup learning led to fewer occurrences of severe medication errors ($p < 0.05$). The researchers concluded that further research needs to be done on the operational impact of turnover so as to better design, fund, and implement appropriate intervention strategies to prevent RN exit from nursing units.

Wagar (2008) suggested that organizations perceived to be employers-of-choice, such as magnet hospitals, retain their employees and are more capable of replacing losses than less-sought-after employers. Therefore, having a healthy work environment provides an advantage in the competition for scarce nursing resources. Research by Kirschling, Colgan, and Andrews (2011) supported this idea, finding that there are definite characteristics of work schedules that can influence a nurse's inclination to stay or leave a position or the profession for that matter. Kirschling et al. suggest that managers can positively impact retention by attempting to match work schedules and hours as closely as possible to employee expectations and by paying attention when nurses request changes in hours.

In addition, Rondeau et al. (2008) found that external labor market forces, including local job markets, have the potential to negate even the most ardent recruitment and retention campaign. Given that these external forces are often beyond the control of the employer, the researchers concluded that employers are better off trying to create positive work environments to be employers-of-choice than trying to control a labor market that is often beyond their control. Clearly, organizations that pay attention to the employee market and understand what people are looking for in the work environment have a better chance to recruit and retain top talent. Retention is a strategic planning priority in high-performing organizations (Hirschkorn et al., 2010).

> CONSIDER THIS Retention of precious nurse resources must be a very real part of the solution to the nursing shortage; health care institutions must make a commitment to improving working conditions for nurses.

## THE CONSEQUENCES OF THE SHORTAGE

What are the consequences of a nursing shortage? To answer this question, it is critical first to recognize that patient outcomes are sensitive to nursing interventions and that, as a result, nurse staffing (total hours of care, as well as staffing mix) affects patient outcomes. This supposition is certainly supported by a review of the literature, which increasingly suggests that RN staffing affects patient outcomes such as inpatient mortality and other measures of quality of hospital care.

Indeed, numerous studies have been conducted to describe the relationship between nurse staffing levels and clinical outcomes of patients at both the hospital and unit levels. Unruh (2008) found that more than 45 U.S. studies and 20 international studies explored the relationship between hospital nurse staffing and patient outcomes, and most studies concluded that there are statistically significant relationships between staffing and patient outcomes and numerous studies have been published since that meta-analysis. A recent example would be research done by Blegen and colleagues (2011) which found that higher nurse staffing was associated with reduced death rates, lower failure-to-rescue incidents, lower rates of infection, and shorter hospital stays.

Certainly though, the most often cited seminal work in this area has been done by Linda Aiken and colleagues at the University of Pennsylvania. Her research team has conducted multiple studies over the past decade demonstrating a significant and quantifiable link between patient-to-nurse ratios and patient mortality, failure-to-rescue (deaths following complications) among surgical patients, and factors related to nurse retention (see Chapter 11).

## ADDITIONAL STRATEGIES FOR SOLVING THE SHORTAGE

Just as the issues that caused the current shortage are complex, so too must be the solutions to the problem. Only some of the solutions that have been presented to address the current nursing shortage are included here, including redesigning the workplace, increasing the number of nursing students in the pipeline, importing foreign nurses, improving nursing's image, increasing the faculty pool, and moving toward a self-service approach to patient care. In addition, Box 5.3 includes

---

### BOX 5.3   STRATEGIES FOR ADDRESSING THE SHORTAGE

- Demonstrate to health care leaders that nurses are the critical difference in the U.S. health care system.

- Reposition nursing as a highly versatile profession in which young people can learn science and technology, customer service, critical thinking, and decision-making skills.

- Construct practice environments that are interdisciplinary and build on relationships among nurses, physicians, other health care professionals, patients, and communities.

- Create patient care models that encourage professional nurse autonomy and clinical decision making.

- Develop additional evaluation systems that measure the relationship of timely nursing interventions to patient outcomes.

- Establish additional standards and mechanisms for recognition of professional practice environments.

- Develop career enhancement incentives for nurses to pursue professional practice.

- Evaluate the effects of the nursing shortage on the preparation of the next generation of nurse educators, nurse administrators, and nurse researchers and take strategic action.

- Implement and sustain a marketing effort that addresses the image of nursing and the recruitment of qualified students into nursing as a career.

- Promote higher education to nurses of all educational levels.

- Develop and implement strategies to promote the retention of RNs and nurse educators in the workforce.

*Source:* Honor Society of Nursing, Sigma Theta Tau International. (n.d.). *Facts on the nursing shortage in North America.* Retrieved June 14, 2011, from http://www.nursingsociety.org/Media/Pages/shortage.aspx. Reprinted with permission.

a list of 11 strategies created by the Honor Society of Nursing, STTI (n.d.), for reducing the current shortage.

## Redesigning the Workplace for an Older Workforce

The age of the current nursing workforce is an important factor in the current nursing shortage because nursing can be both physically and mentally taxing, even to the young. Some experts have suggested that more attention should be given to retaining older workers or bringing retired nurses back into the workforce since these employees are generally more productive, more reliable, and highly experienced. Some adaptations of the working environment may be needed, however, to meet the needs and limitations an aging workforce often experiences (Keller & Burns, 2010). These adaptations may include alternative work shift options, job sharing, time for appointments, childcare and eldercare assistance, and personal days for unexpected home emergencies (Keller & Burns, 2010).

In addition, RNs must be made to feel valued, and physician–nurse relationships reflecting collegiality and collaboration should be fostered. In addition, environments of shared governance should be created in which nurses actively participate in all decision making related to patient care. Staff nurses should feel empowered, and autonomy should be encouraged.

Federwish (2008) described such a program in his description of the Center for Third Age Nurses at Holy Names University in Oakland, California. This center assists nurses aged 45 or older to look at the possibilities for staying engaged in nursing. Instead of talking about retirement, the center encourages the nurses to consider new career pathways and options such as shorter shifts. The program also encourages these experienced nurses to become mentors and to renew their commitment to nursing well into the future. More programs like these will offer older RNs the opportunity to continue to be involved in their professions for many years after they reach the age at which they would be eligible for retirement. Additional strategies for retaining older workers are shown in Box 5.4.

## Changing Nursing's Image

In addition, more efforts must be made to improve the public's image of nursing. Again, this will not be an easy task, given the historical roots of nursing stereotypes and the profession's long history of being unable to effectively change public perceptions regarding professional nursing roles and behaviors (see Chapter 21). It is

### BOX 5.4  STRATEGIES FOR RETAINING OLDER WORKERS

- Flexible shift options with more options for shorter shifts
- Job-sharing
- Work redesign to limit physical energy expenditure
- Using lift teams, special beds, and equipment to reduce work-related injuries and strain
- Benefit packages that recognize the needs of mature workers
- Recognize and use experienced workers as mentors and preceptors

also clear that despite the public's long-standing esteem for RNs, as documented in public opinion polls, this has not translated into an adequate number of individuals wanting to be nurses (Donelan, Buerhaus, Des Roches, Dittus, & Dutwin, 2008).

## A Self-Service Approach to Patient Care

One must also at least consider some fairly radical approaches to the nursing shortage that do not include increasing the number of nurses available. The best known of these is the self-service model. This model suggests that family members can be used as caregivers to supplement RNs by providing most bedside care during the immediate and postacute hospital periods. Indeed, self-service nursing is the preferred model of care in many countries. Sapountzi-Krepia et al. (2008) described such a model as *informal care* and suggested that it is a common phenomenon in Greece as a result of the nursing shortage. Patients' relatives stay by their bedside for long hours and assist with care. This care often reflects specific nursing duties.

Critics of the self-service approach to care suggest that hospitalized patients are far too ill and their needs are too complex to be cared for by a layperson. They also argue that care is too sophisticated, and the technology routinely used for care is not known to individuals outside of health care. Sapountzi-Krepia et al. (2008) agreed, suggesting that it is disquieting to have hospital staff suggest to relatives that there is a need to stay at the patient's bedside or to hire a private paid patient's helper. Instead, they suggest that hospitals should introduce specific staffing policies to reduce this burden on families.

Bern-Klug and Forbes-Thompson (2008), however, in their qualitative study of family members of nursing home residents, found that "family members often hold themselves responsible for overseeing the care of their loved one, representing the resident's perspective and history, and keeping the family connections" (p. 43). They concluded that these role expectations are important to family members but called on nursing staff to "maximize constructive family involvement and minimize the stress families may experience if they are not able to fulfill their role expectations" (p. 43).

## CONCLUSIONS

Many factors have led to the significant professional nursing shortage of the early 21st century. Health care providers, the public, and legislators are beginning to recognize that both the problem and the potential consequences are severe. One would be hard-pressed to find a congressperson or senator who would not identify the current nursing shortage as one of the most serious issues affecting health care today.

Ellenbecker (2010) suggests that the challenges of the current nursing shortage only increase when coupled with the need for national health care reform. Yet efforts to address the shortage have been too few and far between. Short-term solutions to the shortage have been attempted, including importing foreign nurses and increasing federal money for nursing education. The passage of current legislation has encouraged more students to choose nursing as a career and has helped students financially to complete their education. It has also encouraged graduate students to complete their studies and assume teaching positions in nursing schools. Long-term planning and aggressive intervention, however, will be needed for some time at the national and regional levels to ensure that an adequate, highly qualified nursing workforce will be available in the future to meet health care needs in the United States.

More must be done to address the current nursing shortage, and it is increasingly obvious that multiple solutions to the shortage will be needed. These solutions will require the best thinking of experts and will likely reshape fundamental core underpinnings that have been a part of the nursing work world for decades, if not centuries.

## FOR ADDITIONAL DISCUSSION

**1.** In what ways do other professions do a better job of attracting younger workers—both men and women?

**2.** Are salaries a significant driver in the current nursing shortage? At what level would salaries not be a factor?

**3.** How would increasing the educational level for entry into practice affect the current nursing shortage?

**4.** Will the demand for RNs in the future be affected by growing technological developments?

**5.** Why has the nursing workforce historically suffered some degree of a shortage every 10 to 15 years?

**6.** If magnet hospital criteria were to become the baseline for organizational structure and performance, would nursing shortages exist?

**7.** Why are starting salaries for nurses with master's and doctoral degrees in academia so low?

**8.** Why do many health care organizations choose to expend more money on recruitment than on retention strategies? Which is more effective in the short term and in the long term?

**9.** Is implementation of mandatory minimum staffing ratios in acute care hospitals likely to reduce the nursing shortage in California?

## REFERENCES

Aiken, L. H., Sloane, D. M., Clarke, S., Poghosyan, L., Cho, E., You, L., ... Aungsuroch, Y. (2011). Importance of work environments on hospital outcomes in nine countries. *International Journal for Quality in Health Care, 23*(4), 357–364. doi:10.1093/intqhc/mzr022

Allen, L. (2008). The nursing shortage continues as faculty shortage grows. *Nursing Economics, 26*(1), 35–40.

The Alter Group. (2011). *RN turnover costs hospitals an estimated $9.75 billion annually.* Retrieved June 15, 2011, from http://www.altergroup.com/alter-care-blog/index.php/healthcare/rn-turnover-costs/

American Association of Colleges of Nursing. (2010). *Joint statement from the tri-council for nursing on recent registered nurse supply and demand projections.* Retrieved June 7, 2011, from http://www.aacn.nche.edu/Media/NewsReleases/2010/tricouncil.html

American Association of Colleges of Nursing. (2011a). *Fact sheet: Nursing faculty shortage.* Retrieved June 6, 2011, from http://www.aacn.nche.edu/Media/FactSheets/NursingShortage.htm

American Association of Colleges of Nursing. (2011b). *Fact sheet: Nursing shortage.* Retrieved June 13, 2011, from http://www.aacn.nche.edu/Media/FactSheets/NursingShortage.htm

American Association of Colleges of Nursing. (2011c, June 13). AACN partners with the Jonas Center for Nursing Excellence to expand the nation's supply of doctorally prepared nurse faculty (Press release). *Business Wire News Releases.* Retrieved June 16, 2011, from http://financial.businessinsider.com/siliconalleymedia.clusterstock/news/read?GUID=18708705

Auerbach, D. I., Buerhaus, P. I., & Staiger, D. O. (2007). Better late than never: Workforce supply implications of later entry into nursing. *Health Affairs, 26*(1), 178–185.

Baby-boomer nurses are on their way out. Clinical rounds. (2008). *Nursing, 38*(6), 25.

Bae, S., Mark, B., & Fried, B. (2010). Impact of nursing unit turnover on patient outcomes in hospitals. *Journal of Nursing Scholarship, 42*(1), 40–49.

Bern-Klug, M., & Forbes-Thompson, S. (2008). Family members' responsibilities to nursing home residents: "She is the only mother I got." *Journal of Gerontological Nursing, 34*(2), 43–52.

Blegen, M. A., Goode, C. J., Spetz, J., Vaughn, T., & Park, S. H. (2011, April). Nurse staffing effects on patient outcomes: Safety-net and non-safety-net hospitals. *Medical Care, 49*(4), 406–414.

Buerhaus, P. I., Staiger, D. O., & Auerbach, D. I. (2009a). *The future of the nursing workforce in the United States: Data, trends, and implications.* Boston, MA: Jones & Bartlett.

Buerhaus, P., Staiger, D., & Auerbach, D. (2009b). The recent surge in nurse employment: Causes and implications. *Health Affairs, 28*(4), w657–w668.

Caine, R. M. (2011, February 4). *California's nursing shortage hasn't been fixed.* Retrieved June 7, 2011, from http://articles.sfgate.com/2011-02-04/opinion/27100858_1_nursing-shortage-nurse-education-initiative-new-student-enrollments

Calarco, M. M. (2011). The impact of positive practices on nurse work environments: Emerging applications of positive organizational scholarship. *Western Journal of Nursing Research, 33*(3), 365–384.

Donelan, K., Buerhaus, P., Des Roches, C., Dittus, R., & Dutwin, D. (2008). Public perceptions of nursing careers: The influence of the media and nursing shortages. *Nursing Economics, 26*(3), 143–150.

Ellenbecker, C. (2010). Preparing the nursing workforce of the future. *Policy, Politics & Nursing Practice, 11*(2), 115–125.

Elsevier Foundation. (2011). *Preparing nurse educators to confront the nursing shortage.* Retrieved June 14, 2011, from http://www.elsevierfoundation.org/nursing-faculty/stories/text-nurse-shortage.asp

Federwish, A. (2008). Reinventing, not retiring. *NurseWeek (California Edition), 21*(11), 14–15.

Feeg, V., & Nickitas, D. M. (2011, May–June). Doubling the number of nurses with a doctorate by 2020: Predicting the right number or getting it right? *Nursing Economics, 29*(3), 109–110.

Health Resources and Services Administration. (2010). *National sample survey of registered nurses - downloadable data.* Retrieved June 7, 2011, from http://datawarehouse.hrsa.gov/nursingsurvey.aspx

Hirschkorn, C. A., West, T. B., & Hill, K. S. (2010, November). Experienced nurse retention strategies. *Journal of Nursing Administration, 40*(11), 463–467.

Honor Society of Nursing, Sigma Theta Tau International. (n.d.). *Facts on the nursing shortage in North America.* Retrieved from http://www.nursingsociety.org/Media/Pages/shortage.aspx

Issues in nursing. How do we tackle the nurse faculty shortage? (2008). *Nursing, 38*(2), 44–45.

Keller, S., & Burns, C. (2010). The aging nurse: Can employers accommodate age-related changes? *AAOHN Journal, 58*(10), 437–446.

Kirshcling, J. M., Colgan, C., & Andrews, B. (2011, May–June). Predictors of registered nurses' willingness to remain in nursing. *Nursing Economics, 29*(3), 111–117.

Letvak, S. (2008). Retirement or rehirement? *Advance for Nurses (Northern California and Northern Nevada), 5*(15), 21–23.

Marquis, B., & Huston, C. (2012). *Leadership roles and management functions in nursing* (7th ed.). Philadelphia, PA: Lippincott, Williams, & Wilkins.

McNamara, M. (2010). Nursing shortage shows signs of decline. *American Nurse, 42*(6), 12.

Merriam Webster's Online Dictionary. (2011a). *Demand*. Retrieved June 7, 2011, from http://www.merriam-webster.com/dictionary/demand

Merriam Webster's Online Dictionary. (2011b). *Supply*. Retrieved June 7, 2011, from http://www.merriam-webster.com/dictionary/supply

Metzger, M. (2010). What's happened to the nursing shortage? *Bulletin of the Wisconsin Nurses Association, 79*(7), 4.

Mukamel, D. B., Spector, W. D., Limcangco, R., Wang, Y., Shanlian, F., & Mor, V. (2009, October). The cost of turnover in nursing homes. *Medical Care, 47*(10), 1039–1045.

National Council State Boards of Nursing. (2011). *NCLEX examination pass rates*. Retrieved June 11, 2011, from https://www.ncsbn.org/1237.htm

National League for Nursing. (2010, February). *2010 NLN nurse educator shortage fact sheet*. Retrieved June 14, 2011, from http://www.nln.org/governmentaffairs/pdf/NurseFacultyShortage.pdf

PayScale. (2011a). *Hourly rate snapshot for registered nurse (RN) jobs*. Retrieved June 13, 2011, from http://www.payscale.com/research/US/Job=Registered_Nurse_(RN)/Hourly_Rate

Payscale. (2011b). *Salary snapshot for nurse practitioner (NP) jobs*. Retrieved June 16, 2011, from http://www.payscale.com/research/US/Job=Nurse_Practitioner_(NP)/Salary

PR WEB. (2010b, September 23). *National League for Nursing releases faculty census data*. Retrieved June 14, 2011, from http://www.prweb.com/releases/2010/09/prweb4549674.htm

Robert Wood Johnson Foundation. (2010). *New careers in nursing scholarship program*. Retrieved July 27, 2012, from http://www.newcareersinnursing.org/about-ncin

Roman, L. (2008). Nursing shortage: Looking to the future. *RN, 71*(3), 34–36, 38–41.

Rondeau, K. V., Williams, E. S., & Wagar, T. H. (2008). Turnover and vacancy rates for registered nurses: Do local labor market forces matter? *Health Care Management Review, 33*(1), 69–78.

Sapountzi-Krepia, D., Raftopoulos, V., Psychogiou, M., Sakellari, E., Toris, A., Vrettos, A., & Arsenos, P. (2008). Dimensions of informal care in Greece: The family's contribution to the care of patients hospitalized in an oncology hospital. *Journal of Clinical Nursing, 17*(10), 1287–1294.

Texas Organization of Nurse Executives. (2010). *The Texas nursing shortage: Condition critical more graduates needed to close the gap*. Retrieved June 14, 2011, from http://www.texasnurse.org/displaycommon.cfm?an=1&subarticlenbr=44

Tosto, P. (2010, June 9). What's the right number of nurses? *MPR News*. Retrieved June 8, 2011, from http://minnesota.publicradio.org/collections/special/columns/minnecon/archive/2010/06/whats-the-right-number-of-nurses.shtml

Trust for America's Health. (2011). *State data: Nursing shortage estimates*. Retrieved June 7, 2011, from http://healthyamericans.org/states/states.php?measure=nursingshortage

Unruh, L. (2008). Nurse staffing and patient, nurse, and financial outcomes. *American Journal of Nursing, 108*(1), 62–71.

U.S. Department of Labor, Bureau of Health Statistics. (2010-2011). *Occupational outlook handbook* (2010–2011 ed.). Retrieved June 13, 2011, from http://www.bls.gov/oco/ocos083.htm

Williams, S. G. (2011). Nursing faculty shortage. *Advance for Nurses*. Retrieved June 14, 2011, from http://nursing.advanceweb.com/Regional-Content/Articles/Nursing-Faculty-Shortage.aspx

Winter, R. (2009). America's nursing shortage by the numbers. *Soliant Health*. Retrieved June 14, 2011, from http://blog.soliant.com/healthcare-news/americas-nursing-shortage-by-the-numbers/

Wood, D. (2011, June 10). Nurses continue to delay retirement. *Nursezone.com*. Retrieved June 14, 2011, from http://www.nursezone.com/Nursing-News-Events/more-news/Nurses-Continue-to-Delay-Retirement_37086.aspx

## BIBLIOGRAPHY

Carlson, J. (2010). Debating the shortage: Nursing jobs scarce, but experts say that'll change. *Modern Healthcare, 40*(25), 8–9.

Clark, R., & Allison-Jones, L. (2011). Investing in human capital: An academic-service partnership to address the nursing shortage. *Nursing Education Perspectives, 32*(1), 18–21.

Conley, B. (2012). What does "shortage" really mean? *Tennessee Nurse, 75*(1), 5.

Dolan, T. B. (2011). Has the nursing shortage come to an end? *ONS Connect, 26*(8), 8–12.

Fairchild, P., & Mott, S. (2012). Flexible thinking for the future. *Nursing Review,* (1326-0472), 28–29.

Hill, K. S. (2011). Nursing and the aging workforce: Myths and reality, what do we really know? *Nursing Clinics of North America, 46*(1), 1–9.

Hussain, A., Rivers, P. A., Glover, S. H., & Fottler, M. D. (2012). Strategies for dealing with future shortages in the nursing workforce: A review. *Health Services Management Research, 25*(1), 41–47.

Potempa, K., Auerbach, D. I., Buerhaus, P. I., & Staiger, D. O. (2012). A future nursing shortage? *Health Affairs, 31*(3), 652.

O'Reilly, C. (2012). The elephant in the room: Employment for new graduate RNs. *Nevada Rnformation, 21*(1), 17.

Richardson, H., Gilmartin, M. J., & Fulmer, T. (2012). Shifting the clinical teaching paradigm in undergraduate nursing education to address the nursing faculty shortage. *Journal of Nursing Education, 51*(4), 226–231.

Ritter, D. (2011). The relationship between healthy work environments and retention of nurses in a hospital setting. *Journal of Nursing Management, 19*(1), 27–32.

Acks, R., & Epling, E. (2011). New grad economics: What nursing shortage? *Nursing Voice, 16*(1), 12.

Sephel, A. (2011). [Commentary on] Digging deeper: Nurse excess or shortage? The effect on a new nurse. *Journal of Professional Nursing, 27*(6), 390–393.

Shacklock, K., & Brunetto, Y. (2012). The intention to continue nursing: Work variables affecting three nurse generations in Australia. *Journal of Advanced Nursing, 68*(1), 36–46.

Trossman, S. (2011, January–February). The go-to nurses: Finding ways to keep long-time RNs. *American Nurse.* Available at http://www.theamericannurse.org/index. php/2011/02/02/the-go-to-nursesfinding-ways-to-keep-long-time-rns/. Accessed Sept. 14, 2012.

Wilson, L., & Fowler, M. (2012). Leadership needed to address the global nursing and midwifery workforce shortage. *Nursing Outlook, 60*(1), 51–53.

# Chapter **6**

## Importing Foreign Nurses

Carol J. Huston

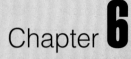

## ADDITIONAL RESOURCES

Visit thePoint for additional helpful resources
- eBook
- Journal Articles
- WebLinks

## CHAPTER OUTLINE

## LEARNING OBJECTIVES

*The learner will be able to:*

1. Examine how the scope of global nurse migration has changed over the last decade.

2. Analyze "push" and "pull" factors that encourage nurses to migrate internationally.

3. Identify primary donor and recipient countries of migrating nurses.

4. Explore potential negative effects of international migration, including "brain drain" from "supplier" countries.

5. Apply the ethical principles of autonomy, utility, and justice in arguing for or against global nurse recruitment and migration.

6. Consider whether embedded *ethos* or *straight thinking* concepts provide an appropriate philosophical foundation for exploring the ethical dimensions of nurse migration.

7. Outline common key components of position statements on nurse migration adopted by professional associations such as the International Council of Nurses (ICN), the International Centre on Nurse Migration, AcademyHealth, and the World Health Organization.

8. Explore national and international efforts to develop best practices or regulatory oversight of international nurse recruitment and migration.

9. Differentiate between the types of work visas foreign nurses use to gain entry for employment in the United States.

10. Outline the certification process required by the Commission on Graduates of Foreign Nursing Schools for migratory nurses to be able to take the NCLEX examination and obtain visas for work in the United States.

11. Discuss the need for ongoing cultural, professional, and psychological support for foreign nurses after their arrival in their importer country to assist them in successful socialization.

12. Reflect on personal beliefs and values regarding the use of widespread international recruitment and nurse migration to address nursing shortages.

Many countries have historically had cyclical shortages of nurses, but typically they were caused by increasing demand outstripping a static or slowly growing supply of nurses. The current situation is more serious. Demand continues to grow while supply decreases as a result of an aging workforce, projected increases in nursing retirements in the coming decade, and an inadequate number of new graduates from nursing education programs. Indeed, almost all of the developed countries in the world are reporting nursing shortages. One increasingly common means of alleviating the current nursing shortage has been to recruit foreign nurses.

International recruitment and *nurse migration*—moving from one country to another in search of employment—has been viewed as a relatively inexpensive, "quick-fix" solution to rapidly increasing health care worker shortages. In fact, hiring nurses from other countries in a global service market is generally seen as a rational choice by recruiting institutions since it typically produces a positive financial outcome in a defined period of time (Habermann & Stagge, 2010).

The current situation, however, is different from those in the past, when nurse migration was mostly based on individual motivation and typically followed previous colonial ties (i.e., Philippines to the United States; South Africa and Australia to the United Kingdom; Kaelin, 2011). Now there is active planning of large-scale international nurse recruitment, often from developing countries that can least afford to lose their most highly educated health care workers.

This recruiting onslaught affects the ability of developing countries to develop sustainable health care systems and provide appropriate care to their citizens. Indeed, few donor nations are prepared to manage the loss of their nurse workforce to such widespread migration, leading to what Barnett, Namasivayam, and Narudin (2010) have called a "crisis in nursing." In addition, developing countries often recruit from each other, even within the same geographical region. Table 6.1 summarizes the current dynamic nature of nurse migration in select countries around the world.

| TABLE 6.1 | Effect of Push–Pull Migration on Select Countries |
|---|---|
| Africa | Clemens and Pettersson (2008) reported that approximately 70,000 African-born professional nurses were working overseas in a developed country in the year 2000. This represents about one tenth of African-born professional nurses, although the fraction of health professionals abroad varies enormously across African countries, from 1% to greater than 70%, depending on the occupation and the country. |
| Australia | Australia has called for a national workforce plan but does have a shortage of nurses, primarily in rural areas. Australia is identified as both a primary donor and a recipient country for migrant nurses and primarily recruits from the United Kingdom and New Zealand. |
| China | Fang (2007) stated that as a result of lack of limited job opportunities, low salary, and low job satisfaction, many Chinese nurses intend to migrate. Commercial recruiters have expressed a strong interest in recruiting Chinese nurses, but there are limited examples of successful ventures. It is likely that China will become an important source of nurses for developed nations in the coming years. |

*continued*

| TABLE 6.1 | Effect of Push–Pull Migration on Select Countries *continued* |
|---|---|
| Canada | Canada is both a source and a destination country for international nurse migration, with an estimated net loss of nurses. The United States is the major beneficiary of Canadian nurse emigration, resulting from the reduction of full-time jobs for nurses in Canada due to health system reforms. Canada faces a significant projected shortage of nurses (Little, 2007). |
| India | Despite an extremely low nurse-to-population ratio in India, large-scale nurse migration to other countries is increasing. Bhalla and Meher (2010) suggest that low wages, heavy workloads, bad working conditions, and a sense of sometimes not being treated with respect have resulted in many Indian nurses migrating to the United States, the United Kingdom, and other countries. |
| Ireland | As late as 25 years ago, Ireland had an abundant pool of nurses. Humphries, Brugha, and McGee (2008) suggested, however, that Ireland began actively recruiting nurses from overseas in 2000 and has recruited almost 10,000 nurses, primarily from India and the Philippines, since that time. Thus, Ireland has moved from being a traditional exporter of nurses to an importer. |
| Israel | Ehrenfeld, Itzhaki, and Michal (2007) suggested that Israel has welcomed large numbers of nurse immigrants but that the nation's expenditures for health care and nursing education have, at times, had to take a back seat to the government's efforts to house new immigrants, to relocate groups, and to defend the nation against politically motivated violence and attacks. All of this has been in the context of regional conflicts and international debates. |
| Lebanon | El-Jardali, Nuhad, Diana, and Mouro (2008) suggested that Lebanon is facing a problem of excessive nurse migration to countries of the Persian Gulf, North America, and Europe. An estimated one in five nurses who receive a bachelor's of science in nursing migrates out of Lebanon within 1 or 2 years of graduation, with the majority of nurses migrating to countries of the Gulf. The main reasons for migration include shift work, high patient–nurse ratios, lack of autonomy in decision making, lack of a supportive environment, and poor commitment to excellent nursing care (El-Jardali et al., 2008). |
| New Zealand | New Zealand has been both a source and destination country since the beginning of the 21st century. As of 2010, almost 25% of the workforce in New Zealand comes from overseas (Questioning the Ethics of Nurse Migration, 2010) with India providing a rapidly increasing number of migrants (Woodbridge & Bland, 2010). The movement of New Zealand RNs to Australia is expedited by the Trans-Tasman Agreement, whereas the entry of foreign RNs to New Zealand is facilitated by nursing being an identified priority occupation. |
| Philippines | Lorenzo, Galvez-Tan, Icamina, and Javier (2007) suggested that the Philippines is a job-scarce environment, and even for those with jobs in the health care sector, poor working conditions often motivate nurses to seek employment overseas. The country is dependent on labor migration to ease a tight domestic labor market. National opinion has generally focused on the improved quality of life for individual migrants and their families and on the benefits of remittances to the nation; however, a shortage of highly skilled nurses and the massive retraining of physicians to become nurses elsewhere has created severe problems for the Filipino health system, including the closure of many hospitals. |
| Saudi Arabia | Saudi Arabia now gets most of its nurses from the Philippines—the same place where most countries, including the United States, are doing the majority of their recruiting. |

| TABLE 6.1 | **Effect of Push–Pull Migration on Select Countries** *continued* |
|---|---|
| United Kingdom | Nichols and Campbell (2010) suggest that an acute shortage of nurses in the mid-1990s, combined with policy initiatives to increase the number of qualified nurses working in the NHS, resulted in an active campaign to recruit nurses from overseas. Since 1997, approximately 100,000 international nurses have been admitted to the nursing register from more than 50 countries worldwide. Outflow has been at a lower level, mainly to other English-speaking developed countries—Australia, the United States, New Zealand, Ireland, and Canada. The United Kingdom is a net importer of nurses. |
| United States | Nurse immigration to the United States has tripled since 1994, to close to 15,000 entrants annually. Foreign-educated nurses are located primarily in urban areas, most likely to be employed by hospitals, and somewhat more likely to have a baccalaureate degree than native-born nurses. |

## GLOBAL MIGRATION OF NURSES: "PUSH" AND "PULL" FACTORS

To understand what is driving the global migration of nurses, it is first necessary to examine what are known as the "push" and "pull" factors of nursing migration. *Push factors* are those factors that push or drive nurses to want to leave their countries to go to another. Low pay, inadequate opportunities for career advancement or continuing education, sociopolitical instability, and unsafe workplaces are examples of push factors. Other factors that act as push factors in some countries include the risk of human immunodeficiency virus and acquired immunodeficiency disease to health system workers, concerns about personal security in areas of conflict, and economic instability.

*Pull factors* are those factors that draw the nurse toward a different country. Pull factors typically include higher pay, more-developed career structures, opportunities for further education and professional development, and, in some cases, safety from the threat of violence (more prevalent in less developed countries). Other pull factors, such as the opportunity to travel or to participate in foreign aid work, also influence some nurses. A summary of push and pull factors for nurse migration is given in Table 6.2.

It is important to remember that developed countries, such as Australia, the United Kingdom, and the United States, are the primary destinations of most migrant nurses, and developing nations are primarily the donors. In fact, in some poor or transitional countries such as Ghana, Malawi, Swaziland, and the Philippines,

| TABLE 6.2 | **Push and Pull Factors for Nurse Migration** | |
|---|---|---|
| **Push Factors** | | **Pull Factors** |
| Low pay (absolute and/or relative) | | Higher pay (and opportunities for remittances) |
| Poor working conditions | | Better working conditions |
| Lack of resources to work effectively | | Better-resourced health systems |
| Limited career opportunities | | Career opportunities |
| Limited educational opportunities | | Provision of postbasic education |
| Impact of HIV and AIDS | | Political stability |
| Unstable/dangerous work environment | | Travel opportunities |
| Economic instability | | Aid work |

*Source:* Buchan, J. (2006). The impact of global nursing migration on health services delivery. *Policy, Politics, & Nursing Practice (Supplement), 7*(3), 16S–25S.

more than half of the registered nurses (RNs) have migrated (Gostin, 2008). In fact, Donkor and Andrews (2011) reported that Ghana has lost half of its nurses in the last 5 years and the Ghanaian Minister of Health estimates this has left only 10,000 nurses in that country to provide care to a population of 20 million people.

---

CONSIDER THIS   Developed countries are often the recipients of migrant nurses and developing countries are often the donors. In essence then, developing countries are supporting the health care infrastructure of more developed countries, often at the expense of their own country.

---

Currently, about 3.1% of the RN workforce in the United States is foreign-born non-U.S. citizens, and 3.3% received their basic education elsewhere. The principal donor countries for foreign nurses in the United States are the Philippines, Canada, India, and England (Schumacher, 2011).

Destination countries are able to recruit nurses as a result of a large number of pull factors. Many internationally recruited nurses suggest they would have preferred to remain in their home country with family and friends and in a familiar culture and environment, but push and pull factors overwhelmingly influenced their decision to migrate.

---

CONSIDER THIS   Nurses migrate for many reasons and the push/pull factors to migrate are in constant imbalance.

---

## THE EFFECT OF GLOBAL MIGRATION ON DEVELOPING COUNTRIES

A review of the literature suggests that different countries have experienced different effects as a result of the push–pull of international nurse migration. In some cases, aggressive recruitment, by which large numbers of recruits are sought, may significantly deplete a single health facility or contract an important number of newly graduated nurses from a single educational institute. This has significant local and regional implications. Gostin (2008) agrees, suggesting that nurse migration often disadvantages societies that are already the poorest

and least healthy and that, because nursing shortages are associated with poor outcomes, not only is critical intellectual capital taken away from the developing country but also the donor country's health outcomes are likely to worsen.

Some national governments and government agencies have, however, actually encouraged the outflow of nurses from their country, including Fiji, Jamaica, India, Mauritius, and the Philippines. For many years, the Philippine government actively endorsed and facilitated initiatives aimed at educating, recruiting, training, and placing nurses around the world. This was likely the result of a financial imperative, to encourage the generation of remittance income. Indeed, labor is the most profitable export of Philippines, with almost 10% of the population working around the globe and generating more than US$15 billion in remittance income annually (Kaelin, 2011). This includes the export of at least 10,000 nurses annually (Kaelin, 2011).

---

CONSIDER THIS   Migrating nurses provide value to source countries, in that health care workers often send remittances back home to support their families and bolster the economy; they may form clinical or educational partnerships between countries; after a time, some workers return home with enhanced skills and experience (Gostin, 2008).

---

The mass export of nurses from the Philippines is a response to a labor market oversupply. The Philippines currently produces 100,000 to 150,000 nurses every year, and less than 5% of them are employed in the Philippines, either by the government or the private sector (Gamolo, 2008). The Philippine Overseas Employment Administration deployed a total of 13,525 licensed nurses around the world in 2006 (James, 2008), and, according to the Trade Union Congress of the Philippines, more than 21,000 new Filipino nurses sought U.S. jobs in 2007 (Gamolo, 2008). The Trade Union continues to encourage the deployment of surplus nurses and other highly skilled workers rather than unskilled workers, whose skills are more easily replaceable.

China, with the second largest nursing workforce in the world (2.2 million nurses), is another country actively seeking to export nurses. Yet Fang (2007) suggested that there is actually a severe shortage of nurses in China, with only 1 nurse per 1,000 population.

Nonetheless, there is a very high level of unemployment and underemployment of nurses. This creates an artificial surplus of nurses who can and do want to migrate. Fang suggested that even if the Chinese government were to increase the nursing jobs available and improve working conditions, some surplus would still exist. He concluded that China will likely become an important source of nurses for developed nations in the coming years.

India is also gaining ground as one of the world's leading nurse exporters. In 2004, for example, India surpassed the Philippines in terms of the number of nurses admitted to the U.K. Registrar for the first time (Brush, 2008) and the World Bank (2011, 2012) reports that India became the world's top receiver of remittances from immigrant workers abroad with US$58 billion flowing into that country in 2011 alone.

Nonetheless, recent reports from South Africa, Ghana, China, the Caribbean, and even the Philippines highlight that such a significant outflow of nurses has had negative effects, including reductions in the level and quality of services and the loss of specialist skills. Indeed, Brush (2010) suggests that the continued exodus of nurses from the Philippines now threatens the public health of that country itself, since so many of the country's most experienced nurses are migrating, leaving the care of the local populace (particularly those in rural communities) in the hands of lesser experienced and lesser qualified personnel.

Similarly, African ministers of health have repeatedly brought resolutions to the World Health Assembly stating that health care worker migration is crippling their health care systems (Kuehn, 2007). Taiwan too has expressed concerns about the brain drain that has occurred as a result of the migration of nurses from there (Brush, 2008).

It is this brain drain that is one of the most critical negative consequences of widespread nursing migration from developing countries. *Brain drain* refers to the loss of skilled personnel and the loss of investment in education that is experienced when those human resources migrate elsewhere. The Federation for American Immigration Reform (FAIR; n.d.) defines brain drain as the flow of skilled professionals from less developed countries to more developed countries and suggests that this practice results in developing countries losing the individuals they can least afford to lose because they are the ones "who are skilled and educated, who perform crucial services contributing to the health and economy of the country, and who create new jobs for others" (para. 1).

> CONSIDER THIS   The positive global economic/social/professional development associated with international migration must be weighed against the substantial brain and skills drain experienced by donor countries.

Complaints of brain drain are heard from donor countries such as India, the Philippines, South Africa, and Zimbabwe. These nations argue that their human health care resources are being extracted at a time when they are needed most. Although these negative effects of international migration on "supplier" countries have been more openly recognized and addressed in the last few years, concerted efforts to address the problem continue to be limited.

In addition, many of the countries that are exporting nurses are also experiencing a nursing shortage. For example, Africa has a significant shortage of RNs in terms of absolute numbers and this is confounded by the fact that RNs (in contrast to lesser educated *enrolled nurses*) are more likely to migrate (IOL, 2011).

> CONSIDER THIS   The majority of countries importing foreign nurses are primarily White, and donor nations typically export nurses of color. The issue of race and the global economics of nursing should be examined in terms of effect on both supplier and donor countries.

It should be noted, however, that brain drain is not just occurring in nursing. Despite Europe's efforts to stop its scientific brain drain, more and more of the continent's brightest young researchers are choosing to pursue careers abroad. In Germany, for example, record numbers of highly qualified individuals are choosing to work abroad, marking the biggest mass exodus in 60 years (Paterson, 2008). Countries in Eastern Europe are reporting the same.

In addition, CSR Europe (2008) suggested that 30% of professionals from African countries work abroad, requiring African countries to invest US$4 billion annually to replace them. In addition, 20,000 skilled professionals, scientists, academics, and researchers leave the African continent annually, "depriving many African countries of the human and intellectual capital they need to develop" (CSR Europe, 2008, para. 1).

Just because the brain drain that occurs in nursing resources also occurs in other disciplines does not make it acceptable. It does, however, suggest that the individual's right to choose cannot be easily negated simply because the donor country does not want to lose its intellectual resources.

Finally, one must consider whether recruiting foreign nurses to solve acute staffing shortages is simply a poorly thought-out quick fix to a much greater problem and whether, in doing so, not only are donor nations harmed but also the issues that led to the shortage in the first place are never addressed. Certainly, one must at least question whether wholesale foreign nurse recruitment would even be necessary if importer nations made a more concerted effort to improve the working conditions, salaries, empowerment, and recognition of the home-born nurses they already employ. Indeed, one must question whether importation occurs in an effort to avoid the costs of doing so. Clearly, many nursing organizations and nursing leaders have begun to recognize the negative effects of international migration on "supplier" countries, but efforts to address the problem have been inadequate.

CONSIDER THIS  Importing foreign nurses to solve the nursing shortage only puts a Band-Aid on the problem. The factors that led to the nursing shortage in the first place still need to be resolved.

## DISCUSSION POINT

If the money that is being spent on recruitment and immigration of foreign nurses was instead spent on resolving the domestic nursing issues that led to a shortage in the first place, would international nurse recruitment even be necessary?

## GLOBAL NURSE RECRUITMENT AND MIGRATION AS AN ETHICAL ISSUE

Controversy regarding the ethics of international recruitment of nurses is not new. Whenever resources are limited, ethical issues regarding their allocation are likely to arise. In the case of global nurse recruitment and migration, the ethical principles of autonomy, utility, and justice seem most relevant. Certainly, there must be some sort of a balance between the right of individual nurses to choose to migrate (autonomy), particularly when push factors are overwhelming, and the more utilitarian concern for the donor nations' health as a result of losing scarce nursing resources.

International law clearly guarantees an individual the right to freedom of movement and residence (as established in the Universal Declaration of Human Rights; United Nations General Assembly, 1948) and the International Covenant on Civil and Political Rights (Office of the United Nations High Commissioner for Human Rights, 1976). The individual's right to migrate is central to self-determination. Jose (2011), in his study of internationally educated nurses working in the United States, confirms that the "dreams of a better life" were central to the decision of these foreign nurses to move to the United States.

## DISCUSSION POINT

Should the right for the individual nurse to migrate (autonomy and self-determination) override what might be best for the donor nation (utilitarianism)?

Justice, or fairness, however, is another ethical principle that seems appropriate to this discussion because it examines how social and material goods are distributed to or withheld from members of a group or society, particularly in relation to fairness. Kaelin (2011) suggests that the uneven distribution of nurses around the globe cannot be just since it deprives so much of the world's population access to professional health care services. Kaelin argues that from the perspective of justice, whether conceptualized universally or from a communitarian framework, unequal distribution of health care is unfair and that this unfairness is increased by nurse migration. He concludes that both receiving and donating countries have strong moral obligations to work toward fairer distributions of health care services as the fate of other communities cannot be ignored.

Donkor and Andrews (2011) agree, arguing that nursing migration from developing countries has resulted in unbearable caseloads, decreased job satisfaction, and emotional fatigue on the part of the remaining nurses. As such, they argue that it is a global concern requiring all stakeholders to move beyond traditional stereotypes and to instead be flexible and forward looking.

The following question then must be asked: Does global recruitment violate the principle of justice, particularly if such migration does not solve the underlying shortage and when such retention is done at the expense of the donor country? Kingma (2007) expressed the same concern in her assertion that injecting migrant nurses into dysfunctional health systems—ones that are not capable of attracting and retaining staff domestically—will not solve the nursing shortage.

Milton (2007) suggested that the ethics of nurse migration become even more complex when nurse leaders must consider whether the issue should be viewed using philosophical frameworks that contain embedded *ethos* or *straight thinking* concepts. She concluded that there are ethical considerations for having an ethos or straight thinking for doing what is right and good for the discipline of nursing and the community, and she argued that the discipline of nursing must focus on creating health policies that value humans and health, as well as human dignity.

Clearly, donor countries have an ethical obligation to do what they can to provide their nurses with a safe, satisfying, and economically rewarding work environment. Importer countries have an ethical obligation to do what is necessary to be more self-reliant in meeting their professional workforce needs and to avoid recruiting nurses from those countries that can least afford to experience brain drain. Finally, professional health care associations must lead the way in addressing how best to respond to these ethical concerns.

## PROFESSIONAL ORGANIZATIONS RESPOND

Given the current extent of nurse migration and the multiplicity of ethical dilemmas associated with it, many professional organizations, representing nurses from around the world, have weighed in on the issue. Some have provided formal position statements to guide both donor and importer countries. Others have attempted to provide guidance to the individual nurse considering global migration.

### The International Council of Nurses

One international agency, the International Council of Nurses (ICN), has issued several position statements arguing for ethics and good employment practices in international recruitment (Box 6.1). The ICN, a federation of more than 130 national nurses' associations, represents millions of nurses worldwide (ICN, 2011). The *ICN Position Statement: Nurse Retention and Migration* authored in 1999 and revised in 2007 confirms the right of nurses to migrate, as well as the potential beneficial outcomes of multicultural practice and learning opportunities supported by migration, but acknowledges potential adverse effects on the quality of health care in donor countries (ICN, 2007a).

---

**BOX 6.1   ICN POSITION STATEMENT ON NURSE RETENTION, TRANSFER, AND MIGRATION (1999)**

ICN and its member associations firmly believe that quality health care is directly dependent on an adequate supply of qualified nursing personnel.

ICN recognizes the right of individual nurses to migrate, while acknowledging the possible adverse effect that international migration may have on health care quality.

ICN condemns the practice of recruiting nurses to countries where authorities have failed to address human resource planning and problems that cause nurses to leave the profession and discourage them from returning to nursing.

In support of the above, ICN does the following:

- Disseminates information on nursing personnel needs and resources and on the development of fulfilling nursing career structures

- Provides training opportunities in negotiation and socioeconomic welfare–related issues

- Disseminates data on nursing employment worldwide

- Takes action to help reduce the serious effects of any shortage, maldistribution, and misutilization of nursing personnel

*continued*

**BOX 18.1    ICN POSITION STATEMENT ON NURSE RETENTION, TRANSFER, AND MIGRATION (1999)**
*continued*

- Advocates adherence nationally to international labor standards
- Condemns the recruitment of nurses as a strike-breaking mechanism
- Advocates for open and transparent migration systems (recognizing that some appropriate screening is necessary to ensure public safety)
- Supports a transcultural approach to nursing practice
- Promotes the introduction of transferable benefits, for example, pension

National nurses' associations are urged to do the following:

- Encourage relevant authorities to ensure sound human resources planning for nursing
- Participate in the development of sound national policies on immigration and emigration of nurses
- Promote the revision of nursing curriculum for basic and postbasic education in nursing and administration to emphasize effective nursing leadership
- Disseminate information on the working conditions of nurses
- Discourage nurses from working in other countries where salaries and conditions are not acceptable to nurses and professional associations in those countries
- Ensure that foreign nurses have conditions of employment equal to those of local nurses in posts requiring the same level of competency and involving the same duties and responsibilities
- Ensure that there are no distinctions made among foreign nurses from different countries
- Monitor the activities of recruiting agencies
- Provide an advisory service to help nurses interpret contracts and assist foreign nurses with personal and work-related problems, such as institutional racism, violence, and sexual harassment
- Provide orientation for foreign nurses on the local cultural, social, and political values and on the health system and national language
- Alert nurses to the fact that some diplomas, qualifications, or degrees earned in one country may not be recognized in another
- Assist nurses with their problems related to international migration and repatriation

*Source:* International Council of Nurses. (2007a). *Position statement: Nurse retention and migration.* Retrieved June 25, 2011, from http://www.icn.ch/images/stories/documents/publications/position_statements/C06_Nurse_Retention_Migration.pdf

The ICN (2007a) position statement also condemns the practice of recruiting nurses to countries where authorities have failed to implement sound human resource planning and to seriously address problems that cause nurses to leave the profession and discourage them from returning to nursing. The position statement also denounces unethical recruitment practices that exploit nurses or mislead them into accepting job responsibilities and working conditions that are incompatible with their qualifications, skills, and experience. The ICN and its member national nurses' associations call for a regulated recruitment process based on ethical principles that guide informed decision making and reinforce sound employment policies on the part of governments, employers, and nurses, thereby supporting fair and cost-effective recruitment and retention practices.

In addition, the ICN adopted a second position paper on ethical nurse recruitment in 2001 that was also revised and reaffirmed in 2007 (ICN, 2007b). This document identifies 13 principles (see Box 6.2) necessary to create a foundation for ethical recruitment, whether international or intranational contexts are being considered. The ICN suggests that all health sector stakeholders—patients, governments, employers, and nurses—will benefit if this ethical recruitment framework is systematically applied.

---

### BOX 6.2   ICN PRINCIPLES OF ETHICAL NURSE RECRUITMENT

1. Effective planning and development strategies must be introduced, regularly reviewed, and maintained to ensure a balance between supply and demand of nurse human resources.

2. Nursing legislation must authorize regulatory bodies to determine nurses' standards of education, competencies, and standards of practice and to ensure that only individuals meeting these standards are allowed to practice as a nurse.

3. Because the provision of quality care relies on the availability of nurses to meet staffing demand, nurses in a recruiting region/country and seeking employment should be made aware of job opportunities.

4. Nurses should have the right to migrate if they comply with the recruiting country's immigration/work policies (e.g., work permit) and meet obligations in their home country (e.g., bonding responsibilities, tax payment).

5. Nurses have the right to expect fair treatment (e.g., working conditions, promotion, and continuing education).

6. Nurses and employers are to be protected from false information, withholding of relevant information, misleading claims, and exploitation (e.g., accurate job descriptions, benefits/allocations/bonuses specified in writing, authentic educational records).

7. There should be no discrimination between occupations/professions with the same level of responsibility, educational qualification, work experience, skill requirement, and hardship (e.g., pay, grading).

8. When nurses' or employers' contracted or acquired rights or benefits are threatened or violated, suitable machinery must be in place to hear grievances in a timely manner and at reasonable cost.

9. Nurses must be protected from occupational injury and health hazards, including violence (e.g., sexual harassment) and made aware of existing workplace hazards.

10. The provision of quality care in the highly complex and often stressful health care environment depends on a supportive formal and informal supervisory infrastructure.

11. Employment contracts must specify a trial period when the signing parties are free to express dissatisfaction and cancel the contract with no penalty. In the case of international migration, the responsibility for covering the cost of repatriation needs to be clearly stated.

12. Nurses have the right to affiliate to and be represented by a professional association and/or union to safeguard their rights as health professionals and workers.

13. Recruitment agencies (public and private) should be regulated, and effective monitoring mechanisms, such as cost-effectiveness, volume, success rate over time, retention rates, equalities criteria, and client satisfaction, should be introduced.

*Source:* Adapted from International Council of Nurses. (2007b). *Position statement: Ethical nurse recruitment.* Retrieved June 24, 2011, from http://www.icn.ch/images/stories/documents/publications/position_statements/C03_Ethical_Nurse_Recruitment.pdf

## The International Centre on Nurse Migration

Another organization, the International Centre on Nurse Migration (ICNM), established in 2005, represents a collaborative project launched by the ICN and the Commission on Graduates of Foreign Nursing Schools (CGFNS). The ICNM serves as a global resource for the development, promotion, and dissemination of research, policy, and information on global nurse migration (ICNM, 2010, para. 1). The ICNM website was redesigned in 2009 and now includes commissioned papers on nurse migration, fact sheets, and e-newsletters. In addition, there are more than 200 titles with links for global nurse migration research, which will be searchable in the near future (ICNM, 2009).

## The Academy Health Project: Achieving Consensus on Ethical Standards of Practice for International Nurse Recruitment

AcademyHealth, a professional society of 4,000 individuals and 125 affiliated organizations throughout the United States and abroad, has also taken an active role in working to assure the ethical recruitment of international nurses (AcademyHealth, 2008). Funded through a grant from the John D. and Catherine T. MacArthur Foundation in collaboration with the O'Neill Institute for National and Global Health Law at Georgetown University, AcademyHealth convened a task force of recruiters, hospitals, and foreign-educated nurses to develop draft standards of practice about global nurse recruitment, as well as recommendations on how to institutionalize these standards. In late 2007, Academy-Health released a report on year 1 of its 2-year project—the International Recruitment of Nurses to the United States: Toward a Consensus on Ethical Standards of Practice (Pittman, Folson, Bass, & Leonhardy, 2007).

In September 2008, AcademyHealth celebrated the formal release of its new Voluntary Code of Ethical Conduct for the Recruitment of Foreign Educated Nurses to the United States. The code is designed to increase transparency and accountability throughout the process of international recruitment and ensure adequate orientation for foreign-educated nurses. It also provides guidance on ways to ensure recruitment is not harmful to source countries. This document was endorsed by the National Council of State Boards of Nursing (NCSBN) in 2008 (NCSBN, 2011a).

## The World Health Organization

Another international organization involved in establishing guidelines for nurse migration is the World Health Organization (WHO). In an effort to balance the right of workers to migrate with a need to assure that global health care needs are met, the WHO launched the Health Worker Migration Policy Initiative in 2007. The initiative brings together professional organizations and other groups to create a code, which emphasizes the positive benefits of health worker migration and minimizes its negative impacts, and to spread the benefits of health worker migration more equitably among developed and developing nations.

The code, as called for by a resolution of the World Health Assembly in 2004, promotes ethical recruitment, protects migrant health workers' rights, and encourages governments in both developed and developing nations to actively address the push and pull factors that promote nurse migration (WHO, 2007). The Code of Practice was the first of its kind on a global scale for migration. In 2011, the Sixty-Third World Health Assembly unanimously passed a resolution to adopt the Code of Practice, acknowledging the global dimension and complexities of the health workforce crisis and the interconnected nature of both the problems and the solutions (Task Force on Migration-Health Worker Migration Policy Initiative, 2011).

In addition, the 2004 WHO Resolution 57.19 urged member states to mitigate the adverse effects of health care worker migration by forming country and regional agreements such as the South Africa/United Kingdom Memorandum of Understanding, the Pacific Code, and the Caribbean Community agreement.

## THE MISTREATMENT OF FOREIGN NURSES

Despite the costs and investment of time and energy that goes into recruiting foreign nurses, some health care organizations treat imported nurses poorly once they arrive. Jose (2011) noted that many migrant nurses reported a difficult journey and a shocking reality upon beginning their employment in another country. In addition, migrant nurses may receive substandard jobs or wages or be subjected to illegal practices by their employers.

For example, Schumacher (2011), using regression analyses, reported that noncitizen (Canadian nurses are an exception) working in U.S. health care agencies earn about 4.5% less than their American counterparts. The wage disadvantage primarily occurs with foreign-born nurses new to the United States. Once a nurse has been in this country for 6 years, the penalty appears to go away (Schumacher, 2011).

In addition, some recruiting firms charge foreign nurses an upfront fee, a practice that has been found illegal in connection with the recruitment of temporary farm workers in the United States and that is prohibited in the U.K. Code of Practice for the International Recruitment of Health Care Professionals. In addition, most recruiters charge migrant nurses a "buyout" or breach fee of up to US$50,000 for resigning before the end of their employment contract.

There are also reports that overzealous recruiters have made false promises to foreign nurses regarding job opportunities and wages and virtually forced the newly migrated RNs to work long hours in substandard working conditions. Part of the reason for this is that private for-profit agencies have increasingly become involved in the search for nursing personnel, and there is generally no designated body that regulates or monitors the content of contracts offered. Internationally recruited nurses may be particularly at risk of exploitation or abuse due to the difficulty of verifying the terms of employment as a result of distance, language barriers, cost, and naiveté.

Indeed, a 1-year study by AcademyHealth suggested that international nurses experience a number of questionable hiring or employment practices, primarily with regard to employment in nursing homes. These are shown in Box 6.3. The study concluded that although it is likely that "only a small group of recruiters and nursing homes engage in abusive practices, the very existence of such practices is indicative of oversight problems" (Pittman et al., 2007, p. 27).

> CONSIDER THIS   Due to the lack of regulatory oversight of global nurse migration contracting, foreign nurses are at increased risk for employment under false pretenses and may be misled as to the conditions of work, remuneration, and benefits.

Pittman et al. (2007) suggested that placement agencies also add to the corruption, in that they often charge health care organizations a standard fee of US$15,000 to US$25,000, depending on the state and the nurse's experience, to bring in a foreign nurse. Staffing agencies,

---

## BOX 6.3   QUESTIONABLE PRACTICES REPORTED BY INTERNATIONAL NURSES

- Denying nurses the right to obtain a copy of the contract at the time of signing
- Altering contracts both before nurses' departure from their home country and on arrival in the sponsor country without their consent
- Imposing excessive demands to work overtime, in some cases with no differential pay, combined with threats that nurses will be reported to immigration authorities if they refuse to comply
- Retention of green cards by employers, delays in processing social security numbers and RN permits, and payment of nurses at lower rates until documentation is complete
- Delaying payments and paying for fewer hours than actually worked
- Paying wages below direct-hire counterparts and in some cases other per-diem nurses
- Providing substandard housing
- Offering insufficient clinical orientation
- Requiring excessively high breach fees and refusing to allow nurses to pay buy-outs in installments

*Source:* Pittman, P., Folsom, A., Bass, E., & Leonhardy, K. (2007, November). U.S. based international nurse recruitment: Structure and processes of a burgeoning industry (Report on year I of the Project International Recruitment of Nurses to the United States: Toward a consensus on ethical standards of practice). Retrieved April 28, 2012, from http://www.intlnursemigration.org/assets/pdfs/Report-on-Year-I.pdf

which also provide foreign nurses, are typically paid on an hourly basis for the nurses they provide, and this rate may be four times greater than the average RN hourly wage in an effort to recover their investment costs (Pittman et al., 2007).

---

### DISCUSSION POINT

Should there be greater regulatory oversight of foreign nurse recruitment? If so, who should be charged with this responsibility?

---

## THE INTERNATIONAL COMMUNITY ADDRESSES THE PROBLEM

The nursing shortage and resulting global migration issues have led several national governments to intervene, and, as a result, some countries have made progress in tackling the ethical issues associated with global recruitment and migration of nurses.

### Some Governments Respond

Within the last few years, many countries, including the United States, have published national nursing strategies for dealing with staff shortages. Norway has issued a policy statement on the ethics of international recruitment. The Netherlands, Ireland, and the Scandinavian countries also have good-practice guidelines on international recruitment or are looking at developing guidelines. The United Kingdom went even further when in August 2006 it began limiting nurse recruitment to the European Union (EU) countries and only granting work permits to nurses from non-EU countries if National Health Services institutions showed that jobs could not be filled by U.K. or EU applications (Depausil, as cited in Brush, 2008).

Other countries have initiated or examined various policy responses to reduce outflow, such as requiring nurses to work in their home countries for a certain amount of time after education completion or by charging the nurse a fee to migrate to another country. For example, the Nurses Association of Jamaica has demanded that the Jamaican government raise salaries in an effort to get nurses to stay (Brush, 2008).

Another response has been to recognize that outflow cannot be halted if principles of individual freedom are to be upheld, but that the outflow that does occur must be managed and moderated. The "managed migration" initiative being undertaken in the Caribbean, which has provided regional support for addressing the nursing shortage crisis and developed initiatives such as training for export and temporary migration, is one example of a coordinated intervention to minimize the negative effects of outflow while realizing at least some benefit from the process (Salmon, Yan, Hewitt, & Guisinger, 2007).

### U.S. Immigration Policy

Currently, foreign nurses who want to work in the United States must have a valid job offer from an employer, and the employer must obtain Department of Labor approval for that hire. In addition, the employer must file a special petition with the U.S. Citizenship and Immigration Services.

In addition, like most national governments, the U.S. government continues to play a pivotal role in the nurse migration issue by virtue of its ability to issue travel visas. The reality is that a finite number of visas are available and caps exist on how many green cards are issued. Clearly, commercial recruiters and employers would like to see fewer restrictions on nurse migration, but labor certification laws and rules regarding the issuance of visas are complex and ever changing.

Labor certification laws in the United States state that under normal circumstances, the Department of Labor is required by law to certify to the Department of State and the Immigration and Naturalization Service (INS) when a foreigner is hired that (1) no U.S. citizens and permanent residents are available or qualified for a given job and (2) the employment of a foreigner will not adversely affect the wages of the concerned profession (LawBrain, 2010). The main purpose of this legal provision has been to protect the domestic labor market; however, the immigration laws have provided preferential provisions for members of certain professions in the national interest of the United States, and, as a result, the government has created a list of occupations and professions, including nursing, that do not require labor certification. Because nursing has been classified as one of the shortage areas in the U.S. economy, a so-called *blanket waiver* of the labor certification is in place.

In addition, from 1962 to 1989, foreign nurses were regarded as "professionals" under U.S. immigration laws and could therefore seek an H-1 temporary work visa in the United States. In 1989, the Immigration Nursing Relief Act (INRA) created a 5-year pilot program. The INRA stipulated that only health care facilities with "attestations" approved by the Department of Health could obtain H-1A occupation visas to employ nurses on a temporary basis. Consequently, other occupations that formerly fell into the H-1 category became part of the new H-1B category. In addition, in 1990, Congress passed the Immigration and Nationality Act, which is the legal foundation for current immigration policies. In this act, nursing continued to be listed as a shortage area.

In 1999, the Nursing Relief for Disadvantaged Areas Act created H-1C occupational visas, which were perceived largely as an effort to renew the INRA of 1989 but with more restrictions. These temporary visas were created for foreign nurse graduates seeking employment in designated U.S. facilities (serving primarily poor patients in inner cities and some rural areas). This visa classification expired in 2005.

Currently, there are no specific nurse visas available in the United States; however, most foreign nurses apply to work under the H-1B visa for skilled workers (open to individuals from countries other than Canada or Mexico) or the TN North American Free-Trade Agreement (NAFTA) work visa (available only to Canadian and Mexican citizens; U.S. Immigration Support, 2011). The H-1B is a nonimmigrant visa which allows recruiting of shortage professionals into jobs that require theoretical and practical application of a body of highly specialized knowledge requiring completion of a specific course of higher education (at least a bachelor's degree). Of particular interest is the fact that many RNs do not qualify for the H-1B visa: A Fifth Circuit Court ruling in February 2000 stated that RN hospital jobs do not currently require a bachelor's degree in nursing, regardless of recruiter requirements. Some nurses can still apply for the H-1B status, however, if they have a specialized skill, particularly in intensive care, management, and specialty nursing areas or if U.S. employers can convince immigration officials that specific jobs do meet the H-1B requirement on a case-by-case basis. H-1B visas are issued for up to 3 years but can be extended up to 6 years although some exceptions to apply (U.S. Citizenship and Immigration Requirements, 2011). The H-1B visa has an annual numerical limit "cap" of 65,000 visas each fiscal year. The first 20,000 petitions filed on behalf of beneficiaries with a U.S. master's degree or higher are exempt from the cap (U.S. Citizenship and Immigration Requirements, 2011).

Still other foreign nurses have sought employment in the United States in accordance with the NAFTA, enacted in December 1993. NAFTA established a reciprocal trading relationship between the United States, Canada, and Mexico and allowed for a nonimmigrant class of admission exclusively for business and service trade individuals entering the United States.

To complicate the matter further, on July 26, 2003, the U.S. Bureau of Citizenship and Immigration Services ruled that foreign-educated health care professionals, including nurses who are seeking temporary or permanent occupational visas, as well as those who are seeking NAFTA status, must successfully complete a screening program before receiving an occupational visa or permanent (green card) visa. This screening, completed by the CGFNS, includes an assessment of an applicant's education to ensure that it is comparable to that of a nursing graduate in the United States, verification that licenses are valid and unencumbered, successful completion of an English-language proficiency examination, and verification that the nurse has either earned certification by the CGFNS or passed the National Council Licensure Examination for Registered Nurses (NCLEX-RN).

Another way nurses get work visas in the United States has been under the immigrant E3 to I-140 status ("green card" or Alien Registration Receipt Card). Green cards are not just work permits; green card holders are required to make the United States their permanent homes and if they do not, they risk losing the card (CGFNS, 2011c). Migrant RNs enter into the United States and become permanent residents through petition to the INS. A problem with this visa status is that it does not require labor certification, so the Department of Labor does not have to certify that the wage offered to the nurse is the prevailing wage. However, the law does state that foreign nurses entering under I-140 cannot have a negative effect on domestic wages.

## ENSURING COMPETENCY OF FOREIGN NURSES COMMISSION ON GRADUATES OF FOREIGN NURSING SCHOOLS AND THE NCLEX-RN EXAMINATION

Nursing is one of the most highly regulated health professions in the United States, and a license is required to practice in all 50 states and U.S. territories. Before 1977, endorsement and taking the State Board Test Pool Examination (SBTPE) were the two ways for foreign nurses to obtain a license. The SBTPE tested the foreign graduate's English-language proficiency and knowledge of U.S. nursing practice, but, alarmingly, only a small percentage (15% to 20%) of foreign RNs typically passed the NCLEX-RN.

---

### DISCUSSION POINT

Does the increased importation of foreign nurses directly or indirectly affect the prevailing wages of domestic RNs?

As a result of this high failure rate and a concern for patient safety, the ANA and the NLN, with collaboration from the Department of Labor and the INS, established CGFNS in 1977 as an independent, nonprofit organization. The mission of CGFNS is "to protect the public by ensuring that nurses and other health care professionals educated in countries other than the United States are eligible and qualified to meet licensure, immigration, and other practice requirements in the United States" (CGFNS, 2011a, para. 4).

The strategies CGFNS uses to accomplish this mission are to evaluate and test foreign graduates via a certification program before they leave their home countries to ensure that there is a reasonable chance for them to pass the NCLEX-RN needed for licensure in the United States. Through a contract with the NLN, which designed the NCLEX-RN, a CGFNS-qualifying examination was developed. The examination consists of two parts to test the applicant's knowledge of nursing and the English language (both written and oral).

To be eligible to take the examination, RNs must have completed sufficient classroom instruction and clinical practice in adult health/medical surgical nursing; maternal/infant (obstetrics) nursing, excluding gynecology; nursing care of children; and psychiatric/mental health nursing, excluding neurology (CGFNS, 2011d). They must also hold an initial as well as current license/registration as a first-level general nurse in their country of education.

In addition, a credentials review of secondary and nursing education, registration, and licensure is required to earn the CGFNS certificate. Earning CGFNS certification meets one of the immigration requirements for securing an occupational visa to work in the United States and helps to meet licensure and NCLEX eligibility requirements in many states (CGFNS, 2011d). Today, the CGFNS qualifying examination is offered in 469 locations around the world (CGFNS, 2011b).

The CGFNS examination, however, should not be mistaken as substitute for the state board licensing examination. Indeed, most states in the United States require foreign nurses to pass the CGFNS certification before they are allowed to take the NCLEX-RN. Just over 9,700 internationally educated nurses took the NCLEX-RN in 2011 with a first-time pass rate of 33.98% (NCSBN, 2012). The exam specifications and passing standards are the same for foreign nurses as they are for students taking the NCLEX in the United States.

The NCSBN has also taken steps to make it easier for foreign RNs to take the NCLEX-RN. Until 2005, the NCLEX-RN was offered only in the United States and its territories. In fact, before 2005, the only option foreign nurses had was to earn the CGFNS certificate, secure a job offer from a U.S. employer, and take the NCLEX-RN

only after they arrived in the United States with their green cards). Now the exam is offered in 11 countries and nonmember board territories including Australia, Canada, England, Germany (temporarily not testing at this location), Hong Kong, India, Japan, Mexico, Philippines, Puerto Rico, and Taiwan (NCSBN, 2011b). These locations were selected based on national security, examination security, and similarity with U.S. Intellectual Property and Copyright Laws.

## ASSIMILATING THE FOREIGN NURSE THROUGH SOCIALIZATION

The ethical obligation to the foreign nurse does not end with his or her arrival in a new country. Woodbridge and Bland (2010) note that travelling to a new country and being viewed as an immigrant is a stressful experience. So too is the move from one cultural context to another. Many migrant nurses are afraid to express dissatisfaction or to ask for help for fear they will no longer have a job or because they fear being sent home. In addition, many of the families left behind in donor countries count on the migrant RN sending money home to improve their living standard. All of these factors place migrated nurses at increased risk for abuse and failure to assimilate. As a result, sponsoring countries must do whatever they can to see that migrant nurses are assimilated into new work environments, as well as new cultures, a process that may take up to 10 years (Habermann & Stagge, 2010).

The importance of appropriate professional and cultural socialization for foreign nurses cannot be overestimated. Aboderin (2007), in an exploratory qualitative investigation, found that Nigerian nurses who had migrated to the United Kingdom in an effort to improve their economic status actually experienced a loss of professional and social status in their host country. This is because the Nigerian nurses come from a national perspective by which "nurses belong not to the poor 'masses' but to a relatively privileged population segment—by virtue of their position as educated professionals. This privilege (as well as their specific choice of profession), makes their global migration possible" (Aboderin, 2007, p. 2244). However, Nigerian nurses who migrate often experience values conflicts in terms of what constitutes a good life: to live well (in due material comfort), among one's people "at home." This supports the idea of a decidedly "local" normative perspective and suggests that country-specific strategies are needed to improve the employment satisfaction and retention of foreign nurses.

Similarly, Deegan and Simkin (2010) reported that migrant nurses in Australia experienced feelings of disempowerment caused by discriminatory practices, professional isolation, and the unrealistic expectations of local nurses. Language and quality of communication also contributed to socialization difficulties. Deegan and Simkin concluded that the migration experience challenged feelings of competence as much as it expanded feelings of competence and the end result for these migrant nurses was often stunted progress toward regaining a full professional identity.

This research supports Xu's (2010) contention that there are typically four broad categories of transitional challenges faced by international nurses who migrate (see Box 6.4). The first is language and communication challenges. Not only do most foreign nurse migrants have an inadequacy of language preparation but they are also unfamiliar with accent, slang, and other language nuances. As a result, they find it difficult to relate to patients, families, and other health care team members, to speak up for themselves, and to advocate for their patients.

The second challenge identified by Xu is the variance in nursing practice across different countries. These include role and expectations of the nurse, scope of practice, legal environment, accountability, professional autonomy, health care technology, and relationships between nurses and physicians.

The third challenge is marginalization, discrimination, and racism. Many migrant nurses experience unfair treatment (such as higher patient loads than others or being passed over for promotions) and racism which results in stereotyping and rejection by patients and peers. In addition, the risk of being bullied is higher in this population.

Finally, the fourth challenge is cultural displacement and adjustment. Cultural uprooting can lead to perceptions of not belonging. In addition, Xu suggests that cultural adjustment often results in communication barriers as well as interpersonal conflicts based on differences in culture-based values, norms, and expectation. Nichols and Campbell (2010) reported similar findings in their study of migrant nurses in the United Kingdom, stating that significant numbers of nurses described not feeling personally or professionally valued by their work peers, resulting in disappointment and unmet expectations.

Xu (2010) suggests that "given the documented transitional challenges facing international nurses and the initial evidence of associated real and potential risks to patient safety and quality of care, transition of international nurses should be regarded as a regulatory requirement" (p. 210). Xu also suggests that such transition programs will likely be required by regulatory agencies in the foreseeable future in the United States as well as the United Kingdom and Australia and that these programs must be qualitatively different from those designed for domestic nurse hires to address the unique transitional needs of foreign migrant nurses.

Tregunno, Peters, Campbell, and Gordon (2009) echo Xu's concerns in their assertion that greater efforts are needed to both understand and address the barriers and challenges internationally educated nurses experience in transitioning into the workforce after having achieved initial registration in their adopted country. Their research suggests that the expectations of professional nursing practice and the role of patients and families in decision making is very different for most migrant nurses between their country of origin and their destination countries. In addition, English-language difficulties often cause work-related stress and cognitive fatigue (see Research Study Fuels the Controversy).

> CONSIDER THIS Recruiting internationally may be a quick-fix solution, but it is far from clear that it is always a cost-effective solution.

---

**BOX 6.4 BROAD CATEGORIES OF TRANSITIONAL CHALLENGES FACING INTERNATIONAL NURSE MIGRANTS**

1. Language and communication
2. Differences in nursing practice
3. Marginalization, discrimination, and racism
4. Cultural displacement and adjustment

*Source:* Xu, Y. (2010). Transitioning international nurses: An outlined evidence-based program for acute care settings. *Policy Politics & Nursing Practice, 11*(3), 202–213.

## RESEARCH STUDY FUELS THE CONTROVERSY

### WHY DO NURSES EMIGRATE?

This empirically grounded study of internationally educated nurses who entered Ontario's workforce between 2003 and 2005 examined the challenges migrant nurses faced as they sought licensure and access to international work.

Internationally educated nurses represented 11.5% of Ontario nurses in 2005 and 34% of the new supply of RNs. Thirty nurses from 20 countries and three health care sectors participated in the study.

*Source*: Tregunno, D., Peters, S., Campbell, H., & Gordon, S. (2009). International nurse migration: U-turn for safe workplace transition. *Nursing Inquiry, 16*(3), 182–190.

### STUDY FINDINGS

The study found that migrant nurses unanimously described nursing as "different" in Canada from their country of origin. Three of the themes (i.e., standards of care, language, and being an outsider) were consistent with previous studies exploring the lived experiences of migrant nurses. Specifically, differences were reported in the expectations of professional nursing practice and the role of patients and families in decision making. In addition, problems with English-language fluency cause work-related stress and cognitive fatigue. Finally, the experience of being an outsider was a reality with many of these nurses reporting racism, aggression, and resentment from their coworkers. The researchers concluded that policy and management decision makers must address and balance the need to ensure there is an adequate supply of safe, competent nurses ready to practice upon registration, whether they are domestically or internationally educated and the delivery of safe patient care.

## CONCLUSIONS

Nurse migration and its associated ethical dilemmas are among the most serious issues facing the nursing profession, and there is little sign that the issue will abate anytime soon. Clearly, developed countries have an advantage in terms of pull factors to recruit migrant nurses from less developed countries, and less developed countries are the ones most likely to suffer the devastating effects of brain drain. One must ask, however, whether this quick-fix solution to the nursing shortage has become too commonplace and too easy. Does it keep recruiter countries from dealing with the issues that led to their shortage in the first place? Does it negatively affect prevailing domestic wages and artificially alter what should be normal supply/demand curves in the health care marketplace? Of even greater concern is the lack of regulatory oversight of contracting with foreign nurses, placing them at risk for unethical, if not illegal, employment practices in their host country.

Some countries and professional nursing organizations are beginning to address these issues. So too are national governments and regulatory agencies in an effort to protect both the migrant nurses and the public those nurses will serve. Yet in the meantime, what may be hundreds of thousands of nurses are migrating internationally, and the potentially negative effects of this increasing trend on both the migrant nurse and the donor nation are becoming ever more apparent. Chopra, Munro, and Lavis (2008) suggested that despite pronounced international concern, little research and few solutions exist regarding the problem. Brush (2008) agreed, suggesting that "despite ongoing debate about how best to manage nurses' international mobility, nurse migration remains relatively unchecked, uncoordinated, and individualized, such that some countries suffer from its effects while others benefit" (p. 23).

## FOR ADDITIONAL DISCUSSION

**1.** Are the requirements for foreign nurses to get visas in the United States adequate?

**2.** Does achieving CGFNS certification and passing the NCLEX-RN examination in the United States assure competency of the foreign nurse graduate?

**3.** As long as international nurse recruitment is a viable option, will the problems that led to a nursing shortage in the first place be addressed?

**4.** Should donor countries develop nurse migration policy efforts that limit human resource exports?

**5.** How can government and professional nursing organizations work together to ensure that recruitment practices of foreign nurses are both ethical and appropriate?

**6.** How does the ethical principle of veracity (truth telling) apply to the zealous recruiting efforts seen, particularly in developing countries?

**7.** Is government regulatory oversight of foreign nurse recruitment efforts in conflict with America's value of capitalistic, free enterprise?

## REFERENCES

Aboderin, I. (2007). Contexts, motives and experiences of Nigerian overseas nurses: Understanding links to globalization. *Journal of Clinical Nursing, 16*(12), 2237–2245.

AcademyHealth. (2008). *About us.* Retrieved June 25, 2008, from http://www.academyhealth.org/about/index.htm

Bhalla, J. S., & Meher, M. A. (2010, March 3). Nursing a foreign dream. *Hindustan Times.* Retrieved April 27, 2012, from http://www.hindustantimes.com/India-news/NewDelhi/Nursing-a-foreign-dream/Article1-514546.aspx

Barnett, T., Namasivayam, P., & Narudin, D. A. A. (2010). A critical review of the nursing shortage in Malaysia. *International Nursing Review, 57,* 32–39.

Brush, B. L. (2008). Global nurse migration today. *Journal of Nursing Scholarship, 40*(1), 20–25.

Brush, B. (2010). The potent lever of toil: Nursing development and exportation in the postcolonial Philippines. *American Journal of Public Health, 100*(9), 1572–1581.

Buchan, J. (2006). The impact of global nursing migration on health services delivery. *Policy, Politics, & Nursing Practice (Supplement), 7*(3), 16S–25S.

Chopra, M., Munro, S., & Lavis, J. N. (2008). Effects of policy options for human resources for health: An analysis of systematic reviews. *Lancet, 371*(9613), 668–674.

Clemens, M., & Pettersson, G. (2008). New data on African health professionals abroad. *Human Resources for Health, 6,* 1. Retrieved April 27, 2012, from http://www.human-resources-health.com/content/6/1/1

Commission on Graduates of Foreign Nursing Schools. (2011a). *About us.* Retrieved June 27, 2011, from http://www.cgfns.org/sections/about/

Commission on Graduates of Foreign Nursing Schools. (2011b). *CGFNS certification program.* Retrieved June 28, 2011, from http://www.cgfns.org/sections/programs/cp/

Commission on Graduates of Foreign Nursing Schools. (2011c). *Immigration and visa questions.* Retrieved June 27, 2011, from http://www.cgfns.org/sections/tools/faq/imm.shtml

Commission on Graduates of Foreign Nursing Schools. (2011d). *The certification program.* Retrieved June 27, 2011, from http://www.cgfns.org/sections/programs/cp/default.shtml

CSR Europe. (2008). *Alleviating brain drain.* Retrieved June 25, 2008, from http://www.csreurope.org/solutions.php?action=show_solution&solution_id=512

Deegan, J., & Simkin, K. (2010). Expert to novice: Experiences of professional adaptation reported by non-English speaking nurses in Australia. *Australian Journal of Advanced Nursing, 27*(3), 31–37.

Donkor, N. T., & Andrews, L. D. (2011). 21st century nursing practice in Ghana: Challenges and opportunities. *International Nursing Review, 58*(2), 218–224.

Ehrenfeld, M., Itzhaki, S., & Michal, B. (2007). Nursing in Israel. *Nursing Science Quarterly, 20*(4), 372–375.

El-Jardali, F., Nuhad, M., Diana, J., & Mouro, G. (2008). Migration of Lebanese nurses: A questionnaire survey and secondary data analysis. *International Journal of Nursing Studies, 45*(10), 1490–1500. Retrieved April 27, 2012, from http://www.ncbi.nlm.nih.gov/pubmed/18242613

Fang, Z. Z. (2007). Potential of China in global nurse migration. *Health Services Research, 42*(3, Pt. 2), 1419–1428.

Federation for American Immigration Reform. (n.d.). *Brain drain.* Retrieved June 25, 2008, from http://www.fairus.org/site/pageserver?pagename=iic_immigrationis suecenterse514

Gamolo, N. O. (2008). RP nurses seen as prime export commodity. *The Manila Times.* Retrieved April 27, 2012, from http://philnurse.com/?p=10

Gostin, L. (2008). The international migration and recruitment of nurses: Human rights and global justice. *Journal of the American Medical Association, 299*(15), 1827–1829.

Habermann, M., & Stagge, M. (2010). Nurse migration: A challenge for the profession and health-care systems. *Journal of Public Health, 18*(1), 43–51.

Humphries, N., Brugha, R., & McGee, H. (2008). *Overseas nurse recruitment: Ireland as an illustration of the dynamic nature of nurse migration.* Retrieved June 25, 2008, from http://epubs.rcsi.ie/ephmart/1/

International Centre on Nurse Migration. (2010). Retrieved June 23, 2011, from http://www.icn.ch/projects/international-centre-on-nurse-migration/

International Centre on Nurse Migration. (2009). *International Centre on Nurse Migration launches redesigned website.* Retrieved June 24, 2011, from http://www.cgfns.org/files/pdf/docs/ICNM_news_release.pdf

International Council of Nursing. (2007a). *Position statement: Nurse retention and migration.* Retrieved June 25, 2011, from http://www.icn.ch/images/stories/documents/publications/position_statements/C06_Nurse_Retention_Migration.pdf

International Council of Nurses. (2007b). *Position statement: Ethical nurse recruitment.* Retrieved April 27, 2012, from http://www.icn.ch/images/stories/documents/publications/position_statements/C03_Ethical_Nurse_Recruitment.pdf

International Council of Nurses. (2011). *About ICN.* Retrieved June 23, 2011, from http://www.icn.ch/about-icn/about-icn

IOL. (2011).*Nursing shortage to ease if colleges reopen.* Retrieved April 28, 2012, from http://www.iol.co.za/business/business-news/nursing-shortage-to-ease-if-colleges-reopen-1.1038914

James, E. (2008). *Global brain drain. Advance perspective: Nurses.* Retrieved April 27, 2012, from http://community.advanceweb.com/blogs/nurses3/archive/2008/04/10/global-brain-drain.aspx

Jose, M. (2011). Lived experiences of internationally educated nurses in hospitals in the United States of America. *International Nursing Review, 58*(1), 123–129.

Kaelin, L. (2011). A question of justice: Assessing nurse migration from a philosophical perspective. *Developing World Bioethics, 11*(1), 30–39.

Kingma, M. (2007). Nurses on the move: A global overview. *Health Services Research, 42*(3, Pt. 2), 1281–1298.

Kuehn, B. M. (2007). Global shortage of health workers, brain drain stress developing countries. *Journal of the American Medical Association, 298*(16), 1853–1855.

LawBrain. (2010, July 13). *Immigration.* Retrieved June 28, 2011, from http://lawbrain.com/wiki/Immigration

Little, L. (2007). Nurse migration: A Canadian case study. *Health Services Research, 42*(3, Pt. 2), 1336–1353.

Lorenzo, F. M. E., Galvez-Tan, J., Icamina, K., & Javier, L. (2007). Nurse migration from a source country perspective: Philippine country case study. *Health Services Research, 42*(3, Pt. 2), 1406–1418.

Milton, C. (2007). The ethics of nurse migration: An evolution of community change. *Nursing Science Quarterly, 20*(4), 319–322.

National Council of State Boards of Nursing. (2011a). *NCSBN partners with group to help prevent unethical recruitment of foreign-educated nurses.* Retrieved June 27, 2011, from https://www.ncsbn.org/1457.htm

National Council of State Boards of Nursing. (2011b). *NCLEX international frequently asked questions.* Retrieved June 27, 2011, from https://www.ncsbn.org/2362.htm#Where_are_the_international_testing_centers_also_known_as_non-member_board_jurisdictions_that_can_administer_the_NCLEX

National Council of State Boards of Nursing. (2012). *Number of candidates taking NCLEX examination and percent passing, by type of candidate.* Retrieved April 27, 2012, from https://www.ncsbn.org/Table_of_Pass_Rates_2011.pdf

Nichols, J., & Campbell, J. (2010). The experiences of internationally recruited nurses in the UK (1995–2007): An integrative review. *Journal of Clinical Nursing, 19*(19/20), 2814–2823.

Office of the United Nations High Commissioner for Human Rights. (1976). *International Covenant on Civil and Political Rights.* Retrieved January 5, 2009, from http://www.unhchr.ch/html/menu3/b/a_ccpr.htm

Paterson, T. (2008). German brain drain at highest level since 1940s. *The New Editor*. Retrieved April 28, 2012, from http://www.theneweditor.com/index.php?/archives/6191-German-Brain-Drain-at-Highest-Level-Since-1940s.html

Pittman, P., Folsom, A., Bass, E., & Leonhardy, K. (2007). U.S. based international nurse recruitment: Structure and practices of a burgeoning industry (Report on year I of the Project International Recruitment of Nurses to the United States: Toward a consensus on ethical standards of practice). Retrieved April 28, 2012, from http://www.intlnursemigration.org/assets/pdfs/Report-on-Year-I.pdf

Questioning the ethics of nurse migration. (2010). *Kai Tiaki Nursing New Zealand, 16*(6), 7.

Salmon, M., Yan, J., Hewitt, H., & Guisinger, V. (2007). Managed migration: The Caribbean approach to addressing nursing services capacity. *Health Services Research, 42*(1), 1354–1372.

Schumacher, E. (2011). Foreign-born nurses in the US labor market. *Health Economics, 20*(3), 362–378.

Task Force on Migration-Health Worker Migration Policy Initiative. (2011). *WHO global code of practice on the international recruitment of health personnel*. Retrieved June 28, 2011, from http://www.who.int/workforcealliance/about/taskforces/migration/en/

Tregunno, D., Peters, S., Campbell, H., & Gordon, S. (2009). International nurse migration: U-turn for safe workplace transition. *Nursing Inquiry, 16*(3), 182–190.

United Nations General Assembly. (1948). *The Universal Declaration of Human Rights*. Retrieved April 28, 2012, from http://www.un.org/en/documents/udhr/

U.S. Citizenship and Immigration Requirements. (2011). *H-1B specialty occupations, DOD cooperative research and development project workers, and fashion models*. Retrieved June 27, 2011, from http://www.uscis.gov/portal/site/uscis/menuitem.eb1d4c2a3e5b9ac89243c6a7543f6d1a/?vgnextoid=73566811264a3210VgnVCM100000b92ca60aRCRD&vgnextchannel=73566811264a3210VgnVCM100000b92ca60aRCRD

U.S. Immigration Support. (2011). *Your online guide to US visas, green cards and citizenship*. Retrieved June 27, 2011, from https://www.usimmigrationsupport.org/nurse-work-visa.html

Woodbridge, M., & Bland, M. (2010). Supporting Indian nurses migrating to New Zealand: A literature review. *International Nursing Review, 57*(1), 40–48.

World Bank. (2011). *India receives world's largest remittance flows*. Retrieved June 21, 2011, from http://www.worldbank.org.in/WBSITE/EXTERNAL/COUNTRIES/SOUTHASIAEXT/INDIAEXTN/0,,contentMDK:20595174~pagePK:141137~piPK:141127~theSitePK:295584,00.html

World Bank. (2012). *Migration and remittances*. Retrieved April 26, 2012, from http://web.worldbank.org/WBSITE/EXTERNAL/NEWS/0,,contentMDK:20648762~pagePK:64257043~piPK:437376~theSitePK:4607,00.html

World Health Organization. (2007). *New initiative seeks practical solutions to tackle health worker migration*. Retrieved April 27, 2012, from http://www.who.int/mediacentre/news/notes/2007/np23/en/index.html

Xu, Y. (2010). Transitioning international nurses: An outlined evidence-based program for acute care settings. *Policy Politics & Nursing Practice, 11*(3), 202–213.

## BIBLIOGRAPHY

Bae, S. H. (2012). Organizational socialization of international nurses in the New York metropolitan area. *International Nursing Review, 59*(1), 81–87.

Bland, M., & Woolbridge, M. (2011). From India to New Zealand—A challenging but rewarding passage. *Kai Tiaki Nursing New Zealand, 17*(10), 21–23.

Lisa, B. (2012). Bridging the gaps. *Canadian Nurse, 108*(2), 5.

Callister, P., Badkar, J., & Didham, R. (2011). Globalisation, localisation and implications of a transforming nursing workforce in New Zealand: Opportunities and challenges. *Nursing Inquiry, 18*(3), 205–215.

Cho, S., Masselink, L. E., Jones, C. B., & Mark, B. A. (2011). Internationally educated nurse hiring: Geographic distribution, community, and hospital characteristics. *Nursing Economics, 29*(6), 308–316.

Cutcliffe, J. R., Bajkay, R., Forster, S., Small, R., & Travale, R. (2011). Nurse migration in an increasingly interconnected world: The case for Internationalization of Regulation of Nurses and Nursing Regulatory Bodies. *Archives of Psychiatric Nursing, 25*(5), 320–328.

Evans, M. M., & Tulaney, T. (2011). Professional issues. Nurse migration: What is its impact? *Medsurg Nursing, 20*(6), 333–336.

Freeman, M., Baumann, A., Blythe, J., Fisher, A., & Akhtar-Danesh, N. (2012). Migration: A concept analysis from a nursing perspective. *Journal of Advanced Nursing, 68*(5), 1176–1186.

Hendel, T., & Kagan, I. (2011). Professional image and intention to emigrate among Israeli nurses and nursing students. *Nurse Education Today, 31*(3), 259–262.

Mercier, C. (2012). The Quebec-France Agreement on the mutual recognition of professional qualifications. *Journal of Nursing Regulation, 2*(4), 53–57.

NMC says Asian nurses may need support with delegating work. (2012). *Nursing Standard, 26*(26), 5.

O'Brien, T., & Ackroyd, S. (2012). Understanding the recruitment and retention of overseas nurses: Realist case study research in National Health Service Hospitals in the UK. *Nursing Inquiry, 19*(1), 39–50.

Rowley, J. (2012). Have skills, will travel. *Nursing Standard, 26*(19), 61.

Shen, J. J., Covelli, M., Yu, X., Torpey, M., Bolstad, A. L., & Colosimo, R. (2012). Effects of a short-term linguistic class on communication competence of international nurses: Implications for practice, policy, and research. *Nursing Economics, 30*(1), 21–28.

Sidebotham, M., & Ahern, K. (2011). Finding a way: The experiences of UK educated midwives finding their place in the midwifery workforce in Australia. *Midwifery, 27*(3), 316–323.

Sidebotham, M. M., & Ahern, K. K. (2011). Factors influencing midwifery migration from the United Kingdom to Australia. *International Nursing Review, 58*(4), 498–504.

Slote, R. J. (2011). Pulling the plug on brain-drain: Understanding international migration of nurses. *Medsurg Nursing, 20*(4), 179–186.

Smith, C. D. A., Fisher, C., & Mercer, A. (2011). Rediscovering nursing: A study of overseas nurses working in Western Australia. *Nursing & Health Sciences, 13*(3), 289–295.

Thekdi, P., Wilson, B. L., & Wu, Y. (2011). Recruitment & Retention Report: Understanding post-hire transitional challenges of foreign-educated nurses. *Nursing Management, 42*(9), 8–14.

Vapor, V. R., & Xu, Y. (2011). Double whammy for a new breed of foreign-educated nurses: Lived experiences of Filipino physician-turned nurses in the United States. *Research & Theory for Nursing Practice, 25*(3), 210–226.

Xu, Y. (2011). A comparison of regulatory standards for initial registration/licensure internationally educated nurses of the United Kingdom, Australia, Canada, and the United States. *Journal of Nursing Regulation, 2*(3), 27–36.

Zhou, Y., Windsor, C., Theobald, K., & Coyer, F. (2011). The concept of difference and the experience of China-educated nurses working in Australia: A symbolic interactionist exploration. *International Journal of Nursing Studies, 48*(11), 1420–1428.

# Chapter 7

# Unlicensed Assistive Personnel and the Registered Nurse

Carol J. Huston

## ADDITIONAL RESOURCES

Visit thePoint for additional helpful resources

- eBook
- Journal Articles
- WebLinks

## CHAPTER OUTLINE

Motivation to Use UAP

Educational Requirements for UAP

UAP Scope of Practice

*Regulatory Oversight of UAP*

UAP and Patient Outcomes

Registered Nurse Liability for Supervision and Delegation of UAP

Registered Nurses Working as UAP: A Liability Issue

Creating a Safe Work Environment

The UAP Shortage

Conclusions

## LEARNING OBJECTIVES

*The learner will be able to:*

1. Identify driving forces leading to the increased use of unlicensed assistive personnel (UAP) in acute care settings beginning in the early 1990s.

2. Name common job titles for UAP.

3. Differentiate between the minimum mandated educational preparation of certified nurses aides (CNAs) and UAP.

4. Analyze current research that explores the effect of increased UAP use on costs and patient outcomes.

5. Discuss how the role of the registered nurse (RN) as delegator has changed with the increased use of UAP.

6. Examine how the role of delegator and supervisor of UAP increases the scope of liability for the RN.

7. Explore strategies for restructuring work environments and clarifying role expectations so that professional nurses spend less time on nonnursing tasks and UAP have role clarity.

8. Identify safeguards that health care organizations can put in place to increase the likelihood that UAP are used both effectively and appropriately as members of the health care team.

9. Outline current efforts seeking to regulate minimum UAP education and competencies.

10. Discuss factors contributing to both the current and projected shortages of UAP, particularly in long-term care settings.

11. Reflect on the self-confidence and skill that an RN might need to successfully delegate to a UAP.

12. Identify the sources of increased legal liability an RN and his or her employer face when health care institutions allow RNs to work beneath their scope of practice as UAP.

In an effort to contain spiraling health care costs, many health care providers in the 1990s restructured their organizations by eliminating registered nurse (RN) positions and/or by replacing licensed professional nurses with unlicensed assistive personnel (UAP). UAP are unlicensed individuals who provide low-risk, assistive care not requiring the judgment or training of a licensed professional, while working under the direct supervision of an RN. The term includes, but is not limited to, nurse aides, nurse extenders, health care aides, technicians, orderlies, assistants, and attendants. Although the term UAP will generally be used throughout this chapter, it is noteworthy that in 2007, the American Nurses Association (ANA) stopped using the term UAP and replaced it with *nursing assistive personnel* (NAP), suggesting that many NAP are now licensed or formally recognized in some manner.

Regardless of nomenclature, unlicensed workers are a significant part of the health care landscape and have been for some time. By the late 1990s, hospitals began actively recruiting the RNs who had been let go just a few years before. RNs who lost their jobs, however, were slow to return to the acute care setting, despite a widespread, worsening nursing shortage. As a result, hospitals again increased their use of UAP early in the 21st century in an effort to supplement their licensed nursing staff.

Both as a result of the restructuring of the 1990s and the current nursing shortage, the skill mix in some hospitals still includes a significant percentage of UAP. According to the U.S. Department of Labor, Bureau of Labor Statistics (2011b), 29% of UAP work in hospitals. In fact, almost all RNs in acute care institutions are involved in some way with the assignment, delegation, and supervision of UAP.

This is even truer in long-term care settings. Stone and Harahan (2010) note that direct care workers form the centerpiece of the formal long-term care system, providing 8 out of every 10 hours of paid care. As such, they have become the "eyes and the ears" of the long-term health care system (p. 110). Indeed, there were an estimated 2.3 million direct care workers—certified nursing aides, home health care aides, and home care/personal care workers providing long-term care to older adults in the United States in 2006 alone (Stone & Harrahan, 2010). This figure likely greatly underestimates the actual direct care worker population because it does not capture many workers hired privately by elderly consumers.

Corrazzini et al. (2010) concur, noting that UAP and licensed practical or vocational nurses (LPNs/LVNs) currently provide more than 90% of the direct care that nursing home residents receive (Corazzini et al., 2010). Randoph and Scott-Cawiezell (2011) also agree, suggesting that the dominant model of care in nursing homes today is CNAs performing under the supervision of licensed nurses (RNs and LVNs).

Several reasons are commonly cited for the increased use of UAP. The primary argument for using UAP instead of licensed personnel is usually cost savings, although the professional nursing shortage may be a contributing factor (Marquis & Huston, 2012). Another widely recognized benefit of using UAP is that they can free professional nurses from tasks and assignments (specifically, nonnursing functions) that can be completed by less well-trained personnel at a lower cost.

So why has the increased use of UAP created so much controversy? The answer is that in many institutions, UAP are not supplements to, but replacements of, professional RN staff. This is of concern because some empirical research exists regarding what percentage of the staffing mix can safely be represented by UAP without negatively affecting patient outcomes. In addition, minimum national educational and training requirements have not been established for UAP, and their scope of practice varies from institution to institution. All of these issues raise serious questions as to whether greater use of UAP represents an effective solution to dwindling health care resources or whether it is an economically driven, short-term response that could lead to compromised patient outcomes.

This chapter, however, does not argue for the elimination of UAP. Instead, it addresses what safeguards must be incorporated in the use of UAP so that safe, accessible, and affordable nursing care is possible.

## MOTIVATION TO USE UAP

UAP can maximize human resources because they free professional nurses from tasks and assignments that do not require independent thinking and professional judgment. This is significant because much of a typical nurse's time is spent on nonnursing tasks and functions. Nonnursing tasks and functions are those routine or standardized activities that can be done by an individual with minimal training and do not require a great deal of individual client assessment, independent thought, or decision making. Examples of nonnursing activities include making a bed, doing vital signs, feeding clients, measuring intakes and outputs, and obtaining a weight or height.

Just how much time is spent by nurses doing nonnursing activities is unclear. Research by Buerhaus, Donelan, Ulrich, DesRoches, and Dittus (2007) suggested that only 41% of the time in a typical RN workweek is spent on direct patient care. The remainder of the time was directed at engaging in patient care documentation (23%), locating supplies and equipment related to patient care (8%), transporting patients (5%), making patient-related telephone calls (8%), engaging in meetings or activities related to patient safety or quality improvement (7%), and engaging in shift changes or other hand-off functions (7%).

Domrose (2008) presented similarly disturbing findings in her study of 767 medical/surgical nurses in 36 hospitals across the country in 2005 and 2006. This study found that nurses spent less than 40% of their time in patient's rooms and that less than 20% of nursing time—about 1 hour and 20 minutes per shift—was spent on patient care activities. In addition, only 7% of time was spent on patient assessment and reading vital signs.

Hendrich, Chow, Skierczynski, and Zhenqiang (2008), in their study of 767 medical surgical nurses at 36 hospitals, found, however, that more than three quarters of the nurses' time was devoted to nursing practice each shift. Activities considered to be waste consumed only 6.6% of each 10-hour shift. Time devoted to nonclinical activities was approximately equivalent for nurse station (20.6 minutes), on the unit (17.8 minutes), and off the unit (18.2 minutes); nonclinical activities accounted for only 11.3 minutes of time spent in the patient room.

---

### DISCUSSION POINT

Why are professional RNs still completing so many nonnursing tasks? Are they reluctant to delegate them to ancillary personnel, or are there inadequate support personnel to take on these tasks?

---

Cost savings associated with UAP use—the second argument for increased UAP use—are less clear. Studies completed early in the 21st century showed conflicting findings with some suggesting significant cost savings with UAP and others suggesting no cost savings as a result of the costs of supervision, high UAP turnover rates, and medical errors. Because so many studies reported that UAP use failed to produce anticipated cost savings, some hospitals have resumed

reliance on RNs as the primary component of their staffing mix.

Mulrooney (2011) cautions though that there is no general consensus among health care professionals as to what constitutes safe staffing. Instead, she suggests it can be broadly defined as

> *having the appropriate number of staff with a suitable mix of skill levels available at all times to ensure that patient care needs are fulfilled and hazard-free working conditions are maintained. In addition, safe staffing optimally requires the absence of negative consequences and minimal errors consistent with benchmarked data.* (Mulrooney, 2011, para. 6)

## EDUCATIONAL REQUIREMENTS FOR UAP

Some monitoring of the regulation, education, and use of UAP has been ongoing since the early 1950s; however, most of this has been for *certified nurse's aides*. The Omnibus Budget Reconciliation Act (OBRA) of 1987 established regulations for the education and certification of nurse's aides (minimum of 75 hours of State-approved theory and practice and successful completion of a competency examination in both areas). No federal or community standards have been established, however, for training the more broadly defined UAP.

Indeed, the health care industry provides many job opportunities for individuals without specialized training. In fact, the U.S. Department of Labor, Bureau of Labor Statistics (2011a) notes that only 47% of workers in nursing and residential care facilities have a high school diploma or less, as do 20% of workers in hospitals.

This does not mean, however, that all UAP are undereducated and unprepared for the roles they have been asked to fill. Indeed, UAP educational levels vary from less than that of a high school graduate to those holding advanced degrees. It does suggest, however, that RNs, in delegating to UAP, must make no assumptions about the educational preparation or training of that UAP. Instead, the RN must carefully assess what skills and knowledge each UAP has or risk increased personal liability for the failure to do so.

The reality is that most UAP training is completed by the employing facility and occurs without formal certification. Formal training programs that do exist are completed at vocational schools and community colleges and typically focus on long-term care, providing certifications only as necessary to meet state requirements. Often, this training is inadequate and does not prepare UAP with the competencies they need to work in a dynamic health care environment, which is very different from that existed even a decade ago. For efficiency and safety, standardized curriculums that address the skill sets needed in the many settings where nurse aides are used should be implemented.

Similar to long-term care, the education and training of UAP in acute care settings is often inadequate. In fact, there are no required educational standards or guidelines for the use of UAP in acute care settings. Instead, UAP educational and training requirements for acute care settings are generally facility based. This is important to remember when UAP transfer from one facility to another because no assumption should be made about UAP competency levels to perform certain tasks, despite their work experience.

---

### DISCUSSION POINT

Can an experienced RN accurately assess an individual UAP's "work experience" of patients as a substitute for formal education and training?

---

## UAP SCOPE OF PRACTICE

In addition to existing state regulations regarding UAP education and training, as well as required competencies, many professional nursing organizations have studied the use and effect of UAP and are adopting position statements regarding their use.

One national effort to define the scope of practice for UAP was undertaken by the ANA in their delineation of tasks appropriate for UAP practice in the early 1990s. Multiple revisions have followed. In 2007, the ANA suggested six actions that should be taken to create a national and/or state policy agenda about the educational preparation of UAP or NAP and the competencies they should have for safe practice. These are shown in Box 7.1. In addition, some state boards of nursing have issued recommendations regarding scope of practice for UAP or attempted to delineate the relationship between RNs and UAP. Few states, however, used the ANA or National Council of State Boards of Nursing (NCSBN) definitions for delegation, supervision, or assignment. Most states also report that there are no standardized curricula in place for UAP employed in acute-care hospitals. The states have not been able to reach a consensus regarding the education,

training, and scope of practice needed for UAP to safely practice either. The end result, then, is that there is no universally accepted scope of practice for UAP.

To address the problem, some state boards of nursing have issued task lists for UAP (lists of activities considered to be within the scope of practice for UAP). However, in creating such a list, an unofficial scope of practice is created, and this suggests that such individuals will be performing activities independently. Task lists also suggest that there is no need for delegation, in that the UAP already has a list of nursing activities that he or she may perform without waiting for the delegation process (Marquis & Huston, 2012).

Yet, despite the efforts by the ANA and state boards of nursing, at the institutional level, most health care organizations interpret regulations broadly, allowing UAP a broader scope of practice than that advocated by professional nursing associations or state boards of nursing. In addition, although some institutions limit the scope of practice for UAP to nonnursing functions, many organizations allow the UAP to perform skills traditionally reserved for the licensed nurse.

---

CONSIDER THIS    Given the lack of national regulatory standards regarding the scope of practice for UAP, many health care institutions allow UAP to complete tasks traditionally reserved for licensed practitioners.

---

In some health care agencies, UAP assist with dressing changes, parenteral therapy, urinary catheter insertion, and perform numerous other tasks typically reserved for licensed personnel. The skill assumed by UAP, however, that has garnered the greatest public outcry, is administering medications. UAP are allowed to administer medications in many states in the United States. In fact, Budden (2011) reported that as of 2009, 34 of the 50 states in the United States permitted UAP or medication technicians to assist with or administer medications. In addition, *Certified medicine aides* (CMAs) have worked in licensed nursing home settings in this country for almost four decades. UAP who administer medications are also known as *unlicensed medication administration personnel* (UMAP), *medication aides* (MAs), or *medication assistant technicians* (MATs).

---

CONSIDER THIS    Two thirds of the states in the United States allow UAP to assist with or administer medications.

## BOX 7.1    AMERICAN NURSES ASSOCIATION (2007)

**Recommendations for a National and/or State Policy Agenda for Nursing Assistive Personnel (NAP)**

1. Recognize that the NAP should never be considered or used as a replacement for RNs or licensed practical nurses.

2. Aggressively promote the understanding that delegation is an integral part of professional nursing practice and not a supervisory act connected to acting on behalf of the employer.

3. Establish recognized competencies for the NAP that will guide the development of a core curriculum.

4. Promote national nursing initiatives to establish criteria and guidelines for the clinical training of the NAP through the use of evidence-based research, preparing the NAP to provide routine care in predictable patient functions.

5. Establish systems for training, certification, registry, and disciplinary monitoring of the NAP.

6. Support continued efforts to implement recommendations related to patient safety and quality and the nursing work environment articulated in reports generated by the Institute of Medicine such as *To Err Is Human: Building a Safer Health System; Crossing the Quality Chasm: A New Health System for the 21st Century;* and *Keeping Patients Safe: Transforming the Work Environment of Nurses.*

*Source:* Excerpted from American Nurses Association. (2007). *Position statement: Registered nurses utilization of nursing assistive personnel in all settings.* Retrieved April 28, 2012, from http://gm6.nursingworld.org/MainMenuCategories/Policy-Advocacy/Positions-and-Resolutions/ANAPositionStatements/Position-Statements-Alphabetically/Registered-Nurses-Utilization-of-Nursing-Assistive-Personnel-in-All-Settings.html

A similarly expanded scope of practice for UAP in assisted living settings was reported by Young, Sikma, Reinhard, Gray, and McCormick (2009), who noted that medications in most assisted living settings are managed primarily by UAP, with limited professional involvement. This is in contrast to skilled nursing facilities (SNFs), where only licensed nurses typically engage in medication administration. Indeed, Barra (2011) noted that UAP are at the forefront in administering medications in assisted living settings in the United States with 32 states currently using MATs, 16 states not using MATs, and two currently exploring pilot programs regarding their use.

UAP also administer drugs in school settings when a school nurse is not present. In fact, Host (2011) reported only 25% of school nurses stated they administered all the medication in their schools. The other 75% said that it was UAP and office workers dispensing medications to students.

School nurses and the organizations which represent them, however, are waging a battle to stop the expansion of UAP practice in terms of the drugs they are allowed to administer (e.g., currently only licensed school nurses can administer insulin). They argue that the administration of medications is much more than dispensing a pill, handing a student an inhaler, or giving a subcutaneous injection. It requires high-level assessment skills; an understanding of drug actions, interactions, and side effects; and the highly developed critical thinking skills needed to intervene when problems occur. In addition, the practice of nursing clearly requires a license under the Nurse Practice Act.

There are those, however, who suggest that the use of UAP to administer drugs to school children is not only appropriate but also essential in today's economic climate. For example, Resha (2010) suggests that delegation to UAP in school settings is necessary due to limited resources and increasing health care needs. She notes that the National Association of School Nurses (NASN; 2010) recommends a nurse-to-student ratio of 1 nurse to 750 well-students, however, most school nurses cover more than one school and have nurse-to-student ratios as high as 1:4,000 (NASN).

Similarly, the American Academy of Pediatrics (AAP), the National Association of School Nurses, and the American Nurses Association suggest that trained and supervised UAP, who have the required knowledge, skills, and composure to deliver specific school health services under the guidance of a licensed RN, should be allowed to do so (American Academy of Pediatrics, 2009). The AAP suggests that UAP can provide standardized, routine health services under the supervision of the nurse and on the basis of physician guidance and school nursing assessment of the unique needs of the individual child and the suitability of delegation of specific nursing tasks. Any delegation of nursing duties must be consistent with the requirements of state nurse practice acts, state regulations, and guidelines provided by professional nursing organizations (AAP).

---

CONSIDER THIS   Many patients given direct care by UAP assume that UAP are licensed nurses. This confusion is promulgated when health care professionals do not include their credentials on their nametags or do not introduce themselves to patients according to their actual job title.

---

The reality, then, is that in many settings, UAP are inappropriately performing functions that are within the legal practice of nursing. This is likely a violation of the state nursing practice act and poses a threat to public safety. The problem, however, is not limited to this country; Dilles, Elseviers, Van Rompaey, Van Bortel, and Vander Stichele (2011) found that 25% of UAP in Belgium participated in preparing medication for administration, a task they were not legally allowed to do in that country.

Clearly, certain professional responsibilities related to nursing care must never be delegated. It is critical, then, that the RN never lose sight of his or her ultimate responsibility for ensuring that patients receive appropriate, high-quality care. This means that although the UAP may complete nonnursing functions such as bathing the patient, taking vital signs, and measuring and recording intake and output, it is the RN who must analyze that information using highly developed critical thinking skills and then use the nursing process to see that desired patient outcomes are achieved. Only RNs have the formal authority to practice nursing, and activities that rely on the nursing process or require

specialized skill, expert knowledge, or professional judgment should never be delegated.

## Regulatory Oversight of UAP

The increased use of UAP, called by some the "deskilling of the nursing workforce," has raised concern among professional organizations, consumers, and legislators alike. In the early 1990s, the ANA took the position that the control and monitoring of assistive personnel in clinical settings should be performed through the use of existing mechanisms that regulate nursing practice. Typically, this includes the state board of nursing, institutional policies, and external agency standards.

Legislation has been introduced at the state level to regulate UAP use and scope of practice. Some states have attempted to regulate UAP practice through registration and certification. Others have proposed direct regulation of UAP by passing legislation that requires UAP to be certified by meeting education and competency requirements. Still others require the state boards of nursing or the department of health to register or certify UAP.

Currently, regulation by state and jurisdiction vary widely. Budden (2011) reported that of the agencies who currently provide regulatory oversight, 43% are boards of nursing, 46% are some other state department, and 11% are a combination of a board of nursing and some other state department or agency. In addition, Budden noted a lack of standardization of UAP roles and regulations by state (see Research Study Fuels the Controversy 7.1).

---

### DISCUSSION POINT

Why has the movement to regulate UAP education and training occurred primarily at the state level? Why has there been no national movement to do the same?

---

Barra (2011) echoed Budden's (2011) concerns, noting the limited consistency between state program requirements for MATs and the extensive variations within classroom, clinical, and experience requirements for UAP administering medications. Barra suggested, "This lack of congruency should be a matter of serious concern for both public protection with providing safe, ethical care and for nurses who are liable" (p. 3).

## RESEARCH STUDY FUELS THE CONTROVERSY 7.1

### THE REGULATION OF MEDICATION AIDES BY STATE

This descriptive study explored medication-aide (MA) regulations by state and jurisdiction by reviewing state websites and legislation and by querying key contacts in each state. Forty-six states provided data. Analyses of regulatory oversight, work setting and supervision, continuing education, and role limitations were conducted.

Budden, J. S. ( 2011). The safety and regulation of medication aides. *Journal of Nursing Regulation*, 2(2), 18–23.

### STUDY FINDINGS

At least 50% of the jurisdictions required MAs to be CNAs, whereas 33% required them to have a specific amount of work experience. At least 39% offered training in facilities such as long-term care and at least 61% offered training in educational institutions such as community colleges. The average number of clinical training hours across jurisdictions was 22.22 hours with a range from 0 to 40 hours. At least 78 of the jurisdictions used a standard written examination after training to verify competency and at least 28% used a manual skills demonstration examination.

Role limitations varied between the states with some states restricting the MA from administering parenteral or injectable medications and other states restricting the MA from administering anything other than oral medications. In addition, some states restricted the administration of controlled substances and others did not allow MAs to given nonroutine medications when the patient's condition was not predictable. Budden concluded that despite calls for more standardization of MA roles and regulations by state, that wide variability continues to exist in the roles and regulations of MAs, and that getting all states to agree to uniform regulations is unlikely.

## UAP AND PATIENT OUTCOMES

Stone and Harahan (2010) suggest that because UAP are so involved in providing activities of daily living, such as bathing, dressing, eating, and toileting, and often have the most direct contact with residents/clients, they directly influence not only the quality of care but also the care recipient's quality of life. A well-trained, caring, and competent UAP then can be a vital and contributing member of the health care team.

Certainly at some point though, given the increasing complexity of health care and the increasing acuity of patient illnesses, there is a maximum representation of UAP in the staffing mix that should not be breached. Those levels have not yet been determined. Considerable evidence does exist, however, that demonstrates a direct link between decreased RN staffing and declines in patient outcomes. Some of these declines in patient outcomes are nurse sensitive and include an increased incidence of patient falls, nosocomial infections, increased physical restraint use, and medication errors.

Outcome data also exist regarding the use of UAP to assist with and administer medications. Young et al. (2009) looked at medication administration errors in assisted living settings (where UAP administer most of the medications) in 12 sites in three states (Oregon, Washington, and

New Jersey). Of their 4,866 observations, there were 1,373 errors (a 28.2% error rate). Of these, 70.8% were wrong time, 12.9% were wrong dose, 11.1% were an omitted dose, 3.5% were an extra dose, 1.5% were an unauthorized drug, and 0.2% were the wrong drug.

Canham et al. (2007) found similar problems with errors in the school setting, where school office staff members (UAP) were typically delegated this task. In that study, five school nurses developed and participated in a medication audit of 154 medications. Audit results showed a wide range of errors and discrepancies, including problems with transcription, physician orders or lack thereof, timing, documentation, and storage.

Another large survey of school nurses showed that nearly half of them reported medication errors in their schools during the previous year (Host, 2011). A major factor in these medication errors was the use of "unlicensed assistive personnel" such as school secretaries, health aides, teachers, parents, and even students, to administer medications, with UAP being three times more likely to make medication errors than their school nurse counterparts. Host also reported that three quarters of the schools had training programs for their UAP administering medications, but in most cases the training was 2 hours or less in length.

Yet Randolph and Scott-Cawiezell (2011), reporting on a pilot program sponsored by the Arizona State Board of Nursing between 2004 and 2008, found no differences in patterns of medication errors before and after the introduction of CNA-trained medication technicians working under the delegation of a licensed nurse. Structured interviews suggested that participants viewed the role favorably with the licensed nurses reporting increased role satisfaction.

## RN LIABILITY FOR SUPERVISION AND DELEGATION OF UAP

Delegation has long been a function of registered nursing, although the scope of delegation and the tasks being delegated have changed dramatically over the last three decades with the increased use of UAP in acute care settings. As a result, the professional nurse (RN) role changed in many acute care institutions from one of direct care provider to one requiring delegation of patient care to others.

This role of delegator and supervisor increased the scope of legal liability for the RN. Although there is limited case law involving nursing delegation and supervision, it is generally accepted that the RN is responsible for adequate supervision of the person to whom an assignment has been delegated. Although nurses are not automatically held liable for all acts of negligence on the part of those they supervise, they may be held liable if they were negligent in the supervision of those employees at the time that those employees committed the negligent acts (Marquis & Huston, 2012).

Liability is based on a supervisor's failure to determine which patient needs could safely be assigned to a subordinate or for failing to closely monitor a subordinate who requires such supervision. Experienced nurses have traditionally been expected to work with minimal supervision. The RN who delegates care to another competent RN does not have the same legal obligation to closely supervise that person's work as when the care is delegated to UAP. In assigning tasks to UAP, then, the RN must be aware of the job description, knowledge base, and demonstrated skills of each person.

---

CONSIDER THIS  The UAP has no license to lose for "exceeding scope of practice," and nationally established standards to state what the limits should be for UAP in terms of scope of practice do not exist. It is the RN who bears the legal liability for allowing UAP to perform tasks that should be accomplished only by a licensed health care professional.

---

### DISCUSSION POINT

Do most UAP believe that they can be held legally liable and accountable for their actions if they are delegated to do something by an RN that is beyond their scope of practice or training?

### DISCUSSION POINT

What happens when the condition of a patient changes? Is the training of UAP adequate to recognize changes in clients' conditions that warrant seeking intervention from the licensed nurse?

---

In addition, communication between the RN-UAP dyad must be "mindful" since it is critical factor in direct patient care and thus patient safety (Anthony & Vidal, 2010). Corazzini et al. (2010) suggest this communication, especially when it involves delegation, can be difficult because of poor partnerships between licensed and unlicensed staff, attitudinal barriers, and a paucity of RN-level clinical leadership. In addition, explicit organizational structures and written guidelines supporting and reinforcing nurses' scope of practice, the translation of UAP role expectations into actual practice, and the effectiveness of communication may be missing in health care organizations (Siegel & Young, 2010; see Research Study Fuels the Controversy 7.2).

The bottom line is that delegating to UAP is similar to delegating to other types of health care workers. RNs are always accountable for the care given and must be responsible for instructing UAP as to who needs care and when. The UAP should be accountable for knowing how to properly perform their segment of assigned care and for knowing when other workers should be called in for tasks beyond the limits of their knowledge and training. As such, the UAP does bear some personal accountability for their actions, despite the legal doctrine of *respondent superior* (the employer can be held legally liable for the conduct of employees whose actions he or she has a right to direct or control).

Regardless of liability issues, the need for nurses to have highly developed delegation skills has never been greater than it is today. The ability to use

## RESEARCH STUDY FUELS THE CONTROVERSY 7.2

### COMMUNICATION BETWEEN RNS AND UAP

This descriptive study analyzed documents from six nursing homes to identify and explore written guidelines for what, how, and when nurses and unlicensed assistive personnel (UAP) are expected to communicate regarding residents' status and care needs.

Siegel, E. O., & Young, H. M. (2010). Communication between nurses and unlicensed assistive personnel in nursing homes: Explicit expectations. *Journal of Gerontological Nursing, 36*(12), 32–37.

### STUDY FINDINGS

Two primary themes emerged. First, extensive and explicit guidelines were identified for UAP-to-nurse communication, in comparison to few corresponding guidelines for nurses. Second, written guidelines for UAP communication were identified in multiple documents, with variations across sites in the situations requiring communication, the level of detail, and the format for how UAP-to-nurse communication should occur (i.e., verbal, written). This study questioned the extent to which explicit organizational structures and written guidelines support and reinforce nurses' scope of practice, the translation of UAP role expectations into actual practice, and the effectiveness of communication to promote quality care.

---

delegation skills appropriately will help to reduce the personal liability associated with supervising and delegating to UAP. It will also ensure that clients' needs are met and their safety is not jeopardized. General principles for RNs to use in delegating to NAP are shown in Box 7.2.

### RNS WORKING AS UAP: A LIABILITY ISSUE

It must also be noted that employers have recently reported hiring new graduate RNs into UAP positions. Boone (2010) suggests this has occurred because of recent national economic woes, the nursing shortage,

---

### BOX 7.2   AMERICAN NURSE ASSOCIATION (2007)

**Recommendations for RNs Who Work With Nursing Assistive Personnel (NAP)**

1. Recognize and use the legal authority that is vested to the RN by the state nurse practice act specific to the delegation of nonprofessional tasks to an adequately trained NAP.

2. Acknowledge and understand the guidance inherent in the professional and specialty nursing scope and standards of practice with regard to the delegation of nonprofessional tasks to an adequately trained NAP.

3. Understand the relevant employer policies, procedures, and position descriptions related to utilization of NAP within the facility.

4. Utilize the right and obligation to know the set of skills that the NAP is competent to perform in order to promote safe patient care. This information should be documented and readily available to the RN.

5. Exercise decision-making authority, based on professional judgment, regarding whether or not to delegate a particular task to the NAP relevant to the patient care situation.

*Source:* Excerpted from American Nurses Association. (2007). *Position statement: Registered nurses utilization of nursing assistive personnel in all settings.* Retrieved April 28, 2012, from http://gm6.nursingworld.org/MainMenuCategories/Policy-Advocacy/Positions-and-Resolutions/ANAPositionStatements/Position-Statements-Alphabetically/Registered-Nurses-Utilization-of-Nursing-Assistive-Personnel-in-All-Settings.html

and health care reform. Many of these transitional employees secured employment in these positions while students in nursing programs.

Though this practice provides employment opportunities for new graduate nurses, Boone suggests it raises several matters of legality. First, these RNs are not able to provide care to the level of their expertise. Instead, they must perform only direct care duties and remain in the scope of practice of an unlicensed person. This violates numerous statutes which govern scope of practice, since these statutes suggest that licensees are held to the level of practice associated with his or her licensure, regardless of employment status. Thus, licensed nurses are held liable to provide care to the level of their existing scope of practice and yet also face risk of charges of negligence or malpractice if they provide care only to the level of the constructs of the assumed position (Boone, 2010). Working then in a capacity beneath the level of licensure appears to greatly increase the potential for legal liability for both the nurse and his or her employer and revocation of license for the nurse.

Boone (2010) also notes that most employers offer few definitive answers about how to address this role discrepancy and, instead, leave these critical decisions to the nurse. He concludes that binding a nurse to the constructs of a job description below their level of licensure not only is ineffective practice but also subjects both employers and RNs working as UAP to greatly increased risks of legal proceedings.

## CREATING A SAFE WORK ENVIRONMENT

There are things that health care organizations can do to increase the likelihood that UAP are used both effectively and appropriately as members of the health care team. First, the organization must have a clearly defined organization structure in which RNs are recognized as leaders of the health care team. This organization structure must facilitate RN evaluation of UAP job performance and encourage UAP accountability to the RN.

Job descriptions must also be developed by health care agencies that clearly define the roles and responsibilities of all categories of caregivers. These descriptions should be consistent with that state's nurse practice legislation, as well as with community standards of care, and should reflect differences between the roles of licensed and unlicensed personnel. Policies should facilitate adequate supervision of UAP by RNs and restrict UAP to simple tasks that can be performed safely. In addition, worker credentials should be readily

apparent on the nametags worn by nursing health care personnel.

Second, uniform training and orientation programs for UAP must be established to ensure that preparation is adequate to provide at least minimum standards of safe patient care. These training and orientation programs should be based on clearly defined job descriptions for UAP. In addition, organizational education programs must be developed for all personnel to learn the roles and responsibilities of different categories of caregivers. In addition, to protect their patients and their professional license, RNs must continue to seek current information regarding national efforts to standardize scope of practice for UAP and professional guidelines regarding what can be safely delegated to UAP.

In addition, there must be adequate program development in leadership and delegation skills for RNs before UAP are introduced. Delegation is a learned skill, and much can be done to better prepare RNs for this role. Educational programs that produce graduate nurses must explore the nature of the RN role, with a focus on professional nurse leadership roles, to better prepare them to meet the challenges of working in restructured health care settings. Practicing RNs should have opportunities for continuing education in the principles of delegation and supervision. This will allow them not only to recognize the limitations of UAP scope of practice but also to gain confidence in differentiating between skills requiring licensure and those that do not.

## THE UAP SHORTAGE

Finally, if all the issues related to the education, training, scope of practice, and delegation to UAP are resolved, there may be an even greater problem. There may not be enough UAP to meet future demand. The U.S. Department of Labor, Bureau of Labor Statistics (2011b) projects that employment needs for UAP will grow 19% between 2008 and 2018, faster than the average for all occupations, predominantly in response to the long-term care needs of an increasing elderly population. In addition, the Labor Department suggests that hospitals will be pressured to discharge patients as soon as possible as a result of diminishing reimbursement and this will boost admissions to nursing and residential care facilities. Modern medical technology will also drive the demand for UAP because as technology saves and extends more lives, the need for long-term care provided by UAP increases.

The unfortunate reality is that the demand for UAP as direct care givers is already growing and the population of persons who have traditionally filled these jobs is declining. Indeed, there is a nationwide shortage of well-trained UAP in all settings, and although many states report recruitment and retention of support personnel as a major area of concern, few are actively addressing the situation. For example, Rider (2011) reported that California will need more than 1 million allied health care workers by 2030 as a result of a growing and aging population, as well as effects of federal health care reform, yet no formalized plan is in place to address this shortfall.

One problem contributing to this shortage is the high turnover rate for nursing assistants, particularly in long-term care. The reasons for this high turnover rate are varied, but long hours, inadequate staffing, and the physical and emotional demands of the job are certainly a part of it. This was borne out in research conducted by McKenzie et al. (2011) who found that UAP working in assistive living facilities experienced high levels of emotional exhaustion, psychiatric distress, and work-related injuries. Providing care to residents with dementia-related behaviors and supporting families were the most frequently reported work stressors.

Low pay is also an issue. The U.S. Department of Labor, Bureau of Labor Statistics (2011b) noted that the median hourly wage of UAP as of May 2008 was US$11.46. The middle 50% earned between US$9.71 and US$13.76 an hour. The lowest 10% earned less than US$8.34, and the highest 10% earned more than US$15.97 an hour. The median hourly wage for UAP employed in general medical and surgical hospitals (US$12.10) was higher than in nursing care facilities (US$11.13) or home health care services (US$10.58).

In addition, Pfefferle and Weinberg (2008) added that many direct care workers encounter negative messages from their managers, supervisors, coworkers, and sometimes residents about the meaning and value of their work. As a result, many unlicensed workers "cast themselves as the last defense for residents, as the ones doing the work that no one else will do" (p. 959).

In addition, few employers provide UAP employer-paid benefits such as health insurance coverage, retirement benefits, or childcare. Furthermore, there are limited career paths or advancement opportunities for UAP who do not want to achieve a licensed job category (e.g., LPN, RN), and they often have little direct input into organizational decision making.

Working conditions are also often less than ideal. Because of high UAP turnover and absenteeism, those UAP who do work must often work short-handed, which leads to greater stress. Long-term care facilities are required to meet only minimum government standards for staffing and few facilities are cited, even when understaffing occurs. In addition, federal regulations are out of date and do not reflect new knowledge on safe staffing levels. For example, minimum standards for RNs require only one licensed nurse in a nursing home, regardless of its size.

The UAP job may also pose hazards related to exposure to infectious diseases and drug-resistant infections. The U.S. Department of Labor, Bureau of Labor Statistics (2011b) noted that nursing aides, orderlies, attendants, and psychiatric aides had some of the highest nonfatal injuries and illness rates for all occupations, in the 98th and 99th percentiles in 2007.

CONSIDER THIS   The brunt of work in long-term care settings typically falls on lowly paid, unlicensed workers who have a tremendous impact on patient satisfaction and the quality of care provided.

To avert an increasing UAP shortage (particularly in long-term care) and to promote worker retention, Stone and Harahan (2010) suggest that action is needed on the part of policy makers, providers, and other stakeholders. They argue that explicit policies should be developed to expand the supply of personnel entering the field, including the

*creation of financial incentives such as grants to foster greater interest among people considering the long-term care field; scholarships, federal traineeships, and residency programs for people preparing for advanced degrees in long-term care; matching grants to fund administrators in-training programs for people interested in management positions; and loan forgiveness programs for people who commit to long-term care careers.* (p. 113)

## CONCLUSIONS

The increased use of UAP presents both opportunities and challenges for the American health care system. Anthony and Vidal (2010) suggest that as the health care system becomes more sensitive to cost escalation, a greater number of unlicensed personnel will be used to provide direct care. They caution though that accountability for outcomes will continue to lie with the professional RN. Clearly, UAP play an increasingly integral role in safe and resource-efficient care delivery in this country (particularly in long-term care settings), and they can be successfully used to augment the health care team.

Nonetheless, the challenge continues to be to use UAP only to provide personal care needs or nursing tasks that do not require the skill and judgment of the RN. With increasing patient loads and the current nursing shortage, many health care organizations and the RNs who work within them are tempted to allow UAP to perform tasks that should be limited to professional nursing practice. Nurses must remember, however, that the responsibility for assuring that patients are protected and that UAP do not exceed their scope of practice ultimately falls to the RN. When UAP are allowed to encroach into professional nursing care, patients are placed at risk. Corazzini et al. (2010) suggests that the nursing profession is

challenged to make delegation content from Nurse Practice Acts central to our discussions of licensed and unlicensed nursing staff care and to view the underlying issues as the core of professional and practical nursing practice.

In addition, the blurring of the lines between the practice of RNs and UAP makes it nearly impossible for patients to make a distinction between providers. "Professional nurses are put in a very powerful and meaningful position of trust as families and friends allow nurses the opportunity to care for their loved ones. However, with such position comes a great deal of responsibility and accountability" (Plawecki & Amrhein, 2010, p. 21). One of the most important roles then for the RN is to be a gatekeeper in assuring that care given by UAP under their supervision is always of high quality. Until answers are found, the likelihood is that UAP will continue to constitute a significant portion of the nursing workforce and the boundary between UAP and RN practice will continue to be blurred.

## FOR ADDITIONAL DISCUSSION

**1.** Is cost or the nursing shortage the greater driving force in increased UAP use in acute care hospitals today?

**2.** Is institutional training and certification of UAP a precursor to future initiatives for institutional licensure of RNs?

**3.** Are the cost savings associated with increased UAP use offset by the need for greater supervision by RNs and potential declines in patient outcomes?

**4.** Should UAP be allowed to administer medications, perform intravenous cannulation, and change sterile dressings?

**5.** Do you believe that patients typically are aware whether it is the UAP or licensed nurse that is caring for them?

**6.** How comfortable do you believe most RNs are in the role of delegator to UAP? Do you believe most RNs feel clarity regarding role differentiation between the RN and the UAP?

**7.** Should the training and certification of UAP fall under the purview of state boards of registered nursing?

## REFERENCES

American Academy of Pediatrics. (2009). *Policy statement—Guidance for the administration of medication in school.* Retrieved June 30, 2011, from http://aap-policy.aappublications.org/cgi/content/full/pediatrics;124/4/1244

Anthony, M. K., & Vidal, K. (2010). Mindful communication: A novel approach to improving delegation and increasing patient safety. *Online Issue of Journals in Nursing, 15*(2). Retrieved June 29, 2011, from http://www.nursingworld.org/MainMenuCategories/ANAMarketplace/ANAPeriodicals/OJIN/TableofContents/Vol152010/

No2May2010/Mindful-Communication-and-Delegation.aspx

Barra, M. (2011). Nurse delegation of medication pass in assisted living facilities: Not all medication assistant technicians are equal. *Journal of Nursing Law, 14*(1), 3–10.

Boone, T. W. (2010).New nurses working as unlicensed assistive personnel. *Advance for Nurses*. Retrieved June 30, 2011, from http://nursing.advanceweb.com/Student-and-New-Grad-Center/Student-Top-Story/New-Nurses-Working-as-Unlicensed-Assistive-Personnel.aspx

Budden, J. S. (2011). The safety and regulation of medication aides. *Journal of Nursing Regulation, 2*(2), 18–23.

Buerhaus, P., Donelan, K., Ulrich, B. T., DesRoches, C., & Dittus, R. (2007). Trends in the experiences of hospital-employed registered nurses: Results from three national surveys. *Nursing Economics, 25*(2), 69–80.

Canham, D. L., Bauer, L., Concepcion, M., Luong, J., Peters, J., & Wilde, C. (2007). An audit of medication administration: A glimpse into school health offices. *Journal of School Nursing, 23*(1), 21–27.

Corazzini, K., Anderson, R. A., Rapp, C., Mueller, C., McConnell, E., & Lekan, D. (2010). Delegation in long-term care: Scope of practice or job description? *Online Journal of Issues in Nursing, 15*(2). Retrieved June 30, 2011, from http://www.nursingworld.org/MainMenuCategories/ANAMarketplace/ANAPeriodicals/OJIN/TableofContents/Vol152010/No2May2010/Delegation-in-Long-Term-Care.aspx

Dilles, T., Elseviers, M. M., Van Rompaey, B., Van Bortel, L. M., & Vander Stichele, R. R. (2011). Barriers for nurses to safe medication management in nursing homes. *Journal of Nursing Scholarship, 43*(2), 171–180.

Domrose, C. (2008). Not enough hours. *Nurse Week (California), 2*(13), 32–33.

Hendrich, A., Chow, M. P., Skierczynski, B. A., & Zhenqiang, L. (2008). A 36-hospital time and motion study: How do medical–surgical nurses spend their time? *Permanente Journal, 12*(3). Retrieved July 6, 2011, from http://xnet.kp.org/permanentejournal/sum08/time-study.html

Host, P. (2011). *School medication administration*. Retrieved June 29, 2011, from http://bipolar.about.com/cs/kids_parents/a/0207_schoolmeds.htm

Marquis, B., & Huston, C. (2012). *Leadership roles and management functions in nursing* (7th ed.). Philadelphia, PA: Lippincott Williams & Wilkins.

McKenzie, G., Teri, L., Salazar, M., Farran, C., Beck, C., & Paun, O. (2011). Relationship between system-level characteristics of assisted living facilities and the health and safety of unlicensed staff. *AAOHN Journal, 59*(4), 173–180.

Mulrooney, G. (2011). A case for improved quality of care through more accurate staffing. White paper: Safe staffing legislation. *API Healthcare*. Retrieved July 6, 2011, from http://www.apihealthcare.com/safe_staffing_legislation/

National Association of School Nurses. (2010). *Healthy children learn better! School nurses make a difference*. Retrieved April 28, 2012, from http://www.dphhs.mt.gov/publichealth/asthma/documents/advisorygroup/SchoolNurseInformation.pdf

Pfefferle, S. G., & Weinberg, D. B. (2008). Certified nurse assistants making meaning of direct care. *Qualitative Health Research, 18*(7), 952–961.

Plawecki, L., & Amrhein, D. (2010). Legal issues. A question of delegation: Unlicensed assistive personnel and the professional nurse. *Journal of Gerontological Nursing, 36*(8), 18–21.

Randolph, P., & Scott-Cawiezell, J. (2010). Developing a statewide medication technician pilot program in nursing homes. *Journal of Gerontological Nursing, 36*(9), 36–44.

Resha, C. (2010). Delegation in the school setting: Is it a safe practice? *Online Journal of Issues in Nursing, 15*(2). Retrieved June 30, 2011, from http://www.nursingworld.org/MainMenuCategories/ANAMarketplace/ANAPeriodicals/OJIN/TableofContents/Vol152010/No2May2010/Delegation-in-the-School-Setting.aspx

Rider, T. (2011). CHA reports possible healthcare worker shortage by 2030. Retrieved June 30, 2011, from http://womenandourhealth.wordpress.com/2011/03/26/cha-reports-possible-healthcare-worker-shortage-by-2030/

Siegel, E. O., & Young, H. M. (2010). Communication between nurses and unlicensed assistive personnel in nursing homes: Explicit expectations. *Journal of Gerontological Nursing, 36*(12), 32–37.

Stone, R., & Harahan, M. (2010). Improving the long-term care workforce serving older adults. *Health Affairs, 29*(1), 109–115.

U.S. Department of Labor, Bureau of Labor Statistics. (2011a). *Healthcare* (2010–2011 ed.). Retrieved June 30, 2011, from http://www.bls.gov/oco/cg/cgs035.htm

U.S. Department of Labor, Bureau of Labor Statistics. (2011b). *Nursing and psychiatric aides* (2010–2011 ed.). Retrieved June 30, 2011, from http://www.bls.gov/oco/cg/cgs035.htm

Young, H. M., Sikma, S. K., Reinhard, S. C., Gray, S. L., & McCormick, W. (2009). Medication monitoring: Research sheds light on medication errors and their clinical significance in assisted living settings in three states. *Advance for Long Term Care Management, 12*(2), 39. Retrieved July 7, 2011, from http://long-term-care.advanceweb.com/Article/Medication-Monitoring.aspx

## BIBLIOGRAPHY

Belcourt, T., & Downie, S. (2012). Ask a practice advisor: What is my responsibility and accountability as an RN working with unregulated care providers (UCPs)? *SRNA Newsbulletin, 14*(1), 8–9.

Buck, D. K. (2011). Nursing assistant and medication aide training program changes. *Oregon State Board of Nursing Sentinel, 30*(2), 12–14.

Carder, P. C. (2012). "Learning about your residents": How assisted living residence medication aides decide to administer pro re nata medications to persons with dementia. *Gerontologist, 52*(1), 46–55.

Flannery, M. (2011). Creating and sustaining an effective coaching culture in home care: One organization's performance improvement related to aides and aide retention. *Home Healthcare Nurse, 29*(5), 275–281. [Erratum, *29*(7), 398]

Griffin, R., & Sines, D. (2012). How nursing support staff contribute to care. *Nursing Times, 108*(11), 18–19.

Kemp, C. L., Luo, S., & Ball, M. M. (2012). "Meds are a real tricky area": Examining medication management and regulation in assisted living. *Journal of Applied Gerontology, 31*(1), 126–149.

Saccomano, S. J., & Pinto-Zipp, G. (2011). Registered nurse leadership style and confidence in delegation. *Journal of Nursing Management, 19*(4), 522–533.

Sanford, P., & Barton, E. (2011). Restructuring non-licensed roles in ambulatory care. *AAACN Viewpoint, 33*(5), 1.

Stonehouse, D. (2011). Management and leadership for support workers. *British Journal of Healthcare Assistants, 5*(10), 507–510.

Thompson, M. A., Horne, K. K., & Huerta, T. R. (2011). Reassessing nurse aide job satisfaction in a Texas nursing home. *Journal of Gerontological Nursing, 37*(9), 42–49.

Timmons, J., & Johnson, S. (2011). To scrub or not to scrub? That is the question. *Journal of Perioperative Practice, 21*(10), 356–358.

Trossman, S. (2011). At the heart of professional practice: ANA, groups continue to fight for control of practice, patient safety. *American Nurse, 43*(6), 1–10.

Vogelsmeier, A. (2011). Medication administration in nursing homes: RN delegation to unlicensed assistive personnel. *Journal of Nursing Regulation, 2*(3), 49–53.

Waters, A. (2012). Survey reveals extent of duties undertaken by support workers. *Nursing Standard, 26*(19), 5.

Zimmerman, S., Love, K., Sloane, P. D., Cohen, L. W., Reed, D., & Carder, P. C. (2011). Medication administration errors in assisted living: Scope, characteristics, and the importance of staff training. *Journal of the American Geriatrics Society, 59*(6), 1060–1068.

# Chapter **8**

# Socialization and Mentoring

Jeanne Madison

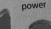

## ADDITIONAL RESOURCES

Visit the Point for additional helpful resources

- eBook
- Journal Articles
- WebLinks

## CHAPTER OUTLINE

## LEARNING OBJECTIVES

*The learner will be able to:*

1. Define socialization, resocialization, and mentoring.

2. Identify common situations that increase nurses' need for socialization and resocialization.

3. Analyze the historical impact of gender socialization and feminism on the advancement of nursing as a profession.

4. Explore the relationship between professional oppression and empowerment.

5. Describe how Kramer's work on reality shock for new graduate nurses influenced socialization research in nursing.

6. Investigate strategies to assist new graduate nurses with socialization to the professional nursing role.

7. Describe why experienced nurses experiencing role transition often need resocialization, and identify specific strategies to promote such resocialization.

8. Provide examples of positive and negative socialization behaviors common in health care workplace settings.

9. Describe characteristics of classic mentoring relationships, as well as stages common to most mentoring relationships.

10. Compare and contrast the roles of mentor, role model, preceptor, coach, and guide in promoting professional socialization and resocialization.

*continued*

11. Contrast the historical availability of mentors for men and women and determine whether these trends have changed over time.

12. Postulate reasons that mentoring was historically less available in "traditionally female" occupations as compared with the situation for women in general.

13. Examine how mentors, preceptors, role models, and guides have influenced his or her own professional development and socialization to professional nursing.

Nurses and nursing are constantly changing. There are *no* nurses who enter and exit their nursing career in the same setting, under the same set of expectations. Indeed, the variety of careers and opportunities available to nurses are some of the most important influential recruitment and retention strategies in health care settings. Nurses can change clinical specialties with ease; leave employers for short- or long-term absences; rarely, if ever, experience lack of employment opportunity; work full- or part-time; and avail themselves of a plethora of specialist training or reentry programs when such potential change seems opportune.

In addition, in keeping with globalization trends, nurses today come from diverse ethnic, religious, and social backgrounds. Many are educated in one country, but practice in several other countries. Given this individual variation, as well as diversity in practice patterns, how these nurses are socialized and resocialized in the health care workplace in the 21st century is of profound importance.

## SOCIALIZATION: ROLES, SKILLS, VALUES, AND CHANGE

*Socialization* is the process by which a person acquires the technical skills of his or her society, the knowledge of the kinds of behavior that are understood and acceptable in that society, and the attitudes and values that make conformity with social rules personally meaningful, even gratifying. Socialization has also been called *enculturation*.

*Resocialization* occurs when individuals are forced to learn new values, skills, attitudes, and social rules as a result of changes in the type of work they do, the scope of responsibility they hold, or in the workplace setting itself (Marquis & Huston, 2012). Individuals who frequently need resocialization include experienced nurses who change work settings, either within the same organization or in a new organization, and nurses who undertake new roles. Some nurses adapt easily to

resocialization, but most experience some stress with role change.

Before the 1970s, little thought was given to how socialization and resocialization occurred in the health care workplace or how new graduates experienced the transition from student to graduate nurse. It was generally believed that because nurses were educated in the hospital environment, they would not be unduly surprised or alarmed by changes in responsibility and accountability on graduation from their nursing program. Kramer's (1974, 1981) work on "reality shock" and issues associated with professional socialization led to a renaissance of this thinking, which continues today.

The latest emphasis on socialization research in nursing occurred, coincidentally, at the same time as another sweeping social phenomenon that profoundly changed nursing and the health care workplace forever: the feminist movement. Research about nursing and women's issues expanded significantly against the backdrop of feminism in the Western world.

Nurses in practice and leadership roles in the 21st century are confronted with a vastly changed workplace from even 5 or 10 years ago. Human resources and the social sciences identify the workplace where Generation Y (1980–2000), Generation X (1965–1980), boomers (1946–1964), and veterans (1925–1945) work together in the new, hopefully egalitarian workplace. Kramer (2010) describes Generation Y as the Net generation or millennial generation, Generation X as closely guarding a work–life balance, boomers as the largest cohort and occupying many leadership positions, and veterans as cautious and conservative. At the same time, Kramer cautions about overgeneralizations and possible stereotyping when considering generational differences. The new workplace creates challenges for workers, managers, and leaders. The concomitant increase in the number of men undertaking nursing education and women undertaking medical education has also established powerful, changed dynamics within the profession(s).

During the 1970s, significant nursing research focused on analyzing the health care workplace in an effort to understand the long-standing mechanisms that disempowered, denigrated, and marginalized nurses and the nursing profession and empowered the predominantly male medical profession. It was evident that the oppressive forces in place were entrenched, powerful, and advantageous to those who were in power. Reversing the trajectory of negative nurse socialization was no simple task and was undertaken by nurses individually and collectively.

> CONSIDER THIS   The oppression of nurses came not only from outside groups, such as medicine and health care administration, but also from within the profession.

## The Health Care Workplace in the 21st Century

Negative and positive socialization patterns in the late 20th century workplace received wide attention in the literature. The expression used for negative socialization is *horizontal violence*, and it includes manifestations such as bullying, harassment, verbal abuse, and intimidation. On the other hand, positive socialization strategies include such behaviors as mentoring, role modeling, and preceptoring.

## Oppression and Horizontal Violence

The literature is clear that horizontal violence is not unique to nursing; rather, it is found in most oppressed groups and professions. Researchers agree that negative socialization and oppressive behaviors had to be eliminated by nurses in order to assume and practice positive socialization strategies, empowering themselves. Understanding typical oppressed-group behavior and horizontal violence was the first step to developing effective change strategies that reduced and eliminate it.

Oppressed groups typically believe they are oppressed because they are deficient in some way and, most importantly, the oppressor defines these deficiencies (Freire, 1968). As this distorted perception is internalized, the oppressed group inadvertently perpetuates the process of oppression. Unsupportive, disempowering, and controlling behaviors *within* the hierarchical nursing structure can easily be identified and demonstrated by horizontal violence. Oppressed-group behavior includes a number of widely accepted characteristics: feelings of inferiority, powerlessness,

inequality, and self-doubt that perpetuate feelings of oppression, which engender feelings of inferiority. Most contemporary workplaces clearly identify themselves as zero tolerant of bullying, harassment, and other associated behaviors.

> CONSIDER THIS   How often do we hear or say, "I'm just a med-surg nurse," or "Oh, you work on a medical floor," or "I just work in a nursing home," rather than hearing or saying, "I am a medical surgical specialist," or "Oh, you're a medical nursing specialist," or "I'm a specialist in caring for the elderly"?

Historically, nurses were exploited by the delegation of tasks that were no longer interesting or challenging to medical practitioners. Just as women can still be marginalized in society, so nurses can find themselves marginalized in the health care workplace. It is imperative that the nursing profession maintains vigilance against outside interference in nursing professional integrity and self-responsibility. In the past, socially and culturally, physicians and health care administrators, mostly male, worked hard to maintain their dominance in health care and to control and restrict nurses and other, until recently, mostly female, health practitioners. Awareness of historical facts and practice is important to the nursing profession as it maintains its autonomy and self-control.

An important and fairly rapid transition occurs when student nurses graduate into the clinical setting as professional registered nurses (RNs). The subtle, somewhat nebulous concepts associated with professionalism and promotion of a positive workplace context contrast with the more mechanical and technical aspects of nursing practice. From novice to early practitioner, nurses are dependent on preceptors in their educational programs to model important socialization strategies. Carlson, Pilhammar, and Wann-Hansson (2010) described the necessity for nurses to self-reflect and to develop and focus on meaning and implications of professionalism. It is important that early in the education of nursing students, curriculum includes strategies that cultivate empowerment and positive personal and professional growth. Early workplace experiences must allow students to see nurses treating each other in professional, positive, and supportive ways.

Positive socialization is exemplified in the various supportive behaviors associated with mentoring, preceptoring, role modeling, coaching, and guiding. Only recently has significant progress been made toward a far more egalitarian workplace where respect for and valuing of a diverse worker and workplace is evident. Positive reinforcement, flexible work hours, recognition of non-work-related responsibilities and equal pay for equal work are no longer "optional" work place strategies.

## Diversity and Equity

Exactly what is the experience of new nurses as they are socialized into the health care environment of the 21st century? Certainly, new nurses are confronted with the challenges associated with difference and diversity and ways to respect, value, and legitimize the "different but equal" employee. Dodd, Saggers, and Wildy (2009) described Generation Y respondents as often leaving employment to travel and change specialties and workplace. Generation X often left their workplace to improve family and travel opportunities. Dodd et al., not surprisingly, found the older "boomers" the most stable employees. As more and more Generation Y nurses enter the workplace, the workplace will need to respond to this group's "live for the moment," multitasking (part-time work/study/leisure) and apparent expectation for fairly rapid career progression, opportunity, and diversity.

Cohen and Veled-Hecht (2010) described the relationship between socialization and commitment and whether (long-term nursing care) health professionals develop and maintain commitment not only to the organization but as well to the workplace colleagues. Building commitment to colleagues *and* the organization is essential to survive and thrive in the sometimes difficult nursing workplace. Acknowledging that new graduates are confronted with a challenging and sometimes negative workplace is critical to progressing the discussion to positive socialization strategies and the ways in which nurses can commit to empowering one another (Clarke, Kane, Rajacich, & Lafreniere, 2012; Duteau, 2012; Rhodes, Schutt, Langham, & Bilotta, 2012).

Significant research exists in the area of toxic organizations and workplace relationships in health care and elsewhere (Chamberlain & Hodson, 2010; MacEachen, Kosny, Ferrier, & Chambers, 2010; Walrafen, Brewer, & Mulvenon, 2012). A full appreciation of the historical subservient and oppressed constraints upon nurses and nursing is important as the profession holds steadfast in its independence and self-monitoring precepts. Without the history and perspective that it brings to nurses and the profession in general, the importance of individual responsibility and accountability could lose its imperative and importance.

---

### DISCUSSION POINT

What and where are some of the resources nurses can access if they need advice and support when attempting to confront issues of inappropriate, unhelpful, and negative workplace behaviors?

---

## SOCIALIZATION AND MENTORING: EMPOWERMENT

*Mentoring* is an intense, positive, discreet, exclusive, one-on-one relationship between an experienced professional and a less experienced novice. The contemporary literature is filled with various definitions and descriptions of mentoring. The mentor relationship is described as similar to the parent–child relationship in that it is usually charged with emotion and is a serious and mutual, nonsexual, loving relationship. The expression "inquisitive teacher" is used when discussing a mentor. From these descriptions, one can assume that mentoring is a high-level human relationship of some significance.

Descriptions of mentors include terminologies such as *caring, trusting, experienced, dedicated*, and almost always some elusive quality frequently called *chemistry*. Clearly, a mentoring relationship is different from the more superficial role model or preceptor that is also discussed in the nursing literature. For Haggard, Dougherty, Turban, and Wilbanks (2010), mentoring is portrayed as containing three essential or "core" attributes; reciprocity, developmental benefits, and regular/ consistent interaction.

---

CONSIDER THIS  Mentoring has been identified as one of the most powerful socialization strategies for professional and career advancement.

---

Perhaps most important for nurses is the research from the late 1970s and 1980s that focused on the unique nature of mentoring among women. Sargent (1977) discussed the many positive aspects of the mentor relationship as described in the literature but emphasized what she considered to be most important. The true value, beyond the teaching, sponsoring, and sharing roles, is the "blessing" in and of itself. To warrant the time and attention ("the blessing") of the mentor is the real worth to the mentee; to have someone believe in them enhances one's belief in self.

The business and management literature contains many references and discussions regarding the mentor–mentee phenomenon. Its value to organizational, as well as personal, development has been clearly established over the last 30 years. Schein (1978, pp. 177–178) discussed the obvious situation that exists in organizations when new employees look to more experienced personnel for advice and information. Schein developed several roles that the willing experienced "mentor" can assume to assist in the development of the new "mentee." The analysis concluded with the observation that the mentor does not necessarily have to be a recognized power figure within the organization, but that experience and willingness to share are important. Other characteristics common to mentoring are shown in Box 8.1.

Kanter (1977) was one of the earliest business-women to identify and use the term *sponsor* to describe the mentor relationship. According to Kanter, the very important role that sponsors play in the power struggle at all levels of the organization has three primary characteristics:

1. The ability to be often in a position to fight for a mentee. The propensity to point out superior performance at important times and promote or support a recommendation from a novice are essential ingredients of the sponsor relationship.

2. The ability to bypass the hierarchy and obtain inside information within the organization.

3. "Reflected power" or support from those with formal or informal power to accelerate the movement of the novice up the organizational ladder. (pp. 181–184)

## Stages of the Mentoring Relationship

Schira (2007) described the phases in mentoring relationships (Box 8.2). The first phase includes finding and connecting with a more experienced person in the workplace. A mentoring relationship can be established when a "chemistry" is present that fosters reciprocal trust and openness. The second phase includes teaching, modeling, and insider knowledge that fosters a sense of competence and confidence. The intensity of the relationship can escalate to high levels during this learning, listening, and sharing phase. The third phase includes a sense of change and growth as the mentoring relationship begins to move to a conclusion. The intensity wanes as the mentee begins to move toward independence. The last stage finds both the mentee and the mentor achieving a different, independent relationship, based (it can be hoped) on positive, collegial characteristics.

---

**BOX 8.1   CHARACTERISTICS OF THE MENTOR**

- *Open:* willing to see multiple perspectives
- *Flexible:* professionally agile and able to try different approaches
- *Perceptive:* insightful and knowledgeable about motives and subtleties
- *Believes:* someone who sees potential, "believes in" the mentee
- *Vision:* sees the possibilities, the big picture
- *Positive:* exudes energy and confidence
- *Motivates:* gives the mentee reason to change and stretch
- *Willing:* available with an "open door" policy
- *Unobtrusive:* steps back while pushing for growth
- *Protects*: able to shield the mentee from workplace danger

---

**BOX 8.2   STAGES OF THE MENTORING RELATIONSHIP**

1. Finding and connecting
2. Learning and listening
3. Changing and shifting
4. Mentoring others

*Source:* Schira, M. (2007). Leadership: A peak and perk of professional development. *Nephrology Nursing Journal, 34*(3), 289–294.

Separation and redefinition are often difficult because the mentor and mentee may share different perceptions about whether it is time to separate and what their new relationship should be. It is critically important for mentees *and* mentors that they should outgrow the need for such intense coaching if the mentor has done a good job of cultivation. Unfortunately, some mentoring relationships get "stuck" and fail to move forward the development of the novice. Personal and workplace circumstances and distractions can cause mentors and protégés to reach a comfort zone that prevents positive and ongoing development of the novice.

Typical mentoring relationships are usually characterized by the participants as intense. Any intense, high-level, interpersonal human relationship that evolves and changes can become a problem and have unfortunate ramifications, particularly in the workplace. As any intense relationship comes to a close, both participants must synchronize the separation or changed relationship. The literature identifies that most mentoring relationships evolve into a warm, lifelong, collegial friendship. Occasionally, however, either the mentor or protégé is unprepared for the end of a mentoring relationship, or an end is foisted on the participants due to job changes; this can cause serious unhappy individual and workplace consequences.

---

### DISCUSSION POINT

What strategies can be used when a mentee or protégé remains grateful and connected to the mentor but also begins to feel confined or restricted by a mentoring relationship?

---

## Mentoring Opportunities for Men and Women: Historical Differences

Before the 1970s, the business world often functioned on "the good ol' boys" network, with mentoring relationships between men an expected, accepted way to progress up the ladder of opportunity and promotion. The older, more experienced males were used to seeking out the younger, newer workplace (male) colleague who they deemed a protégé worthy of "judgment of potential." The golf course, the locker room, and after-work drinks between work colleagues all advanced exclusively male mentoring relationships and, in the meantime, excluded many women from promotional opportunities. This male-to-male mentoring

phenomenon spawned the famous invisible or "glass" ceiling that reduced career advancement opportunities for women and thus affected the predominantly female nursing profession.

---

CONSIDER THIS Mentoring opportunities for all women, and thus for nurses, have been far more limited than for their male counterparts.

---

Historically, then, there were not enough mentors for all the women who wanted one. In the past, far fewer women were in the workplace, and they were usually not at the higher, more visible organizational positions. The lack of emphasis on team sports for many baby boomer women likely contributed to the problem as it may have reduced their effectiveness in later life on a business or professional "team." In addition, solitary activities such as cooking and piano lessons were more common to young girls. Although the socialization of girls has undoubtedly changed in the last 20 years, at least some of these elements continue to exist.

Boys are still traditionally encouraged to participate in football, baseball, and basketball, developing expertise to use in a team effort. Another reason is the potential sexual aspects found in a close personal, albeit business or professional, relationship. Some men may subconsciously wish to avoid the potential complications of close cross-gender work relationships. It is conceivable that many men *still* fail to perceive talent that merits attention in career women.

---

CONSIDER THIS The socialization of young girls and boys has changed in subtle and not so subtle ways over the last 20 years as research has developed new ways of understanding learning and development. The effect of these changes will gradually change the workplace in expected and sometimes unexpected ways.

---

In addition, a shortage of mentors for women may be a result of the still low number of women in top-level business management who are both willing and available to be mentors to other women. Moreover, the emphasis on the affiliative socialization needs of women could affect the mentoring process. "Belonging" is still associated with feminine socialization; "achieving" is often the focus of socialization for men. Because the purpose of mentoring is achievement, it would seem that mentoring would be inconsistent with feminine socialization; however, the skills of cooperation and collaboration could also support and enhance mentoring.

Fortunately, mentoring opportunities for women are increasing. However, the gains are slower for women from diverse backgrounds. Women of color, very young or older women, and women with disabilities have more difficulty finding mentors than their more "traditional," accepted counterparts. Not having an influential mentor or sponsor can slow professional growth and development, reduce opportunities for advancement, and perpetuate the typical male-dominated organizational hierarchy.

> **CONSIDER THIS** It would be the unusual employer in Western society today who does not endeavor to encourage women into leadership roles. Employers are now developing strategies to encourage people from diverse backgrounds (i.e., ethnic, cultural, religious) to achieve promotion and fill leadership roles.

## Mentoring in Nursing

The presence or absence of mentoring within the nursing profession received attention only in the 1970s when the phenomenon became an important researchable topic. So much societal emphasis had been placed on gaining access to male-dominated professions that the predominantly female service-oriented professions remained underdeveloped. The labeling of "traditional" and "female" apparently had been influential in reducing appropriate attention to the mentoring process in these "traditionally female" occupations. Clearly, mentoring was identified and highly regarded in male-dominated workplaces long before it was noted as having potential for women and, later, nurses.

Vance (1977, 1982, 2000) was one of the earliest nurse researchers to explore mentoring in nursing. The mentoring phenomenon and its many permutations are widely acclaimed and largely accepted as an effective strategy for the personal and professional development of nurses in the workplace. It is not an uncommon occurrence to find an editorial or reflective comment in scholarly nursing journals regarding the benefits and positive outcomes associated with mentoring relationships. Interestingly, a 2011 Google search of "nurses" and "mentor" yielded 5,190,000 "hits."

> **DISCUSSION POINT**
>
> What alternatives are available to nurses who are new to a workplace or feel that a professional change is on the horizon, if there do not seem to be any available mentors for advice?

Clearly, nurses must actively seek out and perpetuate mentoring relationships. There is an overwhelming number of positive consequences for nurses who find the supportive interpersonal model that fits their current professional practice and health care workplace. The highly educated professional workforce found in today's health care organizations includes many nurses in powerful positions. Nurses must accept responsibility for individual and collective action to create and maintain an environment that is rewarding and supports positive socialization strategies for themselves and their professional colleagues.

## Increasing Opportunities for Mentoring

Not surprisingly, contemporary nursing literature encourages a more assertive, less passive approach to developing a mentoring relationship. It is not just the employee and the mentor who are advantaged but organizations are advantaged as well (Amagoh, 2009; King-Jones, 2011). Emphasis is placed on the responsibility of leading nurses to bring along, indeed seek out, newer nurses to develop within an area of expertise. Newer nurses are urged to seek out a mentor or mentors to assist them, especially at critical points in their career progress, such as in the beginning or during a change of career direction or promotion. Waiting for a mentor to find a protégé is not always an effective strategy.

As the nursing workforce ages and people remain in the workforce longer, health care organizations need to identify new ways of valuing mature, older, and experienced nurses and other health care professionals. It is not just the novice in a mentoring relationship who benefits. The mentor also receives many advantages. The recognition as a "wise one" is evident for many coworkers to see. The gratitude, challenge, and revitalization of acting in a mentoring role are renewing and pleasurable. Participating in and watching a novice develop confidence, assertiveness, and professional skills are high-level rewards for a mentor.

Additionally and unfortunately, not all nurses are altruistic or interested in the development of other nurses and the nursing profession. Eby, Butts, Durley, and Ragins (2010) describe how bad mentoring experiences can be *very* bad for the mentored. Many nurses can identify colleagues in the workplace who habitually target entry-level and/or vulnerable staff to undertake responsibilities and tasks that benefit the taskmaster. Often, delegation of tasks in this manner is a pattern or habit and can involve a number of dependent, unacknowledged, and exploited staff. Fawning and groveling behavior is encouraged and expected by the taskmaster. This person can abuse his or her (perceived) authority, position, or experience and, in the guise of a pseudo-mentoring bond, encourage the development of an inappropriate workplace relationship. Such relationships should not be confused with mentoring and need to be exposed and named.

CONSIDER THIS  In some cultures, older (less productive and dependent) people were literally or figuratively pushed away to die in isolation. Today, Western cultures are changing the way older people are viewed by placing value and appreciation on the wisdom that comes with experience.

Before the current nursing shortage, research into the mentoring phenomenon was essentially limited to strategies to assist nurses to gain promotion up and away from the bedside. Encouraging nurses to stay in nursing, and particularly at the bedside, became a new and strategically important goal of mentoring and other supportive behaviors. As the shortage of bedside nurses has increased substantially, interest has increased in how mentoring, role modeling, and other supportive behaviors might socialize nurses and improve retention.

## Value of Mentoring in Recruitment and Retention

In an effort to improve recruitment as well as retention, some organizations have initiated programs that "assign" mentors and mentees when the workplace situation does not allow for spontaneous mentoring relationships to develop. Johnson and Andersen (2010) describe the difficulty in establishing and maintaining an effective formal mentoring program in an (military) organization. They describe the problems associated with timing, monitoring, and qualifications of the mentor and

mentored. Much of the current literature identifies the importance of an organization's leaders and high-visibility health professionals to demonstrate the valuing of supportive and positive behaviors. Recognizing the ever more diverse nature of the nursing and health care work environment would seem fundamental to recruitment, retention, and fostering mentoring values.

Kramer (2010) described the current challenge for organizations—an aging, soon-to-retire workforce and the necessity to establish a workplace that is attractive to a younger, perhaps less patient, workforce. She cautions against professionals and organizations ignoring or failing to address the tensions associated with generational diversity. A health care workplace culture of respect and empowerment would seem to be the current imperative of nursing leaders. Kramer also described the important strength that comes with unity and a respect for diversity among RNs. Organizations need to understand differences and ways to approach and motivate based on this understanding. Flexibility in accommodating differences and capitalizing on the strength associated with diversity is an imperative of the organization. Respecting and then actively acknowledging the ever-expanding and different contributions will foster a workplace that enjoys good recruitment and retention statistics.

A culturally competent health care workplace must also understand and appreciate the contribution of racial and ethnic diversity. Bond, Gray, Baxley, Cason, and Denke (2008) explored challenges associated with the socialization of Hispanic nurses into the health care arena. Their interest was in improving the understanding of how Hispanic nurses might view nursing and nursing education differently, in hopes of addressing recruitment and retention, as well as improving health disparities among a large minority.

## Mentoring and Developmental Stages

Nurses should be acquainted with adult developmental issues and life transitions as they relate to wellness and illness. Linking this information to the mentoring phenomenon and workplace socialization is important. It will be clear that establishing a mentoring relationship can be enormously important not only to the novice but also to the mentor.

It was only in the 1970s that Gail Sheehy (1976) in *Passages* and Daniel Levinson (1978) in *The Seasons of Man's Life* connected mentoring and adult developmental theory. They emphasized that people continue to change throughout their adult life. Levinson found, among other information, that in early adulthood (ages 20 to 40 years), several distinct developmental changes occur in a certain sequence. Young people between 22 and 28 years of age enter the adult world. From 28 to 33 years of age, they analyze what has occurred so far and take steps to alter or change what they feel is inappropriate. From 33 years of age to midlife, they invest in realizing their goals or, as Sheehy describes, "climbing the career ladder."

Near age 40 years, people stop to take stock of the first half of their life. The compromises that were necessary in the first half of their life and the realization or lack of realization of their goal(s) are crucial components of the infamous midlife transition. At approximately 45 years of age, a pattern is established that modifies a life structure to accommodate the midlife analysis. Both Levinson and Sheehy identified that for many people the last half of their adult life is the fullest and most satisfying. There was evidence that the same transitional periods as opposed to stable periods continue throughout adulthood.

Both works point out clear life stages marked by internal changes not directly related to external changes, such as divorce, death, marriage, births, and the like. Both Sheehy and Levinson refer to the period of the post-midlife review as being fulfilling, renewing, and satisfying or being full of resignation and stagnation, depending on how one has dealt with previous transitional periods. This conceptual framework is relevant and pertinent for the nurse in the 21st century.

---

CONSIDER THIS Research indicates that internal (life) changes occur despite external or extrinsic changes. Nurses in today's health care environment frequently encounter workplace transfers and employment changes, as well as longer and more diverse careers. The health care workforce has greater differences in age, ethnicity, and gender than ever before.

---

The changes and growth, or lack of growth, demonstrated in the different life stages are interconnected. There are always new heights to be climbed, but the next step is not simply another rung on the same ladder. The top of the first ladder turns out to be the bottom rung on a new ladder (Levinson, 1978, p. 154). During the final thrust toward achievement of success, individuals must devote themselves to that end at the expense of other important parts of themselves. Many believe that if they become the president of the company or the shop steward or whatever their dream might be, they will achieve happiness and contentment forever. At midlife,

an internal mechanism forces most adults to look at the price that has been paid for the place in which they find themselves.

Levinson and Sheehy both described the importance of recognizing the costs and gains and the necessary trade-offs that come to light during midlife analysis. The wisdom that may develop after midlife sets the stage for mentoring. At certain transitional points in life, the mentor relationship has profound and significant value to both participants. Seeing the ladder ahead, one can often see someone ahead who has been climbing.

Schein's (1978) research included the observation that the midlife analysis exposes a career spent as a leader or a key contributor or as dead wood. Levinson stated that the mentor functions primarily as a transitional figure. The mentor "is usually older than the protégé by a half-generation, roughly 8 to 15 years" and is experienced as a "responsible, admirable, older sibling" (Levinson, 1978, pp. 177–178). It would appear that the pre-midlife adult would be most susceptible to the protégé role, just as the post-midlife adult would be most susceptible to the mentoring role. Welcoming, acquainting, guiding, hosting, and counseling roles would serve both adults well.

That said, in their recent meta-analytic investigative research described earlier, Haggard et al. (2010) revealed that mentoring today has evolved and no longer consists of a mentor somewhat older than the mentee and one or two levels higher in the organization. The implication of their findings identify the importance of novice or early career professionals being aware that mentors may be found in diverse settings; across the gender gap, in other professions, and in a wide variety of ages, ethnicity, and experience.

Levinson referred to "generativity," or the sense that one feels for the continuity of life and the concern for the future generations. This can be seen at home, at work, in friendships, in government, and by many nurses. Usually, only after midlife does this sense of responsibility for the development of others take an active form. A clear understanding of adult developmental theory lends credence to the significance and importance of mentoring for the mentor as well as for the protégé.

## CREATING A SUPPORTIVE ENVIRONMENT FOR SOCIALIZATION AND RESOCIALIZATION

The workplace environment is key to nurse satisfaction, retention, and patient care (Porter, Kolcaba, McNulty, & Fitzpatrick, 2010; Spence Laschinger, Leiter, Day, &

Gilin, 2009; Spetz & Herrera, 2010). Employers and nurse leaders have significant responsibility for creating a workplace that genuinely values supportive behaviors, such as mentoring. Many health care organizations encourage and recommend that nurses take advantage of the opportunity to mentor throughout their professional careers. The literature is replete with multiple examples of various forms of formal and informal mentoring programs.

---

CONSIDER THIS   Today's nurses encounter higher workloads and sicker patients than ever before. Energy to combat demeaning and abusive behaviors from workplace colleagues is in short supply because so much energy must be directed to providing safe and competent patient care. This situation encourages workplace and professional "silence," which is an impediment to individual and professional growth.

---

## Leadership

Highly visible organizational leader(s) must "walk the walk," not merely "talk the talk." All leaders and managers in health care facilities need to demonstrate supportive behaviors and identify and support formal and informal mentoring or other supportive programs at individual as well as departmental levels. For positive socialization such as mentoring to flourish, and for the nursing profession to reach its greatest potential, RNs need to be proactive and find ways to facilitate professional and individual growth-producing workplace strategies (Box 8.3).

A workplace culture in which mutual respect is evident in all written and verbal communications is an important strategy for organizations. One of the favorite pastimes of employees everywhere is to observe closely, and then dissect, each word, behavior, and nuance of their managers, supervisors, and leaders. Appropriate acknowledgment, respectful tones, and public positive reinforcement can have long-term and lasting individual and group consequences. However, an impatient, poorly expressed personal or professional observation from a high-visibility person in the organization will be described and embellished throughout the organization for far longer than anyone might anticipate.

Organizational leaders can use a language that creates a positive and supportive work environment. What is included in the language is as important as what is excluded. Seeking out superior performance, knowing

and using people's names, acknowledging the ideas or work of others, and identifying and reducing roadblocks or unnecessary bureaucracy in the workplace need to be everyday occurrences for leaders and managers. However, "constructive criticism" or even "suggestions" can be unhelpful and, more important, go unheeded when presented in front of others. Using these basic interpersonal and professional communication skills is essential in a workplace that hopes to attract and retain high-quality health care professionals.

Organizations are responsible for the ongoing education and training of all employees, including leaders and managers. Poorly trained and performing leaders are the responsibility of the organization's executive and corporate level. Allowing inadequate leaders and leadership to prevail in an organization has long-term serious and negative consequences. Alternatively, an effective, persuasive role model and leader can energize and empower numerous employees and thereby promote a positive, effective workplace. This is particularly important in a health care workplace, where highly educated professionals quite clearly know what they expect from their work environment and organizational leadership (see Research Study Fuels the Controversy).

## Sponsors, Guides, Preceptors, and Role Models

Organizations can also create work environments supportive of socialization through their use of sponsors, guides, preceptors, and role models. Shapiro, Haseltine,

---

### BOX 8.3   TRAITS OF WORK CULTURES THAT PROMOTE POSITIVE SOCIALIZATION

1. Mutual respect is evident in all written and verbal communications.
2. There is appropriate acknowledgment of the ideas and work of others.
3. Superior performance is sought and recognized publicly.
4. Roadblocks to goal achievement or unnecessary bureaucracy in the workplace are identified and addressed promptly.
5. Expectations are clear.
6. Criticism is constructive and given in private.

## RESEARCH STUDY FUELS THE CONTROVERSY

### NURSE LEADER MENTOR AS A MODE OF BEING: FINDINGS FROM AN AUSTRALIAN HERMENEUTIC PHENOMENOLOGICAL STUDY

The purpose of this recent phenomenological research study into the understanding and experiences of mentorship for nurse leaders was to determine how mentorship was conceptualized and whether mentoring contributed to leadership development.

McCloughen, A., O'Brien, L., & Jackson, D. (2011). Nurse leader mentor as a mode of being: Findings from an Australian hermeneutic phenomenological study, *Journal of Nursing Scholarship, 43*(1), 97–104.

### STUDY FINDINGS

The worldwide shortage of RNs has generated substantial research into the phenomenon of nursing socialization, mentoring, and leadership development. This study found that mentoring was a significant factor to the 13 Australian nurse leaders in this study. The researchers found three existential motifs: imagination, journey, and mode of being. *Imagination* allowed nurse mentors to envision all the possibilities that exist for new, less experienced nurses. The unfolding life *journey* of the leader/mentors informed their mentoring attitudes and professional ways of behaving. "Being a mentor was a life position that permeated all intentions and understandings" (p. 99). *Mode of being* reflected their current life position, attitudes, and professional behavior. This research identifies that rather than the classical, spontaneous development of a mentoring relationship, mentors are not living a role; rather the leader describes mentoring "as simply part of their character, an essential and natural aspect of who they were" (p. 103). The study identified participants who could not help but seek ways to develop the potential for leadership. The study illuminated the wide diversity of contexts in which the nurse mentor lived and worked; mentoring was not a simple, singular role; rather it was integrated and deeply embedded in their life and professional work.

and Rowe (1978) suggested that a continuum exists with mentors and peer pals as endpoints and sponsors and guides as internal points on the continuum. At one end are the mentors, who have the most "intense and paternalistic" roles. Sponsors and then guides are at the two-thirds point; sponsors are less powerful in affecting their charges, whereas guides are invaluable in explaining the system. The peer pal, or today's clinical preceptor, is at the other end of the continuum from a mentor. The peer pal or preceptor encourages a relationship between peers as they help each other succeed and progress.

A surprising level of camaraderie can develop between preceptors and students when preceptored clinical experiences are organized. Attention to the socialization of developing nurses in the real world of evening, night, and weekend shifts can be expected to promote a bond between experienced and less experienced nurses. Their experiences do not support the notion that nurses "eat their young." Smedley (2008) explored the development of successful preceptor skills as experienced nurses facilitated the learning, focus, and comfort in the health care workplace of less experienced nurses. She found and identified several characteristics important to successful preceptors; consistent with the literature presented here, three of them were positive attitudes, patience, and the desire to motivate others to learn. Similarly, Hammer and Craig (2008) found that having one specified nurse colleague to answer questions, provide support, and assist the individual nurse in the specific clinical setting was closely linked with ultimately positive experiences and outcomes. The early orientation period was of critical importance to these nurses.

> CONSIDER THIS Clinical coordinators or preceptors are commonly assigned to one or more student nurses during their clinical practice placement. Qualities found in the various supportive roles identified here may or may not be readily available to students in today's health care workplace.

## CONCLUSIONS

Understanding the socialization of novice nurses and the resocialization of nurses in transition or at the peak of their performance is critical to the nursing profession and the health of society. The realization of the full potential of nurses and the nursing profession has a direct effect on patient care and patient outcomes. The history and knowledge available through the nursing research reviewed here authenticate the importance of understanding and developing a range of strategies that enhance positive, supportive socialization among nurses. The continuing evolution toward professionalization and autonomy that sustains and enhances nurse empowerment is the most effective recruitment and retention strategy available.

Nurses comprise the largest group of health professionals, and most nurses practice nursing within an organization. Considering that hospitals are substantial business enterprises with complicated, multifaceted hierarchies and that nurses are largely responsible for significant departmental budgets, one cannot help but see that interest in and research on professional development and positive socialization such as mentoring relationships are important. Today's health care organizations, administrators, health care professionals and particularly nurses, have a vested interest in recognizing and supporting mentoring programs, relationships, and behaviors.

It is within the hospital organization that most nurses develop or grow as individuals and as professionals. Administrators and medical staff need to consider interdisciplinary mentoring relationships because this cross-fertilization will enhance professional relationships in the health care workplace. Altering the workplace to encourage real partnerships among all health professionals with clear appreciation and acknowledgment of the unique contribution of each discipline remains a challenge.

This chapter began with observations about the international contemporary health care workplace and the challenges associated with socialization and mentoring experiences. These experiences are complicated further by issues closely linked to diversity and equity: age, gender, ethnicity, culture, people with disabilities, and life experience differences. Such diversity will find organizations that are rich, vibrant, and resilient. Lack of diversity is monotony, dysfunctional. . . . and ultimately weak. Organizations and professions, who do not welcome debate and differences, will not thrive, grow, and develop to full potential. As professionals, our contribution and the contribution of our diverse colleagues is to be celebrated, nurtured, and potentiated. The strategies outlined in this chapter will contribute to that effort.

## FOR ADDITIONAL DISCUSSION

1. What are some health care workplace behaviors associated with typical oppressed groups?

2. Describe strategies that might be effective in reducing typical oppressed-group behavior.

3. Who is advantaged when negative socialization occurs in the health care workplace? Why?

4. Describe five career changes or transitions that might be facilitated by a mentoring relationship.

5. In what ways does a mentoring relationship provide an advantage to the mentor?

6. What are the advantages and disadvantages to a nursing professional of having positive or negative socialization strategies?

7. Will having increasing numbers of people in nursing from diverse backgrounds and life experience change the frequency or kinds of mentoring relationships that exist in nursing?

8. How can research continue to develop notions associated with positive socialization in the nursing profession?

## REFERENCES

Amagoh, F. (2009). Leadership development and leadership effectiveness. *Management Decision, 47*(6), 989–999.

Bond, M. L., Gray, J. R., Baxley, S., Cason, C. L., & Denke, L. (2008). Voices of Hispanic students in baccalaureate nursing programs: Are we listening? *Nursing Education Perspectives, 29*(3), 136–142.

Carlson, E., Pilhammar, E., & Wann-Hansson, C. (2010). "This is nursing": Nursing roles as mediated by precepting nurses during clinical practice. *Nurse Education Today, 30*(8), 763–767.

Chamberlain, L., & Hodson, R. (2010). Toxic work environments: What helps and what hurts. *Sociological Perspectives, 53*(4), 455–478.

Clarke, C., Kane, D., Rajacich, D., & Lafreniere, K. (2012). Bullying in undergraduate clinical nursing education. *Journal of Nursing Education, 51*(5), 269–276.

Cohen, A., & Veled-Hecht, A. (2010). The relationship between organizational socialization and commitment in the workplace among employees in long-term nursing care facilities. *Personnel Review, 39*(5), 537–556.

Dodd, J., Saggers, S., & Wildy, H. (2009). Retention in the allied health workforce: Boomers, Generation X, and Generation Y. *Journal of Allied Health, 38*(4), 215–219.

Duteau, J. (2012). Making a difference: The value of preceptorship programs in nursing education. *Journal of Continuing Education in Nursing, 43*(1), 37–43.

Eby, L., Butts, M., Durley, J., & Ragins, B. (2010). Are bad experiences stronger than good ones in mentoring relationships? Evidence from the protégé and mentor perspective. *Journal of Vocational Behaviour, 77*, 81–92.

Freire, P. (1968). *Pedagogy of the oppressed.* New York, NY: Seabury Press.

Haggard, D., Dougherty, T., Turban, D., & Wilbanks, J. (2010). Who is a mentor? A review of evolving definitions and implications for research. *Journal of Management, 37*(1), 280–304.

Hammer, V. R., & Craig, G. P. (2008). The experiences of inactive nurses returned to nursing after completing a refresher course. *Journal of Continuing Education in Nursing, 39*(8), 358–368.

Johnson, W., & Andersen, G. (2010). Formal mentoring in the U.S. Military. *Naval War College Review, 63*(2), 113–126.

Kanter, R. (1977). *Men and Women of the Organization.* New York: Basic Books, Inc.

King-Jones, M. (2011). Horizontal violence and the socialization of new nurses. *Creative Nursing, 17*(2), 80–86.

Kramer, L. (2010). Generational diversity. *Dimensions of Critical Care Nursing, 29*(3), 125–128.

Kramer, M. (1974). *Reality shock: Why nurses leave nursing.* St. Louis, MO: Mosby.

Kramer, M. (1981). *Coping with reality shock.* Workshop presented at Jackson Memorial Hospital, Miami, FL.

Levinson, D. (1978). *The seasons of man's life.* New York, NY: Alfred A. Knopf.

MacEachen, E., Kosny, A., Ferrier, S., & Chambers, L. (2010). The "toxic dose" of system problems: Why some injured workers don't return to work as expected. *Journal of Occupational Rehabilitation, 20*(3), 349–366.

Marquis, B., & Huston, C. (2012). *Leadership roles and management functions in nursing* (7th ed.). Philadelphia, PA: Lippincott Williams & Wilkins.

McCloughen, A., O'Brien, L., & Jackson, D. (2011). Nurse leader mentor as a mode of being: Findings from an Australian hermeneutic phenomenological study. *Journal of Nursing Scholarship, 43*(1), 97–104.

Porter, C., Kolcaba, K., McNulty, R., & Fitzpatrick, J. (2010). The effect of a nursing labor management partnership on nurse turnover and satisfaction. *Journal of Nursing Management, 40*(5), 205–210.

Rhodes, M., Schutt, M., Langham, G., & Bilotta, D. (2012). The journey to nursing professionalism: A learner-centered approach. *Nursing Education Perspectives, 33*(1), 27–29.

Sargent, A. G. (1977). *Beyond sex roles.* St. Paul, MN: West.

Schein, E. (1978). *Career dynamics: Matching individual and organizational needs.* Reading, MA: Addison-Wesley.

Schira, M. (2007). Leadership: A peak and perk of professional development. *Nephrology Nursing Journal, 34*(3), 289–294.

Shapiro, E. C., Haseltine, F. P., & Rowe, M. P. (1978). Moving up: Role models, mentors and the "patron system." *Sloan Management Review, 19*(3), 51–58.

Sheehy, G. (1976). *Passages: Predictable crises of adult life.* New York, NY: Bantam.

Smedley, A. (2008). Becoming and being a preceptor: A phenomenological study. *Journal of Continuing Education in Nursing, 39*(4), 185–191.

Spence Laschinger, H., Leiter, M., Day, A., & Gilin, D. (2009). Workplace empowerment, incivility, and burnout: Impact on staff nurse recruitment and retention outcomes. *Journal of Nursing Management, 17*(3), 302–311.

Spetz, J., & Herrera, C. (2010). Changes in nurse satisfaction in California, 2004 to 2008. *Journal of Nursing Management, 18*(5), 564–572.

Vance, C. N. (1977). *A group profile of contemporary influentials in American nursing* (Doctoral dissertation). Teachers College, Columbia University, New York, NY.

Vance, C. (1982). The mentor connection. *Journal of Nursing Administration, 12*(4), 7–13.

Vance, C. (2000). Discovering the riches in mentoring connections. *Reflections on Nursing Leadership, 26*(3), 24–25.

Walrafen, N., Brewer, M., & Mulvenon, C. (2012). Sadly caught up in the moment: An exploration of horizontal violence. *Nursing Economics, 30*(1), 6–13, 49.

## BIBLIOGRAPHY

Anonymous. (2012). Workforce Violence Survey. *Florida Nurse, 60*(1), 13.

Arndt, J., King, S., Suter, E., Mazonde, J., Taylor, E., & Arthur, N. (2009). Socialization in health education: Encouraging an integrated, interprofessional socialization process. *Journal of Allied Health, 38*(1), 18–23.

Bae, S. H. (2011). Organizational socialization of international nurses in the New York metropolitan area. *International Nursing Review, 59*(1), 81–87.

Bednarz, H., Schim, S., & Doorenbos, A. (2010). Cultural diversity in nursing education: Perils, pitfalls and pearls. *Journal of Nursing Education, 49*(5), 252–260.

Bisholt, B. (2012). The professional socialization of recently graduated nurses—Experiences of an introduction program. *Nurse Education Today, 32*, 278–282.

Cleary, B., Hassmiller, S., Reinhard, S., Richardson, E., Veenema, T., & Werner, S. (2010). Uniting state, sharing strategies: Forging partnerships to expand nursing education capacity. *American Journal of Nursing, 110*(1), 43–50.

Cubit, K., & Ryan, B. (2011). Tailoring a graduate nurse program to meet the needs of our next generation nurses. *Nurse Education Today, 31*(1), 65–71.

Currie, D. (2011). The socially just face of public health leadership: Linda Rae Murray. *American Journal of Public Health, 101*(2), 209–211.

Duffy, K. (2012). Mentoring the mentors. *Nursing Standard, 26*(2), 61.

Galperin, B., Bennett, R., & Aquino, K. (2011). Status differentiation and the Protean self: A social-cognitive model of unethical behavior in organizations. *Journal of Business Ethics, 98*, 407–424.

Gustafson, D., & Reitmanova, S. (2010). How are we "doing" cultural diversity? A look across English Canadian undergraduate medical school programs. *Medical Teacher, 32*(10), 816–823.

Hafferty, F., & Hafler, J. (2011). The hidden curriculum, structural disconnects, and the socialization of professionals. *Innovation and Change in Professional Education, 6*(1), 17–35.

Holmes, A. (2011). Transforming education. *Nursing Management, 42*(4), 34–38.

Katz, R. (2011). Larry Meskin: A man of his time with vision beyond his time. *Journal of Dental Research, 90*(2), 154–156.

Lipscomb, M., & Snelling, P. (2010). Student nurse absenteeism in higher education: An argument against enforced attendance. *Nurse Education Today, 30*(6), 573–578.

Mahon, K. (2011). In praise of servant leadership—Horizontal service to others. *Dynamics—Canadian Association of Critical Care Nurses, 22*(4), 5–6.

Mkandawire-Valhmu, L., Kako, P., & Stevens, P. (2010). Mentoring women faculty of color in nursing academia: Creating an environment that supports scholarly growth and retention. *Nursing Outlook, 58*(3), 135–141.

Nairn S., Hardy, C., Harling, M., Parumal, L., & Narayanasamy, M. (2011). Diversity and ethnicity in nurse education: The perspective of nursing lecturers. *Nurse Education Today, 32*(3), 203–207.

Odro, A., Clancy, C., & Foster, J. (2010). Bridging the theory-practice gap in student nurse training: An evaluation of a personal and professional development programme. *Journal of Mental Health Training, Education and Practice, 5*(2), 4–12.

Olinger, B. (2011). Increasing nursing workforce diversity: Strategies for success. *Nurse Educator, 36*(2), 54–55.

Pelletier, K. (2010). Leader toxicity: An empirical investigation of toxic behavior and rhetoric. *Leadership, 6*(4), 373–389.

Phiri, J., Dietsch, E., & Bonner, A. (2010). Cultural safety and its importance for Australian midwifery practice. *Collegian: Journal of the Royal College of Nursing Australia, 17*(3), 105–111.

Sanner, S., Baldwin, D., Cannella, K., Charles, J., & Parker, L. (2010). The impact of cultural diversity forum on students' openness to diversity. *Journal of Cultural Diversity, 17*(2), 56–61.

Sullivan, L., & Suez Mittman, I. (2010). The state of diversity in the health professions a century after Flexner. *Academic Medicine, 85*(2), 246–253.

Toman, C., & Thifault, M. C. (2012). Historical thinking and the shaping of nursing identity. *Nursing History Review, 20*, 184.

Young, S. (2012). Does nursing school facilitate lateral and horizontal violence? *Tennessee nurse, 74*(3), 1, 4.

# Chapter 9

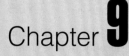

# Diversity in the Nursing Workforce

Carol J. Huston

## ADDITIONAL RESOURCES

Visit the Point* for additional helpful resources
- eBook
- Journal Articles
- WebLinks

## CHAPTER OUTLINE

## LEARNING OBJECTIVES

*The learner will be able to:*

1. Examine the relationship between health disparities and a lack of diversity in the health care workforce.

2. Reflect on personal beliefs and values regarding the assertion that diversity, equity, and parity are both moral imperatives and a corporate social responsibility.

3. Explore factors leading to the lack of ethnic and gender diversity in nursing.

4. Suggest individual, organizational, and professional strategies to increase ethnic and gender diversity in nursing.

5. Identify common barriers faced in both recruiting and retaining minority students and faculty in higher education.

6. Compare opportunity levels for decision making at senior levels of health care management between racial/ethnic minorities and Whites and between men and women.

7. Identify at least three professional nursing associations that are directed at serving the needs of a specific racial or ethnic population.

8. Investigate stereotypes of male nurses that both hinder the recruitment and retention of men into nursing and pose socialization and acceptance challenges for them.

9. Compare economic and advancement opportunities for men and women in nursing.

10. Argue for or against the need for affirmative action to bring more men into the nursing profession.

11. Analyze research exploring generational differences in work values and preferences among registered nurses and explore the challenges inherent in having up to four generations cohabitate in the same profession at the same time.

Diversity has been defined as the differences among groups or between individuals, and it comes in many forms, including age, gender, religion, customs, sexual orientation, physical size, physical and mental capabilities, beliefs, culture, ethnicity, and skin color. Yet, despite increasing diversity (particularly ethnic and cultural) in the United States, the nursing workforce continues to be fairly homogeneous, at least in terms of ethnicity and gender, being White, female, and middle aged. In fact, the Health Resources and Service Administration (HRSA, 2010) reported that as of 2008, Blacks/African Americans, Asians, Hispanics, and American Indian/Alaska Natives together comprised only 16.8% of the nursing workforce, an increase from 12.2% in 2004.

This lack of ethnic, gender, and generational diversity is a concern not only for the nursing profession but also for its clients. Clearly, the nursing workforce should be at least as diverse as the population it serves. Not only is a lack of diversity in the workforce linked to health disparities but also minority health care professionals are more likely than their White peers to work in underserved communities, which, in turn, improves access among underrepresented groups (Giddens, 2008).

In addition, a connection should exist between diversity and corporate social responsibility (CSR). Wiley-Little (2011) defines CSR as "aligning a company's activities with the social, economic, and environmental expectations of its stakeholders" (p. 10). Thus employers have a social responsibility to do what is best for the greater community. Having a diverse employee pool which mirrors the diversity of the population being served and being culturally sensitive to and supportive of all aspects of diversity fosters healthy communities. The same argument could be made for the nursing profession in that there is a responsibility to see that an adequate number of diverse health care providers are available to meet the needs and wants of the population being served because this not only minimizes health disparities but also improves quality of care. Linking diversity and CSP, however, will require an investment of time, talent, and resources for the long term if sustainable change with long-term results is to be achieved (Wiley-Little, 2011).

Indeed, a clamor for greater diversity in the profession continues to occur, and this is readily apparent in a review of the literature. S. K. Banschbach (2008), president of the American Organization of Operating Nurses (AORN), suggested that although some might "marvel at how far we have come in terms of accepting racial and gender differences" (p. 1067), a mixture of professionals with different attributes and skills playing various roles is absolutely essential to an effective organization. Indeed, the Sullivan Commission on Diversity in the Health Care Workforce went so far as to say that "a disproportionately white health care workforce cannot adequately serve a population that is increasingly nonwhite" (Dixon, 2008, para. 6). De Leon Siantz (2008) agrees, suggesting that the elimination of health disparities in the 21st century depends on having nurse leaders who reflect the ethnic and racial diversity of the communities in which they live.

Similarly, the Joint Commission (2008) released a report titled *One Size Does Not Fit All: Meeting the Health Care Needs of Diverse Populations.* This report calls on health care organizations to meet the unique cultural and language needs of a diverse population and provides a tool for organizations to use that promotes patient safety and health care quality for all patients.

In addition, the 2010 Institute of Medicine (IOM) report *The Future of Nursing* suggests that to improve the quality of patient care, more emphasis must be placed on making the nursing workforce diverse, particularly in the areas of gender and race/ethnicity (Lecher, 2011). As a result, the American Assembly for Men in Nursing (AAMN) has launched a campaign (known as 20 × 20) that aims to make 20% of nursing student enrollment men by the year 2020 (Lecher, 2011).

### DISCUSSION POINT

For nursing care to be culturally and ethnically sensitive, must it be provided by a culturally and ethnically diverse nursing population?

Historically, despite this stated need for and appreciation of the benefits of a diverse health care workforce, efforts to increase the number of minority professionals have not been as successful as hoped. The reasons barriers remain are numerous, but the roots can certainly be found in racism, discrimination, and a lack of commitment to changing the situation. Antczak (2011) concurs, suggesting that racism and prejudice from patients and co-workers are still a very real reality for nurses who are not White females. She suggests this is often rooted in a lack of cultural competence and argues that the nursing profession has not evolved as fast as the rest of America's industries in dealing with issues of diversity. This is likely why cultural sensitivity has been identified as one of the eight *Essentials of*

*Baccalaureate Education for Professional Nursing Practice* identified by the American Association of Colleges of Nursing (AACN; 2008).

---

CONSIDER THIS   Barriers to increasing the number of minority health care professionals include, but are not limited to, racism, discrimination, and a lack of commitment to changing the situation.

---

This chapter focuses primarily on three aspects of diversity in the nursing workforce: ethnicity, gender, and age (generational factors). Factors leading to the lack of ethnic and gender diversity in nursing are explored, as are individual and organizational strategies to address the problem. (The importation of foreign nurses as a factor in workforce diversity is discussed in Chapter 6.) In addition, the efforts of current professional nursing organizations to increase diversity in the profession are examined. Finally, the effect of generational diversity on workers and workplace functioning is presented.

## ETHNIC DIVERSITY

### Ethnic Diversity in the United States

Demographic data from the U.S. Census Bureau continues to show increased diversification of the U.S.

population, a trend that began almost 35 years ago. As of 2010, 63.7% of the population was White, not of Hispanic origin (U.S. Census Bureau, 2011). Hispanics continue to be the largest minority group at 16.3% and are the fastest growing population group (U.S. Census Bureau, 2011). Blacks are the second largest minority group (12.6%), followed by Asians (4.8%), American Indians and Alaska natives (0.9%), and native Hawaiians and other Pacific Islanders (0.2%). Wilson, Sanner, and McAllister (2010) note that by 2020, nearly one half of the population of the United States is expected to be a mixture of various ethnic groups.

### Ethnic Diversity in Nursing

There are significant differences between the ethnic and gender demographics of the U.S. population and those of the nursing workforce in the United States (Table 9.1). Whereas the number of nurses from minority backgrounds continues to rise in the United States, it is considerably lower than the minority representation in the general population.

According to the latest National Sample Survey of Registered Nurses (NSSRN) from 2008, nurses from minority backgrounds represent just 16.8% of the registered nurse (RN) workforce, with the RN population comprising 83.2% White, 5.4% African American, 3.6% Hispanic, 5.8% Asian/Native Hawaiian, 0.3% American Indian/Alaskan Native, and 1.7% multiracial nurses (AACN, 2011a). Creating a nursing workforce

---

**TABLE 9.1**   Comparison of U.S. Population and Registered Nurse Workforce in Terms of Ethnicity and Gender

| Characteristic | Year 2010 U.S. Census Data (% Representation) | Year 2004 Registered Nurse Workforce (% Representation) |
|---|---|---|
| Gender: Male | 49.3 | 6.2 |
| Gender: Female | 50.7 | 93.8 |
| White (non-Hispanic) | 63.7 | 83.2 |
| Black/African American | 12.6 | 5.4 |
| Asian/Native Hawaiian/Pacific Islander | 5.0 | 5.8 |
| American Indian/Alaskan native | 0.9 | 0.3 |
| Hispanic/Latino | 16.3 | 3.6 |
| Persons Responding to two or more races | 2.9 | 1.7 |

*Source:* AACN (2011a); U.S. Census Bureau. (2011). *State and county quick facts.* Retrieved July 9, 2011, from http://quickfacts.census.gov/qfd/states/00000.html

that mirrors the degree of diversity in the general population will not be easy. As Dixon (2008) pointed out, "An increase of more than 20,000 minority nurses is needed to increase their proportion of the nursing workforce by just 1%" (para. 10).

Clearly, though, increasing diversity in the nursing profession must begin with the aggressive recruitment and retention of minority students. Ackerman-Barger (2010), in extrapolating data from the *Chronicle of Higher Education* and recent census data, notes that higher education campuses in the United States are not ethnically diverse, with White students dominating campus enrollment at a rate not proportional to White representation in the population. She also notes that when there is enrollment of minority students, it is often in concentrated groups of ethnic minorities. This is especially true for *traditionally underrepresented students* from ethnic backgrounds including, but not limited to, Black, Latino, Native American, and Asian, with these students typically being first-generation college students and low-income students (Ackerman-Barger, 2010).

The AACN's 2010–2011 report *Enrollment and Graduations in Baccalaureate and Graduate Programs in Nursing* is more encouraging, suggesting that 26.8% of nursing students in entry-level baccalaureate programs are now from minority backgrounds (AACN, 2011a). In addition, about 26.1% of master's students and 23.3% of students in research-focused doctoral programs are also from minority backgrounds. Still more must be done to reach equal representation.

It is encouraging to note that according to the 2008 NSSRN, registered nurses from minority backgrounds are, however, more likely than their White counterparts to pursue baccalaureate and higher degrees in nursing (AACN, 2011a). Only 48.4% of White nurses complete nursing degrees beyond the associate degree, in contrast to 52.5% of African Americans, 51.5% of Hispanics, and 75.6% of Asian nurses: "RNs from minority backgrounds clearly recognize the need to pursue higher levels of nursing education beyond the entry-level" (AACN, 2011a, para. 5).

---

### DISCUSSION POINT

Why are RNs from minority backgrounds more likely than their White counterparts to pursue higher education beyond their entry level? What factors might be contributing to this trend?

---

## Recruiting Minority Students Into Nursing

De Leon Siantz (2008) suggests that the key to recruiting more minority students into nursing is the creation of a corporate environment in schools of nursing that integrates diversity and cultural competence across academic programs, research, practice, and public policy to eliminate health disparities in partnership with faculty, students, staff, the university infrastructure, and the community at large. Sequist (2007) concurs, suggesting that financial constraints, as well as a lack of appropriate mentorship, are root causes of the low enrollment of Native American students in medical school and other health-related degree tracks. Sequist suggests that academic institutions can play a vital role in reaching out to provide the appropriate experiences and resources that will engage Native American students and help them take the next step toward a career in health care but cautioned that these programs should always be accompanied by an appropriate evaluation structure that ensures continued improvement and facilitation of particular student needs.

Oscos-Sanchez, Oscos-Flores, and Burge (2008) outlined a different strategy for promoting the recruitment of underrepresented students in health careers in their description of a Teen Medical Academy (TMA) designed to increase career interest in medicine for underrepresented ethnic minority students from economically disadvantaged backgrounds. Students participating in the TMA reported greater interest in medical and allied health careers; confidence in the ability to achieve a health career, to learn surgical skills, and to learn other health career–related technical skills; a sense of belongingness in a health career and among doctors; and commitment to achieve a health career and meaningful work. Higher grade point average and greater involvement in extracurricular health career programs were also reported.

Unfortunately, such positive and nurturing environments for students from underrepresented backgrounds are limited in number, and the end result is that many such students either are never presented the opportunity to pursue nursing as a career or fail to receive the necessary support to successfully complete their nursing education.

In addition, many experts suggest that recruitment and retention rates are low with underrepresented groups because such groups are at greater risk of being economically disadvantaged and this, in turn, places them at greater risk of having received an inferior preparatory education. Students who complete their secondary education in economically disadvantaged communities or institutions may have inadequately developed reading, writing, and critical thinking skills and often lack access to advanced preparation in the natural and physical sciences. This makes them less viable as candidates for admission to a nursing program.

CONSIDER THIS Recruitment and retention of minority nursing students could improve if these students were given solid secondary academic preparation and if the environments in which they are educated were more accepting of and hospitable to students from diverse backgrounds.

## Retaining Minority Students in Nursing

Despite the challenges inherent in recruiting minority students, recruiting them is still often easier than retaining them. The literature overwhelmingly suggests that minority students face more barriers than their White counterparts in completing their nursing education. Some of these barriers are shown in Box 9.1.

For some minority students, it is an inferior secondary education preparation that predisposes them to course and even program failure. In addition, because many minority students are the first in their families to attend college, it might be difficult for family members to understand and be supportive of the challenges of higher education and the rigor of academic coursework. Ackerman-Barger (2010) also notes that students from low-income families or who are first-generation college students may not have learned what it means to be a student or what it means to study. Finances are also often a barrier to minority students, many of whom must work at least part time to subsidize the cost of their college education.

**DISCUSSION POINT**

Should more resources (time, energy, money) be devoted to the recruitment of or retention of minority students? Is a two-pronged approach (emphasizing both recruitment and retention) necessary? Why or why not?

Minority students also tend to experience more difficulty with social adjustment in the college environment, particularly when they are attending a predominantly White institution. In their focus group interviews of 14 Mexican American nursing students from two liberal arts universities, Bond, Gray, Baxley, Cason, and Denke (2008) found that finances, emotional and moral support, professional socialization, mentoring, academic advising, and technical support were important factors contributing to minority student's successful completion of the nursing program requirements. In addition, students identified personal determination as an important component, and the researchers concluded that faculty can play an important role in helping students capitalize on this personal determination.

CONSIDER THIS It is the retention and graduation of minority students that will begin to change the cultural face of nursing.

Wilson et al. (2010) suggest that mentoring by experienced and caring faculty may, in fact, be the key to the

---

**BOX 9.1 COMMON BARRIERS FOR MINORITY STUDENTS IN ACADEMIC NURSING PROGRAMS**

1. Inferior academic preparation
2. Financial problems
3. Inadequate social support
4. A lack of mentoring opportunities
5. Inconsistent faculty and institutional support
6. Inadequate numbers of minority faculty role models

retention of students from minority populations. Wilson et al. described a mentoring program implemented at a southern university with a high percentage of diverse students to address high attrition rates, poor test scores, and a drop in nurse licensing examination scores among minority and English-as-second-language (ESL) students. This mentoring program focused on the academic enhancement of junior- and senior-level nursing students and is detailed in Research Study Fuels the Controversy 9.1.

Perhaps one of the most articulate and well-organized documents for helping culturally diverse students to be successful, regardless of their educational level, is the *2004 Report of the Sullivan Commission on Diversity in the Health Care Workforce for Increasing Diversity in Nursing Education Programs.* Strategies included in the document are shown in Box 9.2.

In addition, the U.S. Health Resources and Services Administration (HRSA) is addressing the need for financial support for individuals from disadvantaged backgrounds by offering the Nursing Workforce Diversity (NWD) program, which was established in 1998 to provide grants or contracts to projects that incorporate retention programs and preentry preparation programs and support student scholarships and/or stipend programs (HRSA, 2011). Applicants are required to address all three program components (retention, preentry preparation, student stipends/scholarships) during each year of the project. The goals of the NWD program are to improve the diversity of the nursing workforce in an effort to provide for culturally sensitive and quality health care, to create a racially and ethnically diverse nursing workforce, and to contribute to the basic preparation of disadvantaged and minority nurses for leadership positions within the nursing profession and the health care community (HRSA, 2011).

To be eligible for an NWD grant, students must come from an educationally or economically disadvantaged background (including students who belong to racial/ethnic minorities underrepresented among nurses) and express an interest in becoming a registered nurse (Rural Assistance Center, 2011). More than US$3.5 million was allocated for these awards in 2011 with the average award estimated to be US$334,000 (Rural Assistance Center, 2011).

## Ethnic Diversity in Education and Health Care Administration

The exact number of minority nurses in leadership positions has not been determined; however, clearly,

## RESEARCH STUDY FUELS THE CONTROVERSY 9.1

### THE IMPACT OF MENTORING ON MINORITY STUDENT RETENTION

The purpose of this program evaluation study was to determine the effectiveness of a formal mentoring program, titled Preparing the Next Generation of Nurses Mentoring Program (NGN), which had been funded by a federal Nursing Workforce Diversity grant. Focus group methodology was used to evaluate the 10 faculty and 30 student respondents' perceptions of the mentoring program.

Wilson, A., Sanner, S., & McAllister, L. (2010). An evaluation study of a mentoring program to increase the diversity of the nursing workforce. *Journal of Cultural Diversity, 17*(4), 144–150.

### STUDY FINDINGS

The major themes which emerged in this study from the faculty mentor focus groups were role modeling, caring, and academic success. Themes emerging from the student mentee focus groups were support system, enhanced perception of the nursing profession, and academic enrichment. The faculty mentors indicated that the mentoring program had a positive influence on the mentee's academic performance. The students perceived that the faculty mentors provided support they had not received prior to entering the mentoring program. They were appreciative of the encouragement they received from their mentors and described their mentors' ability to help them build self-confidence in their ability as critical to achieving success in the nursing program. The one-on-one interactions with their mentors helped sharpen the mentees skills in studying, note taking, and test taking. In addition, as students worked with their faculty mentors, their perceptions of nursing changed for the better. The results supported the need for a formal mentoring program to assist disadvantaged students in being successful in a nursing program.

**BOX 9.2    STRATEGIES IDENTIFIED BY THE SULLIVAN COMMISSION ON DIVERSITY IN THE HEALTH
CARE WORKFORCE FOR INCREASING DIVERSITY IN NURSING EDUCATION PROGRAMS**

1. Diversity program managers should be hired by health profession schools to develop plans to ensure institutional diversity.

2. Colleges and universities should provide an array of support services to minority students, including mentoring, test-taking skills, and application counseling.

3. Schools granting baccalaureate nursing degrees should provide "bridging programs" that help graduates of 2-year programs transition to 4-year institutions.

4. Associate nursing graduates should be encouraged to enroll in baccalaureate programs.

5. Professional organizations should work with schools to promote enhanced admissions policies, cultural competence training, and minority student recruitment.

6. Organizations should provide scholarships, loan forgiveness, and tuition reimbursement programs to remove financial barriers to nursing education.

*Source:* Dixon, M. E. (2008). Diversity in nursing. *Advance for Nurses.* Retrieved July 9, 2011, from http://nursing.advanceweb.com/editorial/content/editorial.aspx?cc=57273

minority nurses are underrepresented in such positions in both academic and service sectors. The National Advisory Council on Nurse Education and Practice suggests there is a need to increase the number of minority nurses in policy/leadership positions in health care administration, academia, and research; to reduce social isolation of minority nurse leaders by increasing opportunities for professional development activities focusing on the development of support systems; and to increase the use of mentors for students and those nurses who are young in their careers (Diversity in Practice, n.d.).

## Minority Nurse Educators

The underrepresentation of minority nurse faculty is well documented. Current data suggest that only 12.6% of all full-time instructional faculty members in baccalaureate and graduate programs are members of racial/ethnic minority groups, and only 6.2% are male (AACN, 2011a). The sad fact is that far too few nurses from racial/ethnic minority groups with advanced nursing degrees pursue faculty careers.

In an effort to increase the number of minority nurse scholars, the American Association of Colleges of Nursing and the Johnson & Johnson Campaign for Nursing's Future launched a national scholarship program in 2007 to increase the number of nursing faculty from ethnic minority backgrounds (AACN, 2011b).

This scholarship program supports full-time nursing students in doctoral or master's degree programs, with a preference given to those completing a doctorate. Scholarship recipients must agree to teach in a U.S. school of nursing after completing their advanced degree. Five scholarship recipients are selected annually, with each receiving a US$18,000 scholarship.

Another opportunity to support minority faculty was described by Jacob and Sanchez (2011) with the Health Resources and Services Administration (HRSA) Minority Faculty Fellowship Program (MFFP) grants. These program grants provide stipends to educational programs to increase the number of faculty representing racial and ethnic minorities. This stipend provides up to 50% of the faculty salary, which is matched or exceeded by the employing institution. Jacob and Sanchez describe how the grant was used at the University of Tennessee Health Science Center (UTHSC) College of Nursing to recruit, mentor, and support a new Hispanic nursing faculty member.

In addition, the School of Nursing at Thomas Edison State College (Llardi, 2010) in New Jersey launched a free online database of minority nurse educators (includes African Americans, Asian Americans, Latinos, Native Americans, and Pacific Islanders) that is available to nursing schools across the country interested in increasing diversity at their institutions and hiring the educators as adjunct faculty. The database, the only one of its kind in the country, includes 52 nurse educators from 24 states in the country who have each completed the School of Nursing's online Minority Nurse Educator certification program and a 12-week mentored online nursing experience at the college under the guidance of an experienced online nurse educator. Educators in the database have agreed to be shared by various institutions in order to increase diversity at nursing schools nationwide.

## Minority Nurse Administrators

The number of minority nurses holding leadership positions in the service sector is less clear. Although there is little disagreement that minorities are underrepresented, perceptions differ as to the degree. Survey data from Witt-Kieffer, an executive search firm for health care leaders, suggested that 20% of minorities believe that minorities are well represented in health care management as compared with 41% of Whites (Moon, 2007). In fact, Moon openly questioned whether any progress has been made since the early 1990s, when an industry study found that just 1% of top hospital management positions were held by minorities, despite the fact that minorities held nearly 20% of the employee positions.

Similarly, M. Evans (2007) reported that a survey by the American College of Health Executives (ACHE) found that despite the nation's increasing diversity, far fewer Blacks, Hispanics, Native Americans, and Asians reported top-tier management jobs than Whites, and a 2007 survey reported that only 6% of ACHE members are Black, 3% are Hispanic, 3% are Asian or Pacific Islander, and fewer than 1% are American Indian or Alaskan.

Similarly, Sloane (2006) suggested that although the number of minorities in executive health care positions may have increased slightly in the last few years, many still find "they bounce off a Teflon ceiling leading to the executive suite" (para. 4). He argued that mentoring is key to addressing the problem so that minorities can experience the same hand up that Whites often report. Only then, he suggests, can Blacks and Hispanics succeed in the largely White world of the executive suite and the boardroom.

Witt-Kieffer (2008) also bemoaned the lack of minorities and women in health care leadership positions and shared research findings that the majority of CEOs report not having enough time to mentor women or minorities for such roles. Minorities fare worse than women, however, with 68% of respondents believing the health care providers fail to effectively develop minority leaders for future CEO roles, whereas only 48% believing that the same is true for women executives.

Even the means through which women and minorities are developed for leadership roles in health care differ. Fifty-five percent of CEOs reported developing future female leaders by exposure to health care provider boards/board members and board committee work, as opposed to 41% who develop minorities in the same manner (Witt-Kieffer, 2008). In addition, nearly three fourths (73%) of respondents said women leaders are developed by enabling them to attend educational conferences, as opposed to 60% who said the same of minorities.

> CONSIDER THIS Increasing the number of ethnic minorities in executive health care positions will require an intentional commitment to do so and a well-planned development program that includes the same type of mentoring activities that White men have long enjoyed and benefited from.

Linda Hill, a professor of business administration at Harvard Business School, suggested in a 2008 interview with *Harvard Business Review* that cadres of globally savvy executives do not currently exist (Hemp, 2008). She suggested that this occurs in part because many organizations fail to view talented people as potential leaders. This may occur because "'demographic invisibles'—people who, because of their gender, ethnicity, nationality, or even age, don't have access to the tools—the social networks, the fast-track training courses, the stretch assignments—that can prepare them for positions of authority and influence" (p. 125).

Hill also suggested that other potential leaders are missed since they are viewed as "'stylistic invisibles'—individuals who don't fit the conventional image of a leader, since they don't exhibit take charge, direction setting behavior" (Hemp, 2008, p. 125). This also may represent cultural differences more than leadership ability. Clearly, then, nursing education programs and health care organizations must be more open-minded about who the profession's future leaders might be and begin to prepare nurses to be effective leaders. This will require the formal education and training that are a part of most management-development programs, as well as a development of appropriate attitudes through social learning (Marquis & Huston, 2012).

Intentional succession planning will be essential to significantly increase the number of minorities and women in health care leadership positions. Greer and Virick (2008) concur, suggesting that "the future of many organizations is likely to depend on their mastery of diverse succession planning given that building bench strength among women and minorities will be critical in the competitive war for talent" (p. 353). They go on to say that direct involvement and commitment by organization leaders are essential threshold requirements for diverse succession planning.

Greer and Virick (2008) also suggest there is a great deal that organizations can do to encourage and support diversity in the workplace, including removing career advancement barriers for women and minorities and actively planning for diverse leadership succession. Although they bemoan the need for special developmental programs for women and minorities, they suggest that they continue to appear to be needed for progress. Wooten (2008) agrees, arguing there is a need to further "identify trigger points for shattering the glass ceiling, removing silos, and erasing boundaries in organizations" (p. 192) before we can move the inclusion journey forward.

## Ethnic Professional Associations in Nursing

There is a professional association for almost every ethnic group in nursing. Several of the many organizations include the National Black Nurses Association, established in 1971; the National Association of Hispanic Nurses, founded in 1975; the Philippine Nurses Association of America, formed in 1979; the National Alaska Native American Indian Nurses Association; and the Asian American/Pacific Islander Nurses Association Incorporated. See Box 9.3 for more information on these groups.

---

### BOX 9.3   ETHNIC PROFESSIONAL ASSOCIATIONS IN NURSING

Support groups and professional associations abound among nurses in the United States. Some of the groups formed to address specific issues related to ethnic diversity in nursing include the following:

**National Black Nurses Association**

The National Black Nurses Association (NBNA), founded in 1971, represents approximately 150,000 Black nurses from the United States (with 76 chartered chapters nationwide), the Eastern Caribbean nations, and Africa (NBNA, 2011). The mission of the NBNA is to provide a forum for collective action by Black nurses to "investigate, define and determine what the health care needs of African Americans are and to implement change to make health care available to African Americans and other minorities that is commensurate with that [health care] of the larger society" (NBNA, 2011, para. 4).

**National Association of Hispanic Nurses**

The National Association of Hispanic Nurses (NAHN) was founded in 1975 by Ildaura Murillo-Rohde and evolved out of the Ad Hoc Committee of the Spanish-Speaking/Spanish Surname Nurses' Caucus, which was formed during the American Nurses Association convention in San Francisco in 1974 (NAHN, 2002–2011). The NAHN strives to serve the nursing and health care delivery needs of the Hispanic community and the professional needs of Hispanic nurses. In addition, it is committed to improving the quality of health and nursing care for Hispanic consumers and to providing equal access to educational, professional, and economic opportunities for Hispanic nurses.

**Philippine Nurses Association of America**

The Philippine Nurses Association of America (PNAA) was formed in 1979 in an effort to address the issues and concerns of Filipino nurses in the United States. Its mission is to uphold and foster the positive image and welfare of its constituent members. In addition, the PNAA seeks to promote professional excellence and contribute to significant outcomes to health care and society (PNAA, 2010).

*continued*

**BOX 9.3   ETHNIC PROFESSIONAL ASSOCIATIONS IN NURSING** *continued*

**National Alaska Native American Indian Nurses Association**

The National Alaska Native American Indian Nurses Association (NANAINA) was founded on its predecessor organization, the American Indian Nurses Association, and, later, the American Indian Alaska Native Nurses Association. The NANAINA is dedicated to supporting Alaska Native and American Indian students, nurses, and allied health professionals through the development of leadership skills and continuing education. It also advocates for the improvement of health care provided to American Indian and Alaska Native consumers and culturally competent health care (NANAINA, 2001–2011). Similar goals exist for the Asian and Pacific Islander population as described by the Asian and Pacific Islander Nurses Association.

**Asian American/Pacific Islander Nurses Association Inc**

The Asian American/Pacific Islander Nurses Association Inc. (AAPINA) obtains current statistics and national information on the health status of Asian Americans and Pacific Islanders (APIs), publishes information on fellowship, grants, and meetings for API nurses, represents API nurses on national and federal groups, and participates in the National Coalition of Ethnic Minority Nurse Associations (AAPINA, 2008–2011).

---

## DISCUSSION POINT

If our goal is to better appreciate and merge cultural and ethnic diversity in nursing, why do culturally and ethnically diverse nurses separate themselves with their own professional nursing organizations?

## GENDER DIVERSITY

### Gender Diversity in Nursing

Diversity goals in nursing are not just directed at ethnicity—they also frequently include increasing the number of men in nursing. Although men have worked as nurses for centuries, just 6.2% of the nation's 3.2 million nurses are men, a percentage that has climbed fairly steadily since the NNSRN was first conducted in 1980 (AACN, 2011a). Indeed, the number of male nurses surged from 45,060 in 1980 to 189,916 in 2008.

Yet, despite a call to increase the number of men in nursing, progress in this regard has been slow for many reasons. Stereotypes of male nurses as being different or effeminate due to their close working relationship with women continue to persist. In addition, most of the public would describe nursing as a female occupation, and young men often report they never even considered a career as a nurse.

The media also perpetuates the image of the nurse as female. Many media sources, and even nursing textbooks at times, refer to the comforting caregiver nurse as "she" and make no mention of men, except as sickly, demanding patients. The difficulty of male nurses socializing into what has long been perceived as a woman's occupation is depicted in Figure 9.1.

The stereotype of the male nurse as homosexual is also prevalent. Harding's (2007) study of New Zealand male nurses found that despite participants' beliefs that most male nurses are heterosexual, many male nurses are exposed to homophobia in the workplace. The heterosexual men reported using strategies to avoid a presumption of homosexuality, including avoiding contact with gay colleagues and overt expression of their heterosexuality. Research by Snyder and Green (2008) suggested that male nurses might also seek employment in areas of nursing they perceive to be "more masculine" in an effort to dispel questions about their sexuality.

---

CONSIDER THIS   Heterosexual male nurses report using strategies to avoid a presumption of homosexuality, including avoiding contact with gay colleagues and overt expression of their heterosexuality. They also tend to seek employment in areas of nursing they perceive to be "more masculine" in an effort to dispel questions about their sexuality.

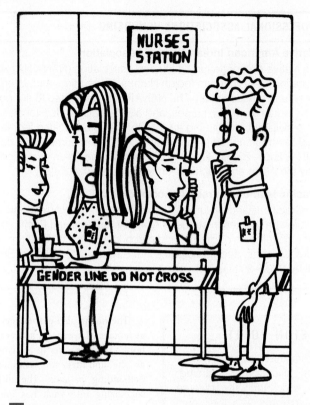

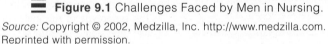

≡ **Figure 9.1** Challenges Faced by Men in Nursing.

*Source:* Copyright © 2002, Medzilla, Inc. http://www.medzilla.com.
Reprinted with permission.

Harding (2007) concluded that a paradox exists between the public call for more men to engage in caring professions such as nursing and the repercussions they often experience as a result of the stereotype of male nurses as gay or sexually predatory. He suggested that these stigmatizing discourses deter men's entry into the profession and likely affect their retention. In addition, the perception that nursing is an occupation only for women deters many men from choosing nursing as a profession.

Equally troubling are the research findings of Harding, North, and Perkins (2008) that whereas touch is important in nursing care, it is problematic for male nurses because women's use of touch is viewed as a caring behavior and men's touch is often viewed sexually. Male nurses in this study described their vulnerability, how they protected themselves from risk, and the resulting stress. The researchers concluded that a paradox

emerges whereby the very measures used to protect both patients and men as nurses exacerbate the perceived risk posed by men carrying out intimate care. Torkelson and Seed (2011) agree, noting that although men in nursing are often portrayed as equal partners in care, contemporary studies still often note gender role distinctions in terms of how nursing tasks are assigned.

CONSIDER THIS  Caregiving is not just a feminine trait.

Clearly, stereotypes that suggest male nurses are less capable of therapeutic caring, compassion, and nurturing than female nurses hurt the profession, as well as society in general. At least partly as a result of these stereotypes, some patients have gender preferences (more commonly female) for their caregivers. This seems to be particularly true for nurses employed in labor and delivery settings.

Dorman (2008) suggested that maternal-newborn nursing is often viewed as women's domain with the exception of physicians and husbands and went on to say that the barriers to men working in this setting are multifaceted. Many male nursing students worry that their care could be interpreted as inappropriately sexual or unprofessional. In some settings, men must still have a woman present when examining patients, and some male students feel comfortable in the labor and delivery setting only when male physicians are present.

Court cases have confused the issue further. In some cases, the courts have ruled that female gender is a legitimate qualification for labor and delivery nurses, yet other courts have found these qualifications to be discriminatory. The Association of Women's Health, Obstetric and Neonatal Nurses (AWHONN) argued that although all clients and families have the right to clinically competent, professional care, the gender of the nurse should not be a factor (Dorman, 2008).

Wolfenden (2011) suggests that the barring of men from specific areas of practice, combined with the education of nurses being increasingly feminized, marginalizes men in nursing. He suggests that if this trend continues, that the result will be less men seeking nursing careers and a gradual erosion of the professional and academic capacity of nursing.

## Is There a Male Advantage in Nursing?

Despite the barriers that male nurses face, their minority status may give male nurses advantages in hiring and promotion, unlike women in male-dominated professions. Walker (2011) agrees, suggesting that despite their minority status, men in nursing rise more rapidly into management positions and earn more money than their female counterparts, all the while being viewed as a disadvantaged group. He argues that this "seems at odds with decades of feminist and cultural diversity scholarship, and it further marginalizes women and ethnic minorities, who continue to experience systematic inequality and disadvantage" (p. 2).

Certainly, male nurses in the United States hold disproportionately more positions of influence and authority than their female counterparts. McMurry (2011) notes that most of the discrimination and prejudice facing men in female professions emanates from outside those professions and that research has found that men in nursing have been given fair, if not preferential, treatment in hiring and promotion. In fact, McMurry suggests that subtle mechanisms are in place to enhance men's position in the nursing profession and that their minority status often results in advantages that promote rather than hinder their careers.

Men in nursing also appear to have an economic advantage. The 2008 Advance Salary Survey showed that male nurses continue to outearn their female counterparts, with an average salary of US$53,792 versus US$50,615 for female nurses (O'Brien, 2008). Similarly, research by Baldwin and Schneller (2008) found that the mean salary for female operating room managers was 93% of the mean salary for men. Male and female nurses in their study had similar education and experience, but men tended to manage more operating rooms, with a higher case volume. In addition, men supervised 50% more personnel than their female counterparts on average, had double the annual budget, and were more likely to work in teaching hospitals. Baldwin and Schneller concluded that there was evidence to suggest gender discrimination in salaries paid to male/female operating room managers, although the unexplained differential was relatively small. In addition, they found evidence of job segregation within this narrowly defined occupation that could not be explained by differences in the average qualifications of male and female nurses.

Some experts have suggested that the more rapid career trajectory and relative higher pay for male nurses likely reflects the historical trend that more men are employed full-time in their career paths whereas women tend to have career gaps related to childbearing or rearing families and often work fewer hours. This was the situation reported by O'Lynn (2008) in his community, where most male RNs worked full-time and most female RNs worked 0.8 positions or less.

A 2008 study, however, disputed this assumption at least in part, arguing that less than 8% of professional women born since 1956 have left the workforce for 1 year or more during their prime childbearing years ("Study Disputes," 2008). In fact, the number of professional women working more than 50 hours each week increased from less than 10% for women born before 1935 to 15% for women born after 1956, and the percentage of mothers with young children working full-time rose from 6% of women born from 1926 to 1935 to 38% for women born from 1966 to 1975. Although the researchers argued that the "opt-out revolution" is merely hype, they did concede that Generation X and late baby boomer women worked less than their male counterparts, although they worked more than the previous cohorts ("Study Disputes," 2008).

> CONSIDER THIS   Many experts suggest that the power of the profession would be elevated if more men were to become nurses. Yet men in nursing hold a disproportionately large share of the high-income jobs and have higher salaries than their female counterparts.

## Why Are Men Leaving Nursing?

McMillian, Morgan, and Arment (2006) suggested that whereas increased numbers of men are joining the nursing profession, disproportionate numbers of male nurses are also leaving, as compared with female nurses. In fact, new male nurses leave the profession within 4 years of graduation at a rate almost twice that of female nurse graduates. McMillian et al. suggested that a lack of social approval, acceptance, and adequate role models beginning in nursing school are to blame. Similarly, a roundtable discussion at the close of the aforementioned October 2007 conference on men in nursing concluded that the "fundamental barrier to gender equality in the field was a lack of positive, visible, and accurate male role models in nursing—both in the classroom and in clinical practice" (S. Evans, 2007, p. 42).

In studying acceptance as a factor for male nurse retention, McMillian et al. (2006) found that the most influential condition on acceptance of male nurses by their female counterparts was length of time worked with a male nurse. In addition, the researchers found that lingering nonacceptance of male nurses continued among some female nurses and that these attitudes were likely the result of early role socialization. They concluded that nursing education could do much to eliminate sexism and discrimination by eliminating any policies that reinforce social- and gender-related segregation, by promoting nursing as a gender-neutral occupation and by the active recruitment of male nursing instructors.

In addition, although the literature has been mixed, the majority of nursing studies that examined gender and job dissatisfaction suggested that male nurses are more dissatisfied than their female counterparts. Some experts argue that more men than women leave nursing because nursing still lacks status and therefore nurses are often demeaned by other health professionals. Male

nurses may be less willing to tolerate this kind of treatment. S. Evans (2007) suggested that the climate was slowly changing for men entering the nursing profession. She suggested, however, that improving support and understanding in both the classroom and practice settings could go far in enhancing the ability to recruit, educate, and retain men in the nursing profession.

> CONSIDER THIS   Recent graduates of the nation's nursing schools are leaving the profession more quickly than their predecessors, with male nurses leaving at a much higher rate than their female counterparts.

## Recruiting Men Into Nursing: Is Affirmative Action Required?

There are efforts underway to increase the number of men in nursing. Some nursing schools are participating in both national and local campaigns to increase gender diversity in the profession.

For example, the School of Nursing at Monterey Peninsula College established a men-only study group and implemented a monthly "Men in Nursing" discussion group to reduce possible feelings of isolation for male students (O'Lynn, 2008). They believed that male students should have a safe setting to share concerns that might interfere with their academic success and obtain guidance from other men who understood their situations. The school then applied for and received a grant from the Regional Health Occupations Resource Center of the Chancellor's Office of the California Community Colleges in 2007 for the purpose of recruiting and retaining men in an academic nursing program and to host a 2008 statewide conference on men in nursing (O'Lynn, 2008).

Other efforts to increase the representation of men in nursing have resulted from corporate partnerships with professional associations. For example, the American Assembly of Men in Nursing received funding from the American Association of Nurse Anesthetists, Kaiser Permanente, the Johnson & Johnson Campaign for Nursing's Future, the Nurses Service Organization, and the Nursing 2006 Foundation to promote a 30-minute film documentary called "Career Encounters: Men in Nursing" (Men in Nursing, 2002–2009). The documentary features male nurses, including students, advanced practice nurses, nurse educators, and staff nurses, in a number of settings, as well as the use of a state-of-the-art simulator to train nurse anesthetists.

Some suggest that such recruitment campaigns are not enough and that affirmative action, similar to the efforts used to increase the number of women in medicine and engineering, will be required before there will be any significant increase in the number of male nurses. O'Lynn (2008) agreed, suggesting that despite a growing recognition in the professional literature that men face unique challenges in nursing school, as well as in transition to professional practice, the response from the profession as a whole has simply been a tacit acknowledgment of the topic. He suggested the need for a national initiative that would enhance the professional climate for men in nursing or promote the large-scale recruitment of men into nursing.

---

### DISCUSSION POINT

Affirmative action has been used successfully to increase the presence of some underrepresented minorities in health care. Should the same be done to increase the number of men in nursing?

---

Walker (2011) disagrees, suggesting that a female profession does not need men to elevate its status. He suggests that if men offer anything to nursing, it is not a function of their maleness—it emerges from our common humanness.

## GENERATIONAL DIVERSITY IN NURSING

Age has become a diversity issue during the last decade. The problem is not that the nursing workforce lacks generational diversity but that typically four generations have not cohabitated at the same time in a profession. This climate offers challenges and opportunities for leaders and also provides opportunities to further diversify a workforce to more closely resemble the clients they serve and to identify the best thinking of so many perspectives.

According to the 2008 NSSRN, the average age of an RN in the United States was 46 years, up from 45.2 years in the year 2000 (AACN, 2011c). With the average age of RNs projected to be 44.5 years by 2012, nurses in their

50s are expected to become the largest segment of the nursing workforce, accounting for almost one quarter of the RN population. Given the current nursing shortage and the need to both retain and recruit older nurses and to bring new, young nurses into the field, generational issues must be examined further.

## Defining the Generations

The research increasingly suggests that the different generations represented in nursing today may have different attitudes and value systems, which greatly impact the settings in which they work. They may also have significantly different career socialization experiences and expectations regarding their chosen profession and employer. In addition, workplace relationships are often influenced by these generational differences.

Most experts identify four generational groups in today's workforce: the veteran generation (also called the *silent generation*), the baby boomers, Generation X, and Generation Y (also called the *millennials*).

The *veteran generation* is typically recognized as those nurses born between 1925 and 1942. Currently, about 9% of employed nurses belong to this age group (Boivin, 2008). Having lived through several international military conflicts (World War II, the Korean War, and the Vietnam War) and the Great Depression, they are often risk averse (particularly in regard to personal finances), respectful of authority, and supportive of hierarchy. They also work well in teams, but require a large amount of verbal communication and rapport building from coworkers and supervisors (Thomas, 2010). They are also called the *silent generation* because they tend to support the status quo rather than protest or push for rapid change. As a result, these nurses are less likely to question organizational practices and more likely to seek employment in structured settings (Marquis & Huston, 2012). Their work values are traditional, and they are often recognized for their loyalty to their employers.

The *boom generation* (born 1943 to 1960) also displays traditional work values; however, they tend to be more materialistic and present oriented and thus are willing to work long hours at their jobs in an effort to get ahead. Forty-seven percent of currently employed nurses and 46% of nurses working in hospitals belong to this generation (Boivin, 2008). In addition, this generation of workers is often recognized as being more individualistic as a result of the "permissive parenting" many of them experienced while growing up. This individualism often results in greater creativity and thus nurses born in this generation may be best suited for work that requires flexibility, independent thinking, and creativity. Yet it also encourages this generation to challenge rules.

In contrast, *Generation Xers* (born between 1961 and 1981), a much smaller cohort than the baby boomers who preceded them or the Generation Yers who follow them, may lack the interest in lifetime employment at one place that prior generations have valued, instead valuing greater work-hour flexibility and opportunities for time off. This likely reflects the fact that many individuals born in this generation had both parents working outside their home as they were growing up and they want to put more emphasis on family and leisure time in their own family units. Thus, this generation may be less economically driven than prior generations and may define success differently than the veteran generation or the baby boomers. Generation Xers are considered to be very comfortable with change, but have a blunt communication style that can be uncomfortable when received by boomers (Thomas, 2010). Forty-two percent of the RN workforce belongs to this generational cohort (Boivin, 2008).

*Generation Y* (born 1982 to 1999) represents the first cohort of truly global citizens. They are known for their optimism, self-confidence, relationship orientation, volunteer-mindedness, and social consciousness. Their team-orientation defies being raised in often highly-scheduled, conformist households. They are also technologically savvy which is why some people call them "digital natives." Generation Y currently represents only 2% of the nursing workforce, but this number will increase rapidly over the coming decade (Boivin, 2008).

Given these attitudinal and value differences, it is not surprising that some workplace conflict results between different generations of workers. For example, Generation Y nurses may test the patience of their baby boomer leaders: "They come to work in flip-flops listening to their iPods and are brash and ready to hit the ground running" ("What Does It Take," 2008, para. 2). They also "often come with a sense of entitlement that can be an affront to older workers. They want to do something meaningful today" and they "don't want to spend days at a desk listening to orientation lectures" ("What Does It Take," 2008, para. 6).

Generation X workers also report higher levels of burnout (specifically feelings of depersonalization and emotional exhaustion) as compared with baby

## RESEARCH STUDY FUELS THE CONTROVERSY 9.2

### VALUE CONFLICTS BETWEEN BABY BOOMER AND GENERATION X NURSES

Canadian nurses ($n = 522$) in three district health authorities in Nova Scotia and two hospitals in Ontario completed a survey assessing various dimensions of work life. For the purpose of generational analysis, the researchers defined Generation X as a birth date from 1963 to 1981. A questionnaire survey of nurses was organized by generation. Analyses of variance contrasted the scores on burnout, turnover intention, physical symptoms, supervisor incivility, coworker incivility, and team civility. A total of 729 completed surveys were received from the 1,600 distributed to nurses for a response rate of 45%.

Leiter, M., Price, S., & Laschinger, H. (2010). Generational differences in distress, attitudes and incivility among nurses. *Journal of Nursing Management, 18*(8), 970–980.

### STUDY FINDINGS

Generation X nurses reported more negative experiences than did baby boomer nurses on all measures. This suggested that newer generations of nurses are significantly less satisfied with their jobs than older generational cohorts and have the largest proportion of nurses experiencing burnout, specifically feelings of depersonalization and emotional exhaustion. Breakdowns in collegiality were integral to the Generation X nurses' greater experience of distress in hospital environments.

Generation X nurses reported high levels of cynicism, which resulted in emotional and cognitive withdrawal and a diminished inclination to identify with the work. The researchers concluded that the social context variables suggest that workplaces are less welcoming than one would expect in a sector eager to recruit new professionals in anticipation of future shortages. They suggest that health care leaders have yet to develop policies and practices that support a fulfilling work life to the day-to-day social environments of health care.

boomers, related to incivility from colleagues and cynicism, which results in emotional and cognitive withdrawal and a diminished inclination to identify with the work (Leiter, Price, & Laschinger, 2010; see Research Study Fuels the Controversy 9.2). Lavoie-Tremblay et al. (2010) also noted conflicts between generational workers related to perceptions of challenge (work environment that allows for the use of a variety of competencies and knowledge), goal achievement, and warmth. Generation Y hospital workers demonstrated significantly lower scores on challenge than did baby boomers but baby boomers were significantly less "warm" than their Generation Y coworkers. In addition, Generation Y nurses expressed a negative perception of the Goal Emphasis scale, compared with baby boomers. The main reason given by workers from Generations Y and X who intended to quit the organization was career advancement. The main reason given by baby boomers was retirement.

Mensik (2007) and Thomas (2010) suggest that although this type of generational diversity poses management challenges, it also provides a variety of perspectives and outlooks that enhance workplace balance and productivity. While the literature often focuses on differences and negative attributes between the generations, particularly for Generations X and Y, a more balanced view is needed.

For example, the literature repeatedly suggests that Generations X and Y may have less loyalty to their employers than the generations who preceded them, but Mensik (2007) cited current research that suggests that their commitment to employment longevity is actually greater than that of the boomers who preceded them. Mensik concluded that instead of focusing on generational differences, nurses should instead move forward and put their energies into seeking collaboration between the generations. In addition, patients should benefit from the optimal outcomes that should occur when all generations of the workforce can work together as a higher-performing team. Lavoie-Tremblay et al. (2010) agrees, suggesting that retention strategies that focus on improving the work climate are beneficial to all generations of hospital workers and nurses.

Boivin (2008) also suggested that the people who benefit the most from such differences and strengths are the patients. She argued that generational diversity allows patients to "have nurses caring for them who have 20 or 30 years of experience under their belts, who are able to use the latest technology to prevent errors, and who are willing to challenge authority and act as patient advocates" (para. 14).

## PROFESSIONAL ORGANIZATIONS SPEAK OUT

In the last decade, many professional nursing organizations have issued position statements or recommendations on diversity. In 1997, the AACN, the national voice for baccalaureate and higher-degree education programs, drafted a position statement that suggests that diversity and inclusion have emerged as central issues for organizations and institutions and that leadership in nursing must respond to these issues by finding ways to accelerate the inclusion of groups, cultures, and ideas that traditionally have been underrepresented in higher education. Moreover, the position statement argues that health care providers and the nursing profession should reflect and value the diversity of the populations and communities they serve.

The ANA issued a position statement on discrimination and racism in health care in 1998 and stated its commitment to working toward the eradication of discrimination and racism in the profession of nursing, in the education of nurses, in the practice of nursing, and in the organizations in which nurses work. The *ANA Code of Ethics for Nurses* advocates diversity in its assertion that the nurse, in all professional relationships, practices with compassion and respect for the inherent dignity, worth, and uniqueness of every individual, unrestricted by considerations of social or economic status, personal attributes, or the nature of health problems.

The American Organization of Nurse Executives also developed a diversity statement in 2005. This statement suggests that the success of nursing leadership as a profession depends on reflecting the diversity of the communities it serves and that diversity is one of the essential building blocks of a healthful practice/work environment.

In contrast, the International Council of Nurses does not have a diversity statement, but rather has embedded *diversity* in its policy and practice. For example, the organization promotes the principles of equal opportunity employment, pay equity, and occupational desegregation.

Some professional organizations have gone beyond simply arguing the need for diversity and have instead given funds to advance the cause. Despite the backlash in the late 1990s over the practice of affirmative action in helping racial and ethnic minorities enter the health professions, the Bureau of Health Professions within the HRSA, U.S. Department of Health and Human Services, has held steadfast to its goal of ensuring representation of underrepresented minorities in the health professions by prioritizing this goal in funding opportunities.

## CONCLUSIONS

Projections suggest that current ethnic minorities are likely, in the not too distant future, to become the majority of the U.S. population. This diversity, however, is not reflected in the nursing workforce or in schools of nursing. Similarly, men are underrepresented in nursing, and efforts to increase the number of men in the nursing profession are even fewer than those directed at increasing ethnic diversity. Finally, generational diversity is occurring in all health care organizations; however, few organizations have directly confronted the implications of how to deal with this diversity or examined the impact it has on the quality of care provided.

Diversity, equity, and parity are business imperatives but should also be moral imperatives. Using "change by drift" strategies to address the lack of ethnic and gender diversity in nursing has been ineffective.

Ackerman-Barger (2010) notes that numerous barriers still exist for minority student success including multiple forms of discrimination, financial restraints, social bonds, lack of minority mentors, and a lack of acknowledgement and understanding of barriers on the part of faculty and university administration. She argues that equity in nursing education cannot be achieved until "faculty, universities, and schools of nursing adopt an attitude of humility to fully understand the situation, foster a cultural desire to learn about and fix the inequities, and find long-term sustainable solutions that are specific to the needs of their students" (p. 681).

In addition, Chavez and Weisinger (2008) argued that contemporary organizations have likely spent millions of dollars on diversity training that has either failed or resulted in less than desired outcomes. Instead, they argued, organizations must create a "culture of diversity" that requires a longer-term, relational approach that emphasizes attitudinal and cultural transformation. Thus, energy is not directed at "managing *diversity*"; instead, it is directed toward "managing *for diversity*" to capitalize on the unique perspectives of a diverse workforce. It is clear that proactive, well-thought-out strategies at multiple levels and by multiple parties will be needed before diversity in the nursing profession mirrors that of the public it serves.

## FOR ADDITIONAL DISCUSSION

1. What are the strongest driving and restraining forces for increasing ethnic diversity in nursing, increasing gender diversity in nursing, and having a multigenerational nursing workforce?

2. Should funding for diversity initiatives come from federal or state governments, or from corporate partnerships?

3. Should the institutions that reap the benefits of a diverse workforce share the costs to make that happen?

4. Should there be different nursing school entry requirements for minority students than for their White counterparts?

5. Is an affirmative action approach needed to increase the number of both men and minorities in the nursing profession?

6. Will having more men in nursing raise the status of the profession?

7. What are the potential barriers to having more men in the nursing profession?

8. Why have women been better able to further their numbers in medicine than men have in nursing?

9. How does the use of mentors assist in both the recruitment and the retention of minority (ethnic and gender) nurses?

10. Does a multigenerational nursing workforce improve patient care? If so, how?

11. Which health disparities do you think would be more positively impacted if the nursing workforce was more diverse?

## REFERENCES

Ackerman-Barger, P. (2010). Embracing multiculturalism learning environments. *Journal of Nursing Education, 49*(12), 677–682.

American Association of Colleges of Nursing. (2008). *The essentials of baccalaureate education for professional nursing practice.* Retrieved April 29, 2012, from http://www.aacn.nche.edu/education-resources/BaccEssentials08.pdf

American Association of Colleges of Nursing. (2011a). *Fact sheet: Enhancing diversity in the nursing workforce.* Retrieved April 29, 2012, from http://www.aacn.nche.edu/media-relations/diversityFS.pdf

American Association of Colleges of Nursing. (2011b). *Johnson & Johnson campaign for nursing's future* (American Association of Colleges of Nursing Minority Nurse Faculty Scholars Program 2011–2012 Academic Year). Retrieved July 9, 2011, from http://www.aacn.nche.edu/Education/scholarships.htm

American Association of Colleges of Nursing. (2011c). *Nursing shortage.* Retrieved July 11, 2011, from http://www.aacn.nche.edu/Media/FactSheets/NursingShortage.htm

Antczak, A. (2011). *Cultural diversity in the nursing profession.* Retrieved July 9, 2011, from http://www.associatedcontent.com/article/6162748/cultural_diversity_in_the_nursing_profession_pg4.html?cat=49

Asian American/Pacific Islander Nurses Association Inc. (2008–2011). *Homepage.* Retrieved April 28, 2012, from http://www.aapina.org/

Baldwin, M. L., & Schneller, E. S. (2008). *Gender discrimination and the salaries of operating room managers* (Workforce issues). Durham, NC: The Fuqua School of Business, Duke University. Retrieved July 25, 2008, from http://ashe2008.abstractbook.org/presentations/228/

Banschbach, S. K. (2008). Diversity equals organizational strength. *AORN Journal, 87*(6), 1067–1069.

Boivin, J. (2008). *Opinion: Nursing enters a new era: Four generations healing under one hospital roof.* Retrieved April 28, 2012, from http://news.nurse.com/apps/pbcs.dll/article?AID=/20080811/FL02/308110018

Bond, M. L., Gray, J. R., Baxley, S., Cason, C. L., & Denke, L. (2008). Voices of Hispanic students in baccalaureate nursing programs: Are we listening? *Nursing Education Perspectives, 29*(3), 136–142.

Chavez, C. I., & Weisinger, J. Y. (2008). Beyond diversity training: A social infusion for cultural inclusion. *Human Resource Management, 47*(2), 331–350.

de Leon Siantz, M. L. (2008). Leading change in diversity and cultural competence. *Journal of Professional Nursing, 24*(3), 167–171.

*Diversity in Practice.* (n.d.). Retrieved July 11, 2011, from http://www.diversitynursing.com/diversity_practice.asp

Dixon, M. E. (2008). Diversity in nursing. *Advance for nurses.* Retrieved April 28, 2012, from http://nursing.advanceweb.com/Article/Diversity-in-Nursing.aspx

Dorman, T. (2008). Guys in LDRP. *Advance for Nurses (Northern California and Northern Nevada), 5*(9), 19.

Evans, M. (2007). Minority execs form groups. *Modern Healthcare, 37*(33), 16.

Evans, S. (2007). Enhancing an image. *Advance for Nurses, Northern California and Northern Nevada, 9*(26), 42. Retrieved April 28, 2012, from http://nursing.advanceweb.com/Article/Enhancing-an-Image.aspx

Giddens, J. (2008). Achieving diversity in nursing through multicontextual learning environments. *Nursing Outlook, 56*(2), 78–83.

Greer, C. R., & Virick, M. (2008). Diverse succession planning: Lessons from the industry leaders. *Human Resource Management, 47*(2), 351–367.

Harding, T. (2007). The construction of men who are nurses as gay. *Journal of Advanced Nursing, 60*(6), 636–644.

Harding, T., North, N., & Perkins, R. (2008). Sexualizing men's touch: Male nurses and the use of intimate touch in clinical practice. *Research and Theory for Nursing Practice, 22*(2), 88–102.

Health Resources and Service Administration. (2010). *HRSA study finds nursing workforce is growing and more diverse.* Retrieved July 11, 2011, from http://www.hrsa.gov/about/news/pressreleases/2010/100317_hrsa_study_100317_finds_nursing_workforce_is_growing_and_more_diverse.html

Health Resources and Services Administration. (2011). *HRSA electronic handbooks for applicants/grantees.* Retrieved July 9, 2011, from https://grants.hrsa.gov/webexternal/FundingOppDetails.asp?FundingCycleId=AF0E72B0-AF4A-4F01-9113-2E49A508FC35&ViewMode=EU&GoBack=&PrintMode=&OnlineAvailabilityFlag=True&pageNumber=1

Hemp, P. (2008). *Where will we find tomorrow's leaders?* A conversation with Linda A. Hill by Paul Hemp. *Harvard Business Review.* Retrieved April 28, 2012, from http://hbr.org/2008/01/where-will-we-find-tomorrows-leaders/ar/1

Jacob, S. R., & Sanchez, Z. V. (2011). The challenge of closing the diversity gap: Development of Hispanic nursing faculty through a health resources and services administration minority faculty fellowship program grant. *Journal of Professional Nursing, 27*(2), 108–113.

Joint Commission. (2008). *Patient safety pulse: Joint Commission releases report on health care and diversity.* Retrieved August 11, 2008, from https://aphid.csuchico.edu/illiad/illiad.dll?SessionID=O065311247Y&Action=10&Form=75&Value=88871

Lavoie-Tremblay, M., Paquet, M., Duchesne, M., Santo, A., Gavrancic, A., Courcy, F., & Gagnon, S. (2010). Retaining nurses and other hospital workers: An intergenerational perspective of the work climate. *Journal of Nursing Scholarship, 42*(4), 414–422.

Lecher, W. T. (2011). *Men in nursing are taking action to improve gender diversity and inclusion.* Retrieved April 28, 2012, from http://blog.rwjf.org/humancapital/2011/10/17/men-in-nursing-are-taking-action-to-improve-gender-diversity-and-inclusion/

Leiter, M., Price, S., & Laschinger, H. (2010). Generational differences in distress, attitudes and incivility among nurses. *Journal of Nursing Management, 18*(8), 970–980.

Llardi, D. (2010). Minority nurse educators: Thomas Edison State College School of Nursing launches nation's first free online database of minority nurse educators. *School Nurse News, 27*(4), 21.

Marquis, B., & Huston, C. (2012). *Leadership roles and management functions in nursing* (7th ed.). Philadelphia, PA: Lippincott Williams & Wilkins.

McMillian, J., Morgan, S. A., & Arment, P. (2006). Acceptance of male registered nurses by female registered nurses. *Journal of Nursing Scholarship, 38*(1), 100–106.

McMurry, T. B. (2011). The image of male nurses and nursing leadership mobility. *Nursing Forum, 46*(1), 22–28.

*Men in nursing.* (2002–2009). Retrieved July 9, 2011, from http://www.discovernursing.com/men-in-nursing

Mensik, J. S. (2007). A view on generational differences from a generation X leader. *Journal of Nursing Administration, 37*(11), 483–484.

Moon, S. (2007). Slow progress seen in promoting nurse executives. *Hospitals & Health Networks, 81*(4), 15–16.

National Alaska Native American Indian Nurses Association. (2001–2011). *History.* Retrieved July 11, 2011, from http://nanainanurses.org/history

National Association of Hispanic Nurses. (2002–2011). *About us.* Retrieved July 11, 2011, from http://www.thehispanicnurses.org/about/

National Black Nurses Association. (2011). *About NBA.* Retrieved July 11, 2011, from http://www.nbna.org/index.php?option=com_content&view=category&id=40&Itemid=59

O'Brien, A. (2008). 2008 Advance Salary Survey. *Advance for Nurses.* Retrieved July 26, 2008, from http://nursing.advanceweb.com/Article/ADVANCE-Salary-Survey-2008.aspx

O'Lynn, C. (2008). Monterey Peninsula College receives grant to retain male nursing students. *Interaction—Official Publication of the American Assembly of Men in Nursing, 26*(1), 1.

Oscos-Sanchez, M. A., Oscos-Flores, L. D., & Burge, S. K. (2008). The Teen Medical Academy: Using academic enhancement and instructional enrichment to address ethnic disparities in the American healthcare workforce. *Journal of Adolescent Health, 42*(3), 284–293.

Philippine Nurses Association of America. (2010). *About PNAA.* Retrieved July 11, 2011, from http://www.mypnaa.org/about-pnaa

Rural Assistance Center. (2011). *Nursing workforce diversity grants.* Retrieved July 9, 2011, from http://www.raconline.org/funding/funding_details.php?funding_id=246

Sequist, T. D. (2007). Health careers for Native American students: Challenges and opportunities for enrichment program design [Supplement 2]. *Journal of Interprofessional Care, 21*, 20–30.

Sloane, T. (2006). Through the Teflon ceiling. *Modern Healthcare, 36*(15), 18.

Snyder, K. A., & Green, A. I. (2008). Revisiting the glass escalator: The case of gender segregation in a female dominated occupation. *Social Problems, 55*(2), 271–299.

Study disputes opt out trend for women. (2008). *Workforce management.* Retrieved July 23, 2008, from http://www.workforce.com/article/20080710/NEWS01/307109995

Thomas, E. (2010). Generational differences and the healthy work environment. *Med-Surg Matters, 19*(6), 20–21.

Torkelson, D. J., & Seed, M. S. (2011). Gender differences in the roles and functions of inpatient psychiatric nurses. *Journal of Psychosocial Nursing & Mental Health Services, 49*(3), 34–41.

U.S. Census Bureau. (2011). *State and county quick facts.* Retrieved July 9, 2011, from http://quickfacts.census.gov/qfd/states/00000.html

Walker, C. A. (2011). Men in nursing: Shock and awe. *Journal of Theory Construction & Testing, 15*(1), 2–3.

Wiley-Little, A. D. (2011). Linking diversity and corporate social responsibility—A lost opportunity. *Insight Into Diversity, 77*(1/2), 10–11.

Wilson, A., Sanner, S., & McAllister, L. (2010). An evaluation study of a mentoring program to increase the diversity of the nursing workforce. *Journal of Cultural Diversity, 17*(4), 144–150.

Witt-Kieffer Executive Search Firm. (2008). *Preparing future leaders in health care.* Retrieved July 27, 2008, from http://www.wittkieffer.com/cmfiles/reports/Future Leaders.pdf

Wolfenden, J. (2011). Men in nursing. *Internet Journal of Allied Health Sciences & Practice, 9*(2). Retrieved April 29, 2012, from http://ijahsp.nova.edu/articles/Vol9Num2/pdf/Wolfenden.pdf

Wooten, L. P. (2008). Guest editor's note: Breaking barriers in organizations for the purpose of inclusiveness. *Human Resource Management, 47*(2), 191–197.

## BIBLIOGRAPHY

Brunetto, Y., Farr-Wharton, R., & Shacklock, K. (2012). Communication, training, well-being, and commitment across nurse generations. *Nursing Outlook, 60*(1), 7–15.

Brox, D. (2012). Nurses for hire: A nationwide look at nursing. *Minority Nurse,* 10–15. Retrieved Sept. 19, 2012 from, http://www.minoritynurse.com/nurses-hire-nationwide-look-nursing.

Burke, J. (2011). Men in nursing. *Registered Nurse Journal, 23*(3), 12–16.

Carver, L., Candela, L., & Gutierrez, A. P. (2011). Survey of generational aspects of nurse faculty organizational commitment. *Nursing Outlook, 59*(3), 137–148.

Codier, E., Freel, M., Kamikawa, C., & Morrison, P. (2011). Emotional intelligence, caring, and generational differences in nurses. *International Journal for Human Caring, 15*(1), 49–55.

Dapremont, J. A. (2011). Success in nursing school: Black nursing students' perception of peers, family, and faculty. *Journal of Nursing Education, 50*(5), 254–260.

Degazon, C., & Mancha, C. (2012). Changing the face of nursing: Reducing ethnic and racial disparities in health. *Family & Community Health, 35*(1), 5–14.

Goldwire, R. (2010). Second opinion: Looking for Black nurse leaders: A call to action. *Minority Nurse,* 43–45.

Gonzalez-Guarda, R. M., & Hassmiller, S. (2011). The IOM/RWJF initiative on the future of nursing: Implications for Hispanic nurses. *Hispanic Health Care International, 9*(1), 3–4.

Ierardi, J., Fitzgerald, D., & Holland, D. (2010). Exploring male students' educational experiences in an associate degree nursing program. *Journal of Nursing Education, 49*(4), 215–218.

Jung, O., & Park, H. (2011). Experience on delivery room practice of male nursing students. *Korean Journal of Women Health Nursing, 17*(1), 64–76.

Kersey-Matusiak, G. (2012). Culturally competent care: Are we there yet? *Nursing, 42*(2), 49–52.

Kouta, C., & Kaite, C. P. (2011). Gender discrimination and nursing: A literature review. *Journal of Professional Nursing, 27*(1), 59–63.

Meadus, R. J., & Twomey, J. (2011). Men student nurses: The nursing education experience. *Nursing Forum, 46*(4), 269–279.

Nairn, S., Hardy, C., Harling, M., Parumal, L., & Narayanasamy, M. (2012). Diversity and ethnicity in nurse education: The perspective of nurse lecturers. *Nurse Education Today, 32*(3), 203–207.

Parker, V. A. (2010–2011). The importance of cultural competence in caring for and working in a diverse America. *Generations, 34*(4), 97–102.

Rambur, B., Palumbo, M., Mclntosh, B., Cohen, J., & Naud, S. (2011). Young adults' perception of an ideal career: Does gender matter? *Nursing Management, 42*(4), 19–24.

Scott, G. (2012). A diverse workplace is a happier workplace. *Nursing Standard, 26*(22), 1.

Torkelson, D. J., & Seed, M. S. (2011). Gender differences in the roles and functions of inpatient psychiatric nurses. *Journal of Psychosocial Nursing & Mental Health Services, 49*(3), 34–41.

Torres, S. (2011). Degrees of success: Online higher education: The key to training, recruiting, and retaining more Hispanic nurses. *Minority Nurse,* 36–38.

University of Medicine and Dentistry of New Jersey. (2012). *Black nurses in history. A bibliography and guide to web resources.* Rowan, NJ: Author. Retrieved Sept. 19, 2012, from http://libguides.rowan.edu/blacknurses

Vigeland, T. (2012, March 21). More men trading overalls for nursing scrubs. *NY Times.* Retrieved April 28, 2012, from http://www.nytimes.com/2012/03/22/your-money/displaced-men-trade-blue-collar-jobs-for-nursing.html?pagewanted=all

# Chapter 10

# New Graduate RN Transition to Practice Programs (Nurse Residencies)

Deloras Jones and Nikki West

## ADDITIONAL RESOURCES

Visit thePoint for additional helpful resources

- eBook
- Journal Articles
- WebLinks

## CHAPTER OUTLINE

## LEARNING OBJECTIVES

*The learner will be able to:*

1. Understand the historical gap between academia and service, and the role that transition to practice programs play in bridging that gap.

2. Identify at least three models of transition to practice programs.

3. List the Institute of Medicine's (IOM) Initiative on the Future of Nursing's four key messages and eight recommendations, and explain how the findings of the IOM report relate to transition to practice programs.

4. Explain the factors creating the current, pressing need for transition to practice programs to retain new graduate nurses and prepare them for employment.

5. Identify the Quality and Safety Education for Nurses (QSEN) competencies and explain their relevance to a new nurse's preparation for clinical practice.

6. Describe the rationale and value of school-based transition to practice programs.

7. Describe potential challenges and threats associated with offering transition to practice programs.

**156**

## THE CONCEPT OF TRANSITION TO PRACTICE PROGRAMS

What are *transition to practice* programs? Multiple types of transition to practice programs exist, but all are focused on helping nursing students bridge from school into employment. There are programs that begin in the final year of nursing school and continue through licensure. Others are structured as employer-based "new graduate classes," typically within a hospital, that take up to a year to complete. Still others are for new graduates who have yet to be hired, so they may gain skills in order to become more employable.

These transition to practice programs have been given various names including "residencies," "externships," and "internships." For purposes of this chapter, the following specific scope and single definition for transition to practice programs (adapted from definitions set forth by the National Council for State Boards of Nursing [NCSBN, 2011a] and the American Association of Colleges of Nursing [AACN]) will be used: A formal program of active learning that includes a series of educational sessions and work experiences for newly licensed registered nurses (RNs) (Krsek & McElroy, 2009). Transition to practice programs are designed to support a newly licensed RN's progression from education to practice as they transition to their first professional nursing role.

This chapter explores the gap between education and service and suggests strategies for closing that gap with transition to practice programs. The chapter suggests that such programs will lower the high turnover rates common to new graduates. In addition, groups leading a national call for transition to practice programs/residencies as an expectation of nursing education are presented. The hiring difficulties new graduates began experiencing in 2009 and the impact that had on transition to nursing practice programs is also discussed. Finally, a current demonstration project that strives to increase the skills, competencies, and confidence of new graduates in community-based transition to practice programs, housed in schools of nursing, is highlighted. This project is put forth as a solution to the hiring dilemma new graduates are experiencing, as it increases their employability. It also adds important evidence regarding the need for transition to practice programs as an expectation of the nursing education process.

## Arguments for Transition to Practice Programs: Closing the Gap Between Education and Practice

Arguments have grown over the last decade regarding the need for transition to practice programs for new graduates of nursing programs. The ever-changing health care delivery care system, with its increasing complexity of patient care, evolving technology, and focus on patient safety, has created expectations from nursing educational systems that are not being met. The practice setting or environment nurses are working in to provide patient care (service), requires nurses with highly developed critical thinking and problem-solving skills, the ability to exercise clinical judgment with the know-how to practice from an evidence-based and outcome-driven perspective, and the ability to develop effectively from a novice to an expert in competency.

Acute care hospitals, which are the traditional employers of new graduates, often report an incongruence between the expectations of education and employers. This difference in expectations and the gap that has resulted between education and practice is not the responsibility of academia alone. Instead, it requires that employers share in creating solutions that provide a bridge from student to practicing nurse. This need to close the gap for new graduates from education to practice fuels arguments for the inclusion of transition to practice programs or residencies as an expectation of the nursing education process.

### Skills/Competencies

New graduates often begin working as an RN with little more than a few weeks of orientation, in contrast to most other professions, which require formal and often standardized internships or residencies. This is largely a residual outcome of the traditional nursing educational system that was grounded in apprenticeship and hospital-based training programs which led to the student receiving a diploma in nursing. A large portion of the education of the diploma-prepared nurse included clinical training by providing direct care to patients in the hospital that sponsored the program. Following graduation, only a few weeks of orientation specific to the hospital or the unit they were assigned was required.

New standards were applied to nursing education in 1965, when the American Nurses Association (ANA) called for a college-based nursing education system. With this change in the standards, the primary focus of nursing education changed from the hospital setting to the university setting, and schools became responsible for preparing students to work in the clinical setting. This resulted in a gap between academia and the practice setting that the profession and employers of nurses continue to grapple with today.

This gap is described in a practice brief completed by Nursing Executive Center, The Advisory Board Company (Nursing Executive Center, The Advisory Board Company, 2006) following interviews with nurse executives from member hospitals. The brief states,

*Many arrive at the hospital unprepared to perform even basic clinical tasks and lacking critical thinking skills to apply their classroom learning to real-life clinical practice. New graduates may also be unprepared for the emotional demands of first-year nursing. The stresses of navigating a new environment, working overnight shifts, and caring for acutely ill patients can take a significant toll . . . (p. viii)*

In addition, Del Bueno (2005) reported that 10-years of performance-based competency testing she completed, suggested that 65% to 75% of new graduates did not meet expectations for entry-level clinical judgment and most had difficulty translating knowledge and theory into practice. Furthermore, a survey conducted for the Advisory Board Company of both hospital nurse executives and leaders of nursing education programs found that only 10% of nurse executives felt that new graduates were fully prepared to provide safe and effective care in hospitals, compared to 90% of nurse educators (Berkow, Virkstis, Stewart, & Conway, 2010).

This academic/practice gap places patient safety and the quality of care at risk if a new graduate does not have the critical thinking skills or competencies needed to apply critical judgments to patient situations. Transition to practice programs bridge the gap by providing the new graduate opportunities to take the learning from nursing school and apply it in an expanded, intensive, and integrated clinical learning situation while providing direct patient care—much in the same way that the internship of physicians is based upon applying academic learning to actual care of patients and transition into the professional role.

A well-designed transition to practice program strengthens new graduates skills and competencies and prepares the new nurse for the demands of caring for patients. Furthermore, a systematic approach to transition not only facilitates "on-boarding" (integration into staffing on the nursing unit to provide direct patient care) but also reduces turnover by decreasing the toll associated with insufficient preparation for the work environment.

> CONSIDER THIS    Other health care professions, including medicine, pharmacy, clinical laboratory scientists, public health, and optometry require residencies or internships to complete their professional training. The costs of medical residencies are largely underwritten by the federal government through Medicare Graduate Medical Education pass-through dollars to hospitals providing training of physicians. Nursing does not have residencies as a requirement nor federal dollars to fund programs. However, arguments seem to be in the favor of requiring residencies or transition to practice programs for nurses as well.

## DISCUSSION POINT

Other professions provide paid internships and residencies as standard practice. Some current new graduate RN transition to practice programs are unpaid, and discussions have taken place suggesting new graduates pay to participate. What do you think of this?

Transition to practice programs should focus on areas where new graduates need additional skills and competencies and not repeat their academic program. According to the Nursing Executive Center, The Advisory Board Company (2006), areas of focus should include organizing work and priority setting; communicating effectively with physicians, team members, families, and patients; clinical leadership skills to include delegating and overseeing the work of others; emergency response; end-of-life care; and technical skills for specific patient care environments.

Krozek (2008) describes transition to practice programs as integrated, interconnected programs hardwired throughout the organization that provide a systematic approach to on-boarding. He goes on to indicate that characteristics of such programs include standardization leading to core training; practical application of knowledge through clinical immersion to hone patient care skills; support systems that include seasoned nurses prepared for roles as preceptors, coaches, and mentors; rigorous evaluation to ensure that expected outcomes are being met; and, continuous improvement based on learning and evolving needs. Major characteristics of employer-based nurse residency programs designed as a transition from nursing school to professional practice are shown in Box 10.1 and goals of exemplary nurse residency programs are displayed in Box 10.2.

## Turnover

Stresses associated with the 1st year of employment, concerns about patient care, and feeling unsupported in their new roles often lead to high turnover rates in new graduates who are more likely than experienced nurses to resign within their 1st year of employment (Nursing Executive Center ,The Advisory Board Company, 2006). The investment made in the high cost of onboarding a new graduate is lost by the hospital/employer when premature turnover occurs. Leaving within 2 years of employment does not allow an effective return on investment (ROI). Studies have reported that turnover rates for new graduates range from 22.6% to 60% (vanWyngeeren & Stuart, n.d.).

---

### BOX 10.1 MAJOR CHARACTERISTICS OF EMPLOYER-BASED NURSE RESIDENCY PROGRAMS

- Designed primarily as a transition from nursing school to professional practice, not primarily to teach specialty-specific skills

- Open only to new graduates or nurses with limited work experience following schooling (e.g., not to nurses returning to practice after years out of the workforce)

- Involve majority of (and preferably all) new graduates hired into the institution

- Focus on building critical thinking and professional practice skills

*Source:* Nursing Executive Center, The Advisory Board Company. (2006). *Transitioning new graduates to hospital practice: Profiles of nurse residency program exemplars.* Washington, DC: Author. Retrieved from www.advisary.com

---

### BOX 10.2 NINE GOALS OF EXEMPLARY NURSE RESIDENCY PROGRAMS

- Bridge gaps in residents' clinical skill set

- Connect "book knowledge" to real-life clinical challenges

- Ensure ongoing support from leadership and peers

- Foster esprit de corps among resident class

- Broaden residents' understanding of health care delivery

- Empower residents to contribute to practice improvement

- Spark continuous professional growth and development

- Demonstrate residency program value

- Facilitate partnerships with area nursing schools

*Source:* Nursing Executive Center, The Advisory Board Company. (2006). *Transitioning new graduates to hospital practice: Profiles of nurse residency program exemplars.* Washington, DC: Author. Retrieved from www.advisary.com

---

High turnover rates result in the "churning of staff," including increased use of temporary staff to fill vacancies, which, in addition to negatively impacting patient care and continuity of care, impacts the stability, and hence the quality, of the work environment; places additional stress on senior nursing staff who are called upon to precept and orient new hires, increases management and supervisory time, and decreases staff productivity (Ulrich et al., 2010). However, residency programs provided by hospitals to new graduates they employ have resulted in a significant drop in turnover.

For example, one large highly respected metropolitan hospital in Western United States reported that 36% of new graduates were leaving within their 1st year and 56% left within 2 years (Ulrich et al., 2010). The hospital implemented a standardized approach for transition to practice programs as a means of increasing retention of new graduates. The 12-month turnover dropped to just over 5%. Versant, the standardized residency program that dramatically decreased the hospital's turnover rate, has continued to produce results in more than 80 hospitals since 1999, providing excellent evidence for the ROI for residencies (Krozek, 2011; Ulrich et al., 2010).

## Cost of Turnover

Estimates of turnover cost per nurse range from US$82,000 to US$88,000 (Jones, 2008). During a typical new nurse training period, which may last anywhere from 2 weeks to 6 months, hospitals essentially pay two nurses (a trainer and a trainee) for the production of one. A recent citing from a survey of hospital CEOs conducted by the audit, tax, and advisory firm KPMG, LLP indicates that the average time to onboard a new graduate is 233 hours, or almost six work weeks (National Association of Travel Healthcare Organizations, 2011).

---

CONSIDER THIS Transition to practice programs can be costly to provide, both in the expense of the faculty and program materials and in the time a new graduate employee spends in class (being paid at full salary), during which time they are not available for staffing and serving patients. For many clinical sites (primarily acute care hospitals), the cost to operate a transition to practice program is justified by the increase in new graduate nurse retention. Turnover rates in facilities that offer programs are often lower than in facilities that do not offer such a program. This results in decreased expense to recruit, hire, and onboard.

---

## NATIONAL CALL FOR TRANSITION TO PRACTICE PROGRAMS

In response to the need to provide a bridge for new graduates from education to practice and to improve retention in the workplace, the movement to provide transition to practice programs is increasing. Groups/organizations who have been most involved in this effort include the following:

1. **The California Institute for Nursing & Health Care** (CINHC), which serves as California's nursing workforce center, has led the dialogue among educators, employers, and professional associations in California about the need to have transition to practice programs as an expectation of nursing education in California, through the development of a

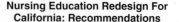

**Nursing Education Redesign For California: Recommendations**

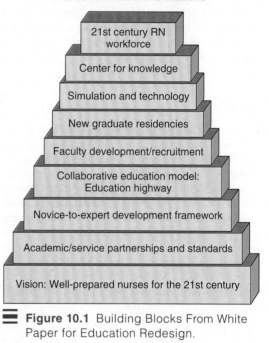

**Figure 10.1** Building Blocks From White Paper for Education Redesign.

*Source*: California Institute for Nursing & Health Care. (2010a).*Education redesign building blocks illustration*. Retrieved from http://www.cinhc.org/wordpress/wp-content/uploads/2010/05/Ed-Redesign-Building-Blocks.pdf

*White Paper for Education Redesign*. This important document, developed in 2008 by thought leaders representing all major stakeholders, serves as a framework for how nursing education needs to be designed to meet the evolving needs of the health care delivery system (CINHC, 2008b; see Figure 10.1).

In the same year, under the leadership of the California Hospital Association (CHA), a statewide workgroup was created with the goal of raising awareness around the importance of residencies for all new graduates within California hospitals. This statewide workgroup continues its efforts and has been identified to carry out the goals of Recommendation No. 3 of the IOM's report on the future of nursing within California (see #8 on page 161).

2. **The National Council of State Boards of Nursing** (NCSBN) has been investigating a regulatory model for transition from education to practice and believes these transition programs are essential and should be postlicensure, not lengthening the time of a nursing

program. In 2010, the NCSBN launched their sponsorship of a multistate, multiyear, and multipractice study on the impact of residencies on patient outcomes (NCSBN, 2011b; Spector & Li, 2007).

3. **The University Health System Consortium and the American Association of Colleges of Nursing** (UHC/AACN) has begun a joint venture on sponsoring residencies for baccalaureate-prepared nurses in academic medical centers. Their position is that new graduates should not be expected to transition into their first jobs without a formal transition to practice program to facilitate bridging the gap between education and practice and that this should be a nationally accredited program. They have been able to demonstrate that after a 1-year residency, the new graduate is able to transition with the skills and knowledge to provide quality, safe care (Goode, Lynn, Krsek, & Bednash, 2009).

4. Patricia Benner and colleagues, in their recent work for the **Carnegie Foundation** (Benner, Sutphen, Leonard, & Day, 2010) called for radical transformation of the nation's education of nurses and identified the development of clinical residencies for all new graduates in their key recommendations. They further recommended that all graduates be required to complete a 1-year residency so that they have the opportunity to develop in-depth knowledge in one clinical area of specialization.

5. **Versant**, a proprietary program developed in 1999 to meet the needs of a major medical center to retain its nurses, has years of experience in implementing transition to practice programs in more than 80 hospitals. Versant leaders have learned that "Implementing the RN residency requires the engagement and active participation of people from throughout the hospital organization including nurses in management, education, administrative and direct care roles; hospital administration; other health care professionals (physicians, pharmacists, social workers); human resource professionals; etc." (Ulrich, 2010, p. 366).

6. **The Advisory Board Company**, which represents 2,900 chief nursing officers, through their Nursing Executive Center, is an important voice of employers on the value of residencies to transition new graduates into practice and increase retention (Pete Simkinson, Senior Director, Member Services, Nursing Executive Center, The Advisory Board Company, personal communication, August 31, 2011).

7. **The Joint Commission (formerly called the Joint Commission on Accreditation of Healthcare Organizations; JCAHO)**, as early as 2002, called for structured postgraduate programs for nurses that would provide the opportunity for skill-building in real clinical setting as do residencies for physicians. These programs would smooth the transition from nursing school and build the confidence and competencies of new graduates (JCAHO, 2002).

8. **The IOM** report on *The Future of Nursing*, released in October 2010, identified transition to practice programs/residencies as one of the eight key recommendations to actualize nursing contributions to the demands of health care reform. The IOM suggested that "State boards of nursing, accrediting bodies, the federal government, and health care organizations should take action to support nurses' completion of a transition-to-practice program (nurse residency) after they have completed a prelicensure or advanced practice degree program or when they are transitioning into new clinical practice areas" (IOM, 2010, p. 280). The report goes on to make specific recommendations to support these programs, including redirecting all graduate medical education funding programs from diploma nursing programs to support the implementation of residencies. They are also calling for programs to be developed outside of the acute care setting, with the expected shift of care from hospitals to community-based settings with health care reform (see Research Study Fuels the Controversy 10.1).

## RESEARCH STUDY FUELS THE CONTROVERSY 10.1

### THE FUTURE OF NURSING

In 2008, The Robert Wood Johnson Foundation (RWJF) and the IOM established a partnership to assess the need to transform the nursing profession to provide higher-quality, safer, more affordable, and more accessible care in the current era of health care reform. They established a 2-year initiative on the future of nursing and assembled a committee to produce a report for an action-oriented blueprint for the future of nursing, including changes in public and institutional policies at the national, state, and local levels. The Initiative on the Future of Nursing Committee includes an impressive group of 18 health care leaders across the nation, chaired by Donna Shalala, president, University of Miami and former secretary of health and human services under President Bill Clinton, and vice chaired by Linda Burnes Bolton, vice president and chief nursing officer of Cedars-Sinai Health System. The committee included a complement of representatives from nursing, medicine, academia, service settings, information technology, business, and public health.

Institute of Medicine. (2010). *The future of nursing: Leading change, advancing health*. Washington, DC: The National Academies. Retrieved from www.futureofnursing.org

## STUDY FINDINGS

As a result of its work, the committee formulated four key messages that structure the discussion and recommendations within the IOM report:

*Key Message 1:* Nurses should practice to the full extent of their education and training.

*Key Message 2:* Nurses should achieve higher levels of education and training through an improved education system that promotes seamless academic progression.

*Key Message 3:* Nurses should be full partners, with physicians and other health professionals, in redesigning health care in the United States.

*Key Message 4:* Effective workforce planning and policy making require better data collection and an improved information infrastructure.

To implement these key messages, the IOM report identifies eight specific recommendations, representing both a major challenge and opportunity for nursing. These recommendations included the following:

*Recommendation 1:* Remove scope of practice barriers.

*Recommendation 2:* Expand opportunities for nurses to lead and diffuse collaboration.

*Recommendation 3:* Implement nurse residency programs.

*Recommendation 4:* Increase the proportion of nurses with baccalaureate degrees to 80% by 2020.

*Recommendation 5:* Double the number of nurses with a doctorate by 2020.

*Recommendation 6:* Ensure that nurses engage in lifelong learning.

*Recommendation 7:* Prepare and enable nurses to lead change to advance health.

*Recommendation 8:* Build an infrastructure for the collection and analysis of interprofessional health care workforce data.

In order to implement the Key Messages and Recommendations within the IOM report, RWJF has leveraged preexisting groundwork and created new collaborations to engage national organizations in guiding implementation. The American Association for Retired Persons' (AARP) Center to Champion Nursing in America, along with state-based Action Coalitions, is moving the recommendations forward at the community and state levels. The Action Coalitions are the driving force of the overall initiative to make progress at the local, state, and national levels and to develop long-term, sustainable means to achieve the goals of the IOM report.

---

CONSIDER THIS   The IOM Report (*The Future of Nursing*) will have a significant impact on nursing education. Identifying the report findings and implications for nursing in the future warrants further explanation.

**DISCUSSION POINT**

What is the outlook for the nursing workforce in the era of health care reform, in terms of types of health care settings where nurses will work, the overall number of nurses needed to serve the population, and roles for nurses in these settings?

**DISCUSSION POINT**

Why do you think interest is building around transition to practice programs and nurse residencies?

## THE HIRING DILEMMA OF NEW GRADUATES—UNANTICIPATED FALLOUT FROM THE NATION'S ECONOMIC RECESSION

The nursing shortage that has long plagued the nation's health care system persists and is likely to worsen in years to come. The 21st century began with the nation preparing for a looming shortage that threatened to result in a public health crisis, driven by 76 million aging baby boomers reaching eligibility for Medicare (sign of the aging of the United States), retirements of an older nursing workforce, and an insufficient number of new nurses to replace those retiring. Analyzing population growth, income, and technology statistics, Buerhaus, Staiger, and Auerbach (2009b) estimated the demand for health care would grow 3% every year in the United States. The "perfect storm" for the nursing shortage crisis was brewing and was expected to begin around 2010 (when the first of the Baby Boomers became eligible for Medicare), reaching a forecasted shortage of 500,000 FTEs by 2025.

Across the country, states responded to this forecasted crisis by building educational capacity to increase the nursing workforce, and a national campaign led by Johnson & Johnson focused on the desirability of nursing as a career. Largely, as a result of these efforts and helped by an influx of foreign-educated nurses and older nurses returning to the workforce, Buerhaus and colleagues (2009a) revised the predicted 2025 shortfall of RNs to 260,000 FTEs.

California's response to the nursing shortage, which was among the worst in the nation, included measures that built educational capacity. In 2004, California ranked 50th out of 50 states for ratio of RNs to population, at 580 RNs per 100,000 population, compared with the nation's average of 825 per 100,000 (Biviano & Spencer, 2004). The state was also forecast to have a shortfall of 116,000 RN FTE by 2020 if the trajectory the state was on at that time continued, meeting only 55% of the state's demand for nurses.

These sobering predictions resulted in a focused and systematic effort, led by the Governor's Task Force for Nursing Education and facilitated by the development of a master plan for building educational capacity under the leadership of CINHC, to increase the state's capacity to educate nurses (CINHC, 2008a). As a result of these efforts, between 2004 and 2010 educational capacity increased 69% and the state rose in RN per capita to 644 per 100,000 (compared with a national average of 860 per 100,000; California Board of Registered Nursing [CBRN], 2009–2010).

However, while these statistics were encouraging, the sudden, severe economic downturn in 2008 created an unexpected "perfect storm" for new RN graduates that resulted in unprecedented difficulty securing employment. In spite of preparing for a looming shortage, several factors changed the employment picture for nurses.

First of all, in late 2008, as the nation's economy began to plummet, fewer patients opted for elective surgeries and other treatments as unemployment resulted in the loss of health plan benefits and uncertainty of income; this led to a decrease in hospital days and revenue and decreased demand for nurses.

Second, as a response to the economic recession, experienced nurses worked more. The majority (68%) of nurses in California were married, and to compensate for a spouse's loss or anticipated loss of employment during the recession, many nurses worked extra hours or took on a second job, part-time nurses transitioned to full-time, and others who were not working returned to the workforce. In addition, older nurses who were eligible for retirement delayed leaving the workforce as the value of their investment accounts dropped.

Hospitals, which were also facing financial hardships during this time, found it easier and less expensive to hire experienced nurses than to bring on new graduates, who were costly to hire since hospitals needed to provide extensive orientation or residencies to prepare them for employment. Thus, experienced nurses held the jobs that new graduates had expected to fill and competed with the new graduates for the fewer jobs that were available. In 2010, California hospital RN vacancy rates dropped to an unprecedented low rate of 3.4% and turnover dropped to 8.2%, compared with 10.2% vacancy rates in 2005 (Hospital Association of Southern California [HASC], 2010).

> CONSIDER THIS  The nursing workforce is elastic. Nurses work less when the economy is good and work more when the economy is bad. Unemployment in California in July of 2011 was 12%, the second highest rate in the country. When the new nurses who were seeking jobs in 2010 and 2011 chose nursing as a career, it was at the height of the shortage of the 2000s, and they were told "You will always have a job" and "Nursing is a recession-proof profession."

The economic climate in the years 2008–2012 temporarily concealed the chronic nurse shortage. These conditions are expected to pass, and once they do, the nation's health care system will again see the consequences of an increasing demand for nurses and a grossly inadequate supply. This demand will further be exacerbated by the demands of health care reform, which calls for a health care delivery system capable of providing care to 32 million more Americans through health plans and the increasing numbers of the aging population requiring more in the way of health care and chronic disease management. Given this prognosis, California cannot afford to lose its invaluable new RNs.

---

### DISCUSSION POINT

Nurses above 50 years of age comprise 50% of California's nursing workforce, and a full 18% are above the age of 60. Retirements have been delayed and nurses are working more because of the economy. The state's unemployment rate is second highest in the country. California is expected to add 4 million individuals to health plans through health care reform. What will happen to the nursing workforce when the economy improves, retirement accounts are rebuilt, unemployment rates drop, and health care reform measures are implemented? How can the state be prepared for what lies ahead?

---

## THE CALIFORNIA
## STORY—A DEMONSTRATION PROJECT

To quantify the extent of the issue of new graduate RNs' inability to secure jobs, a survey of nurse employers, led by CINHC, indicated that approximately 40% of new graduates in 2010 would not be hired in hospitals (CINHC, 2009). A follow-up surveys of new graduate RNs, conducted in 2010 and 2011, validated that 43% had not found jobs in nursing after 6 or more months following graduation (CINHC, 2010, 2012). California's new nurses had fewer opportunities to gain experience and transition successfully into practice.

To address this statewide issue, five regional forums were held across the state to report the survey findings and determine solutions to this hiring dilemma. Participants at these regional forums included health care employers, schools of nursing, state agencies, state nursing organizations, workforce investment boards, and community organizations. After considerable discussion, the solution that resonated was to develop *community-based transition programs for newly graduated RNs, housed in schools of nursing*, to maintain and improve their skills and competencies, and to increase their chances of employability. Santa Rosa Junior College in Santa Rosa, California, led the way in developing this concept with a similar approach, through a partnership with the local workforce investment board (WIB) and community hospitals to address the increased numbers of their new graduates unable to find jobs.

The concept is that programs would be designed in collaboration with service and academic partners to address perceived gaps between nursing school and preparation for practice as a professional nurse. The programs would have schools involved in providing didactic (classroom) instruction, and clinical partners would provide intense clinical instruction with preceptorships in various types of settings. Hospitals would be active partners, yet they would not need to first hire the new nurse in order to provide the experience. This important distinction alleviated the issue of limited job openings, which had been preventing service partners from providing new graduates with traditional transition to practice program experiences.

> CONSIDER THIS  Traditional transition to practice programs (residencies) are funded and provided by employers (usually hospitals). The hospital hires a group of new graduate RNs and provides a curriculum over the first 6 months to 1 year of their employment. The new graduate hires receive full pay, though they do not have a full patient load for some time into their residency. Due to the economy, many hospitals have fewer vacancies for new hires, have had smaller hiring budgets, and have been able to hire experienced nurses who need to work more hours to fill vacancies, and are therefore not employing as many new graduates or training them through residencies.

The school-based transition to practice programs could be customized by each school–clinical partnership providing the education; however, all programs would have standard components. Consistently, leaders involved in designing the school-based transition to practice programs agreed the standard basis for the curriculum should be the Quality and Safety Education for Nurses (QSEN) competencies for professional practice.

## QSEN COMPETENCIES

RWJF has funded the national, multiphase QSEN project to address the challenge of preparing future nurses with the knowledge, skills, and attitudes (KSA) necessary to continuously improve the quality and safety of the health care systems in which they work. QSEN faculty have defined prelicensure and graduate quality and safety competencies for nursing and proposed targets for the KSA to be developed in nursing prelicensure programs for each competency. These are shown in Box 10.3.

QSEN pursues strategies to build and develop effective teaching approaches to assure that future graduates develop competencies in these areas. In terms of new graduate RNs preparing for the workforce, the KSAs in these six competency areas are seen as a solid basis for assessing and creating development plans for nurses as they bridge from student to licensed nurse clinicians serving patients.

---

**BOX 10.3 QUALITY & SAFETY EDUCATION FOR NURSES (QSEN) COMPETENCIES**

- Patient-centered care
- Teamwork and collaboration
- Evidence-based practice
- Quality improvement
- Safety
- Informatics

*Source:* Quality and Safety Education for Nurses. (2011). *Quality and safety competencies.* Retrieved from http://www.qsen.org/competencies.php

---

## SCHOOL-BASED TRANSITION TO PRACTICE PROGRAMS

In mid-September 2009, CINHC partnered with several leading statewide organizations, including the California Hospital Association (CHA), the Association of California Nurse Leaders (ACNL), and philanthropic organizations invested in advancing nursing—the Gordon and Betty Moore Foundation in Palo Alto, California, and the Kaiser Permanente Fund for Health Education at the East Bay Community Foundation, in Oakland, California—to launch these demonstration programs to help new graduates gain skills and experience to become more employable (Jones & West, 2011). As a first step, the group identified common components for all school-based transition to practice programs. Common components were as follows:

- The new graduate must have passed the NCLEX and be licensed.
- The program must be offered through local schools of nursing, which provide liability coverage and workers' compensation, with service partners providing the clinical experience, without the requirement to hire.
- It should award academic credit or continuing education to participants upon completion.
- It should award a common industry recognized certificate of completion.
- It should incorporate clinical, didactic, simulation, skills lab, and e-learning components.
- It should run 12 to 18 weeks in length, with a 24-hour-per-week participant commitment.
- It should follow QSEN competencies for professional practice as an indicator of improved preparation for clinical practice.
- It should use common, QSEN-based evaluation tools to assess participant competence and progress, as well as common evaluation tool for first employers of program participants, in order to determine impact of the program.
- It should provide extended experiential learning opportunities in generalist, acute, specialty, or community health care settings to advance skills.
- It should provide training to program preceptors.
- It should offer generally nonsalaried positions.

Program funders served as thought leaders and partners in developing the concept for these programs. Funding from the Gordon and Betty Moore Foundation, was made available to provide experiences for 250 new graduate RNs within the San Francisco Bay Area. In addition, supplementary funding was used by some programs, provided by the Kaiser Permanente Fund for Health Education at the East Bay Community Foundation and local WIBs. In-kind contributions were made by both school and service partners to offset costs.

In 2009, four pilot or demonstration transition to practice programs were launched, led by the following:

- California State University, East Bay (for a minimum of 81 new graduate RNs)
- Samuel Merritt University (for a minimum of 81 new graduate RNs)
- A collaboration of South Bay schools, including San Jose State University and San Jose/Evergreen Community College District through the Workforce Institute (a division of the San Jose Evergreen Community College District that provides customized education, professional development, and skills upgrade training; for a minimum of 48 new graduate RNs)
- University of San Francisco (for a minimum of 40 new graduate RNs).

The four programs developed their own curriculums based on the core requirements identified above, secured acute and nonacute clinical partners including hospitals, clinics, skilled nursing facilities (SNFs), rehabilitation facilities, and even public schools in some instances (for school nursing), recruited and enrolled new graduate RN participants, and launched their individual programs. Programs admitted a combination of ADN- and BSN-educated nurses from local nursing schools.

> **CONSIDER THIS**  It is expected that more health care will be provided outside of acute care settings as health care reform is implemented. Transition to practice programs focused on nonacute settings, such as primary care clinics, behavior health clinics, long-term care, home health, corrections, school nursing, and public health, provide exposure to career paths that new graduates may not have previously considered and also provide an opportunity for nonacute employers to consider hiring new graduate nurses.

## School-Based Transition to Practice Program Status and Evaluation

The school-based transition to practice programs represent a newly graduated approach to preparing new RNs for the practice setting, as compared with hospital- (employer-) based residencies. These programs do not require clinical sites to hire participants in advance of the program, but do require academia and service to work in a partnership for program design and implementation. The programs are designed within consistent guidelines, resulting in an industry-recognized certificate of completion. Based on their unique characteristics, these programs are receiving attention as a new model for providing nursing education, for implementing Recommendation No. 3 of the IOM Report, and therefore the value of the programs is of interest, both to the funders of the pilots and on a state—even national—level.

Recommendation No. 3 of the IOM Report directly speaks to transition to practice programs: "Implement nurse residency programs." A statewide workgroup within California is meeting regularly to determine goals and action steps for actualizing and defining how to achieve this recommendation. This workgroup has agreed to the goal to strongly recommend that all new graduates have the opportunity to participate in a residency program. The group has developed tools and definitions for residencies (transition to practice programs), which include definitions for "new graduate nurse," "nursing orientation," and "nurse residency/transition to practice programs."

In addition, a certificate of completion has been created, which is expected to build common understanding and industry recognition around these programs. A statewide database on the various models for transition to practice programs and residencies is being created. These programs are also being considered in a variety of new settings and specialties, including home health, long-term care, school health centers, infection control, and primary care clinics. The workgroup is also exploring programs for nurse practitioners.

Interest in the school-based transition to practice programs is growing, and other regions across California are now implementing similar versions. Across the Central Valley, Los Angeles, Orange County, and San Diego, there are now 20 programs using the same model, and evaluation tools.

Kaiser Permanente National Patient Care Services has provided funding to CINHC for evaluation and replication of these school-based transition to practice programs. The evaluation includes working with a university-based research team from the University of San Francisco (USF). At the time of this writing, the evaluation is underway and will include an analysis of the new graduate RN program participant's ability to increase the following:

- perceived self-confidence
- competence
- ability to transition to the workforce—ease of transition and decreased time to independent functioning
- impact on new graduate employability.

Several survey tools have been created to examine the success of the programs, including a competency tool based on QSEN and a survey for the first employers of school-based transition to practice program participants. The First Employer Survey evaluates how the programs have made a difference to employers in terms of the competence, confidence, skills, retention, and overall ability of the new graduate to transition to the workplace. This analysis builds the body of knowledge supporting the importance of transition to practice programs as a sustainable means to assist new graduate nurses and supports transition to practice programs as an expectation of the nursing education process.

CONSIDER THIS Of all the evaluation tools used for the transition programs, the First Employer Survey is arguably the most important. With this tool, managers who have hired and now supervise program participants are asked to identify if there is a difference in this new hire's ability to transition to the workplace, as compared with other nurses they have hired.

## THE FUTURE OF TRANSITION TO PRACTICE PROGRAMS AND ISSUES WITH SUSTAINABILITY

Transition to practice programs have been designed to provide additional clinical experience for new RNs and to meet the needs of health care employers by developing a nursing workforce that is better prepared to bridge the gap between education and practice. In addition, in the case of the school-based programs, the experience is intended to provide access to employment for health care facilities that do not have the resources to fund training programs, especially in nonacute settings. These programs integrate prior academic learning into guided intensive clinical practice in order to transition new graduates to the professional role of the RN. Across California, several schools of nursing and nurse employers support transition to practice programs, and the IOM Report specifically calls for it. The response from the community to

expand programs is encouraging, and we await evaluation data to demonstrate that the programs are meeting the intended goals of increasing new graduates' clinical skills, competence, confidence, employability, and more effectively help bridge the gap from education to practice.

## CHALLENGES AND THREATS

Despite considerable program interest and support, there are factors that make any transition to practice program challenging to sustain. Issues or threats challenging these programs include the following:

- These school-based transition to practice programs are not intended to take the place of employer-based residencies, which often extend to 1 year and have a planned, structured, mentored experience.
- Programs are dependent on the willingness of partners to provide qualified preceptors—Many clinical sites are limited in the number of preceptors they can provide between meeting the needs of both prelicensure students and new graduate nurses.
- Schools of nursing are concerned they will lose clinical sites and preceptors for student nurses to transition to practice programs.
- It may be difficult to secure qualified clinical faculty to supervise the program participants.
- Program development and implementation bears a significant workload on school and clinical site partners, involving many steps, including the following:
  - Gaining approval to offer for credit through colleges and universities for school-based programs
  - Securing faculty and clinical partners
  - Screening applicants and responding to those who were and were not accepted
  - Securing teaching space (classrooms, skills labs, simulation centers)
  - Paying for packaged programs (such as Versant)
- Identifying funding sources to cover program costs, which may include the following:
  - Foundation funding
  - Self-support through tuition paid by participant
  - Employer supplements
- When the economy improves and there is a spike in demand for nurses, employers may forego transition to practice programs as an unnecessary expense in bringing on new nurses.
- As these programs are primarily unpaid experiences, this raises concerns about what is the right thing to do, as some may view the program participants as "free" labor.

## CONCLUSIONS

What is the future of transition to practice programs? Are there models that will become established as norms? Will these programs become an expectation of nursing education? Only time will tell. There is a finite window of time available to build the case and identify evidence of the importance of transition to practice programs for new graduates. There are groups aware of this opportunity, who are actively working to ensure these programs exist into the future, as a way to better prepare tomorrow's nurses.

## FOR ADDITIONAL DISCUSSION

**1.** Schools have voiced concerns that transition to practice programs are taking preceptorship slots that have been historically allocated to prelicensure students. What ideas do you have for ensuring this does not happen?

**2.** Should transition to practice programs/residencies be a requirement for completion of nursing education? Residencies have historically been a cost hospitals have assumed. Should this cost be shared and why?

**3.** Would you participate in a school-based transition to practice program without an associated stipend, if it could help you gain experience? Would you pay to participate?

**4.** How can we make sure transition to practice programs continue to exist once the economy shifts and new graduate nurses have an easier time finding jobs?

## REFERENCES

Benner, P., Sutphen, M., Leonard, V., & Day, L. (2009). *Educating nurses: A call for radical transformation* (Higher and adult education series). San Francisco, CA: Jossey-Bass.

Berkow, P. C., Virkstis, K., Stewart, J., & Conway, L. (2010). Assessing new graduate nurse performance. *Journal of Nursing Administration, 38*(11), 468–474.

Biviano, M., Fritz, M., & Spencer, W. (2004). *What is behind HRSA's projected supply, demand, and shortage of registered nurses?* Rockville, MD: National Center for Health Workforce Analysis, Bureau of Health Professions, Health Resources and Service Administration.

Buerhaus, P. I., Auerbach, D. I., & Staiger, D. O. (2009a). The recent surge in nurse employment: Causes and implication [Abstract] (Web exclusive). *Health Affairs, 28*(4), 658.

Buerhaus, P. I., Staiger, D. O., & Auerbach, D. I. (2009b). *The future of the nursing workforce in the United States.* Sudbury, MA: Jones and Bartlett.

California Board of Registered Nursing.. (2009–2010). *Survey of registered nurses in California 2010.* (Annual School Survey). Retrieved from www.rn.ca.gov/forms/publications

California Institute for Nursing & Health Care. (2008a) *Master Plan for Building Educational Capacity.* Retrieved from http://www.cinhc.org/programs/master-plan

California Institute for Nursing & Health Care. (2008b). *White paper on nursing education redesign.* Retrieved from http://www.cinhc.org/2008/05/nursing-education-redesign-white-paper/

California Institute for Nursing & Health Care. (2009). *New RN graduate workforce regional planning meetings, statewide summary of RN hiring survey.* Retrieved from http://www.cinhc.org/wordpress/wp-content/uploads/2009/07/6_RNJobpresAllRegionsed0809.pdf

California Institute for Nursing & Health Care. (2010). *Education redesign building blocks illustration.* Retrieved from http://www.cinhc.org/wordpress/wp-content/uploads/2010/05/Ed-Redesign-Building-Blocks.pdf

California Institute for Nursing & Health Care. (2012). 2010–2011 *California New Graduate Hiring Survey.* Retrieved from http://www.cinhc.org/wordpress/wp-content/uploads/2012/02/NewGradSurvey Summary-of-FINAL02212012.pdf

Del Bueno, D. J. (2005). A crisis in critical thinking. *Nursing Education Perspectives, 26*(5), 278–282.

Goode, C. J., Lynn, M. R., Krsek, C., & Bednash, G. D. (2009) Nurse residency programs: An essential requirement for nursing. *Nursing Economics, 27*(3), 142–147.

Hospital Association of Southern California. (2010). *Allied for health quarterly turnover and vacancy report* (4th quarter). Los Angeles, CA: Author.

Institute of Medicine. (2010). *The future of nursing: Leading change, advancing health.* Washington, DC: The National Academies.

Joint Commission on Accreditation of Healthcare Organizations. (2002). *Health care at the crossroads: Strategies for addressing the evolving nursing crisis.* Retrieved from http://www.jointcommission.org/assets/1/18/health_care_at_the_crossroads.pdf

Jones, C. B. (2008). Revisiting nurse turnover cost. *Nursing Administration, 38*(1), 11–18.

Jones, D., & West, N. (2011). Community-based transition programs: California's answer to the new-graduate hiring crisis. *Journal of Nursing Regulation, 1*(2), 14–17.

Krozek, C. (2008). The new graduate RN residency: Win/win/win for nurses, hospitals, and patients. *NurseLeader, 5*(6), 41–44.

Krozek, C. (2011). *The Versant team.* Retrieved from http://versant.org/more-about-versant/the-versant-team.html

Krsek, C., & McElroy, D. (2009). *A solution to the problem of first-year nurse turnover.* Retrieved from https://www.uhc.edu/docs/003741626_SolutiontoProblemofNurseTurnover.pdf

National Association of Travel Healthcare Organizations. (2011). *KPMGLLP's 2011 U.S. Hospital Nursing Labor Costs Study.* Retrieved from http://natho.org/kpmgStudy.php

National Council State Boards of Nursing. (2011a). *Goals of NCSBN's transition to practice model.* Retrieved from https://www.ncsbn.org/TransitiontoPractice_goals_081911.pdf

National Council State Boards of Nursing. (2011b). *NCSBN embarks on an innovative multi-site transition to practice study to examine the effects of nurse transition to practice programs on patient outcomes* (Press release). Retrieved from https://www.ncsbn.org/2403.htm

Nursing Executive Center, The Advisory Board Company. (2006). *Transitioning new graduates to hospital practice: Profiles of nurse residency program exemplars.* Retrieved from www.advisory.com

Spector, N., & Li, S. (2007). A regulatory model on transitioning nurses from education to practice. *JONA's Healthcare Law, Ethics, and Regulation, 9*(1), 19–22.

Ulrich, B., Krozek, C., Early, S., Ashlock, C. H., Africa, L. M., & Carman, M. L. (2010). Improving retention, confidence, and competence of new graduate nurses: Results from a 10-year longitudinal database. *Nursing Economics, 28*(6), 363–375.

vanWyngeeren, K., & Stuart, T. (n.d.). Increasing new graduate nurse retention from the student nurse perspective. *RN Journal.* Retrieved from http://www.rnjournal.com/journal_of_nursing/increasing_new_graduate_nurse_retention.htm

## BIBLIOGRAPHY

California Labor and Workforce Development Agency. (2011). *California governor's nurse education initiative.* Retrieved from www.labor.ca.gov/nurseinitindex.htm

Johnson & Johnson. (2011). *Campaign for Nursing.* Retrieved from http://campaignfornursing.com/

Quality and Safety Education for Nurses. (2011). *Quality and safety competencies.* Retrieved from http://www.qsen.org/competencies.php

Randolph, P. K. (2010, Spring). What happened to the nursing shortage? *Leader to Leader: Nursing Regulation & Education Together,* 1–2.

Stowkowski, L. A. (2011). Looking out for our new nurse grads. *Medscape Nurses—Nursing Perspectives.* Retrieved from http://www.medscape.com/viewarticle/744221

U.S. Bureau of Labor Statistics. (2011). *Economic news release: Regional and state employment and unemployment summary.* Retrieved from http://data.bls.gov/cgi-bin/print.pl/news.release/laus.nr0.htm

U.S. Department of Health and Human Services. (2010, March). *The registered nurse population: Initial findings from the 2008 National Sample Survey of Registered Nurses.* Washington, DC: U.S. Department of Health and Human Services, Health Resource and Services Administration.

# Unit 3

# Workplace Issues

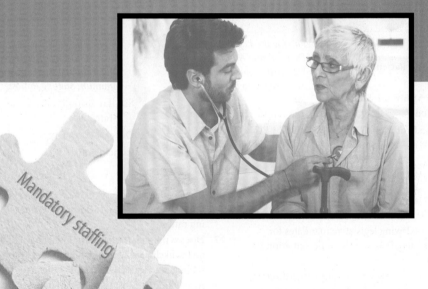

Mandatory staffing

Workplace violence

Entry into practice

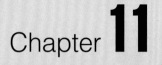

## Chapter 11

# Mandatory Minimum Staffing Ratios
*Are They Working?*

Carol J. Huston

## CHAPTER OUTLINE

## LEARNING OBJECTIVES

*The learner will be able to:*

1. Explore factors driving legislative mandates for minimum registered nurse (RN) representation in the staffing mix.

2. Summarize current research findings regarding the effect of staffing ratios and staffing mix on patient outcomes.

3. Debate driving and restraining forces for legislating minimum licensed staffing ratios.

4. Assess the efficiency and effectiveness of the processes used by the state of California Department of Health Services to determine initial minimum RN–patient staffing ratios for different types of hospital units.

5. Describe challenges to staffing ratio implementation in California, including the need to define "licensed nurses," legal challenges to the "at all times clause," and strategies directed at delaying or rescinding the mandate altogether.

6. Investigate the movement and/or progress of states other than California to adopt minimum RN staffing ratios.

7. Discuss the effect of the current nursing shortage on the likelihood of successful passage of proposed staffing ratio legislation in states other than California.

8. Argue for or against the appropriateness of the "at all times clause" as part of California's staffing ratio mandate.

9. Assess whether California's 2004 implementation of mandatory minimum RN staffing ratios has met its intended goals.

10. Identify alternatives to staffing ratio mandates that seek to assure that staffing resources are adequate to provide safe patient care.

11. Reflect on the staffing ratios used in his or her work setting and assess, using clearly defined criteria, whether they are adequate to provide quality patient care.

For some time now, economics has been the primary driver in dictating changes in the RN skill mix in hospitals. As a result, the trend for at least the last decade has been to reduce RNs in the staffing mix and to replace them with less expensive personnel. Empirical research increasingly concludes, however, that the number of RNs in the staffing mix has a direct effect on quality care and, in particular, patient outcomes. In response, legislators, health care providers, and the public are increasingly demanding adequate staffing ratios of RNs in acute care settings.

Indeed, a national movement to mandate minimum staffing ratios has begun. Many states in the United States, with the backing of some nursing organizations, have moved toward imposing mandatory licensed staffing requirements, and one state (California) has enacted legislation requiring mandatory staffing ratios that affect hospitals and long-term care facilities. In fact, as of 2011, 15 states (California, Connecticut, Illinois, Maine, Minnesota, Nevada, New Jersey, New York, North Carolina, Ohio, Oregon, Rhode Island, Texas, Vermont, and Washington) plus the District of Columbia had enacted legislation and/or adopted regulations addressing nurse staffing and a total of 13 states had staffing laws (American Nurses Association [ANA], 2011a). It should be noted that many of the states that have adopted legislation about staffing originally sought staffing ratio legislation. Seven states (Connecticut, Illinois, Nevada, Ohio, Oregon, Texas, and Washington) now require hospitals to have staffing committees responsible for plans and staffing policy (ANA, 2011b).

This chapter explores both the driving and restraining forces for legislative mandates for minimum RN representation in the staffing mix. California's experience, as the first state to implement minimum staffing ratios, is detailed, as well as its struggle to define appropriate ratios and implement staffing ratios in an era of limited fiscal and human resources. The chapter concludes by looking at the movement of other states toward the adoption of minimum staffing ratios and strategies that have been suggested as alternatives to mandatory staffing ratios.

---

CONSIDER THIS   Evidence exists to suggest that increasing the number of RNs in the staffing mix leads to safer workplaces for nurses and a higher quality of care for patients.

---

## STAFFING RATIOS AND PATIENT OUTCOMES

Numerous studies in the last decade have examined the link between staffing mix and patient outcomes. Indeed, Flynn and McKeown (2009) note that more than 500 papers on nurse staffing levels research were published between 1998 and 2008 with the majority focusing on the impact of "poor" nurse staffing levels on patients and nurses. Many of the studies note a link between the increased representation of RNs in the staffing mix and improved patient outcomes.

For example, a study by Sochalski, Konetzka, Zhu, and Volpp (2008) of acute myocardial infarction (AMI) patients ($n = 348,720$) and surgical failure-to-rescue (FTR) ($n = 109,066$) patients discharged between 1993 and 2001 from 343 California acute care general hospitals found significant cross-sectional associations between higher nurse staffing and reductions in AMI mortality. These improvements, however, were smaller in hospitals with higher baseline staffing. There were no significant cross-sectional associations between higher nurse staffing and FTR. The researchers concluded that strong diminishing returns to nurse staffing improvements and lack of significant evidence that staffing uniformly increases improved outcomes raise questions about the cost-effectiveness of implementing statewide mandatory nurse staffing ratios.

Blegen, Goode, Spetz, Vaughn, and Park (2011) used a cross-sectional analysis of more than 1 million adult patient discharges and staffing for 872 patients from 54 hospitals to determine that total hours of nursing care per patient day were associated with positive patient outcomes including reductions in mortality, failure to rescue, length of stay, and infection rates. In addition, greater RN skill mix was associated with fewer cases of sepsis and failure to rescue (see Research Study Fuels the Controversy).

In addition, Kane, Shamliyan, Mueller, Duval, and Wilt (2007b), in their meta-analysis of 28 studies, found that increased RN staffing was associated with lower hospital-related mortality in intensive care units (ICUs), as well as for patients in surgical and in medical units, when just one additional full-time-equivalent (FTE) RN was added per patient day. Such an increase was also associated with a decreased odds ratio of hospital-acquired pneumonia, unplanned extubation, respiratory failure, and cardiac arrest and with a lower risk of failure to rescue in surgical patients in ICUs. In addition, length of stay was 24% shorter in ICUs and 31% shorter for surgical patients when the additional FTE RN was added.

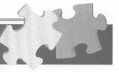

## RESEARCH STUDY FUELS THE CONTROVERSY

### NURSE STAFFING AND PATIENT OUTCOMES

Nurse staffing has been linked to hospital patient outcomes; however, research findings have been inconsistent as a result of the variations in staffing measures used. In this cross-sectional study, data were available for approximately 1.1 million adult patient discharges and staffing for 872 patient care units from 54 hospitals belonging to a University Health System Consortium. Total hours of nursing care (registered nurses [RNs], licensed practical nurses, and assistants) determined per inpatient day (TotHPD) and RN skill mix were the measures of staffing; Agency for Healthcare Research and Quality risk-adjusted safety and quality indicators were the outcome measures.

Blegen, M., Goode, C., Spetz, J., Vaughn, T., & Park, S. (2011). Nurse staffing effects on patient outcomes: Safety-net and non-safety-net hospitals. *Medical Care, 49*(4), 406–414.

### STUDY FINDINGS

TotHPD in general units was associated with lower rates of congestive heart failure mortality ($p < 0.05$), failure to rescue ($p < 0.10$), infections ($p < 0.01$), and prolonged length of stay ($p < 0.01$). RN skill mix in general units was associated with reduced failure to rescue ($p < 0.01$) and infections ($p < 0.05$). TotHPD in ICUs was associated with fewer infections ($p < 0.05$) and decubitus ulcers ($p < 0.10$). RN skill mix was associated with fewer cases of sepsis ($p < 0.01$) and failure to rescue ($p < 0.05$). Safety-net status was associated with higher rates of congestive heart failure mortality, decubitus ulcers, and failure to rescue. Higher nurse staffing then appeared to protect patients from poor outcomes; however, hospital safety-net status introduced complexities in this relationship.

However, Kane, Shamliyan, Mueller, Duval, and Wilt (2007a), in their review of nearly 100 studies by the Agency for Healthcare Quality and Research, found an association between staffing levels, patient mortality, and patient outcomes, but concluded that these relationships are not causal. Flynn and McKeown (2009) agree, suggesting that while there may be an association between models of nurse staffing and outcomes, there is insufficient evidence to establish a causal relationship between these factors. Research by Burnes Bolton et al. (2007) also failed to find the anticipated significant improvements expected in the incidence of falls and the prevalence of hospital-acquired pressure ulcers following the implementation of mandated staffing ratios in California.

A summary of these studies and several other studies completed since 2007 is included in Table 11.1.

Few studies, however, have had as much effect on determining safe staffing ratios as two benchmark research studies published in 2002. The first study was the work of Needleman, Buerhaus, Mattke, Stewart, and Zelevinsky (2002). This study of 799 hospitals in 11 states found a higher prevalence of infections, such as pneumonia and urinary tract infections, failure to rescue, and shock or cardiac arrest when the nurses' workload was high.

The second study, which is often cited as the seminal work in support of establishing minimum staffing ratio legislation at the federal or state level, was completed by Aiken, Clarke, Sloane, Sochalski, and Silber (2002). This study of more than 10,000 nurses and 230,000 patients in 168 hospitals concluded that in hospitals with higher patient-to-nurse ratios, surgical patients had a greater likelihood of dying within 30 days of admission. In addition, they experienced increased odds of failure to rescue (mortality following complications). This occurred because the time nurses have for surveillance, early detection, and timely intervention—particularly with patients who are not at high risk but who are vulnerable to other unfavorable outcomes—has a direct effect on patient outcomes.

CONSIDER THIS  There is wide variation in the skill mix (percentage of licensed to unlicensed workers) and RN-to-patient ratios across the United States.

| TABLE 11.1 | Selected Recent Research on Nurse Staffing Levels and Patient Clinical Outcomes |
|---|---|

| Citation | Description |
|---|---|
| McHugh, M. D., Kelly, L. A., Sloane, D. M., & Aiken, L. H. (2011). Contradicting fears, California's nurse-to-patient mandate did not reduce the skill level of the nursing workforce in hospitals. *Health Affairs, 30*(7), 1299–1306. | This study compared staffing levels in California hospitals with similar hospitals in the United States for the period 1997–2008. The study found that California's mandate did not reduce the nurse workforce skill level as feared. Instead, California hospitals on average followed the trend of hospitals nationally by increasing their nursing skill mix, and they primarily used more highly skilled registered nurses to meet the staffing mandate. In addition, the study found that the staffing mandate resulted in roughly an additional half-hour of nursing per adjusted patient day beyond what would have been expected in the absence of the policy. |
| Needleman, J., Buerhaus, P., Pankratz, V. S., Leibson, C. L., Stevens, S. R., & Harris, M. (2011). Nurse staffing and inpatient hospital mortality. *New England Journal of Medicine, 364*(11), 1037–1045. | A study evaluating nurse staffing for every nursing shift in 43 hospital units at one hospital found that staffing of RNs below target levels was associated with increased mortality. High patient turnover—admissions, discharges and transfers—during a shift also was linked with greater risk of patient deaths. |
| Hickey, P. (2010). The impact of staffing ratios, magnet recognition, and institutional characteristics on risk adjusted mortality, risk adjusted complications, and risk adjusted resource utilization for pediatric cardiac surgery programs in California before and after enactment of the California Safe Staffing Law and relative to other states combined (Doctoral dissertation). University of Massachusetts, Boston. | Hospitals in California made upward adjustments in nursing FTEs and ratios after enactment of AB394. There was a substantial increase in California's charge differential, a decrease in standardized mortality ratio (SMR) and an increase in standardized complication ratio (SCR) after enactment of the legislation. The findings did not reveal a relationship between these changes and individual hospital nursing FTEs or ratios. |
| Kutney-Lee, A., McHugh, M. D., Sloane, D. M., Cimiotti, J. P., Flynn, L., Felber Neff, D., & Aiken, L. H. (2009). Nursing: A key to patient satisfaction. *Health Affairs, 28*(4), 669–677. | Evidence suggests that improving nurse work environments in hospitals could result in improved patient outcomes, including better patient experiences and higher satisfaction ratings. Patient-to-nurse ratios in hospitals do affect patient satisfaction ratings and recommendation of the hospital to others. |
| Sochalski, J., Konetzka, R. T., Zhu, J., & Volpp, K. (2008). Will mandated minimum nurse staffing ratios lead to better patient outcomes? *Medical Care, 46*(6), 606–613. | There were correlations between increased licensed nurse staffing and reduced mortality rates associated with acute myocardial infarction. No relationship was found between increased nurse staffing and failure to rescue in adult surgical patients. |
| Aiken, L. H., Clarke, S. P., Sloane, D. M., Lake, E. T., & Cheney, T. (2008). Effects of hospital care environment on patient mortality and nurse outcomes. *Journal of Nursing Administration, 38*(5), 223–229. | Surgical mortality rates were more than 60% higher in poorly staffed hospitals with the poorest patient care environments than in hospitals with better health care environments, the best nurse staffing levels, and the most highly educated nurses. The researchers conclude that if these three factors could be optimized, the actual number of patient deaths that could be averted annually is somewhere in the range of 40,000. |

*continued*

---

| TABLE 11.1 | Selected Recent Research on Nurse Staffing Levels and Patient Clinical Outcomes *continued* |
| --- | --- |

| Citation | Description |
| --- | --- |
| Kane, R. L., Shamliyan, T., Mueller, C., Duval, S., & Wilt, T. (2007). The association of registered nurse staffing levels and patient outcomes. Systematic review and meta-analysis. *Medical Care, 45*(12), 1195–1204. | Adding just one full-time-equivalent registered nurse (RN) position per patient-day resulted in lower hospital-related mortality in intensive care and medical surgical units. In addition, hospital-acquired pneumonia, unplanned extubation, respiratory failure, and cardiac arrest declined, as did failure to rescue in surgical patients in ICUs. |
| Kane, R. L., Shamliyan, T., Mueller, C., Duval, S., & Wilt, T. (2007). *Nursing staffing and quality of patient care: Evidence Report/Technology Assessment, No. 151* (AHRQ Publication No. 07-E005). Rockville, MD: AHRQ. | More RN hours spent on direct patient was associated not only with a reduction in hospital-related death but also with shorter lengths of stay. Decreased nosocomial bloodstream infections, urinary tract infections, failure to rescue, and other adverse events also were noted when more RN hours were spent on direct patient care. |
| Burnes Bolton, L., Aydin, C., Donaldson, N., Brown, D., Sandhu, M., Fridman, M., & Aronow, H. U. (2007). Mandated nurse staffing ratios in California: A comparison of staffing and nursing-sensitive outcomes pre- and postregulation. *Policy, Politics, & Nursing Practice, 8*(4), 238–250. | Anticipated significant improvements in two key nurse-sensitive indicators of patient care quality and safety—the incidence of falls and the prevalence of hospital-acquired pressure ulcers—were not observed. |
| Thungjaroenkul, P., Cummings, G., & Embleton, A. (2007). The impact of nurse staffing on hospital costs and patient length of stay: A systematic review. *Nursing Economics, 25*(5), 255–265. | Significant reductions in cost and length of stay may be possible with higher ratios of nursing personnel in hospital settings. Sufficient numbers of RNs may prevent patient adverse events that cause patients to stay longer than necessary. Patient costs were also reduced with greater RN staffing because RNs have higher knowledge and skill levels to provide more effective nursing care, as well as to reduce patient resource consumption. |

The study found that staffing at 6 patients per nurse rather than 4 would result in an additional 2.3 deaths per 1,000 patients and an additional 8.7 deaths per 1,000 patients with complications. Staffing at 8 patients per nurse rather than 6 would incur an additional 2.6 deaths per 1,000 patients and 9.5 deaths per 1,000 patients with complications. Uniformly staffing at 8 patients per nurse rather than 4 was expected to entail 5 excess deaths per 1,000 patients and 18.2 complications per 1,000 patients. In addition, patients had a 31% higher chance of dying within 30 days of admission (Aiken, Clarke, Sloane, Sochalski, & Silber, 2002).

Within days of the study's release, Aiken's study results were summarized, repeated, and analyzed in detail in almost all relevant public forums and by most professional health care organizations. The message was clear: There is a direct link between nurse-to-patient ratios and mortality rates from preventable complications, and having an inadequate number of RNs places the public at risk.

---

### DISCUSSION POINT

Why did the study by Aiken et al. (2002) garner so much national attention in so many public forums? Were the findings significantly different than those of earlier studies? Was it timing? Was it how "the message" was managed?

# ARE MANDATORY MINIMUM STAFFING RATIOS NEEDED?

It is little surprise, then, that one proposed solution to Aiken's research findings was the implementation of minimum mandatory RN–patient staffing ratios in acute care hospitals. Numerous articles have appeared in the media attesting to grossly inadequate staffing in hospitals and nursing homes, and professional nursing organizations, such as the ANA, have continued to express concern about the effect poor staffing has both on nurses' health and safety and on patient outcomes.

Indeed, a survey conducted by the ANA (2011b) of almost 220,000 RNs from 13,000 nursing units in more than 550 hospitals found that 54% of nurses in adult medical units and emergency rooms felt they did not have sufficient time with patients, that overtime had increased during the past year with 43% of all RNs working extra hours because the unit was short staffed or busy, and that inadequate staffing affected unit admissions, transfers, and discharges more than 20% of the time.

Proponents of mandated minimum staffing ratios argue that minimum staffing ratios are absolutely essential to assuring that staffing is adequate to promote patient safety and to achieving desired patient outcomes. They also suggest that the use of standardized ratios provides a more consistent approach than acuity-based staffing.

CONSIDER THIS The bottom line is that minimum staffing ratios would not have been proposed if staffing abuses and the resultant decline in the quality of patient care had not occurred in the past.

Critics, however, suggest that the overall cost of care would increase exponentially if mandatory ratios were imposed nationally and that no guarantee of quality improvement or positive outcomes exists with such ratios. In fact, evidence regarding the benefits of staffing ratios is mixed and sometimes contradictory. Mandatory ratios also ignore the education, experience, and skill level of the individual nurse. In addition, there is a risk that staffing may actually decline with ratios because they might be used as the ceiling or as ironclad criteria if institutions are unwilling to make adjustments for patient acuity or RN skill level.

It is cost though that is likely most often cited as a deterrent for implementing minimum staffing ratios. Bobay, Yakusheva, and Weiss (2011) suggested that although increasing RN staffing would likely reduce postdischarge readmissions or emergency department visits, this alternative is not financially attractive to hospitals. Goryakin, Griffiths, and Maben (2011) agree, suggesting that although more intensive nurse staffing is likely associated with better outcomes, it is also more expensive and, therefore, cost effectiveness is not easy to assess.

In fact, Welton (2007) points out that an increase of just 1 hour of additional care by a registered nurse per day at US$40 per hour would increase costs by US$4,000 per day and US$1.4 million dollars annually for a medium-sized hospital that averaged 100 medical/surgical patients per day.

Keeler and Cramer (2007), however, in their review of staffing ratio costs, concluded that hiring more RNs, as would be expected under a federal mandatory staffing policy, would likely not create undue financial burdens in the long term for most urban hospitals. They cautioned, however, that this might not be the case in rural hospitals, and they thus suggested that mandatory staffing policy is better left to the states than the federal government.

Still others argue that it is health care professionals—not legislators or regulators—who understand health care and are best qualified to determine staffing needs. This might be the case, but given that hospitals are no longer exempt from "big business," profit-driven motives, one must question whether what is best for patients can be separated from what is best financially for the institution.

Finally, critics of staffing ratios claim that mandating specific staffing ratios during the current nursing shortage will lead to a reduction in hospital services, increased emergency room diversions, increased unit closures, and increased expenses as hospitals will need to pay additional labor costs for overtime and temporary agency nurses. The dire predictions about hospitals in California having to close doors if mandatory staffing ratio legislation passed, never materialized. In fact, most hospitals in California did not have to hire more contracted RNs to comply with the ratios nor was there a decrease in skill mix as a result. In fact, nurses from all over the country moved to California for jobs when the staffing-ratios legislation passed.

Aiken (2010) agreed, noting that the adverse, unintended consequences of mandatory nurse staffing levels, feared before the implementation of mandated staffing ratios never materialized. Instead, a large proportion of hospitals continued to have more nurses than required, most nurses reported that their workloads had decreased, and when more agency nurses were used, there did not appear to be any negative impacts on quality of care.

## CALIFORNIA AS THE PROTOTYPE FOR MANDATORY MINIMUM STAFFING RATIOS

### Passing the Legislation

California has had a minimum ratio of licensed nurse to patient requirement (Title 22 of the California Code of Regulations) for intensive care and coronary care units for almost three decades; however, no minimums were initially established for other types of acute care units. Given increasing pressure from nursing unions in the state, increasing bad press about poor-quality care, the increased use of unlicensed assistive personnel as direct care providers, and skyrocketing patient loads for licensed nurses in acute care, California stepped forward as the first state in the nation to implement mandatory minimum staffing ratios.

Under Assembly Bill (A.B.) 394 ("Safe Staffing Law"), passed in 1999 and crafted by the California Nurses Association (CNA), all hospitals in California were to comply with the minimum staffing ratios shown in Table 11.2 by January 1, 2004. These ratios, developed by the California Department of Health Services (CDHS) with assistance from the University of California, Davis, represented the maximum number of patients an RN could be assigned to care for, under any circumstance. In addition, this legislation prohibited unlicensed personnel from performing certain procedures such as administering medication, performing venipuncture, providing parenteral or tube feedings, inserting nasogastric tubes, inserting catheters, performing tracheal suctioning, assessing patient conditions, providing patient education, and performing moderately complex laboratory tests.

### Determining Appropriate Ratios

Developing draft regulations for minimum staffing ratios was challenging for the CDHS because data were not readily accessible regarding the distribution of nurse staffing in California hospitals, the number of hospitals likely to be affected by the minimum staffing requirements, or the expected costs of this legislation. In addition, the ratios were meant to supplement valid and reliable patient classification systems (PCS), which had been required in California hospitals since 1996. The problem was that although California hospitals had been required to submit their PCS data to the state, there was no standardization and little guidance about what characterized a valid PCS or what criteria should be used in determining the PCS. Therefore, PCS data yielded little if any helpful information to the CDHS for determining appropriate ratios.

---

**TABLE 11.2** Minimum Registered Nurse Staffing Ratios for Hospitals in California (2004–Present)

| Unit | Registered Nurse–Patient Ratio |
| --- | --- |
| Critical care/ICU | 1:2 |
| Neonatal ICU | 1:2 |
| Operating room | 1:1 |
| Labor and delivery | 1:2 |
| Antepartum | 1:4 |
| Postpartum couplets | 1:4 |
| Postpartum women only | 1:6 |
| Pediatrics | 1:4 |
| Step-down (initial) | 1:4 |
| Step-down (as of 2008) | 1:3 |
| Medical/surgical (initial) | 1:6 |
| Medical/surgical (as of 2005) | 1:5 |
| Oncology (initial) | 1:5 |
| Oncology (as of 2008) | 1:4 |
| Psychiatry | 1:6 |
| Emergency room | 1:4 |

*Source:* National Nurses United. (2010–2011). *Safe RN to patient staffing ratios.* Retrieved August 14, 2011, from http://www.nationalnursesunited.org/issues/entry/ratios

Cost was also not known. Initial projections by the Public Policy Institute of California (PPIC) in July 2001 suggested that many hospitals in California would experience sharp increases in cost associated with the increase in numbers of licensed staff. At least in part as a result of limited empirical data, proposals received by CDHS suggested a wide range of minimum staffing ratios and even more widely differing estimates of cost. The California Hospital Association (CHA), a hospital trade group representing the interests of nearly 500 hospital and health system members in California at that time, called for a minimum staffing ratio of 1 nurse to 10 patients on medical-surgical units, whereas the unions representing the largest numbers of nurses in the state argued for minimum ratios in medical-surgical units of 1 to 4. The CNA recommended a 1-to-3 ratio in medical-surgical units.

Following months of waiting and almost 2 years of wrangling, the final minimum staffing ratios were announced in January 2002. Governor Gray Davis, in a press conference at St. Vincent's Medical Center in Los Angeles, announced that his administration supported a ratio of 1 nurse to every 6 patients in medical-surgical units—twice the number of patients supported by the CNA and 4 fewer than that favored by the CHA. Regulations were released later that spring with 45 days allocated for public comment. Hospitals in California were also required to continue to keep a PCS in place and to staff according to the PCS if it called for a larger number of nurses than the minimum ratios set by the CDHS.

## Delays in Implementation

Implementing the ratio legislation proved to be just as difficult as determining what the ratios should be. The first challenge that arose was interpreting the meaning and intent of the legislation's language in regard to what constituted "licensed nurses." Almost immediately, questions were raised about whether the minimum

mandatory ratios had to reflect RN representation in the staffing mix or whether licensed vocational/practical nurses (LVNs/LPNs) would meet the requirement.

The CNA argued that the intent of the law was to regulate minimum RN staffing, which inflamed the labor unions representing LVNs. Amid much controversy, the issues were aired at a public hearing before the Department of Health Services in San Francisco, and a determination was provided that the ratios referred to RNs only and that LVNs/LPNs would be authorized to practice only under the direction of an RN or licensed physician.

Questions were then raised as to whether hospitals could eliminate or reduce their nonlicensed staff in an effort to save costs, given that the number of RNs would be increased. The CNA argued that the ratios were based on CDHS surveys of existing hospital staffing patterns and that nonlicensed staff should not be cut if safe patient care was to be assured. The state, however, chose not to weigh in, arguing that its position was to regulate minimum RN–patient ratios; as a result, many hospitals immediately began reducing the number of support personnel to offset the increased cost of RN staff, and many registered nurses were forced to assume nonnursing care tasks.

Finally, the CHA, with the help of State Senator Sam Aanestad, introduced new legislation (A.B. 847) to the California State Senate Health and Human Services committee in April 2003 in an attempt to delay implementation of the 1 to 5 minimum nurse–patient staffing ratio on medical-surgical units until it could be ascertained that adequate RNs were available to meet the ratios. Opponents of the delay argued that this was simply an effort to preclude implementation of the mandate altogether. The bill failed.

Then the hospitals persuaded Governor Arnold Schwarzenegger to issue an emergency regulation in November 2004 to overturn emergency room ratios and the improved medical-surgical ratios, citing financial crises (Cortez, 2008). In response, the CNA and the National Nurses Organizing Committee (NNOC) launched more than 100 protests against Schwarzenegger, which resulted in a massive grassroots movement and the stinging defeat of four Schwarzenegger-ballot initiatives in a 2005 special election (Cortez, 2008). The emergency regulation was ruled illegal in March 2005 by a state superior court judge and overturned. The judge argued that the financial state of hospitals did not give the state the right to delay implementing the law because the law's intent was to improve patient safety. Hospitals were told to comply immediately.

Still, resistance to staffing ratio implementation continued. Hospitals were accused of encouraging management staff to undermine and avoid compliance with the new RN staffing ratios. Nursing unions responded with threats to close down units with inadequate staffing, to delay elective surgeries, and to wage a public relations campaign to garner public support for the nurses.

## The Struggle to Implement the Ratios

Despite these efforts and a pervasive, ongoing resistance to staffing ratio implementation, the staffing ratio mandate did become effective January 1, 2004. But were hospitals ready and willing to implement these changes?

By and large, bigger hospitals in the state were ready to meet the mandate by the time of its implementation. Many smaller hospitals, however, had existing budget deficits and had to seek waivers from the CDHS because of their difficulty in meeting ratios. Waivers were allowed; however, hospitals had to be rural and meet very strict conditions.

> ### DISCUSSION POINT
>
> Should small rural hospitals be given waivers for the mandatory staffing ratios? Is this justified by the patient population characteristics, or is it simply an economic incentive to keep these hospitals viable?

## The "At All Times" Clause

In addition, almost immediately after implementation, legal clarification became necessary regarding interpretation of the law with regard to ratio coverage "at all times." A ruling by the CDHS blindsided many hospitals in its strict interpretation that ratios had to be maintained at all times, including breaks and lunches. For many hospitals, this meant hiring additional rotating staff to fill in for nurses when they leave the bedside for short periods (breaks, lunch, transporting patients, etc.) or face being noncompliant.

As a result, the CHA filed a lawsuit on December 30, 2003, challenging the ruling and arguing that the "at all times" ruling was impossible to implement. The motion was heard in a Sacramento court on May 14, 2004. In a 10-page ruling issued on May 26, 2004, the judge dismissed the hospital association lawsuit, saying

that not adhering to the "at all times" clause would make the nurse-to-patient ratios meaningless. Again, the ruling was an effort to maintain the intent of the law—to protect patients.

> ### DISCUSSION POINT
>
> Is an "at all times" ruling necessary to assure quality health care?

## Monitoring Compliance: The Role of the California Department of Health Services

The CDHS is charged with compliance oversight of mandatory minimum staffing ratios in California acute care hospitals and enforces these regulations in the same general manner in which they have enforced intensive care and critical care unit staffing regulations for the last three decades. The CDHS (2010) website details the following procedures for verifying compliance, responding to complaints, and addressing compliance violations:

■ Compliance with the regulations may be verified during a periodic survey or in response to a complaint. Although there is no statutory time frame within which CDHS must initiate an on-site investigation in response to a complaint against an acute care hospital, by existing policy, CDHS will initiate an investigation within 48 hours if a credible allegation of serious and immediate jeopardy to patients is received. If the allegation does not constitute serious and immediate jeopardy, the complaint will be investigated during the next periodic survey or along with the next "serious" complaints.

■ If a violation of the ratio requirements occurs, CDHS will issue a deficiency notice to the hospital and require an acceptable plan of correction. CDHS may verify that the plan of correction has been implemented and the deficiency corrected during any subsequent complaint investigation or periodic survey.

■ There is currently no penalty or monetary fine for a violation of the ratio regulations itself; however, as of 2007, hospitals can be fined up to US$25,000 for staffing violations that result in serious injury or death to patients (Leighty, 2008). If the CDHS concludes that the violation of the ratio regulations is so severe that it poses an immediate and substantial hazard to the health or safety of patients, CDHS may also order the hospital to reduce the number of patients or to close a unit until additional staffing is obtained.

In addition, in 2011, the California Nurses Association sponsored a bill (SB 554) that would allow the state Department of Public Health (DPH) to levy fines on acute care hospitals for violations of nurse staffing mandates (California Healthline, 2011). The bill would have allowed the DPH to impose penalties of up to US$10,000 for each nurse staffing ratio violation after four such violations in a 6-month period. Another US$10,000 fine could have been levied if a hospital did not follow its corrective plan after receiving a penalty. The bill also would have required hospitals to be inspected for compliance at least every 2 years (California Healthline, 2011). The bill, however, was amended in January 2012 and all financial penalties for noncompliance with nurse staffing mandates were removed (Around the Capitol, 2012).

CONSIDER THIS  If there are no monetary fines from the CDHS for noncompliance, what will motivate California hospitals to continue to comply with mandated staffing ratios?

## Has Registered Nurse Staffing and Patient Outcomes Improved in California as a Result of Mandatory Minimum Staffing Ratios?

As of January 1, 2008, California's historic staffing law for registered nurse staffing ratios completed its phase-in period and almost a decade of data now exist regarding compliance with the staffing ratios, as well as changes in patient outcomes. A synthesis by Donaldson and Shapiro (2010) of 12 studies examining the impact of California's ratios on patient care cost, quality, and outcomes in acute care hospitals revealed that the implementation of minimum nurse-to-patient ratios did reduce the number of patients per licensed nurse and increase the number of worked nursing hours per patient day in hospitals. There were, however, no significant impacts of these improved staffing measures on measures of nursing quality and patient safety indicators across hospitals. Donaldson and Shapiro emphasized, however, that adverse outcomes did not increase despite the increasing patient severity reflected in case mix index

and cautiously posited that this finding might actually suggest an impact of ratios in preventing adverse events in the presence of increased patient risk.

In addition, Aiken (2010) and the Center for Health Outcomes and Policy Research at the University of Pennsylvania conducted an independent evaluation of California's mandated nurse staffing requirements. This survey of more than 22,000 registered nurses, working in 604 hospitals in California and two comparison states without legislation—Pennsylvania and New Jersey—found that overall, nurses in California cared for an average of one patient fewer than nurses in the two comparison states. On medical and surgical units, California hospital nurses each took care of two fewer patients.

In terms of patient outcomes, Aiken studied more than 1 million patients who had common surgical procedures in these hospitals in 2006, more than 2 years after mandatory nurse staffing was implemented. She found that California hospitals had significantly lower risk-adjusted mortality and were better at rescuing patients who experienced complications than the comparison states, even after taking into account factors other than differences in nurse staffing.

In contrast, the California HealthCare Foundation released a study in 2009 that suggested that although the state began mandating minimum nurse–patient ratios in 2004, quality of care did not necessarily improve (HC Pro, 2009). The study, based on interviews with health care leaders and data from state quality of care surveys, showed that facilities spent a lot of money hiring new nurses to comply with the minimum ratios, resulting in difficulty balancing hospital budgets later. Facilities also struggled with the requirement to have minimum ratios met "at all times," especially during meal breaks.

In terms of compliance, Conway, Konetzka, Jingsan, Volpp, and Sochalski (2008) reported that nurse staffing ratios in California were relatively unchanged from 1993 to 1999 but increased significantly from 1999 to 2004 in preparation for the implementation of mandated minimum staffing ratios. The largest increase was in 2004. Hospitals most likely to be below minimum ratios had a high Medicaid/uninsured patient population and were government owned, nonteaching, urban, and in more competitive markets.

Clark (2010) suggests that the answer as to whether mandated ratios have improved care or created new cost burdens for California is still not completely clear. She suggests that hospitals and nursing organizations are divided in their perception of how things are going.

*The California Nurses Association says the ratios have improved nurse retention, raised the numbers of qualified nurses willing to work, reduced burnout, and improved morale. Advocates also say narrower ratios in high-intensity areas, such as the emergency room, have improved patient satisfaction and have reduced medical errors, including medication mistakes and falls.* (Clark, 2010, para. 3)

Clark cautions, however, that enforcement of staffing ratios continues to be difficult due to the need for continuous compliance with the "at all times" ruling.

Despite these cautions, Clark (2010) concludes that hospitals in California have moved beyond a one-size-fits-all staffing mentality which is based solely on their bottom-line budget. Instead, a public safety net is in place with hospitals being required to staff up from minimum acuity–based staffing models.

## SIMILAR INITIATIVES IN OTHER U.S. STATES

The U.S. federal government has established minimum standards for licensed nursing in certified nursing homes but not in acute care hospitals. Several attempts have been made in Congress in the past decade to enact hospital nurse staffing laws; however, none have come close to fruition. Section 42 of the Code of Federal Regulations (42CFR 482.23[b]) does require Medicare-certified hospitals to "have adequate numbers of licensed registered nurses, licensed practical (vocational) nurses, and other personnel to provide nursing care to all patients as needed"; however, this "nebulous language and failure of Congress to enact a quality nursing care staffing act to date, has left it to the states to ensure that staffing is appropriate to patients' needs" (ANA, 2011b, para. 10).

Many states are in fact actively pursuing minimum staffing ratio legislation. For example, in June 2008, Governor Ted Strickland of Ohio signed safe nurse staffing legislation into law (ANA, 2011b). This legislation established hospital-wide nursing care committees at each hospital that must recommend a nursing services staffing plan that is at minimum, consistent with current standards established by private accreditation organizations or governmental entities. The legislation also called for at least annual evaluation of the staffing plan in terms of patient outcomes, clinical management, and costs.

Similarly, in May 2008, Governor Mary Jodi Rell of Connecticut signed legislation requiring the establishment of hospital-wide staffing plans, by committees

with membership comprising at least 50% direct care RNs, at hospitals in that state. The plan must include the minimum professional skill mix for each patient care unit in the hospital; identify the hospital's employment practices concerning the use of temporary and traveling nurses; set forth the level of administrative staffing for each patient care unit that ensures direct care staff are not used for administrative functions; establish a process review of the staffing plan; and include a mechanism for obtaining input from direct care staff and other members of the patient care team in the development of the staffing plan (ANA, 2011b).

More recently (June 2009), the Texas governor signed into law, nurse staffing protections that required governing bodies of hospital adopt, implement, and enforce a written nurse staffing policy to ensure adequate number and skill mix of nurses available to met patients needs by unit and shift, using a staffing committee (ANA, 2011b). There were also provisions for whistleblower protections and mandatory overtime prohibition.

Similarly, Nevada enacted staffing legislation in 2009 overriding the governor's veto. This legislation requires hospitals in counties with a population of 100,000 more and greater than 70 beds to establish a staffing committee comprising 50% direct care nurses who will develop staffing plans with management (ANA, 2011b). It is expected that plans will be flexible enough to accommodate for changes in patients, staff, unit design, and technology.

## OTHER ALTERNATIVES

Efforts are also under way, in both California and the rest of the nation, to explore alternatives to improving nurse staffing that do not require legislated minimum staffing ratios. The staffing plans outlined earlier in this chapter are examples of such efforts.

The reality is that many leading health care and professional nursing organizations do not support the need for legislated minimum staffing ratios. For example, the Joint Commission, one of the most powerful accrediting bodies for hospitals in the United States, has been reluctant to endorse nationally mandated minimum staffing ratios, suggesting that this would not be flexible enough to encompass the diversity represented in hospitals across the United States.

In addition, the ANA does not support fixed nurse–patient ratios. Instead, it advocates a workload system that takes into account the many variables that exist to ensure safe staffing. Instead of staffing ratios, the ANA has recommended three general approaches to assure sufficient nurse staffing at the state level (see Table 11.3). The ANA (2011b) argues that this type of approach better accommodates changes in patients' needs, available technology, and the preparation and experience of staff. In addition, the ANA argues that what may be established through legislation today as an appropriate minimum nurse to patient ratio may be obsolete by the next shift or 2 years from now and that disclosure of staffing plans without evaluation and recourse for inadequate levels are futile.

Buerhaus (2010) agrees, suggesting that efforts to establish mandated staffing ratios are shortsighted, and, that although proponents may have the best intentions, insufficient quality outcome evidence exists to support the imposition of mandated nurse staffing ratios. Buerhaus goes on to suggest that there are high opportunity costs with mandated staffing ratios which force employers to ignore the dynamic interactions of economic, technology, capital, and labor supply variables, and thus needlessly impose the effect of increased labor costs on hospitals, taxpayers, and nurses themselves.

## CONCLUSIONS

The literature suggests that increasing RN representation in the staffing mix improves at least some patient outcomes. What is less clear is what the optimal staffing levels are for various patient populations and when costs associated with staffing mix become unreasonable in terms of attempting to improve patient outcomes. In addition, given the lessons that have already been learned with the "RN/LVN debate" and the "at all times" requirement, more thought must be given to how strictly staffing ratio regulations are to be interpreted and how enforcement can be effective when there are no monetary consequences for breaking rules. In addition, the intermingling roles of state government as a legislator of minimum staffing ratios, compliance officer, disciplinary enforcer, and potential funding source to assist

with mandated ratio implementation needs further examination and clarification.

Finally, it must be recognized that patient acuity is continuing to rise, and the mandatory minimum staffing ratios adopted in California in 2003 were arguably inadequate just 5 years later, especially when hospitals refused to staff above the ratios when census and acuity call for it (Cortez, 2008). In fact, the CNA and the NNOC proposed even lower ratios as part of the CNA/NNOC's Hospital Patient Protection Act in 2008 (CNA, 2008). Although not implemented, these ratios would have posed even greater fiscal and human resource challenges to California hospitals in terms of their implementation (Table 11.4).

The implementation and subsequent evaluation of mandatory staffing ratios in California should, however, provide some insight into these ongoing issues that will be helpful to other states that choose to follow in California's footsteps. Clearly, the enactment of California's nurse-to-patient ratio law was far from smooth, and concerns continue about whether there are enough registered nurses to meet the ratios, the costs of hiring additional licensed staff, and the need to meet the "at all times" clause.

It is not clear yet whether California has the resources (both human and fiscal) it needs to sustain successful staffing ratio implementation. Some of the implementation struggles may have been related to the normal issues that arise whenever a new law takes effect; however, the reality is that California may lack some of the nursing resources needed to implement and oversee its law. The struggles California has experienced thus far in implementing the mandate have been significant. The fact that it took 5 years from passage of the legislation to mandated implementation is telling. What is even more telling are the number of hospitals in California that continue to report difficulty in meeting staffing ratio requirements and the pervasive resistance that continues to be a part of its implementation.

---

**TABLE 11.3** Three General Approaches Recommended by the American Nurses' Associations to Maintain Sufficient Staffing

1. The formation of nurse-driven staffing committees to create staffing plans that reflect the needs of the patient population and match the skills and experience of the staff.
2. Legislators mandate specific nurse to patient ratios in legislation or regulation.
3. Facilities are required to disclose staffing levels to the public and/or a regulatory body.

TABLE 11.4 Proposed (Not Enacted) California Nurses Association (CNA)/ National Nurses Organizing Committee (NNOC) Minimum Registered Nurse Staffing Ratios for Hospitals in California as Part of the CNA/NNOC's Hospital Patient Protection Act

| Unit | Registered Nurse–Patient Ratio |
| --- | --- |
| Critical care/ICU | 1:2 |
| Neonatal ICU | 1:2 |
| Operating room | 1:1 |
| Labor and delivery | 1:1 |
| Antepartum | 1:3 |
| Postpartum couplets | 1:3 |
| Postpartum women only | 1:4 |
| Pediatrics | 1:3 |
| Step-down and telemetry | 1:3 |
| Medical/surgical | 1:4 |
| Other specialty care units | 1:4 |
| Psychiatry | 1:4 |
| Rehab unit and skilled nursing | 1:5 |
| Emergency room | 1:4 |
| ICU patient in emergency room | 1:2 |
| Trauma patient in emergency room | 1:1 |

*Source:* California Nurses Association. (2008). *CNA/NNOC RNs across the nation take up the fight.* Retrieved July 30, 2008, from http://www.calnurses.org/assets/pdf/ratios/ratios_booklet.pdf

## FOR ADDITIONAL DISCUSSION

**1.** Given rising patient acuity levels and increased scope of responsibility for registered nurses, at what point should California reexamine the adequacy of the staffing ratios adopted in 2003?

**2.** In an effort to cut the costs associated with implementing minimum RN staffing ratios, many hospitals have eliminated their support staff. Have RNs gained anything when this is the case?

**3.** Should LVNs be counted to meet minimum mandatory staffing ratio requirements?

**4.** Is allowing hospitals to determine their staffing needs a little like having the "fox guard the chicken coop"?

**5.** Does the implementation of mandatory staffing ratios in the midst of a severe national nursing shortage make sense? Why or why not?

**6.** At what point does cost related to staffing mix become so prohibitive that society will be willing to accept some increase in patient morbidity and mortality?

**7.** What critical lessons should other states learn from California's experience thus far in implementing mandatory staffing ratios?

## REFERENCES

Aiken, L. (2010). Safety in numbers. *Nursing Standard,* 24(44), 62–63.

Aiken, L. H., Clarke, S. P., Sloane, D. M., Lake, E. T., & Cheney, T. (2008). Effects of hospital care environment on patient mortality and nurse outcomes. *Journal of Nursing Administration,* 38(5), 223–229.

Aiken, L. H., Clarke, S. P., Sloane, D., Sochalski, J., & Silber, J. (2002). Effects of nurse-staffing on nurse burnout and job-dissatisfaction and patient deaths. *Journal of the American Medical Association, 288,* 1987–1993.

American Nurses Association. (2011a). *Safe staffing saves lives.* Retrieved August 12, 2011, from http://www.safestaffingsaveslives.org/WhatisANADoing/StateLegislation.aspx.

American Nurses Association. (2011b). *Nurse staffing plans and ratios.* Retrieved August 12, 2011, from http://nursingworld.org/MainMenuCategories/Policy-Advocacy/State/Legislative-Agenda-Reports/State-StaffingPlansRatios.

Around the Capitol. (2012). *California legislation > SB 554 (Yee): Health facilities: Direct care nurses.* Retrieved April 29, 2012, from http://www.aroundthecapitol.com/billtrack/text.html?bvid=20110SB55498AMD.

Blegen, M., Goode, C., Spetz, J., Vaughn, T., & Park, S. (2011). Nurse staffing effects on patient outcomes: Safety-net and non-safety-net hospitals. *Medical Care,* 49(4), 406–414.

Bobay, K. L., Yakusheva, O., & Weiss, M. E. (2011). Outcomes and cost analysis of the impact of unit-level nurse staffing on post-discharge utilization. *Nursing Economics,* 29(2), 69–87.

Buerhaus, P. (2010). What is the harm in imposing mandatory hospital nurse staffing regulations? *Nursing Economics,* 28(2), 87–93.

Burnes Bolton, L., Aydin, C., Donaldson, N., Brown, D., Sandhu, M., Fridman, M., & Aronow, H. U. (2007). Mandated nurse staffing ratios in California: A comparison of staffing and nursing-sensitive outcomes pre- and postregulation. *Policy, Politics, & Nursing Practice,* 8(4), 238–250.

California Department of Health Services. (2010). *Nurse-to-patient staffing ratios for general acute care hospitals: Frequently asked questions.* Retrieved July 30, 2008, from http://www.cdph.ca.gov/services/DPOPP/regs/Documents/R-37-01_FAQ2182004.pdf.

California Healthline. (2011). *Nurses group pursues stringent penalties for staffing violations.* Retrieved August 15, 2011, from http://www.californiahealthline.org/articles/2011/3/3/nurses-group-pursues-stringent-penalties-for-staffing-violations.aspx.

California Nurses Association. (2008). *CNA/NNOC RNs across the nation take up the fight.* Retrieved July 30, 2008, from http://www.calnurses.org/assets/pdf/ratios/ratios_booklet.pdf.

Clark, C. (2010). *Does mandating nurse-patient ratios improve care?* Retrieved August 14, 2011, from http://www.healthleadersmedia.com/content/NRS-245408/Does-Mandating-NursePatient-Ratios-Improve-Care##

Conway, P. H., Konetzka, T. R., Jingsan, Z., Volpp, K. G., & Sochalski, J. (2008). Nurse staffing ratios: Trends and policy implications for hospitalists and the safety net. *Journal of Hospital Medicine,* 3(3), 193–199.

Cortez, Z. (2008). *California's nurse-patient ratio law: Saving lives, reducing the nursing shortage.* Retrieved July 29, 2008, from http://www.californiaprogressreport.com/2008/01/californias_nur.html.

Donaldson, N., & Shapiro, S. (2010). Impact of California mandated acute care hospital nurse staffing ratios: A literature synthesis. *Policy, Politics & Nursing Practice,* 11(3), 184–201.

Flynn, M., & McKeown, M. (2009). Nurse staffing levels revisited: A consideration of key issues in nurse staffing levels and skill mix research. *Journal of Nursing Management,* 17(6), 759–766.

Goryakin, Y., Griffiths, P., & Maben, J. (2011). Economic evaluation of nurse staffing and nurse substitution in health care: A scoping review. *International Journal of Nursing Studies,* 48(4), 501–512.

HC Pro. (2009). Study: Although CA nurse-patient ratios have increased, quality of care not necessarily improved. *Patient Safety Monitor Alert.* Retrieved August 15, 2011, from http://www.hcpro.com/QPS-228772-873/Study-Although-CA-nursepatient-ratios-have-increased-quality-of-care-not-necessarily-improved.html.

Hickey, P. (2010). *The impact of staffing ratios, magnet recognition, and institutional characteristics on risk adjusted mortality, risk adjusted complications, and risk adjusted resource utilization for pediatric cardiac surgery programs in California before and after enactment of the California Safe Staffing Law and relative to other states combined* (Doctoral dissertation). University of Massachusetts, Boston.

Kane, R. L., Shamliyan, T., Mueller, C., Duval, S., & Wilt, T. (2007a). *Nursing staffing and quality of patient care: Evidence Report/Technology Assessment, No. 151* (AHRQ Publication No. 07-E005). Rockville, MD: AHRQ.

Kane, R. L., Shamliyan, T., Mueller, C., Duval, S., & Wilt, T. (2007b). The association of registered nurse staffing levels and patient outcomes: Systematic review and meta-analysis. *Medical Care, 45*(12), 1195–1204.

Keeler, H. J., & Cramer, M. E. (2007). *Journal of Nursing Administration,* 37(7/8), 350–356.

Leighty, J. L. (2008). The final phase: California implements the last stages of its landmark RN-to-patient ratios law. *NurseWeek California,* 21(2), 24–25.

McHugh, M. D., Kelly, L. A., Sloane, D. M., & Aiken, L. H. (2011).Contradicting fears, California's nurse-to-patient mandate did not reduce the skill level of the nursing workforce in hospitals. *Health Affairs,* 30(7), 1299–1306.

National Nurses United. (2010–2011). *Safe RN to patient staffing ratios.* Retrieved August 14, 2011, from http://www.nationalnursesunited.org/issues/entry/ratios.

Needleman, J., Buerhaus, P., Mattke, S., Stewart, M., & Zelevinsky, K. (2002). Nurse-staffing levels and the quality of care in hospitals. *New England Journal of Medicine, 346,* 1715–1722.

Sochalski, J., Konetzka, R. T., Zhu, J., & Volpp, K. (2008). Will mandated minimum nurse staffing ratios lead to better patient outcomes? *Medical Care, 46*(6). Retrieved April 29, 2012, from http://www.ncbi.nlm.nih.gov/pubmed/18520315.

Thungjaroenkul, P., Cummings, G., & Embleton, A. (2007).The impact of nurse staffing on hospital costs and patient length of stay: A systematic review. *Nursing Economics, 25*(5), 255–265.

Welton, J. M. (2007). Mandatory hospital nurse to patient staffing ratios: Time to take a different approach. *OJIN: The Online Journal of Issues in Nursing, 12*(3). Retrieved April 29, 2012, from http://nursingworld.org/MainMenuCategories/ANAMarketplace/ANAPeriodicals/OJIN/TableofContents/Volume122007/No3Sept07/MandatoryNursetoPatientRatios.html.

## BIBLIOGRAPHY

Anderson, E., Frith, K. H., & Caspers, B. (2011). Linking economics and quality: Developing an evidence-based nurse staffing tool. *Nursing Administration Quarterly,* 35(1), 53–60.

Diya, L., Koen, Sermeus, W., & Lesaffre, E. (2011). The use of "Lives Saved" measures in nurse staffing and patient safety research: Statistical considerations. *Nursing Research,* 60(2), 100–106.

Diya, L., Van den Heede, K., Sermeus, W., & Lesaffre, E. (2012). The relationship between in-hospital mortality, readmission into the intensive care nursing unit and/or operating theatre and nurse staffing levels. *Journal of Advanced Nursing,* 68(5), 1073–1081.

Duffin, C. (2012). RCN says the case for mandatory staff levels is now overwhelming. *Nursing Standard,* 26(29), 5.

Esparza, S., Zoller, J., White, A., & Highfield, M. (2012). Nurse staffing and skill mix patterns: Are there differences in outcomes? *Journal of Healthcare Risk Management,* 31(3), 14–23.

Hickey, P. A., Gauvreau, K., Jenkins, K., Fawcett, J., & Hayman, L. (2011). Statewide and National Impact of California's Staffing Law on Pediatric Cardiac Surgery Outcomes. *Journal of Nursing Administration,* 41(5), 218–225.

Kalisch, B., Friese, C., Choi, S., & Rochman, M. (2011). Hospital nurse staffing: Choice of measure matters. *Medical Care,* 49(8), 775–779.

Kong, F., Cook, D., Paterson, D., Whitby, M., & Clements, A. (2012). Do staffing and workload levels influence the risk of new acquisitions of meticillin-resistant Staphylococcus aureus in a well-resourced intensive care unit? *Journal of Hospital Infection,* 80(4), 331–339.

Mark, B. A., & Harless, D. W. (2011). Adjusting for patient acuity in measurement of nurse staffing: Two approaches. *Nursing Research,* 60(2), 107–114.

Mchugh, M. D., Brooks C., Sloane, D. M., Wu, E., Kelly, L., & Aiken, L. H. (2012). Impact of nurse staffing mandates on safety-net hospitals: Lessons from California. *Milbank Quarterly,* 90(1), 160–186.

Myny, D., Van Hecke, A., De Bacquer, D., Verhaeghe, S., Gobert, M., Defloor, T., & Van Goubergen, D. (2012). Determining a set of measurable and relevant factors affecting nursing workload in the acute care hospital setting: A cross-sectional study. *International Journal of Nursing Studies,* 49(4), 427–436.

Needleman, J., Buerhaus, P., Pankratz, V., Leibson, C., Stevens, S., & Harris, M. (2011). Nurse staffing and inpatient hospital mortality. *New England Journal of Medicine,* 364(11), 1037–1045.

Petty, J. (2012). Nurse:patient ratios influence the achievement of oxygen saturation targets in premature infants. *Evidence Based Nursing,* 15(1), 15–16.

Reiter, K., Harless, D., Pink, G., Spetz, J., & Mark, B. (2011). The effect of minimum nurse staffing legislation on uncompensated care provided by California hospitals. *Medical Care Research & Review,* 68(3), 332–351.

Schwab, F., Meyer, E., Geffers, C., & Gastmeier, P. (2012). Understaffing, overcrowding, inappropriate nurse:ventilated patient ratio and nosocomial infections: Which parameter is the best reflection of deficits? *Journal of Hospital Infection*, 80(2), 133–139.

Tong, P. (2011). The effects of California minimum nurse staffing laws on nurse labor and patient mortality in skilled nursing facilities. *Health Economics*, 20(7), 802–816.

Twigg, D., Duffield, C., Bremner, A., Rapley, P., & Finn, J. (2011). The impact of the nursing hours per patient day (NHPPD) staffing method on patient outcomes: A retrospective analysis of patient and staffing data. *International Journal of Nursing Studies*, 48(5), 540–548.

Wood, D. (2012). Searching for a magic number. *Nurse. Com (New York/New Jersey Metro)*, 24(7), 22–23.

# Chapter 12

# Mandatory Overtime in Nursing
## *How Much? How Often?*

Carol J. Huston

## ADDITIONAL RESOURCES

Visit thePoint for additional helpful resources

- eBook
- Journal Articles
- WebLinks

## CHAPTER OUTLINE

**Mandatory Overtime as a Way of Life in the United States**

**Legislating Mandatory Overtime**
*The Fair Labor Standards Act*

*Recent Changes to Federal Overtime Rules*
*Legislating Limits on Nursing Overtime*

**The Consequences of Mandatory Overtime**

**Professional Duty and Conscience**

**Patient Abandonment**

**Unions and Mandatory Overtime**

**Conclusions**

## LEARNING OBJECTIVES

*The learner will be able to:*

1. Identify the strengths and the limitations of the Fair Labor Standards Act (FLSA) of 1938 in terms of protecting workers against mandatory overtime.

2. Identify how 2004 changes to federal overtime rules and more recent court rulings have affected traditional "white collar" employees, including salaried nurses in the United States.

3. Investigate current federal and state legislative efforts to regulate overtime limits for nurses.

4. Explore the current extent of mandatory overtime in nursing as identified in the literature.

5. Identify consequences of mandatory overtime in nursing, including fatigue, increased error rates,

increased legal liability, threats to the nurse's personal safety, and increased staff turnover rates.

6. Know and understand the provisions of the Nurse Practice Act in his or her state, as well as the position statements or advisory opinions that have been issued by his or her state board of nursing regarding mandatory overtime and patient abandonment.

7. Discuss the limits of the nurse's professional duty and assess how much risk a professional nurse should assume in fulfilling a professional duty.

8. Reflect on the number of hours he or she can safely work before quality of care is potentially compromised.

One short-term means of dealing with the current nursing shortage has been to require nurses to work extra shifts, often under threat of "patient abandonment" or punitive measures. *Mandatory overtime*, also called *compulsory* or *forced overtime*, occurs when employees are required to work more hours than are standard (generally 40 hours per week) or risk employer reprisals as a result of their refusal to do so. Mandatory overtime may result from a number of unexpected events such as natural or human-caused disasters, sudden job vacancies, staff absences due to illness, or rapid changes in patient care requirements or it may be a standard staffing practice.

A review of the literature suggests that the use of mandatory overtime in nursing varies greatly from institution to institution and from state to state. Kauffman (2011) identified a psychiatric hospital in Connecticut where employees were often forced to do the work of two full-time employees. While they earned the wages of three full-time workers, they were constantly exhausted and worried about the safety of their patients. In fact, about one in 10 full-time employees at that hospital doubled their base salaries in 2010 through overtime, shift differentials, bonuses, or other additional pay and at least a dozen nurses and mental health assistants tripled their salaries, with the top 25 overtime earners adding a total of more than US$3.5 million to their base pay.

In addition, Magnet status appears to impact the use of mandatory overtime as a staffing tool. Trinkoff et al. (2011) found that nurses in Magnet hospitals were significantly less likely to be required to work mandatory overtime than in non-Magnet hospitals, although the total numbers of hours nurse worked in the two types of institutions did not differ.

Some health care employers have suggested that nursing shortages are the cause of mandatory overtime in their facilities. Increasingly, however, nurses are reporting that mandatory overtime has become standard operating procedure instead of a last resort to short staffing. In fact, in some hospitals, mandatory overtime is routinely used in an effort to keep fewer people on the payroll, as well as to alleviate immediate shortage needs.

Indeed, a recent national survey found that nurses are working an average of 6.5 hours of overtime a week, or 8.5 weeks of overtime a year, with nurses in California working an additional 11 weeks of overtime on average per year (Service Employees International Union [SEIU], 2011). Bae and Brewer (2010) noted that about half of all nurses in the 2004 *National Sample Survey of Registered Nurses* reported working more than 40 hours per week, with nurses working in states regulating mandatory overtime reporting less overtime than states without

such restrictions. Nurses working in nursing homes reported higher levels of the percentage of mandatory overtime hours worked than those working in hospitals.

Some nursing specialty units are known, however, to have more mandatory overtime than others, such as the operating room and postanesthesia care units. In fact, Garrett (2008) reported that many nurses in perioperative units consider it normal to work a 40-hour week and then take mandatory call for an additional 4 to 72 hours each week. Garrett suggested that the fatigue of nurses working in this setting and under these conditions might actually approximate that of being under the influence of alcohol. She noted research done by Rosekind and colleagues that demonstrated that after 17 hours without sleep, performance degrades to the equivalent of having a blood alcohol concentration of 0.05%, and after 24 hours without sleep, the effect on performance is equivalent to having a blood alcohol level of 0.10%. Garrett concluded that although mandatory overtime is commonplace in the perioperative setting, it leads to staff-member fatigue that might adversely affect patient safety.

In an effort to create guidelines for safe practice in the perioperative setting, the Association of Perioperative Registered Nurses (AORN) created a Position Statement on Safe Work/On-Call Practices in 2007 (AORN, 2011). Excerpts from this document are shown in Box 12.1.

---

### DISCUSSION POINT

Is mandatory overtime simply part of the work culture in the operating room or postanesthesia care units? Should there be different expectations or rules regarding mandatory overtime in these units?

---

## MANDATORY OVERTIME AS A WAY OF LIFE IN THE UNITED STATES

Although nurses bemoan mandatory overtime in the profession, the reality is that mandatory overtime is not new, nor is it restricted to nursing. Gelb (2008) suggested that Americans typically work more hours and take fewer vacations than workers in other advanced economies. In fact, the International Labor Organization (ILO) suggested that about 80% of Americans work 40 hours or more each week, as compared with fewer than half of Danes, Finns, the French, or Germans (Gelb, 2008). Moreover, the ILO states that "Americans

## BOX 12.1   EXCERPTS FROM THE 2007 AORN POSITION STATEMENT: SAFE WORK/ON-CALL PRACTICES

The AORN, recognizing the potential negative consequences of sleep deprivation and sustained work hours and further recognizing that adequate rest and recuperation periods are essential to patient and perioperative personnel safety, suggests the following strategies:

1. Perioperative registered nurses should not be required to work in direct patient care more than 12 consecutive hours in a 24-hour period and not more than 60 hours in a 7-day period.

2. Sufficient transition time is required for appropriate patient handoff and staff relief. Under extreme conditions, exceptions to the 12-hour limit may be required (e.g., disasters). Organization policy should outline exceptions to the 12-hour limitation. All worked hours (i.e., regular hours and call hours worked) should be included in calculating total hours worked.

3. Off-duty periods should be inclusive of an uninterrupted 8-hour sleep cycle, a break from continuous professional responsibilities, and time to perform individual activities of daily living.

4. Arrangements should be made, in relation to the hours worked, to relieve a perioperative registered nurse who has worked on-call during his or her off shift and who is scheduled to work the following shift to accommodate an adequate off-duty recuperation period.

5. The number of on-call shifts assigned in a 7-day period depends on the type of facility and should be coordinated with the number of sustained work hours and adequate recuperation periods mentioned above.

6. An individual's ability to meet the anticipated work demand should be considered for on-call assignments. Limited research indicates older people are more likely than younger people to be adversely affected by sleep deprivation; however, there is no research specific to the effects of on-call assignment and a person's age.

*Source:* Reprinted with permission from Association of Perioperative Registered Nurses. (2011). *AORN position statement: Safe work/on-call practices* (April 2005/Sunset Review March 2010). Denver, CO: Author. Retrieved August 17, 2011, from http://www.aorn.org/PracticeResources/AORNPositionStatements/

spend about 1,800 hours a year at work, compared to 1,600 hours or fewer in Belgium, Denmark, France, Germany, the Netherlands and Sweden" (Gelb, 2008, para. 14). In contrast, South Koreans work about 2,400 hours per year (Gelb, 2008).

Gelb (2008) suggested that for many Americans, hard work is a badge of honor. However, it may well be that Americans are working this hard because they are afraid not to. In the United States, unlike most European countries, employment is *at will*, meaning that employers can dismiss employees for any reason (aside from those of gender, race, age, or disability) or for no reason at all. Thus, employees who refuse to work overtime can lose their jobs or face other reprisals.

Nurses argue, however, that mandatory overtime in nursing is not comparable with mandatory overtime in other fields because the consequences of being overly fatigued for the nurse may literally have life-and-death

consequences. Proponents of mandatory overtime argue that it is an economic reality, given how limited labor health care resources are, particularly in light of the international nursing shortage. The problem is that both positions are correct.

> **CONSIDER THIS**  Many nurses report a dramatic increase in the use of mandatory overtime to solve staffing problems and fear potential consequences for safety and quality of care for their patients.

This chapter will define mandatory overtime, examine the extent of its use in nursing, and discuss the consequences of mandatory overtime in nursing as identified in the literature.

## LEGISLATING MANDATORY OVERTIME

### The Fair Labor Standards Act

The definition of what constitutes overtime in the United States or how it should be calculated has historically varied from state to state and from industry to industry. There are, however, national standards in terms of the *Fair Labor Standards Act* (FLSA) of 1938. This act, which regulates overtime, imposes no limits on overtime hours, nor does it prohibit dismissal or any other sanction for declining overtime work. It does, however, require that payroll employees (those who are not "exempt" from the overtime requirements of the FLSA) be paid an overtime premium of at least one and one-half times the regular rate of pay for each hour worked more than 40 in a week (U.S. Department of Labor, 2011).

CONSIDER THIS  Labor laws such as the FLSA need to be amended to protect workers against excessive work hours and mandatory overtime and to protect the public from the dangers of an overburdened, stressed workforce.

The FLSA does, however, contain language which permits the health care industry to use a different overtime standard than the 40-hour work week.

*Hospitals and residential care facilities are permitted to utilize an overtime standard in which overtime is paid after either eight hours in a day or 80 hours in a 14-day pay period. This is used in health care primarily because of the weekend scheduling pattern in hospitals. It permits employees to work more than 40 hours in a week and not be paid overtime provided they do not work more than eight hours in a shift or if they work fewer than 40 hours in the next week.* (Breslin, 2010, p. 10)

To use this standard, employers are required to have an agreement with the unions representing employees before work is performed. Breslin also notes that employers are permitted to use both the 40-hour and the 80-hour standards in the same facility depending on the scheduling patterns for employees, but they must use one standard for individual employees and it must be applied consistently.

Lyncheski (2010) notes that while the FLSA has changed little since its inception, health care has become the target industry for a surge in FLSA cases. Lyncheski

suggests this has occurred because overtime is often a "normal operational requirement" in facilities which have 24-hour, 7-day-a-week staffing needs. In addition, Lyncheski notes that most FLSA violations in health care occur because of acts and omissions "on the floor" and not from actions in payroll, human resources, or the executive suite.

### Recent Changes to Federal Overtime Rules

There have been changes, however, to the federal overtime rules in the last decade. These changes, which became effective August 23, 2004, defined exemptions from the FLSA for what were traditionally called "white-collar" employees. The new rules increased the amount of money employees could earn before they were no longer eligible to receive overtime pay; however, employees who directed and supervised two or more other full-time employees fell under the executive exemption (Overtime Pay and White-Collar Exemptions, 2008).

Similarly, the new rules excluded employees from the FLSA who have the authority to hire, fire, and promote employees or if their primary duties involve the performance of office or nonmanual work and the exercise of discretion and independent judgment (Overtime Pay and White-Collar Exemptions, 2008). In addition, employees who have primary duties requiring knowledge of an advanced type were excluded because the rules no longer distinguished advanced knowledge from "knowledge obtained from a general academic education, an apprenticeship or from training in the performance of routine, manual, or physical process" (Overtime Pay and White-Collar Exemptions, 2008, para. 4).

Almost immediately, nursing leaders expressed concern that the language in the new rules opened the door for employer attempts to reclassify nurses as exempt from overtime protections historically given to workers under the FLSA. This occurred because under the new regulations, "learned professionals" earning fairly low salaries (anything above US$455 per week) could not earn overtime pay.

Nurses meet the criteria of *learned professional*, which is defined in part as "employees who perform work that requires advanced knowledge (work which is predominantly intellectual in character and which includes work requiring the consistent exercise of discretion and judgment)" (U.S. Department of Labor, 2011, para. 6). In addition, the learned professional must have advanced knowledge in a field of science or learning, and the advanced knowledge must be customarily acquired by a prolonged course of specialized intellectual instruction (U.S. Department of Labor, 2011).

Concerns about the exemption of health care workers from protection under the FLSA were borne out in a June 2007 Supreme Court ruling that the U.S. Department of Labor had acted appropriately in denying FLSA protection to 10 home care workers even when employed by large, third-party home care agencies (Dawson, 2007). In the case of *Long Island Care at Home, LTD. v. Coke,* "the Court ruled that Ms. Evelyn Coke, a home care aide from Queens, New York, deserved neither overtime pay nor minimum wage, although she was frequently asked to work up to 70 hours per week" (Dawson, 2007, para. 1).

The *Legal Eye Newsletter* (Bergman, 2008) suggested that this ruling occurred because of an exemption to the FLSA that applies to companions and housekeepers who work in the homes of their clients. The *Newsletter* went on to note that the U.S. District Court for the Southern District of Florida recently clarified the law, suggesting that licensed staff who go into clients' homes to perform nursing assessments and to provide treatments are not home companions or housekeepers and thus are entitled to overtime.

In addition, it is important to note that nurses are eligible for overtime pay and protection under the FLSA if they are classified by employers as hourly—not salaried—employees, because salaried employees are not eligible for overtime. Thus, salaried employees and nurses who are considered to be exempt under the FLSA have virtually no rights under these new overtime rules. They are entitled only to their base salary, less deductions, by law and may be held to whatever schedule an employer demands because there are no restrictions on mandatory overtime in the FLSA.

Lyncheski (2010) notes that the most expensive violations of the FLSA typically involve the misclassifications of individuals exempt from overtime compensation pursuant to these new federal overtime rules. The most frequent violation, however, is the miscalculation of the "regular rate." Overtime compensation must be calculated based on the employee's regular rate of pay, which may differ from his or her base rate because of other forms of compensation which must be included in the rate and which can vary from work week to work week, but it is the least consequent in terms of liability.

## Legislating Limits on Nursing Overtime

Despite multiple efforts over the last decade to introduce national legislation directed at prohibiting employers from requiring licensed health care employees to work more than 8 hours in a single workday or 80 hours in any 14-day work period—except in the case of a natural disaster or declaration of emergency by federal, state, or local government officials—no such legislation has passed.

States are, however, increasingly taking a role in both defining mandatory overtime and putting limits to its use. Every nurse should know and understand the provisions of the Nurse Practice Act in his or her state, as well as the position statements or advisory opinions that have been issued by the state board of nursing on mandatory overtime and patient abandonment.

---

### DISCUSSION POINT

What position statement or advisory opinion has your state board of nursing issued regarding mandatory overtime and patient abandonment? Do you feel that it is adequate to protect both nurses and patients from unsafe working conditions?

---

In addition, the ANA has added the mandatory overtime issue to its Nationwide State Legislative Agenda, supporting the enactment of mandatory overtime legislation by state legislatures and the attention to such issues by regulatory agencies. As of 2011, 16 states had restrictions on the use of mandatory overtime for nurses, 14 states by enacting legislation (Alaska, Connecticut, Illinois, Maryland, Minnesota, New Jersey, New Hampshire, New York, Oregon, Pennsylvania, Rhode Island, Texas, Washington, and West Virginia) and 2 by including such provisions in regulations (California and Missouri; ANA, 2011a).

Six states introduced legislation in the 2011/2012 year alone, including Florida, Illinois, Massachusetts, New York, Pennsylvaina, and Vermont (ANA, 2011a). Some of these bills are attached to Patient Protection Acts or broader bills related to staffing and safe patient handling.

Alaska passed mandatory overtime restrictions for nurses in health care settings in 2010 preceded by Texas in 2009. Pennsylvania enacted the Prohibition of Excessive Overtime in Health Care Act (HB 834) in October 2008. This law states that a health care facility could not require an employee to work in excess of an agreed to, predetermined, and regularly scheduled daily work shift unless there was an unforeseeable declared national, state, or municipal emergency or a catastrophic event which was unpredictable or unavoidable and which substantially affects or increases the need for health care services (ANA, 2011a). This law did not preclude employees from voluntarily accepting overtime, and it did not apply to those workers compensated for "on call" time.

New York also enacted legislation in 2008 prohibiting health care employers (excluding home care facilities) from forcing nurses to work overtime, except during health care disasters that increased the need for health care personnel unexpectedly or when a health care employer determined that there was emergency and had made a good faith effort to have overtime covered on a voluntary basis (ANA, 2011a). Another exception included an ongoing medical or surgical procedure in which the nurse is actively engaged, such as in surgery, and whose continued presence through completion is essential to the health and safety of the patient (ANA, 2011a).

Although the New York legislation provides a good example of how states can reduce the risk of mandatory overtime for nurses, it should be noted that the New York Nurses Association first proposed legislation to ban mandatory overtime in 2000. Eight years were required to gain enough support from patient advocacy groups and other unions that represent nurses (such as the New York State Public Employees Federation and the New York State United Teachers) for the legislation to pass (Nurses Welcome Agreement, 2008).

Minnesota also successfully passed legislation in 2007 that prohibited nurses from being required to work more than a "normal work period," meaning 12 or fewer consecutive hours, consistent with their predetermined work shift, but again excludes an emergency (ANA, 2011a):

*The definition of emergency refers to a period when replacement staff are not able to report for duty for the next shift or increase patient need, because of unusual, unpredictable, or unforeseen circumstances such as, but not limited to, an act of terrorism, a disease outbreak, adverse weather conditions, or natural disasters which impact the continuity of patient care.* (para. 5)

Similar legislation became effective in New Hampshire in 2008. This legislation prohibited an employer from disciplining or removing any right, benefit, or privilege of a registered nurse, licensed practical nurse, or licensed nursing assistant for refusing to work more than 12 consecutive hours, except under specific circumstances, such as those identified in the New York and Minnesota legislation (ANA, 2011a). A nurse might be disciplined for refusing to work mandatory overtime in these situations.

## THE CONSEQUENCES OF MANDATORY OVERTIME

Research on the effects of overtime has largely focused on studies of individuals working scheduled 12-hour shifts. However, when staff *plan* to work 12-hour shifts or additional shifts on a volunteer basis, they are more likely to get plenty of rest immediately before working the extended shift. Overtime mandated by an employer, however, occurs with little or no prior notice, so higher levels of fatigue may occur. In addition, many nurses report working far more than 12 hours when mandatory overtime is involved.

How long can nurses work safely? Given the variability in each situation, there is no one answer to this question. There is little doubt, however, that after a certain point of protracted worktime, fatigue becomes a factor and the likelihood of errors, near errors, mistakes, and lapses in judgment increases.

Other industries, such as airlines and trucking, have recognized this for years and have limited the hours employees in these industries can work without breaks. The ANA authored a position statement in 2006, arguing that nursing employers should do the same by ensuring that sufficient system resources exist to (1) provide the individual registered nurse in all roles and settings with a work schedule that provides for adequate rest and recuperation between scheduled work and (2) provide sufficient compensation and appropriate staffing systems that foster a safe and healthful environment in which the registered nurse does not feel compelled to seek supplemental income through overtime, extra shifts, and other practices that contribute to worker fatigue (ANA, 2006).

---

CONSIDER THIS   Federal regulations have used transportation laws to place limits on the amount of time that can safely be worked in aviation and trucking. It seems appropriate that Congress needs to go beyond the FLSA and at least examine the need to create safety parameters around mandatory overtime in nursing.

The reality, however, is that mandatory overtime is very much a part of contemporary nursing practice, and the literature increasingly suggests that fatigue can result in a whole host of negative consequences including occupational injury, illness, burnout, and errors. For example, research conducted by de Castro et al. (2010) found that mandatory overtime resulted in potential risks for nurses' safety and health (see Research Study Fuels the Controversy 12.1).

Similarly, a study by Warren and Tart (2008) at a not-for-profit magnet community hospital found that fatigue caused by long work hours, working on call, and insufficient rest periods led to perioperative documentation errors. When a reduced call schedule was implemented, a significant reduction in nursing documentation errors was observed, with the greatest reduction in errors seen among nurses working 12-hour or call shifts.

In another recent study of 2,273 registered nurses in the United States, Geiger-Brown found that adverse work schedules negatively affect sleep quality and work performance (Study Reveals Sleep Problems, 2008). The research analyzed work schedule variables including hours per day, days per week, weekends per month, quick returns (less than 10 hours off between shifts), mandatory overtime, on-call, and circadian mismatch, and found that the worse the schedule, the worse was the sleep for most nurses. Geiger-Brown suggested that the inadequate sleep that occurs as a result of adverse work schedules has both short-term (needle-stick injuries and musculoskeletal disorders) and long-term (cardiovascular and metabolic diseases) health consequences for nurses and possibly for the patients for whom they care (Study Reveals Sleep Problems, 2008).

These findings reinforce those of a report of the Board on Health Care Services (HCS) and the Institute of Medicine (IOM), *Keeping Patients Safe: Transforming the Work Environment of Nurses*, which said that nurses' long working hours pose a serious threat to patient safety. In fact, the report argued that "limiting the number of hours worked per day and consecutive days of work by nursing staff, as is done in other safety-sensitive industries, is a fundamental safety precaution" (PA Nurses Also Address, 2007, para. 3). Similarly, Marquis and Huston (2012) argued that certain minimum criteria should always be met for safe staffing. These criteria are shown in Box 12.2.

---

## DISCUSSION POINT

How many hours can the typical nurse work before she or he might be considered unsafe? How much individual leeway is feasible in making this determination?

---

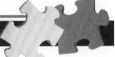

## RESEARCH STUDY FUELS THE CONTROVERSY 12.1

### THE IMPACT OF WORK SCHEDULE ON OCCUPATIONAL INJURY AND ILLNESS

In this cross-sectional study, using questionnaire data, of 655 registered nurses in the Philippines, the researchers investigated whether regular work shifts and mandatory overtime (i.e., employer-imposed work time in excess of one's assigned schedule) posed potential risks for nurses' safety and health. Multiple logistic regression was used to assess associations of shift work and mandatory overtime with four work-related health outcomes.

de Castro, A., Fujishiro, K., Rue, T., Tagalog, E., Samaco-Paquiz, L., & Gee, G. (2010). Associations between work schedule characteristics and occupational injury and illness. *International Nursing Review, 57*(2), 188–194.

---

### STUDY FINDINGS

After accounting for weekly work hours, shift length, and demographic variables, nonday shifts were associated with work-related injury and work-related illness. Also, the frequency of working mandatory overtime was associated with work-related injury, work-related illness, and missing more than 2 days of work because of a work-related injury or illness. The researchers concluded that nonday shifts and mandatory overtime may negatively impact nurses' health, independent of working long hours, and suggested that mechanisms through which these work characteristics affect health, such as circadian rhythm disturbance, nurse-to-patient ratios, and work–family conflict, be examined in future studies.

## BOX 12.2 MINIMUM CRITERIA FOR STAFFING DECISIONS

- Decisions made must meet state and federal labor laws and organizational policies.

- Staff must not be demoralized or excessively fatigued by frequent or extended overtime requests.

- Long-term as well as short-term solutions must be sought.

- Patient care must not be jeopardized.

*Source:* Marquis, B., & Huston, C. (2012). *Leadership roles and management functions* (7th ed.). Philadelphia, PA: Lippincott Williams & Wilkins.

### DISCUSSION POINT

Is increasing the use of mandatory overtime perpetuating the nursing shortage? Do you think nurses who no longer work in nursing roles would be more apt to return to work if they felt they had more control over the hours they worked (mandatory overtime was banned)?

## PROFESSIONAL DUTY AND CONSCIENCE

Mandatory overtime and patient abandonment must also be examined in terms of professional duty. A *professional duty* is the direct result of others having welfare rights, such as the right to safe care. Because people have a right to such care, nurses have an associated duty to ensure that they accept patient care assignments only if they are mentally and physically able to provide, at minimum, safe care.

The problem is that there is great variability in terms of how many hours a nurse can work and still provide competent safe care. For example, the practice of mandatory overtime is grounded in the commitment to prevent harm to patients by guaranteeing adequate nurse–patient ratios, yet the overfatigued nurse may pose even greater risk of harm to patients by agreeing

to work. The ANA (2011a) agreed, suggesting that "regardless of the number of hours worked, each registered nurse has an ethical responsibility to carefully consider his/her level of fatigue when deciding to accept any assignment extending beyond the regularly scheduled work day or week, including mandatory or voluntary overtime assignment."

### DISCUSSION POINT

Who bears the risk or the consequences of risk when an overworked nurse makes errors that contribute to patient harm?

Cady (2008) added that there are many reasons why a nurse might refuse to care for a patient. She suggested that nurse managers must be aware of the nexus between moral dilemmas in health care and the right of providers to refuse a patient care assignment.

Cady went on to say that one option nurses should consider if they do not want to work mandatory overtime is to file for *conscientious objection*. The purpose of conscientious objection is to protect the rights of employees who refuse to participate in procedures on the basis of conscience. The issue of whether a nurse can refuse mandatory overtime on the basis of conscience, however, has limited case law precedent.

The ANA's *Code of Ethics* (ANA, 2001) might also be helpful to some nurses in resolving potential ethical conflicts between their professional duty to provide care and conscience, or the realization that providing such care may actually place patients at risk for harm. The *Code of Ethics*, however, might actually potentiate the dilemma because it states that nurses should care for all people without discrimination and maintain and foster nursing competence and professional development. The problem is that it also says that the nurse is to maintain conditions of employment that are conducive to high-quality nursing care.

The ANA also recommends a Bill of Rights as a tool for dialogue to resolve concerns that nurses may have about work environments that might not support professional practice. The Bill of Rights was actually conceived to support nurses in an array of workplace situations, including mandatory overtime, and suggests that nurses must bring these workplace issues to the attention of employers to meet their responsibilities to their patients and to themselves (ANA, 2011b).

## PATIENT ABANDONMENT

One of the most common reasons nurses cite for working mandatory overtime is the threat that refusal to do so could be construed as *patient abandonment*, a charge that can result in loss of licensure. Therefore, many nurses believe that they have no choice when confronted by a request for overtime, despite the fact that they might be working a shift in excess of 12 hours.

---

CONSIDER THIS   In some facilities, nurses are being threatened with dismissal or with the charge of patient abandonment if they refuse to accept overtime.

---

Despite this perception, the ANA does not support the forced overtime of nurses, and their position is that a nurse should not be held accountable for patient abandonment if the nurse turned down an assignment that could be unsafe to patients or self. In fact, generally speaking, most state boards of nursing suggest that refusal to work mandatory overtime is not patient abandonment; in a situation in which a nurse has accepted a patient or assignment, the nurse must simply notify the supervisor that he or she is leaving and report off to another nurse.

Usually, however, nurses have less likelihood of losing their license or being reprimanded if an assignment (mandatory overtime) is never accepted in the first place than if the assignment is accepted and then the nurse changes his or her mind. This is because accepting the assignment suggests that a nurse–patient relationship has been established. Cady (2008) agreed, suggesting the following:

> When the nurse accepts a patient assignment, the nurse maintains responsibility for that patient until the nurse–patient relationship is ended by the patient's discharge, the transfer of responsibility to another nurse, or the patient's refusal of the nurse's services. If no nurse is available for the transfer of responsibility, then the presently assigned nurse is legally and morally obligated to continue to care for the patient until the time that another nurse becomes available to take over that patient assignment. (para. 15)

In addition, boards of nursing in several states have developed clear statements differentiating patient abandonment from *employee abandonment*. Typically, these statements define *employment abandonment* as nurses leaving their places of work to avoid injury to patients or to themselves.

Cady (2008) also distinguished between the refusal to accept a patient assignment and patient abandonment. Cady suggested that patient abandonment occurs when the nurse engages in a patient assignment and ceases to provide nursing care without appropriately transferring the responsibility for the patient to another professional nurse.

This definition is similar to language used by the Maryland Board of Registered Nursing (BRN) in defining patient abandonment; however, the Maryland BRN (2011) suggested that there are many variables to be examined in determining whether patient abandonment has actually occurred. The definition of patient abandonment and these variables are shown in Box 12.3.

---

**BOX 12.3    THE LINK BETWEEN NURSE–PATIENT RELATIONSHIPS AND PATIENT ABANDONMENT AS OUTLINED BY THE MARYLAND BOARD OF REGISTERED NURSING**

*Abandonment* occurs when a licensed nurse terminates the nurse–patient relationship without reasonable notification to the nursing supervisor for the continuation of the patient's care.
*The nurse–patient relationship* begins when responsibility for nursing care of a patient is accepted by the nurse. Nursing management is accountable for assessing the capabilities of personnel and delegating responsibility or assigning nursing care functions to personnel qualified to assume such responsibility or to perform such functions.

**The Variables That Need to Be Examined in Each Alleged Incident of Abandonment Include but Are not Limited to:**

1. What were the licensee's assigned responsibilities for what time frame? What was the clinical setting and resources available to the licensee?

*continued*

**BOX 12.3 THE LINK BETWEEN NURSE–PATIENT RELATIONSHIPS AND PATIENT ABANDONMENT AS OUTLINED BY THE MARYLAND BOARD OF REGISTERED NURSING** *continued*

2. Was there an exchange of responsibility from one licensee to another? When did the exchange occur, that is, shift report and so on?

3. What was the time frame of the incident, that is, time licensee arrived, time of exchange of responsibility, and the like?

4. What was the communication process, that is, whom did the licensee inform of his or her intent to leave, and was it lateral, upward, downward, and so forth?

5. What are the facility's policies, terms of employment, and/or job description regarding the licensee and call-in, refusal to accept an assignment, reassignment to another unit, mandatory overtime, and the like?

6. What is the pattern of practice/events for the licensee and the pattern of management for the unit/facility, that is, is the event of a single isolated occurrence, or is it one event in a series of events?

7. What were the issues/reasons why the licensee could not accept an assignment, continue an assignment or extend an original assignment, and so forth?

*Source:* Maryland Board of Registered Nursing. (2011, July 1). *Abandonment.* Retrieved August 16, 2011, from http://www.mbon.org/main.php?v=norm&p=0&c=practice/abandonment.html

CONSIDER THIS Although boards of nursing often rule that refusing mandatory overtime is not patient abandonment and thus is not cause for loss of licensure, they have no jurisdiction over employment and contract issues. Refusing to work mandatory overtime may still result in termination of a nurse's employment.

## UNIONS AND MANDATORY OVERTIME

Because collective bargaining agreements can require greater protections beyond those outlined in the FLSA, the position of most collective bargaining agents is that the practice of mandatory overtime should be eliminated entirely. However, there are differences among union contracts, and the strategies used by unions to reduce mandatory overtime vary greatly.

The American Federation of Teachers (AFT, n.d.) has been working with its state affiliates to ban the practice of mandatory overtime through a twofold approach—legislation and contract language: At the federal level, AFT is working with legislators on a proposal that would require facilities receiving Medicare funding to stop mandating overtime. In addition, many local unions have negotiated contract language limiting the practice of mandatory overtime (AFT, n.d.).

The Service Employees International Union (SEIU) has also consistently spoken out against mandatory overtime. In addition, the SEIU, in partnership with the Nurse Alliance, created an Overtime Report Form for nurses, union or nonunion, to document mandatory or pressured overtime. The American Federation of State, County and Municipal Employees (AFSCME) is also working to eliminate mandatory overtime in response to inadequate staff to operate public agencies such as prisons, veterans homes, and mental health and developmental centers (AFSCME, 2011).

## CONCLUSIONS

The AFSCME suggests that while many hospital administrators believe that the imposition of mandatory overtime saves money by limiting recruitment and benefit expenses, multiple studies have "shown mandatory overtime to be perhaps the single worst practice to emerge from the era of downsizing and managed care" (AFSCME, 2011, para. 1). In the end, the mandatory overtime dilemma, like so many in nursing, comes down to a conflict regarding how best to use limited resources (fiscal and human) to provide safe, quality health care. Most nurses and administrators can agree on two goals: (1) staffing should be at least minimally adequate to assure that all patients receive safe care and

(2) nursing staff should not be placed at personal or legal risk to provide that care.

The problem is that the onus is on management to ensure that there is appropriate staffing, and most health care institutions state that there simply are not enough resources to meet the first goal without jeopardizing the second. Clearly, more alternatives such as shift bidding and pay enhancement programs need to be explored. Neither health care administrators nor nurses should have to choose between meeting the needs of patients and meeting the needs of nurses.

The bottom line is that workers should have the right to refuse overtime without fear of repercussion, especially when staffing shortages and mandated overtime are the norm and not the exception. Unfortunately, as long as nursing shortages exist, mandatory overtime will continue to be used as a means of meeting minimum staffing needs.

## FOR ADDITIONAL DISCUSSION

**1.** How does the presence of a collective bargaining agreement affect a hospital's ability to require mandatory overtime? How much power do unions have in negotiating this aspect of working conditions?

**2.** Would passage of a national ban on mandatory overtime tie the hands of hospitals to assure that staffing is at least minimally adequate during periods of acute nursing shortages?

**3.** Does the use of mandatory overtime really save hospitals money in terms of recruitment and benefits?

**4.** How do the rates of mandatory overtime in nursing compare with those in other professions?

**5.** Are other healthcare professionals at risk for loss of licensure if they are found guilty of patient abandonment?

**6.** Are charges of patient abandonment legally and morally appropriate if a nurse works his or her required shift but refuses to stay and work longer?

**7.** Given the severity and scope of the nursing shortage, what is the likelihood that mandatory staffing will continue to be used for both emergency and routine staffing needs?

## REFERENCES

American Federation of State, County and Municipal Employees, AFL–CIO. (2011). *Worst practices. Mandatory overtime.* Retrieved September 4, 2011, from http://www.afscme.org/news/publications/healthcare/solving-the-nursing-shortage/worst-practices-mandatory-overtime

American Federation of Teachers. (n.d.). *Ban on mandatory overtime.* Retrieved September 4, 2011, from http://www.aft.org/issues/healthcare/overtime/index.cfm

American Nurses Association. (2001). *Code of ethics for nurses with interpretive statements.* Washington, DC: Author. Retrieved May 1, 2012, from http://www.nursingworld.org/MainMenuCategories/EthicsStandards/CodeofEthicsforNurses.aspx

American Nurses Association. (2006). *Position statement: Assuring patient safety: The employers' role in promoting healthy nursing work hours for registered nurses in all roles and settings.* Retrieved September 3, 2011, from http://www.nursingworld.org/MainMenuCategories/EthicsStandards/Ethics-Position-Statements/AssuringPatientSafety.aspx

American Nurses Association. (2011a). Mandatory overtime. *Nursing World.* Retrieved May 1, 2012, from http://ana.nursingworld.org/MainMenuCategories/ANAPoliticalPower/State/StateLegislativeAgenda/MandatoryOvertime.aspx

American Nurses Association. (2011b). *Bill of rights FAQs.* Retrieved September 5, 2011, from http://www.nursingworld.org/MainMenuCategories/WorkplaceSafety/Work-Environment/NursesBillof-Rights/FAQs.html

Association of Perioperative Registered Nurses. (2011). *AORN position statement: Safe work/on-call practices* (April 2005/Sunset Review March 2010). Denver, CO: Author. Retrieved August 17, 2011, from http://www.aorn.org/PracticeResources/AORNPosition-Statements/

Bae, S., & Brewer, C. (2010). Mandatory overtime regulations and nurse overtime. *Policy, Politics & Nursing Practice, 11*(2), 99–107.

Bergman, V. (2008). Home health: Professional staff get overtime pay. *Legal Eagle Eye Newsletter for the Nursing Profession, 16*(4), 4.

Breslin, T. (2010). Fair Labor Standards Act: Federal protections for overtime work. *Massachusetts Nurse Advocate, 81*(7), 10.

Cady, R. F. (2008). Refusal to care. *JONA's Healthcare Law, Ethics, & Regulation, 10*(2), 46–47.

Dawson, S. L. (2007). Taking a cue from the Supreme Court. *Nursing Homes: Long Term Care Management, 56*(10), 8–10.

de Castro, A., Fujishiro, K., Rue, T., Tagalog, E., Samaco-Paquiz, L., & Gee, G. (2010). Associations between work schedule characteristics and occupational injury and illness. *International Nursing Review, 57*(2), 188–194.

Garrett, C. (2008). The effect of nurse staffing patterns on medical errors and nurse burnout. *AORN Journal, 87*(6), 1191–1192, 1194, 1196–2000.

Gelb, M. (2008). *For many Americans, hard work is badge of honor: Americans skimp on vacations; economists say work ethic can pay off.* Retrieved August 1, 2008, from http://www.america.gov/st/econenglish/2008/July/20080703151840berehellek0.7706415.html

Kauffman, M. (2011). *State spends millions on forced OT at Connecticut Valley Hospital.* Retrieved September 4, 2011, from http://articles.courant.com/2011-04-03/health/hc-cvhot-0403-20110403_1_mandatory-overtime-cvh-workers-double-shift

Lyncheski, J. E. (2010). Old law—new problem: The surge in FSLA lawsuits. *Long-Term Living: For the Continuing Care Professional, 59*(9), 32–33.

Marquis, B., & Huston, C. (2012). *Leadership roles and management functions* (7th ed.). Philadelphia, PA: Lippincott Williams & Wilkins.

Maryland Board of Registered Nursing. (2011). *Abandonment.* Retrieved August 16, 2011, from http://www.mbon.org/main.php?v=norm&p=0&c=practice/abandonment.html

Nurses welcome agreement to ban mandatory overtime, New York. (2008). Retrieved July 31, 2008, from http://www.medicalnewstoday.com/articles/112051.php

Overtime pay and white-collar exemptions: Seeking clarification in light of recent revisions. (2008). *Illinois Business Law Journal.* Retrieved August 1, 2008, from http://www.law.illinois.edu/bljournal/post/2008/02/21/Overtime-Pay-and-White-Collar-Exemptions-Seeking-Clarification-in-Light-of-Recent-Revisions.aspx

PA nurses also address mandatory overtime [Abstract]. (2007). *American Nurse, 39*(3), 4.

Service Employees International Union Local 7. (2011). *Federal mandatory overtime bill will improve patient care, prevent medical errors.* Retrieved September 4, 2011, from http://seiu7.org/appResources/scPages/mandatoryovertimeindepth.cfm

Study reveals sleep problems with shiftwork. (2008). *Lamp, 65*(6), 13.

Trinkoff, A., Johantgen, M., Storr, C., Han, K., Liang, Y., Gurses, A., & Hopkinson, S. (2010). A comparison of working conditions among nurses in magnet and non-magnet hospitals. *Journal of Nursing Administration, 40*(7–8), 309–315.

U.S. Department of Labor. (2011). *Overtime pay.* Retrieved September 4, 2011, from http://www.dol.gov/dol/topic/wages/overtimepay.htm

Warren, A., & Tart, R. C. (2008). Fatigue and charting errors: The benefit of a reduced call schedule. *AORN Journal, 88*(1), 88–95.

## BIBLIOGRAPHY

Bae, S., Brewer, C. S., & Kovner, C. T. (2012). State mandatory overtime regulations and newly licensed nurses' mandatory and voluntary overtime and total work hours. *Nursing Outlook, 60*(2), 60–71.

Barker, L. M., & Nussbaum, M. A. (2011). Fatigue, performance and the work environment: a survey of registered nurses. *Journal of Advanced Nursing, 67*(6), 1370–1382.

Chalupka, S. (2012). Overtime work as a predictor of a major depressive episode. *Workplace Health & Safety, 60*(4), 192.

Frellick, M. (2012). Balancing act. *Nurse.Com (New York/New Jersey Metro), 24*(4), 20–21.

Geiger-Brown, J., Trinkoff, A., & Rogers, V. E. (2011). The impact of work schedules, home, and work demands on self-reported sleep in registered nurses. *Journal of Occupational & Environmental Medicine, 53*(3), 303–307.

Harrison, R. (2012). Mandatory overtime. *Nurse.Com (West), 12*(3), 12.

Increasing registered nurse staffing, reducing overtime hours can improve patients' experience. (2011). *Nursingmatters, 22*(5), 20.

Ludwig, G. (2010). Leadership sector: Mandatory overtime: Workin' nine to . . . ? *Journal of Emergency Medical Services, 35*(4), 26.

Medical interns who work extended-duration shifts double their risk of car crashes when driving home from the hospital. (2005). *ISNA Bulletin, 31*(3), 20–21.

Pinkham, J. (2011). Executive director's column: Are you owed overtime pay? *Massachusetts Nurse Advocate, 82*(4), 3.

Raso, R. (2012). Leadership Q&A: The legality of mandatory vaccination and overtime. *Nursing Management, 43*(2), 56.

Soares, M. M., Jacobs, K., Estryn-Béhar, M., Beatrice, I. J. M., & Van der, H. (2012). Effects of extended work shifts on employee fatigue, health, satisfaction, work/family balance, and patient safety. *Work: A Journal of Prevention, Assessment and Rehabilitation, 41*(1),4283–4290.

Stanley, S. (2011). You can refuse to do unpaid overtime. *Nursing Times, 107*(18), 9.

Twarog, J. (2011). Realities of mandatory overtime on the patient and the nurse. *Massachusetts Nurse Advocate, 82*(3), 10–11.

Unruh, L., Agrawal, M., & Hassmiller, S. (2011). The business case for transforming care at the bedside among the "TCAB 10" and lessons learned. *Nursing Administration Quarterly, 35*(2), 97–109.

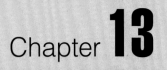

## Chapter 13

# Violence in Nursing
## *The Expectations and the Reality*

Charmaine Hockley

## ADDITIONAL RESOURCES

Visit thePoint* for additional helpful resources
- eBook
- Journal Articles
- WebLinks

## CHAPTER OUTLINE

## LEARNING OBJECTIVES

*The learner will be able to:*

1. Identify common terms used to describe workplace violence, including horizontal violence, bullying, and mobbing.

2. Explore the prevalence of workplace violence in nursing as compared with other professions.

3. Recognize workplace violence as both a national and a global problem.

4. Differentiate among the different categories of violence in the health care sector, generally, and nursing, specifically.

5. Compare the incidence, most frequent types, and common consequences of workplace violence for men and women.

6. Identify antisocial workplace behaviors that may lead to nurses causing each other harm.

7. Analyze common reasons that nurses are reluctant to report workplace violence.

8. Recognize potential long-term consequences of workplace violence, including physical, emotional, and financial repercussions.

9. Delineate specific strategies that can be undertaken by individuals, employers, organizations, and governments to reduce workplace violence.

10. Integrate ethical and moral codes of professional practice as guides for developing best practices to guard against and respond to workplace violence.

11. Reflect on personal behaviors or attitude that might create a threatening workplace environment for others.

Violence in nursing continues to be one of the major professional issues facing nurses in the 21st century. After the slow acceptance in the 1990s that violence in nursing was occurring, research has evolved rapidly. Until recently, research has focused on the nature and extent of bullying. This was important work. We now have a good understanding of the nature of violence in nursing and that it is not rare or isolated to a single setting but is experienced by nurses in a wide variety of geographical locations and service areas. Research has shown that nurses can be targeted by other nurses, or by other health professionals, patients, visitors, or strangers. In other words, the violence that nurses experience may occur wherever they may live, work, or the position they hold.

This chapter moves beyond an understanding of the nature and extent of workplace violence by introducing strategies that have the potential to reduce the violence nurses experience. However, it is important to briefly revisit what is meant by violence in nursing, the language that is used to describe this behavior, and the types of violence that nurses experience. Therefore, this chapter is divided into two sections. The first section begins by providing an overview of violence in nursing. The second section introduces strategies to consider in addressing this behavior. Contemporary and wide-ranging violence in nursing is research and showcased throughout the chapter.

---

### DISCUSSION POINTS

How does violence in nursing affect patient care?
How does violence in nursing affect your private life?

---

## WHAT IS VIOLENCE IN NURSING?

Over the years, violence in nursing has often been a difficult concept to grasp, in part because of people's misunderstanding of what the term *violence* implies, as well as because of the language used to describe this behavior. The language issues often derive from a reluctance to expand the meaning of violence to being more than a physical act, or it could be the result of an erroneous perception that such things do not happen to nurses. For example, the use of the term *bullying* to describe and define workplace incidents may conjure up a perception of schoolyard bullying and therefore minimize the effect that this behavior can have on the person involved. Furthermore, when people consider violence, they often ignore the nonphysical aspects, such as the emotional, financial, sexual, and psychological harm, which are experienced by many people who are abused.

Another reason violence in nursing is often misunderstood is the lack of an agreed upon definition. One reason put forward recently is that it is difficult to differentiate concepts such as workplace and horizontal violence because there are other terms such as *bullying* and *mobbing* that are all used interchangeably and their definitions coincide with each other (Kirkhorn, Stehle Werner, & Heintz, 2010).

## TERMINOLOGY

Historically, different countries have used different terms to describe this violent behavior. For example, the nursing literature in the United States led the way by referring to this behavior as *horizontal violence*. Although the term horizontal violence continues to be used (Walrafen, Brewer, & Mulvenon, 2012), this term appears to be overtaken with the use of *bullying* or *lateral violence* (American Nurses Association, 2012) as the preferred term. In Europe, the preferred term has been *mobbing*, and in the United Kingdom, the literature refers to this behavior as *bullying*. Although the Australian nursing literature initially used the term horizontal violence in other contexts, bullying became the term of choice during the 1990s.

The term *workplace violence* has gradually become the preferred term in many countries, particularly since the release of papers from internationally recognized organizations such as the International Council of Nurses (ICN), the World Health Organization (WHO), the Honor Society of Nursing, Sigma Theta Tau International (STTI), the Royal College of Nursing (RCN), and the Royal College of Nursing, Australia (RCNA).

Research into workplace aggression constructs, such as *abusive supervision, bullying, incivility, social undermining*, and *interpersonal conflict*, was recently undertaken but the author concluded that the manner in which these terms have been differentiated did not add greatly to our knowledge of workplace aggression (Hershcovis, 2011).

---

CONSIDER THIS   Violence has penetrated every sector of society, including the workplace, and yet there continues to be difficulty defining these incidents.

## THEORY

The theory underpinning violence in nursing has generally received less attention than the practical manifestation of violence in nursing. One of the earliest references is from Roberts (1983), who, in examining horizontal violence, argued compellingly that some of the salient aspects of nursing subculture and behaviors came within the framework of oppression theory. Since then, different theoretical frameworks and developing new instruments to measure workplace bullying (Simons, Stark, & De Marco, 2011) have been used to research violence within the health care sector. This theory-based research has the ongoing potential to considerably reduce the amount of violence experienced by nurses by assisting nurses to develop informed strategies to manage the violent behavior.

## SPECIALIZED AREAS OF RESEARCH

In recent years, violence in nursing has been researched from different geographical locations, for example Italy (Magnavita & Heponiemi, 2011) and Chile (Burgos & Paravic, 2010). There has also been a growing research interest in nursing specialty areas such as midwifery (Martin & Martin, 2010), dementia care (Boström, Squires, Mitchell, Sales, & Estabrooks, 2012), and HIV/AIDS patients (Ndou & De Villiers, 2010). There has also been a growing interest in student incivility and student–faculty relationships (Robertson, 2012) and exploring the vulnerability of faculty (Dal Pezzo & Jett, 2010). A review of the violence in the health care sector literature shows that this violent behavior is not unique to any specific country or any specific nursing location and can impact on all levels of nursing.

Each of these perspectives and nursing services bring forward language that is unique to them and highlights that although there is a common theme—violence in nursing—how this behavior is defined or the language used depends on the researchers' or practitioners' perspective.

## WHAT TYPES OF VIOLENCE DO NURSES EXPERIENCE?

Nurses experience different types of violence, often depending on the location, the service provided, and the perpetrator. Moreover, what one person considers being harmed may not be perceived as such by another. Therefore, every person's experience with or perceptions about violence are unique to that person. However, it is possible to categorize the different types of violence that nurses might experience. Over the years, there have been various taxonomies (Hutchinson, Vickers, Wilkes, & Jackson, 2010) put forward to categorize workplace violence in general and nurses in particular. Box 13.1 lists seven basic categories specific to nursing and Box 13.2 and Box 13.3 expand on the non-physical and physical aspects of violence.

Recent research continues to focus on nurse-to-nurse violence and organizational violence. However, a literature review showed that there is a gap in research into the impact of mass trauma or natural disaster on nurses and third-party violence. All of these types of violence have the potential to lead to physical, emotional, and financial harm.

---

**BOX 13.1  TYPOLOGY OF VIOLENCE IN NURSING**

1. Nurse-to-nurse violence (horizontal violence)
2. Patient-to-nurse violence
3. Organization-to-nurse violence (vertical violence)
4. External perpetrators (strangers, visitors)
5. Third-party violence (colleagues/family members)
6. Impact of mass trauma or natural disasters on nurses (earthquakes, tornadoes, tsunamis)
7. Nurse-to-patient violence

### BOX 13.2   TYPES OF NONPHYSICAL VIOLENCE INVOLVING NURSES

1. Being uncivil, such as exhibiting rudeness, impoliteness, and silence
2. Condoning improper behavior by being unsupportive and uncooperative
3. Setting someone up for failure, imposing ideas, taking someone's ideas, undermining, embarrassing someone
4. Exhibiting threatening behavior—making someone feel intimidated, threatened, or fearful
5. Spreading rumors, making defamatory online statements, improperly taking credit, assigning blame or fault
6. Stalking
7. Defaming
8. Cyber bullying

There are many nonphysical types of violence experienced by nurses. Research shows that verbal abuse, such as yelling, swearing, and threats, were one of the most common forms of abuse experienced by nurses irrespective of the geographical location (e.g., Australian studies by Pich, Hazelton, Sundin, & Kable, 2011; Palestinian study by Ali, 2010). Being shouted at, making unreasonable demands, and intimidation were the most commonly reported forms of verbal abuse in the Australian study (Pich et al., 2011). Seventy-four percent of respondents in Ali's (2010) study reported verbal abuse compared with 34.3% who had experienced physical abuse in a 12-month period.

The majority of the physical forms of violence such as slapping, hitting, lashing out, stabbing, kicking, and spitting from patients occurred mainly in specialized areas, particularly in psychiatric nursing (Needham, Frauenfelder, Gianni, Dinkel, & Hatcher, 2010).

In addition, the American Nurses Association (ANA; 2011) reported the physical forms of violence over a 6-year period (2003–2009) as shown in Box 13.4. In 2009, there were 2,050 assaults and violent acts reported by RNs requiring an average of 4 days away from work (ANA, 2011).

### DISCUSSION POINT

Do you believe that there is an increasing trend in physical violence in the workplace or is there better reporting of these events?

### BOX 13.3   TYPES OF PHYSICAL VIOLENCE INVOLVING NURSES

1. Hitting/punching/pinching
2. Spitting
3. Kicking
4. Sexual assault/rape
5. Assault
6. Homicide

## BOX 13.4 THE SPREAD OF EXTREME PHYSICAL WORKPLACE VIOLENCE INVOLVING NURSES

- 8 registered nurses were FATALLY injured at work: 4 RNs received gunshot wounds (RNs) leading to their death and 4 RNs received other fatal injuries.

- 8 of 8 RNs were working in private health care facilities (not state or local government).

- 8 of 8 RNs were 35 to 54 years of age.

*Source:* American Nurses Association. (2011).*Workplace violence.* Retrieved May 5, 2012, from http://ana.nursingworld.org/workplaceviolence

Box 13.5 summarizes the nonfatal assaults and violent acts of the 2,050 assaults experienced by nurses.

## WHO ARE THE VICTIMS?

Although the true extent of violence in nursing is considered to be greater than the statistics indicate, studies show that violence against female nurses is greater than that against male nurses (e.g., Motamedi, 2010). A Canadian study revealed that men viewed workplace violence as less of an issue than did women (Back et al., 2010).

Studies into violence against men in other contexts tend to focus on rites of initiation of apprentices, college fraternity rites of passage (hazing), and armed service "bastardization" practices. However, the question of whether workplace violence against male nurses is an outcome of the same forces identified in studies into workplace violence between female nurses is open to further research. Because the statistics show that men are often the major perpetrators of violence in society and in the workplace (except possibly for *internal* violence in nursing), that is violence that comes from within the organization, the very fear that some male nurses may experience violence could also create more violent incidents in the workplace, generating a recurring cycle of violence.

## ADDRESSING VIOLENCE IN NURSING

Violence in nursing is an emotive phenomenon to all involved. It can affect families and other service providers as well as those who are being targeted. Even strangers can be victims of violence in the workplace, often because they are in the wrong place at the wrong time. It is not surprising that violence in nursing raises complex problems that will not be solved with simple solutions. One size does not fit all. It is vital therefore for a broad and sustained approach be considered to address this issue.

Although less so, violence in nursing continues to be perceived as a part of the job (Carmody, 2010), and

## BOX 13.5 NONFATAL ASSAULTS AND VIOLENCE INVOLVING NURSES

- 1,830 were inflicted with injuries by patients or residents.

- 80 were inflicted by visitors or people other than patients.

- 520 RNs were hit, kicked, or beaten.

- 130 RNs were squeezed, pinched, or scratched requiring days away from work.

- 30 RNs were bitten.

- In 2009, the Emergency Nurses Association reported that more than 50% of emergency center (EC) nurses had experienced violence by patients on the job and 25% of EC nurses had experienced 20 or more violent incidents in the past 3 years.

*Source:* American Nurses Association. (2011). *Workplace violence.* Retrieved May 5, 2012, from http://ana.nursingworld.org/workplaceviolence

there remains reluctance for some nurses to report this issue for management to intervene. Why this view remains despite research, education, legislation, and other strategies that explain and inform nurses that this behavior is not acceptable is difficult to explain.

---

CONSIDER THIS  The law often imposes definitions that are under- or overinclusive and demands uniform treatment that fit the definition, despite the recognition that addressing workplace violence is complex.

---

Discussing violence in nursing challenges many of the traditional views of nurses and nursing as trustworthy and caring. The two main ethical and legal principles that apply to nurses are that they (1) should do no harm and (2) have a duty of care to persons in their care. The legal requirements of nurses may vary, but they must consider the consequences of their actions to ensure that they have not breached their legal obligations toward their colleagues as well as to those in their care. For example, from an individual perspective, nurses must be aware of the laws that relate to negligence, defamation, discrimination, assault, and homicide. Organizations also have a duty of care to their employees, for example, occupational health and safety legislation which requires them to take reasonable precautions to protect the health and safety of its employees. This provision includes protecting employees from the risk of workplace violence and extends to those in their care such as patients, residents and visitors.

## GOVERNMENT RESPONSES TO WORKPLACE VIOLENCE

Many countries have legislation which specifically focuses on workplace violence and considers this behavior as an occupational health and safety hazard. Invariably, there is a statutory responsibility to meet standards, provide training and education, as well as requiring reports relating to workplace injuries or deaths.

### United States of America

Under the *Occupational Safety and Health Act of 1970* (OSH Act), employers are responsible for providing safe and healthful workplaces for their employees. The role of the *Occupational Safety and Health Administration* (OSHA) is to ensure these conditions for all workers by setting and enforcing standards, as well as providing training, education and assistance.

The OSHA mandates that "in addition to compliance with hazard-specific standards, all employers have a general duty to provide their employees with a workplace free from recognized hazards likely to cause death or serious physical harm" (OSHA, 2004). The General Duty Clause of the OSH Act (1970), Section 5(a)(1), states, "Each employer shall furnish to each of his employees employment and a place of employment which are free from recognized hazards that are causing or are likely to cause death or serious physical harm to his employees" (OSH Act, 1970). This act requires employers to comply with OSHA standards. Therefore, when there is a high risk of violence that is recognized as a serious hazard, then under Section 5(a)(1) of the OSH Act, the employer is required to take steps to minimize the risks (OSH Act 1970). If the employer fails to implement reasonable steps to address the hazard, such as violence in nursing, this failure could result in the finding of an OSHA violation.

The OSHA investigates and reports on these events leading to injuries and death. For example, in 2011 one hospital was fined US$4,500

> *after a nurse at the hospital was attacked and severely injured while performing normal duties that included providing group therapy sessions to psychiatric patients. The OSHA Administration inspectors found that her employers had failed to implement adequate measures to protect employees from assault in the workplace.* (U.S. Department of Labor, 2011)

The U.S. Census of Fatal Occupational Injuries Summary, 2009, released on 19 August 2010, reports that health care practitioners and technical occupations showed that 54 fatalities ($n = 4,340$) occurred, of which 19 were homicides. It is not possible to differentiate just how many of this number were nurses (U.S. Department of Labor, 2010). However, following the death in 2010 of a nurse who was attacked by an inmate at a county prison, the president of the California Nurses Association was reported to have stated that "Statistics have shown that over 2 million cases set forth by the labor department say that 49% of those occur in the healthcare setting. So our nurses are really at risk and so are our other healthcare workers" (Mabuhay, 2010).

Box 13.6 provides examples of legislation enacted for workplace violence prevention in various states of the United States such as California, Illinois, and New Jersey (ANA, 2011). Some of these states have increased their penalties whereas others have broadened the scope of potential victims.

Over the past 6 or 7 years, other states have approached the issue of workplace violence by elevating

## BOX 13.6 STATE PENALTIES FOR VIOLENCE INVOLVING NURSES

- **ARIZONA** (HB 1759) increases aggravated assault to a Class C felony.

- **NEW JERSEY** (AB1512/AB 2309/SB 911/SB1044) upgrades the offense of simple assault to aggravated assault if the victim is a health care worker or health care professional who is clearly identifiable as being engaged in his or her duties.

- **TENNESSEE** (HB 1586/SB 134) expands the scope of the present law to allow "any employer or employee who has suffered unlawful violence or a credible *threat* of violence" to seek such a temporary restraining order or injunction and broadens the definition of "unlawful violence" to include "intimidation or extortion" in addition to assault, aggravated assault, or stalking (ANA, 2011).

*Source:* American Nurses Association. (2011). *Workplace violence.* Retrieved May 5, 2012, from http://ana. nursingworld.org/workplaceviolence

the category for the offense and subsequent penalty—for example, Colorado (2005), Illinois (2003), Nevada (2003), and New Mexico (2006; ANA, 2011).

## Canada

The Canadian provinces, such as Quebec, British Columbia, and Ontario, have their respective occupational health and safety legislation. For example, Ontario workplaces that are subject to their Occupational Health and Safety Act, as of June 15, 2010, define workplace violence as

- the exercise of physical force by a person against a worker, in a workplace, that causes or could cause physical injury to the worker;

- an attempt to exercise physical force against a worker, in a workplace, that could cause physical injury to the worker; or

- a statement or behavior that it is reasonable for a worker to interpret as a threat to exercise physical force against the worker, in a workplace, that could cause physical injury to the worker.

Some of the types of violence that workers could experience in the workplace include hitting, pushing, physical assault, sexual assault, stalking, criminal harassment, robbery, or threats of violence (Ontario Ministry of Labor, 2010).

## Australia

In comparison, the various Australian state laws tend to avoid the term *violence* when describing these types of workplace behaviors, preferring the terms *inappropriate*

*behavior* or *bullying*. For example, the South Australian Occupational Health, Safety & Welfare Act, 1986 (SA) (SA OHS Act) has section 55A, which reads as follows:

*55A—Inappropriate behaviour towards an employee*

*(1) For the purposes of this section, bullying is behaviour*
  *(a) that is directed towards an employee or a group of employees, that is repeated and systematic, and that a reasonable person, having regard to all the circumstances, would expect to victimize, humiliate, undermine or threaten the employee or employees to whom the behaviour is directed; and*
  *(b) that creates a risk to health or safety.*

*(2) However, bullying does not include*
  *(a) reasonable action taken in a reasonable manner by an employer to transfer, demote, discipline, counsel, retrench or dismiss an employee; or*
  *(b) a decision by an employer, based on reasonable grounds, not to award or provide a promotion, transfer, or benefit in connection with an employee's employment; or*
  *(c) reasonable administrative action taken in a reasonable manner by an employer in connection with an employee's employment; or*
  *(d) reasonable action taken in a reasonable manner under an Act affecting an employee.* (Occupational Health, Safety & Welfare Act (South Australia) (1986))

This definition clearly shows the fundamental difference between what is considered bullying and other inappropriate behaviors and what the employers' fundamental legal rights are to manage their organization effectively.

Since these amendments were presented in 2005, further amendments have been made. In 2010, the South Australian Government introduced the *Occupational Health, Safety and Welfare (Industrial Manslaughter) Amendment Bill* 2010—as an amendment to the SA OHS Act. This Bill created an offence where an employer "breaches their duty of care, or knows or is recklessly indifferent or creates a substantial risk of serious harm to a person and that breach causes a person's death" (Franks, 2010).

---

## DISCUSSION POINT

Is legislation the best approach to addressing violence in nursing?

---

Since 2011, Australian states introduced, or are planning to introduce, laws to criminalize bullying. For example, following the suicide of a 19-year-old waitress who had been bullied at work and in response to public outcry, the Victorian (an Australian state) Parliament passed an act entitled *Crimes Amendment (Bullying) Act* 2011.

The Victorian government also expanded the definition of mental harm in Section 21A (8) into the Victorian *Crimes Act 1958* as follows:

*(8) In this section—*

*mental harm includes—*
  *(a) psychological harm; and*
  *(b) suicidal thoughts.*

South Australia is also reviewing legislation relating to various forms of bullying including abuse through social media websites such as *Facebook* and *Twitter* as well as by emails and text messages via mobile phones (Willis, 2011).

## NURSES LEGISLATION

In Australia, the Nurses Act gives the Australian Health Professional Registering Agency (AHPRA) legislative power for the registration of nurses, similarly to the California Nurses Practice Act. In general, a typical board of nurses' role is to endorse professional standards and ensure that the highest standards are achieved

and maintained. Disciplinary powers can range from requiring mediation and education to address the problem (e.g., managing aggressiveness) to requiring registration restrictions—in very severe cases, the power of deregistration.

Although each country has its own processes for undertaking disciplinary action against a nurse, generally if a criminal action arises from the behavior of a nurse, this action would initially override any other disciplinary action. For example, in Australia, if a nurse assaults a patient, he or she could be charged with the criminal offense of assault, occasioning actual bodily harm. If the nurse is found guilty, the appropriate disciplinary nursing body can take action by making a complaint to the respective Tribunal. The role of the Tribunal is primarily protective but it also has the role of "maintaining public confidence in the profession and maintain the reputation of the profession. Orders of the Tribunal may operate to have a general deterrent effect for other members of the profession" (*HCCC v. Gillies*, 2010, Nurses and Midwives Tribunal of New South Wales [NSWNMT] 7). In the case of *HCCC v. Gilles*, the case was heard before the NSWNMT.

The orders of the Tribunal may vary depending on the complaint, but one example may be for the name of the nurse to be removed from the register and not be entitled to apply for reregistration for a period of 1 or more years.

---

CONSIDER THIS   Is enforcing the law the best approach to addressing violence in nursing?

---

## INTERNATIONAL HUMAN RIGHTS

It is a basic human right to work in a safe and healthy workplace, no matter where the person works, the work performed, or the position held. For more than a decade, various researchers have stated that workplace violence is a human rights issue (e.g., Di Martino, 2002; Hockley, 2002). However, it is not an area that is well recognized as a process to be considered when addressing violence in nursing.

The Universal Declaration of Human Rights (UDHR) was adopted by the United Nations General Assembly on December 10, 1948. Article 23 of the UDHR does not explicitly refer to workplace violence. However, Article 23(1) of the UDHR refers to "everyone" having the right to "just and favorable conditions" at work.

There are two UN treaties, relevant to workplace violence—the International Covenant on Economic, Social and Cultural Rights (ICESCR) (http://www2.ohchr.org/english/law/cescr.htm) and the International Covenant on Civil and Political Rights (ICCPR) (http://www2.ohchr.org/english/law/ccpr.htm).

Article 7 of the ICESCR states,

> The State Parties to the ICESCR recognize the right of everyone to the enjoyment of just and favourable conditions of work which ensure, in particular: Safe and healthy working conditions (Office of the United Nations Commissioner for Human Rights).

### DISCUSSION POINT

Although the United States has not ratified the ICESCR, does it have any obligations as a signatory of this Covenant in respect to human rights into workplace violence?

The ICESCR opened for signature, ratification, and accession on December 19, 1966 and entered into force January 3, 1976. The United States and South Africa signed the treaty, but have not ratified it. Although it has been more than thirty years since the United States signed it in 1979, the Covenant is not fully binding until it is ratified by the U.S. Senate. Canada acceded to the treaty on May 19, 1966, and Australia ratified this treaty on December 10, 1975.

The Optional Protocol to the ICESCR, which opened for signature on December 10, 2008, is yet to be enforced by the United Nations. Until this occurs, an individual who has had their treaty rights violated cannot proceed any further than domestic law currently allows.

The preamble to the International Covenant on Civil and Political Rights (ICCPR) state that these rights derive from the inherent dignity of the human person. These rights include the right to dignity and respect in the workplace.

The ICCPR has an Optional Protocol (ICCPROP) where an individual can make a complaint to the United Nations Human Rights Commission (HRC) as long as the complainant has exhausted domestic remedies first.

## RESEARCH STUDY FUELS THE CONTROVERSY

### STUDYING GOVERNMENT INTERVENTION TO ADDRESS WORKPLACE VIOLENCE AND BULLYING IN THE WORKPLACE: AN INTERNATIONAL PERSPECTIVE

*Aim*: This study reviewed legislation and other legal approaches introduced to respond to violence and other inappropriate behavior in the workplace.

*Background*: In less than a decade, the states, territories, and provinces of countries such as Australia, Canada, and the United States have introduced new laws or made amendments to their current legislation in an attempt to address workplace violence and bullying.

*Data sources*: The literature, Austlii, and World Legal Information Institute databases were searched from 2001 to 2011 using keywords *occupational health and safety legislation, crimes act, workplace violence, bullying*, and *nurses act*. Professional nursing organizations and health professionals' registration bodies' websites were included.

*Findings*: This study is a work in progress. To date, the literature shows that there is not a uniform pattern in any of the countries studied. Each of their respective states, territories, and provinces has introduced different approaches at different times.

Hockley, C. (2011). *Studying government intervention to address workplace violence and bullying in the workplace: An international perspective.* Unpublished manuscript.

Research Study Fuels the Controversy refers to the research currently being undertaken by the author exploring government intervention as a strategy to address workplace violence and bullying from an international perspective. The work is still in progress but early data show the scope of potential victims has broadened in recent years. Also, there has been an increase in penalties to match the elevation of the category of offense.

## ORGANIZATIONAL APPROACH

Organizations have a legal and moral duty of care to their employees. Through OHS legislation, organizations can proactively address violence in nursing through policies and procedures, education, and training, as well as by having an organizational culture that does not condone this behavior. There continues to be an ever increasing focus on organizational culture in the research literature in exploring and developing strategies to addressing violence in nursing. The concept of trust/mistrust has been reported from many of these studies (St. Pierre & Holmes, 2010). For example, although many of these services are provided with the best of intentions, staff offered these services, particularly if they relate to nurse-to-nurse violence, are wary and concerned that the information will "get back to the workplace" (S. K. P., personal communication, 29 September 2011). When counseling is not successful, some complaints can be addressed through conciliation. If the perpetrator is a nurse, he or she may be referred to an appropriate statutory organization for disciplinary action.

## RESEARCH INTO WORKPLACE VIOLENCE

### International Recognition

One of the earliest and most significant international studies on workplace violence was written in 2002 by the International Labour Office (ILO), International Council of Nurses (ICN), World Health Organization (WHO), and Public Services International (PSI) and was entitled "Framework Guidelines for Addressing Workplace Violence in the Health Sector: Joint Program on Workplace Violence in the Health Sector" (ICESCR, 2002).

Since then, there has been a rapid growth into researching violence in the health care in general and nursing in particular. Successful international joint projects sponsoring conferences such as the biannual International Workplace Violence in Health Care Conference to be held in Canada in 2012 is one example. Nursing organizations such as the Honor Society of Nursing, Sigma Theta Tau International and the International Council of Nurses who sponsor such conferences, assist nurses in promoting their research.

### Under-Researched Issues

As was discussed throughout this chapter, studies have consistently shown that violence in nursing continues to be a major issue within the nursing profession. Studies show that there is a consistency about the prevalence rate of workplace violence. Recent studies show that there is a plethora of legal, ethical, organizational, and individual strategies in place to address this phenomenon. Yet there are still underresearched areas where the information is mainly ad hoc. Suicide and self-harm behaviors among nurses and other health professionals is one such topic. One of the difficulties in researching sensitive topics such as suicide is in part because it remains undetected until the event occurs. Then the problem would be to identify if there was a causal relationship between the death and workplace violence and bullying behavior.

Another important area that appears to be missing in the literature is nurses who have been accused of bullying. This may also be a difficult area to research because many perpetrators do not see themselves as bullies, only as "doing their job." In other words, why do nurses act inappropriately in the workplace? How can nurses become self-aware of their inappropriate behavior? What causes nurses to act in this way? What can be done to prevent this behavior?

One approach is to move the focus away from the individual and to consider that most people who bully have wide organizational support or tacit approval. Without that support, these people would not be tolerated as long as they are. Therefore, it is important to examine why this behavior is tolerated and what strategies should be implemented to counter organizational support.

## CONCLUSIONS

There has been a growing interest in violence in nursing as researchers interested in the health care sector have become increasingly aware that this phenomenon is not only an individual or organizational problem but also a public health and human rights issue. Although many changes have been made to minimize this unconscionable behavior in the health care culture and environment, much more work is needed. Current evidence continues to highlight the need for more research and a better understanding of the strategies required to address violence in nursing.

## FOR ADDITIONAL DISCUSSION

**1.** Why does violence in nursing exist?

**2.** How important is the language used to address violence in nursing?

**3.** What are the advantages and disadvantages of having general definitions of violence included in legislation?

**4.** Is it possible to experience violence in nursing without being professionally or personally harmed?

**5.** Are education and training programs the most cost-effective approach to addressing violence in nursing?

**6.** How can legislation or organizations assist third-party witnesses, such as family members, when they are harmed by the outcome of violence in nursing?

**7.** What role do professional nursing organizations play in addressing violence in nursing?

**8.** Should nurses take civil action against patients that attack them?

**9.** Is it paradoxical that those whose responsibility it is to provide care and promote an environment in which the human rights, values, customs, and spiritual beliefs of those in their care are respected should commit heinous crimes against those individuals?

**10.** Is zero tolerance of violence in nursing achievable?

## REFERENCES

Ali, N. J. (2010, October). *Violence against health professionals in Palestinian Hospitals: Prevalence and prevention*. Presented at the International Conference on Violence in the Health Sector—From Awareness to Sustainable Action, Amsterdam, Netherlands.

American Nurses Association. (2011). *Workplace violence*. Retrieved May 5, 2012, from http://ana.nursingworld.org/workplaceviolence

American Nurses Association. (2012). *Bullying in the workplace: Reversing a culture*. Retrieved May 7, 2012, from http://nursesbooks.org/Main-Menu/eBooks/General/Bullying-in-the-Workplace-Reversing-a-Culture.aspx

Back, C., Larsen, T., Acheson, L., Sagar, M., Lovick, M., Rahmat, A., & Thompson, J. (2010, October). *Social marketing campaign—A violence prevention pilot project*. Presented at the International Conference on Violence in the Health Sector—From Awareness to Sustainable Action, Amsterdam, Netherlands.

Boström, A.-M., Squires, J. E., Mitchell, A., Sales, A. E., & Estabrooks, C. A. (2012). Workplace aggression experienced by frontline staff in dementia care. *Journal of Clinical Nursing, 21*(9/10), 1453–1465.

Burgos, M., & Paravic, T. (2010, October). *The hospital's role in the violence of patients*. Presented at the International Conference on Violence in the Health Sector—From Awareness to Sustainable Action, Amsterdam, Netherlands.

Carmody, C. (2010). Not "part of the job." *American Nurse*. Retrieved April 28, 2011, from http://www.theamericannurse.org/?p=181

Crimes Act 1958 (Victoria). (1958). Retrieved May 7, 2012, from http://www.austlii.edu.au/au/legis/vic/consol_act/ca195882/

Crimes Amendment (Bullying) Act (Victoria). (2011). Retrieved May 7, 2012, from http://www.austlii.edu.au/cgi-bin/sinodisp/au/legis/vic/bill/cab2011266/cab2011266.html?stem=0&synonyms=0&query=bullying

Dal Pezzo, N. K., & Jett, K. T. (2010). Nursing faculty: A vulnerable population. *Journal of Nursing Education, 49*(3), 132–136.

Di Martino, V. (2002). *Workplace violence in the health sector—Country case studies* (Brazil, Bulgaria,

Lebanon, Portugal, South Africa, Thailand, and an additional Australian study). Geneva, Switzerland: Synthesis report, ILO, WHO, ICN, and PSI.

Franks, T. A. (Hon.). (2010). Occupational Health Safety and Welfare (Industrial Manslaughter) Amendment Bill 2010, (South Australia) Hansard, Legislative Council, Second Reading, p. 1196.

HCCC v. Gillies (2010). NSWNMT 7. Retrieved May 6, 2012, from http://www.austlii.edu.au/au/cases/nsw/NSWNMT/2010/7.html

Hershcovis, M. S. (2011). Incivility, social undermining, bullying . . . oh my!: A call to reconcile constructs within workplace aggression research. *Journal of Organizational Behavior, 32*(3), 499–519.

Hockley, C. (2002). *Silent hell: Workplace violence and bullying*. Norwood, Australia: Peacock.

Hutchinson, M., Vickers, M. H., Wilkes, L., & Jackson, D. (2010). A typology of bullying behaviours: The experiences of Australian nurses. *Journal of Clinical Nursing, 19*(15/16), 2319–2328.

International Covenant on Civil and Political Rights. (n.d.). Retrieved May 5, 2012, from http://www2.ohchr.org/english/law/ccpr.htm

International Covenant on Economic, Social and Cultural Rights (ICESCR) Retrieved 24 September, 2012 http://www2.ohchr.org/english/law/cescr.htm

International Labour Office (ILO), International Council of Nurses (ICN), World Health Organization (WHO), and Public Services International (PSI) (2002). Report: Framework Guidelines for Addressing Workplace Violence in the Health Sector: Joint Program on Workplace Violence in the Health Sector. Geneva, Switzerland.

Kirkhorn, L. E., Stehle Werner, J., & Heintz, M. (2010, October). *Review of evidence regarding workplace violence*. Presented at the International Conference on Violence in the Health Sector—From Awareness to Sustainable Action, Amsterdam, Netherlands.

Mabuhay. (2010). *Inmate kills Filipina prison nurse in California*. Retrieved May 7, 2012, from http://mabuhaycity.com/forums/pinoys-north-america/13081-inmate-kills-filipina-prison-nurse-california.html

Magnavita, N., & Heponiemi, T. (2011). Workplace violence against nursing students and nurses: An Italian experience. *Journal of Nursing Scholarship, 43*(2), 203–210.

Martin, C. J. H., & Martin, C. (2010). Bully for you: Harassment and bullying in the workplace. *British Journal of Midwifery, 18*(1), 25–31.

Motamedi, B. (2010, October). *Situation and contributing factors of workplace violence among nurses.*

Presented at the International Conference on Violence in the Health Sector—From Awareness to Sustainable Action, Amsterdam, Netherlands.

Ndou, N. D., & De Villiers, L. (2010, October). *South African professional experiences of caring for HIV/AIDS patients*. Presented at the International Conference on Violence in the Health Sector—From Awareness to Sustainable Action, Amsterdam, Netherlands.

Needham, I., Frauenfelder, F., Gianni, C., Dinkel, J., & Hatcher, R. (2010, October). *The psychological impact of aggression on a sample of psychiatric nurses in Germany and Switzerland*. Presented at the International Conference on Violence in the Health Sector—From Awareness to Sustainable Action, Amsterdam, Netherlands.

Occupational Health and Safety Act (Ontario). (1990). *R.S.O. 1990, CHAPTER O.1*. Retrieved May 7, 2012, from http://www.e-laws.gov.on.ca/html/statutes/english/elaws_statutes_90o01_e.htm

Occupational Health, Safety & Welfare Act (South Australia). (1986). Retrieved May 7, 2012, from http://www.austlii.edu.au/au/legis/sa/consol_act/ohsawa1986336/

Occupational Health, Safety and Welfare (Industrial Manslaughter) Amendment Bill. (2010). Retrieved May 7, 2012, from http://www.legislation.sa.gov.au/

Occupational Safety and Health Act of 1970 (United States). Retrieved May 7, 2012, from http://www.osha.gov

Occupational Safety and Health Administration. (2004). *Guidelines for preventing workplace violence for health care & social service workers*. Retrieved May 7, 2012, from http://www.osha.gov

Ontario Ministry of Labour. (2010). *Violence in the workplace*. Retrieved May 7, 2012, from http://www.labour.gov.on.ca/english/hs/pubs/wvps_guide/guide_4.php

Pich, J., Hazelton, M., Sundin, D., & Kable, A. (2011). Patient-related violence at triage: A qualitative descriptive study. *International Emergency Nursing, 19*(1), 12–19.

Roberts, S. (1983). Oppressed group behavior: Implications for nursing. *Advances in Nursing Science, 5*(4), 21–30.

Robertson, J. E. (2012). Can't we all just get along? A primer on student incivility in nursing education. *Nursing Education Perspectives, 33*(1), 21–26. Retrieved from http://www.highbeam.com/doc/1G1-280855787.html

Simons, S. R., Stark, R. B., & De Marco, R. F. (2011). A new, four-item instrument to measure workplace bullying. *Research in Nursing & Health, 34*(2), 132–140.

St. Pierre, I., & Holmes, D. (2010). *Broadening the understanding of intra/inter professional aggression: A nursing managers' perspective.* Presented at the International Conference on Violence in the Health Sector—From Awareness to Sustainable Action, Amsterdam, Netherlands.

U.S. Department of Labor. (2011). *40 OSHA QuickTakes 19(6). OSHA cites hospital for failing to protect staff from workplace violence.* Retrieved May 5, 2012, from http://www.osha.gov/as/opa/quicktakes/qt03152011.html

U.S. Department of Labor, Bureau of Labor Statistics. (2010). *Census of Fatal Occupational Injuries, 2009.* Retrieved May 5, 2012, from http://www.bls.gov/news.release/cfoi.t03.htm

U.S. Department of Labor, Occupational Safety and Health Administration. (2011). *Quick Takes.* Retrieved May 7, 2012, from http://www.osha.gov/as/opa/quicktakes/qt03152011.html

Walrafen, N., Brewer, M. K., & Mulvenon, C. (2012). Sadly caught up in the moment: An exploration of horizontal violence. *Nursing Economics, 30*(1), 6–12, 49.

Willis, D. (2011, April 26). Send bullies to jail. *Advertiser, South Australia.*

## BIBLIOGRAPHY

Aasland, M. S., Skogstad, A., Notelaers, G., Nielsen, M. B., & Einarsen, S. (2010). The prevalence of destructive leadership behaviour. *British Journal of Management, 21*(2), 438–452.

Bechtoldt, M. N., & Schmitt, K. D. (2010). It's not my fault, it's theirs: Explanatory style of bullying targets with unipolar depression and its susceptibility to short-term therapeutical modification. *Journal of Occupational and Organizational Psychology, 83*(2), 395–417.

Fitzgibbons, H. (2011). *Victoria to criminalise workplace bullying: Lateline television, Australian Broadcasting Corporation.* Retrieved May 5, 2012, from http://www.abc.net.au/lateline/content/2011/s3183259.htm

Hogh, A., Carneiro, I. G., Giver, H., & Rugulies, R. (2011). Are immigrants in the nursing industry at increased risk of bullying at work? A one-year follow-up study. *Scandinavian Journal of Psychology, 52*(1), 49–56.

Hospital's History of Violence Leads to OSHA Fine. (2010). Retrieved May 5, 2012, from http://ohsonline.com/articles/2010/07/20/hospitals-history-of-violence-leads-to-osha-fine.aspx

Hutchinson, M., Wilkes, L., Jackson, D., & Vickers, M. H. (2010). Integrating individual, work group and organizational factors: Testing a multidimensional model of bullying in the nursing workplace. *Journal of Nursing Management, 18*(2), 173–181.

Laschinger, H. K. S., & Grau, A. L. (2012). The influence of personal dispositional factors and organizational resources on workplace violence, burnout, and health outcomes in new graduate nurses: A cross-sectional study. International Journal of Nursing Studies, 49(3), 282–291.

Laschinger, H. K. S., Grau, A. L., Finegan, J., & Wilk, P. (2010). New graduate nurses' experiences of bullying and burnout in hospital settings. *Journal of Advanced Nursing, 66*(12), 2732–2742.

Lindy, C., & Schaefer, F. (2010). Negative workplace behaviours: An ethical dilemma for nurse managers. *Journal of Nursing Management, 18*(3), 285–292.

Matsunaga, M. (2011). Underlying circuits of social support for bullied victims: An appraisal-based perspective on supportive communication and postbullying adjustment. *Human Communication Research, 37*(2), 174–206.

National Institute for Occupational Safety and Health. (2011a). *Occupational violence, research on occupational violence and homicide.* Atlanta, GA: Centers for Disease Control and Prevention. Retrieved March 2, 2011, from http://www.cdc.gov/niosh/topics/violence/traumaviol_research.html#community

National Institute for Occupational Safety and Health. (2011b). *Safety and occupational health study section, survey of work-related assaults treated in hospital emergency departments.* Atlanta, GA: Centers for Disease Control and Prevention. Retrieved March 2, 2011, from http://www.cdc.gov/niosh/topics/violence/traumaviol_research.html#er

O'Donnell, S., MacIntosh, J., & Wuest, J. (2010). A theoretical understanding of sickness absence among women who have experienced workplace bullying. Qualitative Health Research, 20(4), 439–452.

# Chapter 14

# Technology in the Health Care Workplace

## Benefits, Limitations, and Challenges

Carol J. Huston

## ADDITIONAL RESOURCES

Visit thePoint for additional helpful resources

- eBook
- Journal Articles
- WebLinks

## CHAPTER OUTLINE

## LEARNING OBJECTIVES

*The learner will be able to:*

1. Describe emerging opportunities for robotic technology in health care, including surgery, diagnostics, and therapy, the provision of direct care, assistance with pharmaceutical applications/dispensing, and as couriers in supply chain automation.

2. Reflect on the degree to which technologically sophisticated, emotion-sensing, mental service robots will be able to replace professional nurse caregivers in the future.

3. Discuss how different types of biometric technology can be used to increase the likelihood that access

to health care information is both targeted and appropriate.

4. Identify current "smart object" applications in health care.

5. Detail how point-of-care bar coding is being implemented and potential benefits for its use.

6. Explore the effect of computerized physician/prescriber order entry on the reduction of medication errors and adverse drug events, as well as current barriers to widespread implementation of its use.

7. Provide examples of expanding electronic and wireless communication technologies that assist in personal organization, as well as data management.

8. Identify how electronic health records (EHRs), telehealth/telenursing, and point-of-care testing can be used to overcome geography-of-care issues.

9. Identify barriers to the widespread implementation of EHRs despite governmental encouragement to develop this technology.

10. Analyze how the Internet has changed the relationship between providers and their patients in terms of the power of information.

11. Recognize emerging roles for nurse informaticists (also known as clinical nurse informaticists).

12. Engage in futuristic thinking regarding how technology will further alter 21st-century health care and the roles of health care providers.

13. Examine his or her degree of "technophobia" and complete a personal assessment of technology skills deficits and strengths.

---

Technology is everywhere, and it is continually transforming health care, particularly nursing care. Indeed, both consumer and provider expectations of health care continue to be shaped by experiences with more technologically advanced enterprises. With advances in technology come new challenges, opportunities, and problems. Technology can cut costs, improve patient outcomes, streamline workflow, and improve information accessibility. It can also be costly, require ongoing training, and bring about new moral dilemmas. Determining what technology should be developed in an era of limited resources and how it should be used raises all kinds of issues. In addition, many questions exist as to how to educate health care providers about using new technology.

> CONSIDER THIS  Technology is like a rolling freight train—it is very difficult to stop it and even more dangerous to get in the way.

This chapter addresses many of the technological advances being used in 21st-century health care, including robotics, computers, and wireless communication, to improve the utilization of human resources. Biometrics, point-of-care testing, and computerized data access/entry are presented as technological approaches for improving documentation and knowledge acquisition. Electronic health records (EHRs) and telehealth are recognized as strategies for overcoming geography-of-care issues, and computerized provider order entry and clinical decision support (CDS) systems are discussed both as strategies for improving existing care processes and as a means for high-quality clinical decision making. Finally, the Internet's effect on both patients and providers is explored, including the concept of "expert patient" and the resultant need for nurses trained in consumer health informatics.

## NEW TECHNOLOGIES IN HEALTH CARE

Most baby boomers remember the TV show *Star Trek*, in which the spaceship crew and aliens dematerialized into tiny atoms for transport between locations and sensors were waved over patients in the sick bay, rendering an immediate diagnosis and treatment. Although technology has not yet fully reached this point, much of the futuristic thinking envisioned on *Star Trek* may someday become a reality in health care.

### Biomechatronics

*Biomechatronics*, which creates machines which replicate or mimic how the body works, will continue to increase in prominence in the future. This interdisciplinary field encompasses biology, neurosciences, mechanics, electronics, and robotics to create devices that interact with human muscle, skeleton, and nervous systems to establish or restore human motor or nervous system function. For example, Global Architects Guide (GlobalArchitectsGuide.com, 2011) suggests biomechatronic devices can accomplish all the steps needed to lift a foot to walk with biosensors being inserted to detect what the user wants to do (his or her intentions) in terms of motion. Future Biomechatronics applications are innumerable and will likely include such things as functional stimulation of paralyzed limbs, pancreas pacemakers for diabetics, wireless active capsule endoscopy, and mentally controlled electronic muscle stimulators for patients with brain injuries.

> ### DISCUSSION POINT
>
> Do you believe that technology will someday eliminate "disease" as we know it today? If so, what are the implications in terms of life span and the prevalence of chronic disease?

# Robots and Health Care

## Robots in Surgery

The use of robotics in health care is no longer science fiction. The first robotic-assisted surgery dates back to the mid-1980s when a robot was used to place a needle for brain biopsy using computed tomographic guidance. Robotic-assisted heart bypass surgery followed in the late 1990s, and the first unmanned robotic surgery took place in May 2006 in Italy.

Several years later, engineers at Duke University, using novel three-dimensional technology and a basic artificial intelligence program, guided the actions of a rudimentary tabletop robot to perform surgery (McNicol, 2008). The engineers suggested this technology would eventually allow robots to perform surgery on patients in dangerous situations or in remote locations, such as on the battlefield or in space, with minimal or no human guidance.

On a more immediate-level, technology such as this immediately began making certain contemporary medical procedures safer for patients. For example, robots already perform cataract surgery. With Femto-second laser, approved by the Food and Drug Authority (USA) in December 2010, a cone is placed on the eye and the laser light is fired at the target in a pre-determined manner. Since this is computer controlled, accuracy can be achieved with almost utmost precision (Bhalla, 2011).

Surgical robotics are not, however, cheap. Saver (2010) notes that getting into robotics requires a large capital investment in addition to ongoing costs. "A robot costs $1.7 million to $2.2 million, with maintenance costs of about $150,000 annually and additional disposable equipment costs of $1,500 to $2,000 per procedure" (p. 13). In addition, special instrumentation is needed to do consecutive cases at a start-up of typically close to US$200,000.

Questions have also been raised about whether need is driving surgical robotics or whether the introduction of such robotics is creating a need where one did not exist before. For example, a new study shows that after Wisconsin hospitals acquired robotic surgery technology, the number of prostate removals they performed doubled within 3 months. In contrast, the number of prostate surgeries stayed the same at hospitals that did not purchase the new US$2-million technology ("Do Robots Drive Up," 2011). One must question whether surgeons at hospitals with robots are recommending surgery for men with prostate cancer because the outcomes (potential reductions in incontinence and impotence) are better or whether the new technology is simply more exciting than alternative treatments like radiation or "watchful waiting" ("Do Robots Drive Up," 2011).

## Robots in Diagnostics and Therapy

In addition, robots are increasingly being used in diagnostics and therapy because their accuracy and steadiness often exceed those of human caregivers (Brumson, 2008). For example, Brumson discussed the use of robotics with linear accelerators in treating tumors: "Linear accelerators are small devices mounted on the end of the robot to direct a thin beam of radiation into a tumor. Using the robot, doctors can precisely place high dose radiation inside a tumor" (para. 9).

Similarly, although still in prototype development, robotic technology in cardiology is being developed that will allow a snake-like device to be inserted through a small incision below the sternum, which can then adhere to a patient's beating heart. A robot is able to access areas of the heart that normally require the patient's lungs to be deflated. "The hope for this type of robot is to inject medication, attach pacemakers or target specific points for cauterization as a treatment for cardiac arrhythmia into areas of the heart that are difficult to access" (Brumson, 2008, para. 10).

## Robots as Direct Care Providers

Robots are also being developed to provide direct patient care. Indeed, Greenemeier (2011) suggests that this is a pivotal time for the development of the underlying technology that will enable safe and reliable automated elder care, not to mention other services that robots are expected to perform in the coming decade. In fact, robots are already being used as caregivers, particularly for the elderly. This is especially true in Japan, known as the "Robot Kingdom," as a result of a burgeoning elderly population and a low birth rate, which has resulted in a severe shortage of caregivers.

According to Takanori Shibata, a senior research scientist at the National Institute of Advanced Industrial Science and Technology, "Robot caregivers can be divided into *physical service* and *mental service* robots. The former are designed to help with tasks such as washing or carrying elderly people, although given the limitations of current technology, not to mention safety concerns, they are still quite a long way from commercialization" (McNicol, 2008, para. 5).

Thanks, however, to a standardized personal robot platform introduced in 2010, known as *PR2*, roboticists are making rapid strides in creating robots that can provide a much high level of assistance than ever before (Greenemeier, 2011). The PR2 *includes a mobile base, two arms for manipulation, a suite of sensors and two computers, each with eight processing cores, 24 gigabytes of RAM and two terabytes of hard-disk space. The out-of-the-box robot, which costs US$400,000, also features an operating system that handles the robot's computation and hardware manipulation functions.* (Greenemeier, 2011, para. 2)

Mental service robots, however, are being commercially produced, and have been in use for some time. One of the best known is *Paro*, an interactive robot designed by Shibata himself to help people relax and reduce their stress levels. The sophisticated robot, which is the 8th generation of a design that has been in use since 2003, is shaped like a baby harp seal, can remember its name, and can change its behavior depending on how it is treated. It has been used extensively in homes for elderly people and with autistic children. In 2011, Paro was used to provide comfort and reduce stress in nursing home residents located near the tsunami-crippled nuclear power plant leaking radiation in Fukushima (Kyung-hoon, 2011). Residents named two of the Paro robots "Love" and "Peace" and treated them more like real animals than robots.

Guizzo (2009) notes that short-term experiments in Japan and the United States have shown that Paro can positively impact the mental health of some elderly people and long-term studies are under way in Europe. Paro has become commercially available in the United States at a cost of about US$6,000 each (Guizzo, 2009).

Many consumers and health care providers have expressed concern, however, about the lack of emotion in robots, suggesting that this is the element of human caregivers that can never be replaced. New technology developed by scientists at Meiji University in Tokyo, however, has resulted in a kind of robot intelligence known as *kansei*, which means "emotion or feeling" (McNicol, 2008). *Kansei* robots use vision systems to monitor human expressions, gestures, and body language and voice sensors to pick up on intonation and individual words and sentences. In addition, *kansei* robots sense human emotion through wearable sensors that monitor pulse rate and perspiration.

When the *kansei* robot hears a word, it searches through its database of more than 500,000 words to find common associations and matches an appropriate emotional expression on its polyurethane face. For example, the word *sushi* elicits a smile, whereas the word *war* brings about a frown.

### Robots as Couriers

Service robots are also being used as robot couriers for mundane, repetitive jobs such as supply chain automation. Aethon Inc. has produced mobile robots called *TUGs* that can locate assets as well as transport them, including medications, supplies, equipment, and other goods that rely on scarce, valuable human resources for pushing carts (Ben Franklin Technology Partners, 2011). Indeed, Aethon suggests that most hospitals can save the work done by 2.4 employees over 21 shifts for every TUG in use and that the average return on investment is better than 30%. The TUG can haul up to 500 pounds and transport a variety of hospital carts. "The hospital worker simply attaches a delivery to the cart, presses a button to select the destination and pushes the "go" button. The TUG has been programmed to "remember" and navigate the layout of the facility. It automatically travels to its destination, announces that the delivery has arrived and returns to its home base, where it waits on its charger for the next delivery" (Ben Franklin Technology Partners, 2011, para. 5).

### Biometrics

The health care environment continues to be rapidly transformed by new technology as a result of the need to provide confidentiality and security of patient data and to comply with the Health Insurance Portability and Accountability Act of 1996 (HIPAA). HIPAA calls for a tiered approach to data access in which staff members have access only to the information that they need to know to perform their jobs, and so new technology to assure that access is both targeted and appropriate is being developed.

One such new technology is *biometrics*, the science of identifying people through physical characteristics such as fingerprints, handprints, retinal scans, voice recognition, facial structure, and dynamic signatures. Fingerprint biometrics is still the most common type of biometrics in health care, primarily because of its ease of use, small size, and affordable price. Detection of facial geometry, however, is also beginning to make inroads into health care as a biometric measure. Facial geometry

---

**DISCUSSION POINT**

To what degree can nurses be replaced by technology? Can therapeutic "caring" be demonstrated by robots? Do you feel that you could have a therapeutic conversation with a robot?

captures facial landmarks such as approach angles, eyebrow and mouth contours, skin texture analysis, and hairstyles which can then be confirmed later by facial recognition software.

Palm vein patterns are also now being used as biometric identifiers. Using near infrared light to capture each individual's unique palm vein pattern bypasses the need to have quality fingerprints. After implementing palm vein reader technology at ValleyCare Health System in Pleasanton, California, outpatient lab wait times of 7 minutes or less increased from 75% to 92% within 2 years ("Natural Next Step," 2011). The cost to implement palm veining biometrics ranges from US$100,000 to US$150,000 for a 200-bed hospital and training is typically a 30-minute session ("Natural Next Step," 2011).

## Smart Cards and Smart Objects

Health care organizations are also increasingly integrating biometrics with *smart cards* to ensure that an individual presenting a secure ID credential really has the right to use that credential. Smart cards are credit card–sized devices with a chip, stored memory, and an operating system that record a patient's entire clinical history. Although still in the early development stage, the integration of biometrics with smart cards eliminates the need for multiple identification requirements.

*Smart objects* are everyday objects injected with easy-to-use software that give devices some degree of intelligence. For example, "smart hospital rooms" typically include computer screens that pull up patient records, display vital signs, medications, and other personal information, and identify health professionals who enter a patient's room (Silvey, 2011). In addition, the computer system can remind patients to ask for help in getting out of bed if they are at risk for falls and focuses a spotlight on the hand sanitizer dispenser when people enter or leave, reminding them to wash their hands.

Hatler (2008) described the use of "smart beds" at St. Joseph's Hospital and Medical Center in Phoenix. The smart bed offers "continuous, noncontact, noninvasive, real time monitoring of heart and respiratory rate and potential early detection of bed exit" (p. 21). The smart bed actually consists of two components: a passive sensor array embedded in a coverlet that zips over the existing matter and a bedside unit: "The bedside unit accommodates digital signal processing algorithms used to calculate heart and respiratory rates and displays the data" (Hatler, 2008, p. 21).

Preliminary outcomes from the smart bed use at St. Joseph's Hospital and Medical Center suggest that smart bed use did not result in lower fall rates on the unit; however, when fall rates were compared with those of other patients receiving care in the unit, the fall rate did show a significant downward trend. Hospital length of stay and costs were also not significantly affected by use of the vigilance system. Hatler (2008) reported, however, that there were a significantly smaller number of emergent returns to the intensive care unit, declining from 11% to 1% during the study period. This was attributed to the enhanced ability of the smart bed to detect early changes in patients' conditions.

In addition, hospitals are increasingly turning to so called *smart pumps* for intravenous (IV) therapy infusions. These smart pumps have safety software inside an advanced infusion therapy system that prevents IV medication errors by setting minimum and maximum dose limits, as well as preset limits that cannot be overridden at a clinician's discretion.

> **CONSIDER THIS**   Smart pumps cannot outsmart the provider who decides to override them.

## Point-of-Care Testing

Point-of-care testing (POCT), which has evolved into a multibillion-dollar industry, is another technological advance that is improving bedside care and promoting more positive outcomes, as a result of more timely decision making and treatment. The College of American Pathologists (2012) defines POCT as testing designed to be used at or near the site where the patient is located, that does not require permanent dedicated space, and that is performed outside of the physical facilities of the clinical laboratories. Two primary types of POCT instruments exist: small bench-top analyzers (e.g., blood gas and electrolyte systems) and handheld, single-use devices (such as urine albumin, blood glucose, and coagulation tests).

In POCT, caregivers gather and test specimens near the patient or at the bedside using handheld analyzers, pulse oximeters, and blood glucose monitoring systems. Then, by networking via the Internet and downloading results to a central clinical lab, manual documentation of test results can be eliminated. POCT also works for consumer use in the home. Patients can precisely monitor their laboratory values, submit them electronically to the lab, and then have results in minutes. POCT represents only a small portion of clinical laboratories' total testing volume, however, and evaluation challenges exist for all POCT programs in terms of accuracy, ease of use, quality control, and accurate data management. Indeed, delivering diagnostic tests at the bedside may be prone to errors as a result of failure to follow procedures, inappropriate documentation, improper patient identification, and failure to perform required quality control tests. More pilot programs are needed to evaluate the use of POCT.

## Medication Administration: Bar Coding

Bar coding has been developed to help caregivers ensure the right medication, in the right dose, is given to the right patient at the right time and by the right route (the *five rights*). Bar coding works by requiring the nurse to match, with a handheld scanner, his or her name tag, the bar code on the patient's identification band, and the medication to be given. When one of the five "rights" does not match, an alert is issued or the medication will not be dispensed from its storage system.

Goldstein (2008) reported that about one third of the nation's hospitals currently have a bar-code medication-dispensing system, but most, if not all, hospitals are expected to install such a system within a few years. The cost to implement such a system is hundreds of thousands of dollars, so the cost may be prohibitive for smaller rural hospitals.

---

### DISCUSSION POINT

Given that rural hospitals often cannot afford the expensive technological innovations that larger hospitals can, will this limitation result in a two-tiered system of health care quality?

---

In addition, implementation of point-of-care bar coding is not without problems. One study by the *Journal of the American Medical Informatics Association* found that nurses often develop workarounds that undermine bar coding's safeguards. For example, if a nurse needed to go to another unit or floor to pick up a drug for several patients, he or she might choose to just scan all the patients' barcodes to pick up the doses, even though these scans would be done far from the patients' bedsides (Goldstein, 2008). In fact, research by Koppell found that "nurses overrode patient ID scans 4.2 percent of the time, often

because bar codes were unreadable for reasons ranging from the child who chewed on hers to the patient with dementia who tore his off to the ones smudged and soggy from blood, urine or feces" (Goldstein, 2008, para. 20). In addition, caregivers encountered numerous other obstacles, including wireless dead spots, dead batteries in handheld scanners or on the computer, and an inability to take the handheld scanner into rooms where contagious diseases are an issue.

Nurses also frequently disable, silence, or ignore alarms due to what is known as "alarm fatigue." Because alarms are such a normal part of the equipment on many critical care units, there is great risk that nurses will become desensitized to the sound of these alarms. When this happens, the risk of harm to patients clearly increases.

Conversely, Browne and Cook (2011) warn that nurses may have inappropriate levels of trust in the technological equipment they use, leading to inadequate monitoring and potentially serious consequences to patients. Browne and Cook conclude that further research is needed to identify direct evidence of this complacency and its consequences (see Research Study Fuels the Controversy 14.1).

## Computerized Physician/Provider Order Entry

Computerized physician/provider order entry (CPOE) is also a rapidly growing technology. Part of this growth has occurred as a result of its designation as one of the three key patient safety initiatives by the Leapfrog Group, a conglomeration of non–health care *Fortune 500* company leaders committed to modernizing the current healthcare system. In addition, the Institute of Medicine study *To Err Is Human* recommended the use of CPOE to address medical errors.

CPOE is a clinical software application designed specifically for providers to write patient orders electronically rather than on paper. With CPOE, providers produce clearly typed orders, reducing medication errors based on inaccurate transcription.

CPOE also gives providers vital clinical decision support (CDS) via access to information tools that support a health care provider in decisions related to diagnosis, therapy, and care planning of individual patients. For example, physicians might access evidence-based medicine databases electronically for CDS when writing medication orders. If the provider has ordered a test or treatment that is contraindicated for a particular patient or condition, the CDS will inform that provider of the potential danger at the time the order is entered.

## RESEARCH STUDY FUELS THE CONTROVERSY 14.1

### TECHNOLOGY AND COMPLACENCY

Research from other occupations, such as airline pilots, suggests that experienced operators of highly reliable automation may display inappropriately high levels of trust in the automation, and this can lead to inadequate monitoring of the equipment by the operator. Inadequate monitoring means that the operator may fail to notice that the equipment is not functioning correctly which may have serious consequences.

Browne, M., & Cook, P. (2011). Inappropriate trust in technology: Implications for critical care nurses. *Nursing in Critical Care, 16*(2), 92–98.

### STUDY FINDINGS

This literature review of multiple databases including Academic Search Premier, CINAHL, Pubmed, and Science Direct suggested there is significant potential for critical care nurses to display complacency, defined as a mismatch between the trust that an operator has in a piece of equipment and its actual trustworthiness. If nurses fail to recognize the potential and actual consequences of inappropriate trust, patients may suffer harm as a result. The researchers concluded there is an urgent need for more research to identify the extent of technology complacency in nursing and its consequences. There is also a need for these issues to be highlighted in the training of intensive care nurses, and there are implications for intensive care unit practice protocols and equipment manufacturers.

---

### DISCUSSION POINT

Should health care organizations require prescribing providers to write their orders electronically, or should this be left to the discretion of the provider?

---

Translating CPOE into action has not been without challenges. Although many health care organizations see the value in CPOE technology, they do not consider it an immediate necessity. As of 2009, only 17% of hospitals in the United States had functional CPOE systems in place (Maslove, Rizk, & Lowe, 2011). In some cases, new error types have arisen with the use of CPOE and intensive care unit workflow and staff relationships have been affected by CPOE, often in unanticipated ways such as changes in workflow and staff roles (Maslove et al., 2011).

There may also be cultural obstacles to CPOE; for example, a physician might prefer to write orders by hand instead of using a computer. This may be due to the normal resistance experienced with almost any change or it may reflect a reluctance to take on the increased cognitive workload associated with the use of CPOE. Either way, the design of CPOE software has a strong impact on user acceptance (Maslove et al., 2011).

In addition, the requirements to fully meet Leapfrog's CPOE standards are stringent (Box 14.1). Still, institutional and clinician adoption of CPOE is crucial to helping caregivers reduce medical errors and enhance patient safety, and health care institutions must commit the necessary human and financial resources to make this technological innovation a reality.

## Clinical Decision Support

*Clinical decision support* is defined broadly as "a process for enhancing health-related decisions and actions with pertinent, organized clinical knowledge and patient information to improve health and healthcare delivery" (Healthcare Information and Management Systems Society, 2011, para. 2). Like CPOE, CDS will likely be commonplace by 2020, giving providers the promise for access at the point of care to cutting-edge research, best practices, and decision-making support to improve patient care.

## Electronic and Wireless Communication

Electronic communication technologies are also expanding at an exponential pace. Computers are increasingly a part of interdisciplinary team communication and care documentation in acute care hospitals,

**BOX 14.1 REQUIREMENTS FOR FULL COMPLIANCE WITH LEAPFROG'S CPOE STANDARD**

1. Hospitals must ensure that physicians enter at least 75% of medication orders via a computer system with prescribing error-prevention software.

2. Hospitals must demonstrate that their inpatient CPOE system can alert physicians to at least 50% of common, serious prescribing errors, using Leapfrog's CPOE Evaluation Tool.

*Source:* Leapfrog. (2011). *Leapfrog fact sheet: Computerized physician order entry.* Retrieved May 8, 2012, from http://www.leapfroggroup.org/media/file/FactSheet_CPOE.pdf

although futurists predict that computers in the not-too-distant future will essentially be invisible, replaced with smart objects.

Computerized charting is the norm, with more institutions moving toward the use of tablet personal computers—flat-panel laptops that use a stylus pen or touch-screen technology. In addition, personal digital assistants (PDAs), which are mobile handheld devices, give users access to text-based information and the latest computer and cellular applications. With institution-wide documentation systems, everyone uses the same documentation software, and the information is transferred to and retrieved from a central server via "hot synching" (putting the PDA into a cradle or connecting it via cable to the central server). In addition, the PDA can serve as a reference library, especially for drug information, and as a calculator for computing drug doses.

PDAs, however, are not cheap, typically costing between US$100 for a barebones glorified calculator and up to US$800 for a device that uses Microsoft or Palm operating systems. In addition, PDAs can be lost or stolen, posing concerns about patient confidentiality. Finally, some nurses feel uncomfortable using such technology in front of patients and some just feel uncomfortable with the technology itself. However, the quality and number of PDA applications continue to grow, as does their use.

The use of wireless local area networking (WLAN) is also growing rapidly. WLAN uses a spread-spectrum radio frequency to link two or more computers or devices without using wires. This allows caregivers to access, update, and transmit critical patient and treatment information despite moving between or being located at multiple sites of care. The area of outreach in the network is called the *basic service set.*

Similarly, Bluetooth technology creates a small wireless network (called a *piconet*) between two pieces of hardware through short-range radio signals. This allows devices such as keyboards to link with personal computers and headsets to link with cell phones.

## Electronic Health Records (EHRs)

Even health records have changed as a result of technology. The EHR is a digital record of a patient's health history that may be made up of records from many locations and/or sources, such as hospitals, providers, clinics, and public health agencies. For example, an EHR might include immunization status, allergies, patient demographics, lab test and radiology results, advanced directives, current medications taken, and current health care appointments. The EHR is available 24 hours a day, 7 days a week and has built-in safeguards to assure patient health information confidentiality and security.

In May 2003, the U.S. Department of Health and Human Services asked the Institute of Medicine (IOM) to provide guidance on the key care delivery–related capabilities of an EHR system. According to Bordowitz (2008), the IOM report stated that an EHR system has eight core functions (Box 14.2) and should include the following:

■ Longitudinal collection of electronic health information for and about people, in which health information is defined as information pertaining to the health of an individual or health care provided to an individual

■ Immediate electronic access to person- and population-level information by authorized users only

■ Provision of knowledge and decision support that enhance the quality, safety, and efficiency of patient care

■ Support of efficient processes for health care delivery. Critical building blocks of an EHR system are the EHRs maintained by providers (e.g., hospitals, nursing homes, ambulatory settings) and by individuals (also called personal health records).

In addition, in January 2004, President George W. Bush set a goal that most Americans would have an EHR by 2014. This goal was endorsed by President Barack

## BOX 14.2   EIGHT CORE FUNCTIONS OF AN EHR

1. Health information and data
2. Results management
3. Order entry/management
4. Decision support
5. Electronic communication and connectivity
6. Patient support
7. Administrative processes
8. Reporting and population health management

*Source:* Bordowitz, R. (2008). Electronic health records: A primer. *Laboratory Medicine, 39*(5), 301–307.

operations; however, further research is needed to examine the benefits and the drawbacks of using EHRs.

Physicians have been especially slow to adopt EHRs. A study by DesRoches et al. (2008) of 2,758 physicians revealed that only 4% had an extensive, fully functional electronic records system as part of their practice and only 13% reported having a basic system. Primary care physicians and those practicing in large groups, in hospitals or medical centers, and in the Western region of the United States were more likely to use EHRs. Financial barriers were viewed as the most significant variable affecting the adoption of EHRs.

In addition, Bordowitz (2008) noted that some studies have suggested that the use of an EHR may interfere with the patient–provider encounter, preventing quality information from being attained. Patients felt less satisfied when providers were using a computer in the examination room because the visits typically took longer and seemed less personal to them.

CONSIDER THIS   The electronic record is not a single panacea for solving problems related to confidentiality or continuity of medical data access.

Obama and supported financially with US$30 billion in stimulus funds to support hospital implementation over the next several years. As a result, this optional improvement has become a near-mandatory initiative (Haughom, Kriz, & McMillan, 2011).

Similarly, Canada Health Infoway (2011), an independent not-for-profit corporation, is working hard to foster and accelerate the development and adoption of EHR systems with compatible standards and communications technologies throughout Canada. Indeed, most developed countries are actively moving toward the establishment and implementation of EHRs. Australia has proposed a strategy known as Health Connect to facilitate the adoption of common standards by all e-health systems in the Australian national, state, and territorial governments. The National Health Service in the United Kingdom began an EHR system in 2005 and has developed a national system to transfer records directly and securely from one general practitioner (GP) to another.

It is not easy, however, to make such systemwide changes. Cost, debates about ownership of data, and communication across computer systems pose relentless challenges. Indeed, a review of the literature suggests limited success regarding the use of EHR. Perhaps this simply reflects normal resistance to change, given the number of behavioral and procedural changes required to rework such a fundamental aspect of normal

## Other Electronic Data Repositories and Intranets

Many electronic data repositories have been created within organizations as a way of cataloging internal reference materials, such as policy and procedure manuals. This increases the likelihood that staff will be able to find such resources when they need them and that they are as up to date as possible. In such a system, references are typically converted to the portable document format and launched electronically via an Intranet. *Intranets* are internal networks (not normally accessible from the Internet) that allow workers and departments to share files, use websites, and collaborate.

### IS TECHNOLOGY WORTH THE COSTS?

Most health care economists would agree that the rapid introduction of new technologies is a significant factor in high health care costs. However, it also has the potential to significantly improve the quality of health care. In a study of 98 Florida hospitals, Menachemi, Chukmaitov, Saunders, and Brooks (2008) found that hospitals that had adopted a greater number of IT applications were significantly more likely to have desirable quality outcomes on seven inpatient quality indicators.

Not all critics agree, however. Some argue that technology not only is expensive (both initially and in terms of maintenance and technical support) but also needs constant upgrades, and the education needed to truly be competent in the use of all these technologies is never ending.

In addition, not all nurses embrace technology. This may simply represent a resistance to change, or it might be that nursing input has not historically been used in technology acquisition decisions. In addition, it is possible that many health care providers, including nurses, have received inadequate orientation to the technology in place. One must also remember that not all technology is worth the cost. Cost must always be weighed against possible benefits of the technology, effect on health care provider satisfaction, and projected utilization patterns.

## TELEHEALTH AND TELENURSING

Given declining insurer reimbursement, the current nursing shortage, and an increasing shift in care to outpatient settings, home care agencies are increasingly exploring technology-aided options that allow them to avoid the traditional 1:1 nurse–patient ratio with face-to-face contact. *Telehealth*, also called remote monitoring technology, telemedicine, telenursing, telecare, telehomecare, telemanagement, e-health, and telephone care, allows nurses to care for patients over a distance, using a combination of telecommunication and multimedia technologies.

> CONSIDER THIS   If the benefits of telemedicine are to be fully realized, providers need to be able to merge telehealth data with information from other clinical systems. EHRs may be one means of accomplishing this goal.

For nurses, telehealth has meant greater ubiquity—nurses can now practice across geographic boundaries and be directly involved in patient care, even when they are not directly on site with patients. For patients, telehealth has meant increased flexibility and, often, more personalized care. For health care providers, telehealth has typically resulted in improved quality of care and lower costs. It has also provided new strategies for dealing with the health disparities created by geographic location, age, and homebound status.

> CONSIDER THIS   Telehealth provides greater opportunities for nurse–patient encounters, particularly for homebound, geographically isolated individuals.

## How Telehealth Works

In more advanced telehealth, providers interact with patients through computer stations hooked up in the patient's home that typically include a video monitor, a moveable color video camera, a speakerphone and microphone, and one or more medical peripherals for patient self-monitoring, such as blood pressure and pulse meter, stethoscope, pulse oximeter, scale, and glucometer. Patients record their heart rates, blood pressures, blood glucose levels, and other readings periodically and then transmit these data to a provider with a computer station similar to theirs. This gives the provider a real-time picture of the patient's health status. In less sophisticated telehealth programs, assessment, intervention, and evaluation occur by fax, e-mail message, or simply by telephone.

> ### DISCUSSION POINT
>
> What, if anything, is "lost" when there is no face-to-face meeting between the nurse and the patient? Can technology overcome this loss? What does technology offer that face-to-face visits do not?

## Telehealth and Telenursing Outcomes

Because telehealth and telenursing are relatively new, performance indicators and appropriate measures of quality are still being determined. More research is also needed to determine what telehealth system—or mix of telehealth and in-home visits—adds the most value both clinically and financially.

Desired patient outcomes for telehealth nursing are a little better defined. They include patient satisfaction, increased involvement in health care decision making, reduced travel time and expense, increased time with health care providers, improved health care, improved quality of life, and increased medical record data for clinical decision making.

> CONSIDER THIS   The practice of telehealth nursing
> has not yet been standardized, but efforts are occurring to
> develop standardized tools to assess outcomes.

Despite a need to continue to further clarify what constitutes quality in telenursing, researchers are examining outcomes. The literature reflects numerous studies supporting the use of home telehealth in caring for multiple medical issues including diabetes, foot ulcers, lung transplants mental health, high-risk pregnancy monitoring, heart failure, other cardiac conditions, and smoking cessation.

## THE INTERNET AND HEALTH CARE

## The Exponential Growth of the Internet

The growth of the Internet as an information source for all types of information, including health, has been exponential, and will continue to be so. Gobry (2011) points out that the Internet as a sector now produces about 3% of the U.S. gross domestic product, more than agriculture or energy, representing more than 20% of the economic growth in the country in the past 5 years.

## The Internet and Expert Patients

Historically, health care providers were recognized as the keepers of medical information. This allowed them to be the primary health care decision maker, often relegating patients to a somewhat passive and dependent role. The Internet has, however, changed these dynamics because it has expanded the power and control of health information from providers alone to patients themselves. Indeed, the Internet, which is growing faster than any other medium in the world, has great potential to improve Americans' health by enhancing communications and improving access to information for care providers, patients, health plan administrators, public health officials, biomedical researchers, and other health professionals.

Indeed, thousands of health information websites currently exist for consumers to explore in attempting to answer their health-related questions and more are launched daily. The end result is that patients have electronic access to medical information on virtually any topic, any time. This suggests that many consumers have at least the opportunity to be better informed about their health care problems and needs than in the past. In fact, this increased opportunity for consumers

to access information has resulted in the creation of what is known as the *expert patient*—a patient who has the confidence, skills, information, and knowledge to participate in his or her health care.

Theoretically, expert patients are better informed and thus better able to be active participants in decision making. Although most providers appreciate well-informed patients who have demonstrated the initiative to learn more about their health care needs and problems, there are concerns regarding the accuracy and currency of information patients find on the Internet. In addition, many patients do not fully understand the information that is available to them, even when it is accurate. Some providers are concerned that patients will inappropriately self-diagnose, leading them to seek inappropriate treatment or no treatment at all. A smaller number of providers simply do not want to share decision-making power with patients. Students in health care programs must be taught to not only recognize patient expertise but also to actively encourage and support it.

> **DISCUSSION POINT**
>
> Empowering patients and involving them in their health care decision making is a socially encouraged value in health care today. Do you believe that most providers value and appreciate having increased numbers of "expert patients"?

In addition, little research has been done to validate the currency or accuracy of the information on health care Internet sites. Krotoski (2011), citing a recent study of more than 12,000 people across 12 different countries, noted that more people than ever are using the Web to find out more about an ailment before or instead of visiting the doctor. Alarmingly, only a quarter of the people surveyed checked the reliability of health information they found online by looking at the credibility of the source. In addition, Krotoski suggests that "a typical medical consultation follows this trajectory: 1) you discover a growth, 2) do a Google search, 3) believe the first result that confirms your expectations" (para. 6). Krotoski concludes then that while the wealth of health information online has contributed to a more informed public, the expertise of the professional should not be undermined by the leveling power of the Web.

Clearly, patients need to become experts at retrieving health care information and deciphering it to better empower themselves in health care decision making.

## Nursing Informatics

Handling access to virtually unlimited information via the Internet has been a challenging transition for both patients and providers. As a result, new nursing specialties have emerged, including *nursing informatics* (NI). NI is a specialty that integrates nursing science, computer science, and information science to manage and communicate data, information, and knowledge in nursing practice. *Nurse informaticists*, also known as *clinical nurse informaticists*, are often involved in the implementation of information technology initiatives such as the EHR.

The competency of the informatics nurse is critical. Such competency has not, however, historically been guaranteed by advanced education. Before the American Nurses Associations' designation of NI as a specialty in 1992, most nurses involved in informatics were self-educated. Many NI specialists simply adopted the title when they were appointed to serve as a nurse member of a hospital information system team. In 1988, however, the first graduate program in nursing informatics was established at the University of Maryland School of Nursing in Baltimore, and numerous other graduate programs have proliferated since then.

Most nurse informaticists, however, do not hold graduate degrees. Many do hold an informatics nurse specialist certification, which became available from the American Nurses Credentialing Center in 1995. Requirements to take the certification exam include a baccalaureate or higher degree; an active registered nurse license with at least 2 years of professional practice; and experience of at least 2,000 hours of NI within the last 3 years, or 12 hours of graduate work and 1,000 hours of NI practice, or completion of a graduate program in NI that includes at least 200 clinical hours of practicum (ANCC, 2011).

> CONSIDER THIS  Informatics theories and competencies are now being incorporated into many basic nursing curriculums.

## CONCLUSIONS

Evolving technologies offer great opportunities to improve the quality of patient care, but technology alone is not the answer. Regardless of the system that is deployed, health care organizations must consider what technology can best be used in each individual setting and how it should be used. In addition, successfully adopting and integrating new technology requires care providers to understand that technology's limitations as well as its benefits.

Debates about how best to merge the human element of care (caring) and emerging technology will undoubtedly continue. Historically, machines have been unable to demonstrate caring, although the development of new robotic devices is challenging this long-held belief.

Nurses also need to overcome their "technophobia" because, clearly, care can be improved with the appropriate use of technology and, ironically, it is technology that will likely give nurses more time to do "nursing." Nurses must therefore keep the improvement of patient care first and foremost in their technology-development agenda. In addition, nurses must embrace the use of technology as part of the skill set that will be expected of nurses in the 21st century.

## FOR ADDITIONAL DISCUSSION

1. Is there a place for technology development in health care, even when it does not contribute to the improvement of patient outcomes? In other words, should the technology itself ever be the desired goal?

2. Are nursing schools adequately preparing students with the skill sets and competencies they will need to function successfully in a progressively more technological workplace?

3. How should organizations deal with "technophobic" nurses? Should health care employers let nurses decide what level of expertise they wish to acquire?

*continued*

4. What safeguards are in place to assure confidentiality of the EHR? Do you believe confidentiality is greater with electronic or paper records?

5. What technology do you believe has the greatest potential to reduce the current nursing shortage? Why?

6. What technologies currently in use would you predict to be obsolete in 10 years?

7. What barriers exist in health care environments that will impede the development of technology in years to come?

8. What safeguards do consumers have that the health information they find on the Internet is accurate and appropriate?

## REFERENCES

American Nurses Credentialing Center. (2011). *Informatics nursing certification eligibility criteria.* Retrieved September 4, 2011, from http://www.nursecredentialing.org/Informatics-Eligibility.aspx

Ben Franklin Technology Partners. (2011). *Aethon: Robotic tugs deliver improved care and cost savings for hospitals.* Retrieved September 5, 2011, from http://benfranklin.org/news/aethon-robotic-tugs-deliver-improved-care-and-cost-savings-for-hospitals

Bhalla, J. S. (2011, August 12). Eye doctors trying out robotic surgery to cure cataracts. *Hindustantimes.* Retrieved September 4, 2011, from http://www.hindustantimes.com/Eye-doctors-trying-out-robotic-surgery-to-cure-cataracts/Article1-732723.aspx

Bordowitz, R. (2008). Electronic health records: A primer. *Laboratory Medicine, 39*(5), 301–307.

Browne, M., & Cook, P. (2011). Inappropriate trust in technology: Implications for critical care nurses. *Nursing in Critical Care, 16*(2), 92–98.

Brumson, B. (2008). *Robots for life: Laboratory, medical and life science applications.* Retrieved August 12, 2008, from http://www.robotics.org/content-detail.cfm/Industrial-Robotics-Feature-Articles/Robots-for-Life:-Laboratory-Medical-and-Life-Science-Applications/content_id/605

Canada Health Infoway. (2011). *About Canada Health Infoway.* Retrieved September 5, 2011, from https://www.infoway-inforoute.ca/lang-en/about-infoway

College of American Pathologists. (2012). *Point of care testing toolkit.* Retrieved May 8, 2012, from http://www.cap.org/apps/cap.portal?_nfpb=true&cntvwrPtlt_actionOverride=%2Fportlets%2FcontentViewer%2Fshow&_windowLabel=cntvwrPtlt&cntvwrPtlt{actionForm.contentReference}=committees%2Fpointofcare%2Fpoc_toolkit_definition.html&_state=''' maximized&_pageLabel=cntvwr

DesRoches, C. M., Campbell, E. G., Rao, S. R., Donelan, K., Ferris, T. G., Jha, A., . . . Blumenthal, D. (2008). Electronic health records in ambulatory care—A national survey of physicians. *New England Journal of Medicine, 359*(1), 50–60.

Do robots drive up prostate surgeries? (2011, July 20). *FoxNews.com.* Retrieved September 5, 2011, from http://www.foxnews.com/health/2011/07/20/do-robots-drive-up-prostate-surgeries/

GlobalArchitectsGuide.com. (2011). *Biomechatronics information.* Retrieved September 5, 2011, from http://www.globalarchitectsguide.com/library/Biomechatronics.php

Gobry, P.-E. (2011). The Internet is 20% of economic growth. *Business Insider.* Retrieved September 3, 2011, from http://www.businessinsider.com/mckinsey-report-internet-economy-2011-5

Goldstein, J. (2008, July 1). Hospital bar codes not a perfect Rx. *Philadelphia Inquirer.* Retrieved September 23, 2012. http://www.healthleadersmedia.com/content/QUA-214351/Hospital-bar-codes-not-a-perfect-Rx.html

Greenemeier, L. (2011, January 4). 2011: The year of the personal robot? *Scientific American.* Retrieved September 3, 2011, from http://www.scientificamerican.com/article.cfm?id=personal-robot-research

Guizzo, E. (2009, May). Paro the robotic seal could diminish dementia. *IEEE Spectrum.* Retrieved September 3, 2011, from http://spectrum.ieee.org/robotics/home-robots/paro-the-robotic-seal-could-diminish-dementia

Hatler, C. (2008). How intelligent are smart beds? *Nursing Management, 39*(2), 20–26.

Haughom, J., Kriz, S., & McMillan, D. (2011). Overcoming barriers to EHR adoption. *Healthcare Financial Management, 65*(7), 96–100.

Healthcare Information and Management Systems Society. (2011). *Clinical decision support.* Retrieved September 5, 2011, from http://www.himss.org/ASP/topics_clinicalDecision.asp

Krotoski, A. (2011, January 9). What effect has the Internet had on healthcare? *Guardian.co.uk*. Retrieved September 5, 2011, from http://www.guardian.co.uk/technology/2011/jan/09/untangling-web-krotoski-health-nhs

Kyung-hoon, K. (2011, August 8). *Robot Paro comforts the elderly in Fukushima*. Retrieved September 3, 2011, from http://blogs.reuters.com/photo/2011/08/08/robot-paro-comforts-the-elderly-in-fukushima/

Leapfrog. (2011). *Leapfrog fact sheet: Computerized physician order entry*. Retrieved May 8, 2012, from http://www.leapfroggroup.org/media/file/FactSheet_CPOE.pdf

Maslove, D.M., Rizk, N. & Lowe, H. J. (May/June 2011). Computerized physician order entry in the critical care environment: A review of current literature. *Journal of Intensive Care Medicine, 26*(3),165-71.

McNicol, T. (2008). *Robots lend a hand in Japan*. Retrieved September 4, 2011, from http://www.roboticstrends.com/article/print/robots_lend_a_hand_in_japan

Menachemi, N., Chukmaitov, A., Saunders, C., & Brooks, R. G. (2008). Hospital quality of care: Does information technology matter? The relationship between information technology adoption and quality of care. *Health Care Management Review, 33*(1), 51–59.

"Natural next step" for access: Biometrics. (2011). *Hospital Access Management, 30*(6), 70–72.

Saver, C. (2010). Considering robotics? Plan for a program, not just procedures. *OR Manager, 26*(8), 1, 13–15.

Silvey, J. (2011, January 6). Hospital room gets "smart." *Columbia Daily Tribune*. Retrieved September 5, 2011, from http://www.columbiatribune.com/news/2011/jan/06/hospital-room-gets-smart/

## BIBLIOGRAPHY

Aylott, M. (2011). Blurring the boundaries: Technology and the nurse–patient relationship. *British Journal of Nursing (BJN), 20*(13), 810–816.

Brusco, J. (2012). The business of technology. *AORN Journal, 95*(2), 279–285.

Cipriano, P. (2012). The importance of knowledge-based technology. *Nursing Administration Quarterly, 36*(2), 136–146.

Cvitkovic, M. (2011). Point-of-care testing. *Critical Care Nursing Quarterly, 34*(2), 116–127.

Day, K., & Kerr, P. (2012). The potential of telehealth for "business as usual" in outpatient clinics. *Journal of Telemedicine & Telecare, 18*(3), 138–141.

Early, C., Riha, C., Martin, J., Lowdon, K. W., & Harvey, E. M. (2011). Scanning for safety: An integrated approach to improved bar-code medication administration. *CIN: Computers, Informatics, Nursing, 29*(3), 157–164.

Goldberg, M. R. (2011). In depth: Rehabilitation Robotics. *PN, 65*(7), 22–25.

Haring, K. S., Mougenot, C., Ono, F., & Watanabe, K. (2012, May 22–25). *Cultural differences in perception and attitude towards robots*. Paper presented at the International Conference on Kansei Engineering and Emotional Research (KEER 2012), Penghu, Taiwan.

Khajouei, R., Wierenga, P., Hasman, A., & Jaspers, M. (2011). Clinicians satisfaction with CPOE ease of use and effect on clinicians' workflow, efficiency and medication safety. *International Journal of Medical Informatics, 80*(5), 297–309.

Nouskalis, G. (2011). Biometrics, e-identity, and the balance between security and privacy: Case study of the passenger name record (PNR) system. *ScientificWorld Journal, 11*, 474–477.

Overmyer, M. (2011). Robotics offers good outcomes, but cost remains a factor. *Urology Times, 39*(6), 1–21.

Pillemer, K., Meador, R. H., Teresi, J. A., Chen, E. K., Henderson, C. R., Lachs, M. S., ... Eimicke, J. P. (2012). Effects of electronic health information technology implementation on nursing home resident outcomes. *Journal of Aging & Health, 24*(1), 92–112.

Soares, M. M., Jacobs, K., Samaras, E. A., Real, S. D., Curtis, A. M., & Meunier, T. S. (2012). Recognizing nurse stakeholder dissonance as a critical determinant of patient safety in new healthcare information technologies. *Work, 41*, 1904–1910.

Spetz, J., Burgess, J. F., & Phibbs, C. S. (2012). What determines successful implementation of inpatient information technology systems? *American Journal of Managed Care, 18*(3), 157–162.

Stone, S., & Munoz, J. (2012). Barcoding: The way to patient safety. *MLO: Medical Laboratory Observer, 44*(4), 46.

Suter, P., Suter, W., & Johnston, D. (2011). Theory-based telehealth and patient empowerment. *Population Health Management, 14*(2), 87–92.

Thornby, D. (2011). Working with new or unfamiliar technology. *Critical Care Nurse, 31*(1), 99–103.

Welch, J. (2011). An evidence-based approach to reduce nuisance alarms and alarm fatigue. *Biomedical Instrumentation & Technology*, 4546–4552.

Wood, J. L., & Burnette, J. S. (2012). Enhancing patient safety with intelligent intravenous infusion devices: Experience in a specialty cardiac hospital. *Heart & Lung, 41*(2), 173–176.

Chapter **15**

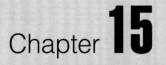

# Medical Errors
## An Ongoing Threat to Quality Health Care

Carol J. Huston

## ADDITIONAL RESOURCES

Visit thePoint for additional helpful resources
- eBook
- Journal Articles
- WebLinks

## LEARNING OBJECTIVES

*The learner will be able to:*

1. Differentiate among the terms *medical error, medication error*, and *adverse event*.

2. Describe highly publicized patient cases from the mid- to the late 1990s as well as seminal research studies that brought national attention to the problem of medical errors in the United States.

3. Identify current research studies examining the scope, common causes, and financial/human costs of medical errors in the United States.

4. Summarize key findings of the 1999 Institute of Medicine (IOM) report *To Err Is Human*, as well as the multipronged approach identified by the IOM to address the problem of medical errors in the United States.

5. Identify national committees and groups formed as a result of governmental or legislative intervention to address the problem of medical errors.

6. Describe the intent and impact of Medicare's Pay for Performance (P4P) initiatives, as well as Medicare's 2008 decision to no longer reimburse health care providers for care needed as the result of "never events" or other preventable errors.

7. Differentiate between workplaces that emphasize a "culture of blame" and those that seek to provide a "just culture" or a "culture of safety management."

8. Identify the meaning of a six-sigma error failure rate and determine how error rates in health care compare with other industries such as banking and the airlines.

9. Analyze the effect of the medical liability system on systematic efforts to uncover and learn from mistakes that are made in health care.

10. Differentiate among the three evidence-based standards identified by Leapfrog as having the greatest potential to reduce medical errors: computerized physician order entry (CPOE),

evidence-based hospital referral (EHR), and intensive care unit (ICU) physician staffing (IPS).

11. Track current federal and state legislative efforts that encourage the voluntary reporting of health care errors by affording confidentiality protections for such reports.

12. Review current research to determine whether organizational, governmental, and national efforts to reduce the incidence of medical errors in the United States have resulted in desired outcomes.

13. Reflect on the likelihood that he or she would self-report his or her medical errors to his or her employer, as well as to the involved patients and families.

Quality health care has emerged as a critically important yet underachieved goal in the United States. Among the most significant threats to achieving quality health care are the scope and prevalence of medical errors. Although medical errors have surely occurred since medicine began, the problem did not receive nationwide attention in the United States until several highly publicized cases between the late 1990s and early 2000s.

One such case involved Betsy Lehman, a *Boston Globe* reporter who died following multiple chemotherapy administration errors. The news media jumped on the story because it demonstrated repeated widespread communication and dispensing errors, despite multiple safeguards in place to keep them from happening.

Libby Zion's case occurred about this same time. Zion, an 18-year-old, died 8 hours after entering a New York emergency department with seemingly minor complaints of fever and earache. Her death from drug interactions brought attention both to the all-too-narrow range between effective and toxic doses of some drugs and the danger of drug–drug interactions, even when all drugs are administered in doses that are considered safe when administered individually. The case also brought attention to the lack of supervision of residents and interns in the United States, as well as the excessive work hours forced on them and the errors that occur as a result.

There was also the story of Willie King, a diabetic man from Tampa, Florida, who had the wrong leg amputated. This case, which became known as the "wrong leg" case, captured the collective dread of wrong-site surgery, but it is a medical error that occurs too frequently as a result of the symmetry of the human body.

Finally, there was the story of Lewis Blackman, a healthy, gifted 15-year-old, who slowly bled to death after undergoing a minor surgical procedure at a major university medical center. Despite multiple warning signs, those caring for him repeatedly missed signs and symptoms that he was bleeding internally from a perforated ulcer.

### DISCUSSION POINT

Do you believe that the public considers itself to be at risk for harm when receiving health care? Do you personally know someone who has been harmed by a medical error?

Perhaps it was the clustering of these high-profile cases that made Americans stop and look at the problem of medical errors, or maybe it was just time to do so. The result was that an unprecedented number of seminal research studies delving into medical errors were undertaken in the past 10 to 15 years to discover how many errors were occurring, what was causing them, and what their financial and human costs were.

The results were disconcerting, to say the least. Most studies highlighted multiple concerns about quality of care, including high rates of provider-induced injury, unnecessary care, and inappropriate care. Many studies found the number of errors in health care to be unacceptably high. The seminal study of this time, *To Err Is Human*, published in 1999 by the Institute of Medicine

(IOM), a congressionally chartered independent organization, provided evidence that the public was highly vulnerable to human error in U.S. health care institutions, an arena in which many thought they were safe.

In addition, unlike most health care research, which generally receives little if any national press, medical error research findings in the late 1990s were published and analyzed in almost every media forum in the country. Consumers were barraged with study findings suggesting that the quality of health care was inadequate and that medical errors were a significant problem leading to increased morbidity and mortality.

---

### DISCUSSION POINT

Do you believe that the quality of health care has declined in the last few decades, or is it simply better monitored and more openly reported today?

---

As a result, consumers, providers, and legislators stepped forward to voice their concerns and to demand, at minimum, a safer health care system. The government listened and directed providers to reexamine how quality health care was provided, measured, and monitored so that cultures of safety could be developed in all health care organizations.

This chapter examines seminal and current research on medical errors, medication errors, and adverse events, as well as the directives that emerged as a result of their findings. Mechanisms for achieving four goals put forth by the IOM as part of *To Err Is Human* are identified. Finally, strategies for creating a culture of safety management in health care are identified, as are the challenges of changing a system that all too often focuses on individual errors rather than on the need to make systemwide changes.

## DEFINING TERMS: MEDICAL ERRORS, MEDICATION ERRORS, AND ADVERSE EVENTS

In reviewing the literature on medical errors, medication errors, and adverse events in health care, it is helpful to first define common terms. *Medical errors* are defined by the *Encyclopedia of Surgery* (2011) as adverse events that could be prevented given the current state of medical

knowledge. In addition, the Quality Interagency Coordination Task Force (QuIC) suggests that medical errors are "the failure of a planned action to be completed as intended or the use of a wrong plan to achieve an aim. Errors can include problems in practice, products, procedures, and systems" (Encyclopedia of Surgery, 2011, para. 3).

Medication errors are the most common type of medical error and are a significant cause of preventable adverse events. *Medication errors* are defined by the National Coordinating Council for Medication Error Reporting and Prevention (NCC MERP) as follows:

*Any preventable event that may cause or lead to inappropriate medication use or patient harm while the medication is in the control of the health care professional, patient, or consumer. Such events may be related to professional practice, health care products, procedures, and systems, including prescribing; order communication; product labeling, packaging, and nomenclature; compounding; dispensing; distribution; administration; education; monitoring; and use.* (NCC MERP, 1998–2011, para. 1)

Finally, *adverse events* are defined as adverse changes in health that occur as a result of treatment. When medications are involved, these are known as *adverse drug events* (ADEs).

## SEMINAL RESEARCH ON MEDICAL ERRORS: 1990 TO 2000

The last decade of the 20th century was marked by a rapid increase in research on medical errors. One of the earliest large-scale studies suggesting that medical errors were a significant problem in health care was published by Brennan et al. (1991) in the *New England Journal of Medicine*. This benchmark study involved more than 30,000 hospitalized patients in New York State. Nearly five of every 100 patients suffered an adverse event caused by a medical error of omission or commission. Of these adverse events, approximately one in four involved negligence. The overwhelming majority of iatrogenic occurrences, however, resulted from organization, system, or process failures. This study, extrapolated to the national population, suggested that 1.3 million people were injured each year in hospitals; of that number, 180,000 would die from those injuries. Providing additional cause for alarm, the report suggested that most of those injuries were actually preventable.

Leape et al. (1991) also reported that drug complications represented 19% of these adverse events and that 45% of these adverse events were caused by medical errors. In this study, 30% of the individuals with drug-related injuries died.

In another study, Leape (1994) reported that the average intensive care unit (ICU) patient experienced almost two errors per day. One of five of these errors was potentially serious or fatal. In fact, this translates into a level of proficiency of approximately 99%, which seems reasonable. However, if performance levels of 99.9%—substantially better than those found in the ICU by Leape—were applied to the airline and banking industries, it would equate to two dangerous landings per day at Chicago's O'Hare International Airport, or 32,000 checks deducted hourly from the wrong account (Leape, 1994).

CONSIDER THIS   The safety record in health care is a far cry from the enviable record of the similarly complex aviation industry.

Another seminal study in the late 1990s involving medical errors was completed by Thomas et al. (1999). Their research, based on a chart review of 14,732 medical records from 28 hospitals in Colorado and Utah, found that 265 of 459 (57%) adverse events were preventable. The total cost of adverse events was US$661,889,000, with preventable adverse events costing an additional US$308,382,000. In addition, the study estimated the national costs of all preventable adverse events to be just under US$17 billion (in 1996 dollars).

A recent study by Van Den Bos et al. (2011) suggests these costs were relatively unchanged a decade later with the annual cost of measurable medical errors that harm patients being US$17.1 billion in 2008. Pressure ulcers were the most common measurable medical error in Van Den Bos et al.'s study, followed by postoperative infections and postlaminectomy syndrome, a condition characterized by persistent pain following back surgery. Since 10 types of errors account for more than two thirds of the total cost of errors, Van Den Bos et al. suggested these errors should be the first targets of prevention efforts.

CONSIDER THIS   Nearly 1 million patient safety incidents occurred among Medicare patients in 2009, a figure that matches what happened in the years 2006, 2007, and 2008. These errors cost the federal Medicare program nearly US$8.9 billion and resulted in 96,402 potentially preventable deaths from 2006 through 2008 (Claims Journal, 2010).

## To Err Is Human

Many of the studies done in the 1990s laid the foundation for what is perhaps the best known and largest study ever done on the quality of health care: *To Err Is Human* (Kohn, Corrigan, & Donaldson, 2000). This report, which represented a compilation of more than 30 studies completed by the IOM, found the following:

- At least 44,000 Americans die each year as a result of medical errors, and the number may be as high as 98,000.

- Even when using the lower estimate, deaths due to medical errors could be considered the eighth-leading cause of death in 1999.

- More people die in a given year as a result of medical errors than from motor vehicle accidents, breast cancer, or AIDS.

The IOM study also examined the types of errors that were occurring. Many of the adverse events were associated with the use of pharmaceutical agents and were potentially preventable. Medication errors alone, both in and out of the hospital, were estimated to account for more than 7,000 deaths in 1993, and one of every 854 inpatient hospital deaths was the result of a medication error. Children experienced harmful medication errors three times more often than adults (5.7% of medication orders for pediatric patients), and the rate was higher yet for neonates in the neonatal ICU. In addition, ICU patients suffered more life-threatening medication errors than any other patient population.

CONSIDER THIS   "Experts agree that medication errors have the potential to cause harm within the pediatric population at a higher rate than in the adult population. For example, medication dosing errors are more common in pediatrics than adults because of weight-based dosing calculations, fractional dosing (e.g., mg vs. Gm), and the need for decimal points" (Joint Commission, 2008, para. 1).

Within a short time of the IOM report's release, some people began to question the numbers, asking whether the problem of medical errors could be as serious as it seemed. The first study to reliably confirm the IOM figures was a 2004 study by the health care ratings company HealthGrades (2004). This study looked at 3 years of Medicare data in all 50 states and Washington, D.C., and reported that approximately 1.14 million patient safety incidents (PSIs) occurred among the 37 million hospitalizations in the Medicare population for the study period. The most commonly occurring PSIs were failure to rescue, decubitus ulcer, and postoperative sepsis.

Of the total 323,993 deaths among Medicare patients who developed one or more patient-safety incidents, 263,864, or 81%, of these deaths were directly attributable to the incidents (HealthGrades, 2004). In addition, one in every four Medicare patients who were hospitalized from 2000 to 2002 and experienced a patient-safety incident died. Perhaps most startling, however, was the conclusion that the United States loses more lives to patient safety incidents every 6 months than it did in the entire Vietnam War. This also equates to three fully loaded jumbo jets crashing every other day for the last 5 years. Finally, the study noted that if the Centers for Disease Control and Prevention's annual list of leading causes of death included medical errors, it would show up as number six, ahead of diabetes, pneumonia, Alzheimer disease, and renal disease (HealthGrades, 2004).

A follow-up report by the IOM in 2006 also confirmed the scope of medical errors identified in *To Err Is Human*. This report, *Preventing Medication Errors*, suggested that medication errors were surprisingly common and costly to the nation. The report concluded that at least 1.5 million preventable adverse drug events occur in the United States each year and that "changes from doctors, nurses, pharmacists, and others in the health care industry, from the Food and Drug Administration (FDA) and other government agencies, from hospitals and other health-care organizations, and from patients" would be necessary to decrease the prevalence of these errors (National Conference of State Legislatures, 2008, para. 1).

---

### DISCUSSION POINT

Is the U.S. public aware of the prevalence of medical errors? If not, what could be done to galvanize them to take action?

---

## The Response to the Institute of Medicine Report

Within weeks of the release of *To Err Is Human*, the Senate held its first hearings on the issue, and additional hearings were conducted by committees of both the House of Representatives and the Senate. Local, state, and national leaders, as well as private and public sector leaders, took immediate action. The significance of the IOM report as a catalyst for change cannot be overstated.

That said, however, it is important to note that the problems of medical errors and patient safety were not completely unrecognized before *To Err Is Human* was published. Perhaps the most significant aspect of the IOM study was that it summarized the high human cost of medical errors in language that was understandable by the general public. In addition, previously, an assumption was made that most patient injuries were the result of negligence, incompetence, or corporate greed. The IOM report indicated, however, that errors are simply a part of the human condition and that the health care system needed to be redesigned so that fewer errors would occur.

As a result of these findings, the IOM recommended a national goal of reducing the number of medical errors by 50% over 5 years (Kohn et al., 2000). To that end, it outlined a four-pronged approach to reducing medical mistakes nationwide (Box 15.1). The strategies needed to achieve this national goal and attend to each of the four approaches are numerous, however, and only a few are detailed in this chapter.

## WORKING TO ACHIEVE THE INSTITUTE OF MEDICINE GOALS

The first of the IOM's four-pronged approach to reducing medical errors was to "establish a national focus to create leadership, research, tools, and protocols to enhance the knowledge base about safety" (Kohn et al., 2000, p. 6). The second was to "raise standards and expectations for improvements in safety through the actions of oversight organizations, group purchasers, and professional groups" (Kohn et al., 2000, p. 6). Work to achieve both of these goals began almost immediately after the IOM report was published. Indeed, a number of national committees and groups were formed as a result of governmental or legislative intervention. Some of the committees, groups, and legislative efforts spearheading the task to reduce medical errors are outlined here.

## BOX 15.1 THE IOM'S FOUR-PRONGED APPROACH TO REDUCING MEDICAL MISTAKES NATIONWIDE

- Establish a national focus to create leadership, research, tools, and protocols to enhance the knowledge base about safety.

- Identify and learn from medical errors through both mandatory and voluntary reporting systems.

- Raise standards and expectations for improvements in safety through the actions of oversight organizations, group purchasers, and professional groups.

- Implement safe practices at the delivery level.

*Source:* Kohn, L. T., Corrigan, J. M., & Donaldson, M. S. (Eds.). (2000). Executive summary. In *To err is human: Building a safer health system* (pp. 1–6). Retrieved May 20, 2012, from https://www.premierinc.com/safety/topics/patient_safety/downloads/01_exsum-iom_1toerr.pdf

## Quality Interagency Coordination Task Force

The Quality Interagency Coordination (QuIC) Task Force was established by President Bill Clinton in 1998 to coordinate federal agencies that provided health care services. In December 1999, the task force began to evaluate the IOM recommendations and develop strategies for identifying threats to patient safety and reducing medical errors.

The final report, *Doing What Counts for Patient Safety: Federal Actions to Reduce Medical Errors and Their Impact*, was delivered to the president in February 2000. The report proposed taking strong action on all of the IOM recommendations to reduce errors, implementing a system of public accountability, developing a robust knowledge base about medical errors, and changing the culture in health care organizations to promote the recognition of errors and improvement in patient safety.

## The National Forum for Health Care Quality Measurement and Reporting

Consistent with the QuIC's recommendations, the National Forum for Health Care Quality Measurement and Reporting was launched by Vice President Al Gore in 2000. Known as the National Quality Forum (NQF), it is a broad-based, private, not-for-profit body that establishes standard quality measurement tools to help people better ensure the delivery of quality services. The mission of the NQF is to improve the quality of American health care by building consensus on national priorities and goals for performance improvement and working in partnership to achieve them, endorsing national consensus standards for measuring and publicly reporting on performance, and promoting the attainment of national goals through education and outreach programs (NQF, 2011a, para. 1).

Since its inception, the NQF has endorsed hundreds of performance measures and practices, and many more are either in the early stages of development or moving through the NQF endorsement process. NQF was also the first to create a list of 27 *serious reportable events*, a list that was expanded to 28 events in 2006. In 2011, the NQF board approved for endorsement a list of 29 serious reportable events (SREs) in health care (Box 15.2). Of the events, 25 were updated from their earlier endorsement in 2006 and 4 new events were added to the list.

In addition, the NQF board of directors approved expansion of their mission in 2008 to include working in partnership with other leadership organizations to establish national priorities and goals for performance measurement and public reporting. The first draft of their core set of national priorities is shown in Box 15.3. Finally, the NQF was identified as the consensus-based entity for implementation of the Affordable Care Act (ACA; launched in late 2011), including convening a multistakeholder group to provide annual input to the Department of Health and Human Services on the development of a National Quality Strategy (NQF, 2011b). The resultant National Priorities Partnership (NPP) includes representatives from 48 major national organizations "representing public and private sector stakeholder groups in a forum that balances the interests of consumers, purchasers, health plans, clinicians, providers, communities, states, and suppliers" (NQF, 2011b, para. 5). Structurally, the full partnership will accomplish its work through three subcommittees: Healthy People/Healthy Communities, Better Care, and Affordable Care.

## Floyd D. Spence National Defense Authorization Act of 2001

In October 2000, President Clinton signed into effect the Floyd D. Spence National Defense Authorization Act (NDAA) of fiscal year 2001, specifically requiring the Department of Defense to establish a centralized

**BOX 15.2   SERIOUS REPORTABLE EVENTS IN HEALTH CARE (NQF 2011 UPDATE)**

1. Surgical or invasive procedure events
   - Surgery or other invasive procedure performed on the wrong site
   - Surgery or other invasive procedure performed on the wrong patient
   - Wrong surgical or other invasive procedure performed on a patient
   - Unintended retention of a foreign object in a patient after surgery or other invasive procedure
   - Intraoperative or immediately postoperative/postprocedure death in an ASA Class 1 patient
2. Product or device events
   - Patient death or serious injury associated with the use of contaminated drugs, devices, or biologics provided by the health care setting
   - Patient death or serious injury associated with the use or function of a device in patient care, in which the device is used or functions other than as intended
   - Patient death or serious injury associated with intravascular air embolism that occurs while being cared for in a health care setting
3. Patient protection events
   - Discharge or release of a patient/resident of any age, who is unable to make decisions, to other than an authorized person
   - Patient death or serious injury associated with patient elopement (disappearance)
   - Patient suicide, attempted suicide, or self-harm that results in serious injury, while being cared for in a health care setting
4. Care management events
   - Patient death or serious injury associated with a medication error (e.g., errors involving the wrong drug, wrong dose, wrong patient, wrong time, wrong rate, wrong preparation, or wrong route of administration)
   - Patient death or serious injury associated with unsafe administration of blood products
   - Maternal death or serious injury associated with labor or delivery in a low-risk pregnancy while being cared for in a health care setting
   - (NEW) Death or serious injury of a neonate associated with labor or delivery in a low-risk pregnancy
   - Patient death or serious injury associated with a fall while being cared for in a health care setting
   - Any Stage 3, Stage 4, and unstageable pressure ulcers acquired after admission/presentation to a health care setting
   - Artificial insemination with the wrong donor sperm or wrong egg
   - (NEW) Patient death or serious injury resulting from the irretrievable loss of an irreplaceable biological specimen
   - (NEW) Patient death or serious injury resulting from failure to follow up or communicate laboratory, pathology, or radiology test results
5. Environmental events
   - Patient or staff death or serious injury associated with an electric shock in the course of a patient care process in a health care setting

*continued*

**BOX 15.2 SERIOUS REPORTABLE EVENTS IN HEALTH CARE (NQF 2011 UPDATE)** *continued*

- Any incident in which systems designated for oxygen or other gas to be delivered to a patient contains no gas, the wrong gas, or is contaminated by toxic substances
- Patient or staff death or serious injury associated with a burn incurred from any source in the course of a patient care process in a health care setting
- Patient death or serious injury associated with the use of physical restraints or bedrails while being cared for in a health care setting

**6.** Radiologic events
- (NEW) Death or serious injury of a patient or staff associated with the introduction of a metallic object into the MRI area

**7.** Potential criminal events
- Any instance of care ordered by or provided by someone impersonating a physician, nurse, pharmacist, or other licensed health care provider
- Abduction of a patient/resident of any age
- Sexual abuse/assault on a patient or staff member within or on the grounds of a health care setting
- Death or serious injury of a patient or staff member resulting from a physical assault (i.e., battery) that occurs within or on the grounds of a health care setting

*Source:* National Quality Forum. (2011c). *NQF releases updated serious reportable events.* Retrieved November 7, 2011, from http://www.qualityforum.org/News_And_Resources/Press_Releases/2011/NQF_Releases_Updated_Serious_Reportable_Events.aspx

process for reporting, compiling, and analyzing errors in health care within the defense health program. It also mandated the creation of a Patient Safety Center at the Armed Forces Institute of Pathology to analyze patient care errors and to develop and execute plans to reduce and control those errors.

## The National Patient Safety Foundation

*The National Patient Safety Foundation (NPSF) was also formed in response to the IOM report. The mission of the NPSF, as amended in 2003, is to measurably improve patient safety in the delivery of health care by its efforts*

**BOX 15.3 THE NATIONAL QUALITY FORUM'S NATIONAL PRIORITIES PARTNERSHIP GOALS**

**1.** Engage patients and their families in managing their health and making decisions about their care.

**2.** Improve the health of the population.

**3.** Improve the safety and reliability of America's health care system.

**4.** Ensure patients received well-coordinated care within and across all health care organizations, settings, and levels of care.

**5.** Guarantee appropriate and compassionate care for patients with life-limiting illnesses.

**6.** Eliminate overuse while assuring the delivery of appropriate care.

*Source:* National Quality Forum. (2008). *National priorities and goals.* Retrieved November 5, 2011, from http://www.nationalprioritiespartnership.org/uploadedFiles/NPP/About_NPP/ExecSum_no_ticks.pdf

*to identify and create a core body of knowledge; identify pathways to apply the knowledge; develop and enhance the culture of receptivity to patient safety; raise public awareness and foster communications about patient safety; and improve the status of the Foundation and its ability to meet its goals.* (NPSF, 2011, para. 1)

Basic tenets of the NPSF are shown in Box 15.4.

---

CONSIDER THIS   Although few organizations would argue against the benefits of well-developed and well-implemented quality control programs, quality control in health care organizations has evolved primarily from external effects and not as a voluntary monitoring effort.

---

### BOX 15.4   BASIC BELIEFS: NATIONAL PATIENT SAFETY FOUNDATION

- Patient safety is central to quality health care as reflected in the Hippocratic Oath: "Above all, do no harm."

- Prevention of injury, through early and appropriate response to evident and potential problems, is the key to patient safety.

- Continued improvement in patient safety is attainable only through establishing a culture of trust, honesty, integrity, and open communication.

- An integrated body of scientific knowledge and the infrastructure to support its development are essential to advance patient safety significantly.

- Patient involvement in continuous learning and constant communication of information among caregivers, organizations, and the general public will improve patient safety.

- The system of health care is fallible and requires fundamental change to sustainably improve patient safety.

*Source:* National Patient Safety Foundation. (2011). *About us.* Retrieved May 20, 2012, from http://www.qualityforum.org/About_NQF/Mission_and_Vision.aspx

## The Joint Commission

New organizations were not the only ones that responded to the recommendations of the IOM. The Joint Commission (formerly known as the Joint Commission for Accreditation of Healthcare Organizations [JCAHO]), in existence since 1951, accredits hospitals, long-term care facilities, psychiatric facilities, ambulatory care programs, and home health operations.

The Joint Commission's National Patient Safety Goals, implemented in January 2003, set forth clear, evidence-based recommendations to focus health care organizations on significant documented safety problems. These goals are updated annually for ambulatory care settings, behavioral health settings, hospitals, home care disease-specific care, laboratories, home-based care, and office-based surgery. The goals for hospitals in 2011 are shown in Box 15.5.

The Joint Commission also maintains one of the nation's most comprehensive databases of sentinel (serious adverse) events by health care professionals and their underlying causes. A *sentinel event* is defined by the Joint Commission (2011b) as "an unexpected occurrence involving death or serious physical or psychological injury, or the risk thereof. Serious injury specifically includes loss of limb or function. The phrase, 'or the risk thereof' includes any process variation for which a recurrence would carry a significant chance of a serious adverse outcome" (para. 2). Such events are called *sentinel* because they signal the need for immediate investigation and response. Information from the JCAHO sentinel database is regularly shared with accredited

---

### BOX 15.5   JOINT COMMISSION 2011 NATIONAL PATIENT SAFETY GOALS FOR HOSPITALS

1. Identify patients correctly.
2. Improve staff communication.
3. Use medicines safely.
4. Prevent infection.
5. Identify patient safety risks.
6. Prevent mistakes in surgery.

*Source:* Joint Commission. (2011a). *2011 Hospital national patient safety goals.* Retrieved November 6, 2011, from http://www.jointcommission.org/assets/1/6/HAP_NPSG_6-10-11.pdf

organizations to help them take appropriate steps to prevent medical errors.

Another JCAHO priority is the development of a *root cause analysis* with a plan of correction for the errors that do occur. The Joint Commission's (2011c) Sentinel Event Policy provides that organizations that are either voluntarily reporting a sentinel event or responding to the Joint Commission's inquiry about a sentinel event submit their related root cause analysis and action plan electronically to the Joint Commission whenever such events occur. The sentinel event data are then reviewed, and recommendations are made. The Joint Commission defends the confidentiality of the information, if necessary, in court.

Similarly, some organizations use a *failure mode and effects analysis* (FMEA) to examine all possible failures in a design—including sequencing of events, actual and potential risk, points of vulnerability; and areas for improvement (American Society for Quality, n.d.).

---

CONSIDER THIS  National legislation designed to keep such error analyses confidential is a critical but still-unrealized step. This discourages error reporting.

---

## Centers for Medicare and Medicaid Services

The Centers for Medicare and Medicaid Services (CMS), formerly the Health Care Financing Administration (HCFA), also plays an active role in setting standards and measuring quality of health care. With the introduction of the Medicare Quality Initiatives (MQIs) in November 2001, a new era of public reporting on quality began. These diverse initiatives encouraged the public reporting of quality measures for nursing homes, home health agencies, hospitals, and kidney dialysis facilities. These data are then made available to consumers on the Medicare website to assist them in making health care choices or decisions.

Medicare also established *pay for performance* (P4P), also known as *quality-based purchasing*, in the middle of the first decade of the 21st century. Because research conducted in the past decade has suggested little relationship between quality of care provided and the cost of that care, P4P initiatives were created to align payment and quality incentives and to reduce costs through improved quality and efficiency.

As part of P4P, the Physician Quality Reporting Initiative (PQRI), which was launched in 2007, allowed

for payments to eligible professionals (EPs) who satisfactorily reported quality information to Medicare on at least 3 of 74 individual quality measures on 80% of the cases from July 1, 2007 through December 31, 2007. Those who met the criteria for submitting quality data were eligible to earn a lump-sum incentive payment equivalent to 1.5% of their total estimated allowable charges for Medicare Part B Physician Fee Schedule (PFS: American Academy of Orthopaedic Surgeons, 1995–2011).

The Medicare Improvements for Patients and Providers Act of 2008 (MIPPA) made the PQRI program permanent, with incentive payments increased to 2.0% and authorized through 2010. There were 153 individual quality measures and 7 measure groups for reporting under the program in 2009. For 2010, there were 175 individual measures and 13 measure groups (American Academy of Orthopaedic Surgeons, 1995–2011).

With the introduction of the Affordable Care Act in 2011, the PQRI was changed to the Physician Quality Reporting System (PQRS) and incentive payments of 1.0% were established for successfully reporting the current 190 individual PQRS measures. An additional 0.5% incentive payment is possible for providers who qualify for or maintain board certification status, participate in a maintenance of certification program, and successfully complete a qualified maintenance of certification program practice assessment (American Academy of Orthopaedic Surgeons, 1995–2011).

Critics of the P4P incentive system suggest, however, that the system has failed to yield the desired results. They state this has occurred for many reasons including a focus on provider improvement and not achievement, the risk adjustment of provider scores supposedly being imprecise or even inapplicable to certain pay-for-performance metrics, sample sizes being small resulting in too few patients who are eligible to be scored for a given metric, and patients being treated often by multiple physicians (Pay for Performance, 2011). In addition, they suggest that

*P4P may result in better documentation of care, without a concurrent improvement in actual care. In addition, physicians may move their practices to areas where they believe patients can more effectively manage their own care; coordination of care could decline, especially for patients with multiple illnesses; physicians might focus on improving care only in areas addressed by financial rewards; and practice administrative costs could increase. (Pay for Performance, 2011, para. 13)*

In addition, in an effort to reduce the number of preventable medical errors, including *never events* (errors that should never happen, such as removing the wrong limb in surgery, leaving a foreign object inside a patient during surgery, or sending a baby home with the wrong parents), Medicare announced that effective October 1, 2008, it would no longer pay for care that was required as a result of eight specific preventable errors or never events (Box 15.6). Medicaid followed suit in 2011.

In 2008, Medicare also stopped reimbursing hospitals for treating conditions, infections, or illnesses that were acquired in the hospital, and for any readmissions associated with treating those hospital-acquired conditions (Walker, 2011). The Affordable Care Act (ACA) extended the ruling to Medicaid in 2011 by prohibiting states from making Medicaid payments to providers for conditions that are deemed "reasonably preventable" (Walker, 2011).

Private insurance companies are following suit. For instance, Aetna no longer reimburses for eight hospital-acquired infections or for three never events and Cigna does not pay for never events, reduces payments for

---

**BOX 15.6   EIGHT "NEVER ERRORS" THAT WERE NO LONGER PAID FOR BY MEDICARE AS OF OCTOBER 1, 2008**

1. Pressure ulcers
2. Preventable injuries such as fractures, dislocations, and burns
3. Catheter-associated urinary tract infections
4. Vascular catheter–associated infections
5. Certain surgical-site infections
6. Objects mistakenly left inside surgical patients
7. Air emboli
8. Blood incompatibility reactions

---

hospital-acquired infections in certain cases, and offers payment incentives for hospitals that follow standardized protocols to improve patient safety (Walker, 2011). These new policies require hospitals to maintain meticulous documentation about what conditions are present on admission to differentiate between preexisting conditions and those that are acquired during the hospital stay.

## Institute for Healthcare Improvement

The Institute for Healthcare Improvement (IHI), established in the late 1980s by Donald Berwick, is an independent not-for-profit organization focused on "motivating and building the will for change; identifying and testing new models of care in partnership with both patients and health care professionals; and ensuring the broadest possible adoption of best practices and effective innovations" (IHI, 2011, para. 2). During the annual National Forum on Quality Improvement in Health Care conference, the IHI highlights evidence-based best practices in an effort to more rapidly translate research into practice. For example, IHI launched the "Ventilator Bundle," a collection of effective care processes reliably combined to eliminate ventilator-associated pneumonia (IHI, 2010).

In addition, IHI maintains disciplined research and development processes and prototyping projects to pursue health care quality improvements. This work typically happens in collaboratives based on a breakthrough series model whereby participating organizations work together for 9 to 12 months to achieve sustainable change within a specific topic area (IHI, 2010).

For example, one IHI initiative was the identification of "triggers" (or clues) to identify patients with adverse events. This research in turn led to the "Idealized Design of the Medication System" and later to applications which supported the elimination of harm levels across entire systems (IHI, 2010).

In addition, IHI has facilitated further research, adaptation, and adoption of quality improvement strategies such as rapid response teams and medication reconciliation at health care institutions worldwide. Dissemination of best practice improvement knowledge occurs through the IHI Improvement Map (an interactive, web-based tool), the IHI Open School for Health Professions, the IHI website, and Fellowship programs sponsored by the George W. Merck family, the Health Foundation, and the Commonwealth Fund (IHI, 2010).

## Health Care Report Cards

In response to the demand for objective measures of quality, including the number and type of medical errors, many health plans, health care providers, employer purchasing groups, consumer information organizations, and state governments have begun to formulate health care quality report cards. Most states have laws requiring providers to report some type of data. The Agency for Healthcare Research and Quality (AHRQ) also is exploring the development of a report card for the nation's health care delivery system, and the National Committee for Quality Assurance's (NCQA) Health Plan Report Card lets an individual create a health plan report card online. In addition, CMS released a proposed rule in June 2011 that would make Medicare information regarding provider cost and quality available to certain organizations.

It is important to remember, however, that many report cards do not contain information about the quality of care rendered by specific clinics, group practices, or physicians in a health plan's network. In addition, most report cards focus on service utilization data and patient satisfaction ratings and have minimal data regarding medical errors. Critics of health care report cards also point out that health plans may receive conflicting ratings on different report cards. This results from using different performance measures, as well as how each report card pools and evaluates individual factors. Report cards might also not be readily accessible or might be difficult for the average consumer to understand. Still, there is no doubt that consumers want more access to meaningful quality-of-care information and it is apparent that such data, which have long been kept secret, are now becoming public.

## CONTEMPORARY RESEARCH ON MEDICAL ERRORS

Despite all the interventions that came out of the IOM study, current literature suggests that only minimal progress has been made in addressing the problem and that medical errors continue to occur at an alarming rate. Only some of the current studies are discussed here due to space constraints.

A large study by HealthGrades (2008) that reviewed 41 million Medicare patient records between 2004 and 2006 in virtually all of the nation's nearly 5,000 nonfederal hospitals reported 238,337 potentially preventable deaths. The overall incident rate was approximately 3% of all Medicare admissions, accounting for 1.1 million patient safety incidents during the 3 years studied. Medicare patients who experienced a patient safety incident had a one-in-five chance of dying as a result of the incident. The study concluded that if all of the hospitals had performed at the level of Distinguished Hospitals for Patient Safety, approximately 220,106 patient safety incidents and 37,214 Medicare deaths could have been prevented, saving the US$2.0 billion during the study period.

Similarly, a study by Garrouste-Orgeas et al. (2010) found that while ICUs are created for patients with life-threatening illnesses, the ICU environment generates a high risk of iatrogenic events. An observational prospective multicenter cohort study of medical errors found that 1,192 errors were reported for 1,369 patients, and 367 (26.8%) patients experienced at least one medical error (2.1/1,000 patient-days). The most common errors were insulin administration errors (185.9/1,000 days of insulin treatment). Of the 1,192 medical errors, 183 (15.4%) in 128 (9.3%) patients were adverse events that were followed by one or more clinical consequences ($n = 163$) or that required one or more procedures or treatments ($n = 58$). Having two or more adverse events was an independent risk factor for ICU mortality. The researchers concluded that the impact of medical errors on mortality indicated an urgent need to develop prevention programs.

Similarly disturbing, a study by Classen et al. (2011) found that as many as one in three patients in the United States encounter a medical error during a hospital stay. The most common errors were medication errors, followed by surgical errors, procedural errors, and nosocomial infections. The study also compared three different methods of detecting adverse events: voluntary reporting of sentinel events (as mandated by state and other oversight bodies), the commonly used AHRQ's Patient Safety Indicators (which rely on automated review of discharge codes to detect adverse events), and the Global Trigger Tool pioneered by the Institute for Healthcare Improvement (which uses specific methods for reviewing medical charts that lead to further investigation into whether an adverse event occurred and how severe it was). The chart-review methodology picked up at least 10 times more confirmed serious event cases (90% of 393) than did the other two methods (10% or 39 events). This finding suggests that the two currently used methods for detecting medical errors in the United States are unreliable, underestimate the real burden, and also risk misdirection of present efforts to improve patient safety.

A 2010 study by Landrigan et al. (2010) also found medical errors in U.S. hospitals to be a serious problem even in places where local governments have made efforts to improve safety of inpatient care. Landrigan et al. noted 588 harms among 2,341 admissions, a rate of 25.1 harms per 100 admissions in 10 hospitals in North Carolina, despite efforts to implement error reduction strategies over the 5-year period between 2002 and 2007. Similarly, a November 2010 document from the Office of the Inspector General of the Department of Health and Human Services reported "that, when in hospital, one in seven beneficiaries of Medicare (the government-sponsored health-care program for those aged 65 and older) have complications from medical errors, which contribute to about 180,000 deaths of patients per year" (Medical Errors in the USA, 2011, para. 3).

## CREATING A CULTURE OF SAFETY MANAGEMENT

In response to public forces and professional concerns, patient safety has become one of the nation's most pressing challenges and a mandate for every health care organization. Indeed, the final recommendation of the IOM report was to implement safe practices at the delivery level. The strategies that have been recommended to achieve this goal are overwhelming both in scope and quantity.

Strategies discussed in this chapter include the "six-sigma" approach (a customer-based, management philosophy) to error management; the mandatory/voluntary reporting of errors; attempts to increase confidentiality of reporting to reduce the fear of legal liability for reporting errors that do occur; the Leapfrog recommendations; the use of bar coding; a change in organizational cultures from that of "individual blame" to error identification and system modification; and the development of patient safety solutions by the World Health Organization's World Alliance for Patient Safety.

---

CONSIDER THIS  Because quality health care is a complex phenomenon, the factors contributing to quality in health care are as varied as the strategies needed to achieve this elusive goal.

---

## A Six-Sigma Approach

One approach that has been taken to create a culture of safety management at the institutional level has been the implementation of the "six-sigma" approach. *Sigma* is a statistical measurement that reflects how well a product or process is performing. Higher sigma values indicate better performance. Historically, the health care industry has been comfortable striving for three-sigma processes (all data points fall within three standard deviations) in terms of health care quality instead of six. This is one reason why health care has more errors than the banking and airline industries, in which achieving six sigmas is the expectation. Organizations aim for this lofty target by carefully applying six-sigma methodology to every aspect of a particular product or process.

---

### DISCUSSION POINT

Should the health care industry be willing to accept higher error rates than the banking or airline industries? Why or why not? Is the public willing to do so?

---

### DISCUSSION POINT

Is a six-sigma failure rate a reasonable goal for all health care organizations? Should some health care organizations be expected to have higher failure (defect) rates than others? What variables might affect an organization's ability to achieve this goal?

---

## Mandatory Reporting of Errors

The third prong of the IOM's four-pronged approach to creating a safer health care system is "to identify and learn from medical errors through both mandatory and voluntary reporting systems" (Kohn et al., 2000, p. 6). To accomplish this, the IOM report recommended developing a mandatory reporting system for medical errors and adverse events at both the state and national levels.

State mandates for reporting medical errors and adverse events have been slow to materialize, although as of 2011, at least 27 states required hospitals and/or other medical facilities to report serious medical errors and 17 states mandated that pharmacies implement continuous quality improvement (CQI) programs (National Association of Boards of Pharmacy, 2011). Some states also have reporting mandates that apply only to specific types of error, such as hospital-acquired infections (HAIs). It is important to note that the IOM report did suggest, in addition to mandatory reporting, that more options be created for limited voluntary reporting systems in all 50 states. The IOM also recommended that more research be conducted on how best to develop voluntary reporting systems that complement proposed mandatory reporting systems.

Increased mandatory and voluntary reporting must also occur at the institutional level, as well as by individual providers. As a result, the IOM report suggested that mandatory adverse event reporting should initially be required of hospitals and eventually of other institutional and ambulatory care delivery facilities. This was the impetus for the subsequent JCAHO action for sentinel event reporting as part of the accreditation process.

It is difficult, however, to enforce greater disclosure and reporting at the individual provider level. Ethical and professional guidelines suggest that providers have a responsibility to disclose medical errors. Yet the literature continues to suggest that this does not happen because of fear of legal suits or disciplinary measures by employers. The ironic part is that full disclosure after errors occur often reduces the likelihood of legal suit or the extent of patient retribution.

> ### DISCUSSION POINT
>
> Do you believe that error disclosure rates differ between nurses and physicians? If so, which professional group is more likely to disclose errors and why?

Perhaps this failure to disclose medical errors is a major contributor to the disconnect that exists between consumers' perceptions of the quality of their health care and the actual quality provided. Even consumers who are aware of medical error statistics often report that they believe medical errors to be a problem but believe that such errors will not happen to them because they trust and believe in their health care provider.

> ### DISCUSSION POINT
>
> Do you consider the care you receive from your primary care provider to be of high quality? Are your perceptions subjective, or do you have objective data to back up your impression? Have you actively searched for such data on your primary care provider?

## Legal Liability and Medical Error Reporting

If quality health care is to be achieved, the medical liability system and our litigious society must be recognized as potential barriers to systematic efforts to uncover and learn from mistakes that are made in health care. One recommendation of the IOM panel was to encourage learning about safety from cross-institutional reporting systems for errors. This reporting is inhibited by fears that such data will be discovered in liability lawsuits.

> ### DISCUSSION POINT
>
> Have you ever encouraged a family member, friend, or colleague to seek compensation for medical errors? If so, do you think this was the most appropriate means of redress?

The provision of stronger confidentiality protections likely would improve the voluntary sharing of data. In 2002, the Patient Safety Improvement Act was introduced in the House of Representatives. This bill provided legal protections for medical error reporting, stating that error information voluntarily submitted to patient safety organizations could not be subpoenaed or used in legal discovery. It also generally required that the information be treated as confidential. After multiple revisions, the final legislation, called the Patient Safety and Quality Improvement Act of 2005, was signed into law by President George W. Bush in July 2005.

Federal legislation has also been proposed to protect the voluntary reporting of ordinary injuries and "near misses"—errors that did not cause harm this time but easily could the next time. This would be like what is done in aviation, in which near misses are confidentially reported and can be analyzed by anyone.

### DISCUSSION POINT

Given the known incidence of medical errors and adverse events that result in patient injury and the challenges inherent in tracking errors that have already been made, how difficult will it be to track "near misses"? What resources would be needed to accomplish this goal?

## Leapfrog Group

The Leapfrog Group is a conglomeration of non–health care *Fortune 500* leaders dedicated to reducing preventable medical mistakes and improving the quality and affordability of health care (Leapfrog Group, 2011a). The group has advised the health care industry that big leaps in patient safety and customer value can occur if specific evidence-based standards are implemented, including (1) computerized physician (or prescriber) order entry (CPOE), (2) evidence-based hospital referral (EHR), and (3) ICU physician staffing (IPS).

CPOE, which was discussed in Chapter 14, is a promising technology that allows physicians to enter orders into a computer instead of handwriting them:

> Recent research shows that if this Leapfrog practice was implemented in all urban hospitals in the U.S., we could prevent as many as 3 million serious medication errors each year. Studies have also shown that CPOE reduces length of stay; reduces repeat tests; reduces turnaround times for laboratory, pharmacy and radiology requests; as well as delivering cost savings. (Leapfrog, 2011c, para. 1)

EHR involves making sure that patients with high-risk conditions are treated at hospitals whose characteristics are associated with better outcomes. Indeed, HealthGrades' (2008) analysis of 41 million Medicare patient records found that patients treated at top-performing hospitals had, on average, a 43% lower chance of experiencing one or more medical errors compared with the poorest performing hospitals.

Similarly, a recent HealthGrades (2011) study found that patients had a 46% lower risk of experiencing a patient safety incident at a top-rated hospital compared with a poorly rated hospital. For example, the study suggested that while some hospitals have made rapid progress in reducing infection rates, other hospitals continue to show wide variation in their rates. Patients treated at those hospitals performing in the top 5% in the nation for patient safety were, on average, 30% less likely to contract a hospital-acquired bloodstream infection and 39% less likely to suffer from postsurgical sepsis than those treated at poor-performing hospitals. The significance of this finding is clear given that one in six patients who acquired a bloodstream infection while in the hospital died.

IPS considers the level of training of ICU medical personnel. Evidence suggests that quality of care in hospital ICUs is strongly influenced by whether "intensivists" (those familiar with ICU complications) are providing care and how the staff is organized (Leapfrog Group, 2011b). "Mortality rates are significantly lower in hospitals with ICUs managed exclusively by board-certified intensivists. Research has shown that in ICUs where intensivists manage or co-manage all patients versus low intensity there is a 30% reduction in hospital mortality and a 40% reduction in ICU mortality" (Leapfrog, 2011b, para. 1).

## Bar Coding Medications

In addition, Leapfrog has endorsed the use of bar coding to reduce point-of-care medication errors (see Chapter 14 for a further discussion of bar coding medications). Per a U.S. Food and Drug Administration (FDA) rule adopted in April 2004, all prescription and over-the-counter medications used in hospitals must contain a national drug code number. The FDA suggested that a bar code system, coupled with a CPOE system, would greatly enhance the ability of all health care workers to follow the "five rights" of medication administration—that the *right* person receives the *right* drug, in the *right* dose, via the *right* route, at the *right* administration time.

In addition, JCAHO originally proposed in its 2005 National Patient Safety Goals and Requirements that accredited organizations would have to implement bar code technology to identify patients and match them to their medications or other treatments by January 2007. Because of implementation concerns, especially in terms of costs, this proposal was abandoned by JCAHO in July 2004. See Chapter 14 for additional discussion on bar coding medications at the point of care.

## Changing Organizational Cultures

Nurses are likely the health care providers with the greatest potential to change organizational cultures by the early identification, interruption, and correction of medical errors. As a result, the Quality and Safety Education for Nurses (QSEN) project (funded by Robert Wood Johnson Foundation) began in 2005 with the goal of preparing future nurses who will have the knowledge, skills, and attitudes (KSAs) necessary to continuously improve the quality and safety of the health care systems within which they work (QSEN, 2011). When nurses have these KSAs, they are better able to identify potential errors and intervene before errors occur. Indeed, this was the case in research conducted by Henneman et al. (2010) which found that nurses in critical care settings actually used 17 different strategies to identify, interrupt, and correct medical errors (see Research Study Fuels the Controversy 15.1).

> CONSIDER THIS  Henneman et al. (2010) found that the ability of nurses to interrupt an error was influenced by their experience and confidence.

Perhaps though, the most significant change that must occur before a nationwide culture of safety management can exist is that organizational cultures must be created that remove blame from the individual and instead focus on how the organization can be modified to reduce the likelihood of such errors occurring in the future.

Gaskill (2008) agrees, suggesting that the implementation of a "just culture" in work settings will be needed to encourage voluntary reporting and reduce the prevalence of errors. Just cultures exhibit "giving constructive feedback and critical analysis in skillful ways, during assessments based on facts, and having respect for the complexity of the situation" (p. 14). This type of intervention encourages people to reveal the errors they have made so that the organization can learn from them. In addition, the just culture philosophy suggests rewarding staff who report errors or near-errors to help them overcome the fear of reporting (Gaskill, 2008).

Clearly, a punitive approach to medical errors is not productive, and errors will not be reported if workers fear the consequences. Employees and patients need to feel comfortable and without fear of personal risk in reporting hazards that can affect patient safety.

> CONSIDER THIS  Ignoring the problem of medical errors, denying their existence, or blaming the individuals involved in the processes does nothing to eliminate the underlying problems.

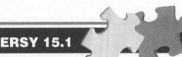

## RESEARCH STUDY FUELS THE CONTROVERSY 15.1

### THE NURSE'S ROLE IN IDENTIFYING, INTERRUPTING, AND CORRECTING MEDICAL ERRORS

Nurses are uniquely positioned to identify, interrupt, and correct medical errors and to minimize preventable adverse outcomes. Only recently, however, have their error-recovery strategies been described.

Henneman, E., Gawlinski, A., Blank, F., Henneman, P., Jordan, D., & McKenzie, J. (2010). Strategies used by critical care nurses to identify, interrupt, and correct medical errors. *American Journal of Critical Care, 19*(6), 500–509.

### STUDY FINDINGS

This study using focus group surveys of 20 nurses from 5 critical care units at 2 urban university medical centers and 2 community hospitals on the East and West coasts of the United States revealed that these nurses used 17 strategies to identify, interrupt, and correct errors. Eight strategies were used to identify errors: knowing the patient, knowing the "players," knowing the plan of care, surveillance, knowing policy/procedure, double-checking, using systematic processes, and questioning. Three strategies were used to interrupt errors: offering assistance, clarifying, and verbally interrupting. Nurses used six strategies

to correct errors: persevering, being physically present, reviewing or confirming the plan of care, offering options, referencing standards or experts, and involving another nurse or physician. Many participants discussed the need to correct system failures by using appropriate communication channels with administrative and clinical leaders.

The researchers concluded that critical care nurses play a critical role in the recovery of medical errors and ensuring patient safety. In addition, they recommended further study to identify approaches to interrupting error that maximize positive outcomes and satisfaction for all involved parties.

## Patient Safety Solutions

Recognizing that health care errors affect at least one in every 10 patients around the world, the World Health Organization's (WHO) World Alliance for Patient Safety and the Collaborating Centre packaged nine effective solutions, called *patient safety solutions,* to reduce such errors. A patient safety solution was defined as "any system design or intervention that has demonstrated the ability to prevent or mitigate patient harm stemming from the processes of health care" and is based on interventions and actions that have reduced problems related to patient safety in some countries (WHO Collaborating Centre for Patient Safety Solutions, 2008, para. 2).

In 2006 and 2007, more than 50 recognized leaders and experts in patient safety from around the world came together to identify and adapt the nine solutions to different needs. An international field review of the solutions was then conducted to gather feedback from leading patient safety entities, accrediting bodies, ministries of health, international health professional organizations, and other experts. In April 2008, the International Steering Committee approved the inaugural solutions and initiated the process for developing the second round of patient safety solutions (WHO Collaborating Centre for Patient Safety Solutions, 2008). The patient safety solutions adopted in 2008 are shown in Box 15.7.

---

### BOX 15.7   WHO'S COLLABORATING CENTRE'S PATIENT SAFETY SOLUTIONS (2008)

Patient safety solutions that demonstrate the ability to prevent or mitigate patient harm stemming from the processes of health care include the following:

1. *Look-alike, sound-alike medication names:* Look-alike and sound-alike drug names are among the most common causes of medication errors and is a worldwide concern.

2. *Patient identification:* Failure to correctly identify patients often leads to medication, transfusion, and testing errors; wrong-person procedures; and the discharge of infants to the wrong families.

3. *Communication during patient handovers:* Gaps in handover (or hand-off) communication can cause serious breakdowns in the continuity of care and result in inappropriate treatment and patient harm.

4. *Performance of correct procedure at correct body site:* Cases of wrong procedure or wrong-site surgery are largely the result of miscommunication and unavailable or incorrect information.

5. *Control of concentrated electrolyte solutions:* Biologics, vaccines, and contrast media have a defined risk profile, and concentrated electrolyte solutions that are used for injection are especially dangerous.

6. *Ensuring medication accuracy at transitions in care:* Medication reconciliation is a process designed to prevent medication errors at patient transition points.

7. *Avoiding catheter and tubing misconnections:* The design of tubing, catheters, and syringes currently in use is such that it is possible to inadvertently cause patient harm through connecting the wrong syringes and tubing and then delivering medication or fluids through an unintended wrong route.

8. *Single use of injection devices:* One of the biggest global concerns is the spread of human immunodeficiency virus (HIV), the hepatitis B virus (HBV), and the hepatitis C virus (HCV) because of the reuse of injection needles.

9. *Improved hand hygiene to prevent health care–associated infection:* Effective hand hygiene would prevent many of the infections acquired by more than 1.4 million people worldwide at any given time.

*Source:* WHO Collaborating Center for Patient Safety Solutions. (2008). *Patient safety solutions.* Retrieved May 20, 2012, from http://www.ccforpatientsafety.org/Patient-Safety-Solutions/

## CONCLUSIONS

Medical errors are not the only indicator of quality of care. They are, however, a pervasive problem in the current health care system and one of the greatest threats to quality health care.

Efforts to reduce medical errors over the last decade have not resulted in the achievement of desired outcomes. There is a plethora of current studies that suggest that the health care system continues to be riddled with errors and that patient and worker safety are compromised. Yet movement toward the IOM goals is occurring. It is likely that there has never been another time when the public, providers, and government have worked together so closely to achieve a shared health care goal.

Much, however, remains to be done. Sustained public interest will be needed to create the momentum necessary to systematically change the health care system in a way that reduces patients' vulnerability to medical errors. In addition, although there has been a great deal of talk about using a systems approach to address the problem of medical errors, there has not been much discussion regarding exactly how this integration is to be accomplished. The bottom line is that significant and continuous reform of the health care system will be needed before the problem of medical errors shows any resolution.

## FOR ADDITIONAL DISCUSSION

1. If cost containment and quality goals conflict, which do you think will take precedence in health care organizations today?

2. Why do so many providers, despite stated dissatisfaction levels, state that they feel helpless about reducing medical errors and improving the quality of health care?

3. Why have quality control efforts in health care organizations evolved primarily from external requirements and not as voluntary monitoring efforts?

4. Where does individual provider responsibility and accountability begin and end in a culture in which medical errors are recognized as being a failure of the system?

5. How common is it that medical error documentation is used against employees as part of the performance appraisal process? If so, does this discourage reporting?

6. Does the average consumer have access to and an accurate understanding of health care report cards?

7. Given that most individuals can quickly identify medical errors that have happened to them, a friend, or a family member, why does the U.S. public seem so reluctant to accept that medical errors constitute a threat to the quality of their health care?

8. Has your fear of legal liability ever influenced your decision to report a medical error?

## REFERENCES

American Academy of Orthopaedic Surgeons. (1995–2011). *Physician quality reporting system (PQRS)*. Retrieved November 7, 2011, from http://www.aaos.org/research/committee/evidence/pqri_intro.asp

American Society for Quality. (n.d.). *Quality tools: Failure modes and effects analysis (FMEA)*. Retrieved November 6, 2011, from http://asq.org/learn-about-quality/process-analysis-tools/overview/fmea.html

Brennan, T. A., Leape, L. L., Laird, N. M., Hebert, L., Localio, A. R., Lawthers, A. G., . . . Hiatt, H. H. (1991). Incidence of adverse events and negligence in hospitalized patients: Results of the Harvard Medical Practice Study 1. *New England Journal of Medicine, 324*(6), 370–376.

Claims Journal. (2010). *One million Medicare patients experience medical errors*. Retrieved October 2, 2011, from http://www.claimsjournal.com/news/national/2010/04/01/108648.htm

Classen, D. C., Resar, R., Griffin, F., Federico, F., Frankel, T., Kimmel, N., . . . James, B. C. (2011). "Global trigger tool" shows that adverse events in hospitals may be ten times greater than previously measured [Abstract]. *Health Affairs, 30*(4), 581–589. Retrieved from http://content.healthaffairs.org/content/30/4/581.abstract

Encyclopedia of Surgery. (2011). *Medical errors: Introduction and definitions.* Retrieved October 2, 2011, from http://www.surgeryencyclopedia.com/La-Pa/Medical-Errors.html

Garrouste-Orgeas, M., Timsit, J. F., Vesin, A., Schwebel, C., Arnodo, P., Lefrant, J. Y., et al. (2010). Selected medical errors in the intensive care unit: Results of the IATROREF study: Parts I and II. *American Journal of Respiratory & Critical Care Medicine, 181*(2), 134–142.

Gaskill, M. (2008). Learning from mistakes: "Just culture" is replacing blame in some California hospitals. *NurseWeek (California), 21*(8), 14–15.

HealthGrades. (2004). *HealthGrades quality study: Patient safety in American hospitals.* Retrieved August 15, 2008, from http://www.healthgrades.com/media/english/pdf/hg_patient_safety_study_final.pdf

HealthGrades. (2008). *Medical errors cost U.S. $8.8 billion, result in 238,337 potentially preventable deaths according to HealthGrades Study.* Retrieved August 15, 2008, from http://www.healthgrades.com/media/DMS/pdf/HealthGradesPatientSafetyRelease2008.pdf

HealthGrades. (2011). *Patient safety excellence award.* Retrieved November 1, 2011, from http://www.healthgrades.com/cms/ratings-and-awards/2011-Patient-Safety-Excellence-Award-Announcement.aspx

Henneman, E., Gawlinski, A., Blank, F., Henneman, P., Jordan, D., & McKenzie, J. (2010). Strategies used by critical care nurses to identify, interrupt, and correct medical errors. *American Journal of Critical Care, 19*(6), 500–509.

Institute for Healthcare Improvement. (2011). *About IHI.* Retrieved November 7, 2011, from http://www.ihi.org/about/pages/default.aspx

Institute for Healthcare Improvement. (2010). *Closing the quality gap: An introduction to IHI.* Retrieved November 6, 2011, from http://www.ihi.org/about/Documents/IntroductiontoIHIBrochureDec10.pdf

Joint Commission. (2008). *Preventing pediatric medication errors.* Retrieved November 6, 2011, from http://www.jointcommission.org/assets/1/18/SEA_39.PDF

Joint Commission. (2011a). *2011 Hospital national patient safety goals.* Retrieved November 6, 2011, from http://www.jointcommission.org/assets/1/6/HAP_NPSG_6-10-11.pdf

Joint Commission. (2008). *Sentinel event.* Retrieved August 16, 2008, from http://www.jointcommission.org/sentinel_event.aspx

Joint Commission. (2011b). *Sentinel event.* Retrieved November 6, 2011, from http://www.jointcommission.org/sentinel_event.aspx

Joint Commission. (2011c). *Sentinel event policy and procedures.* Retrieved November 6, 2011, from http://www.jointcommission.org/Sentinel_Event_Policy_and_Procedures/

Kohn, L. T., Corrigan, J. M., & Donaldson, M. S. (Eds.). (2000). Executive summary. In *To err is human: Building a safer health system* (pp. 1–6). Retrieved May 20, 2012, from https://www.premierinc.com/safety/topics/patient_safety/downloads/01_exsumiom_1toerr.pdf

Landrigan, C., Parry, G., Bones, C., Hackbarth, A., Goldmann, D., & Sharek, P. (2010). Temporal trends in rates of patient harm resulting from medical care. *New England Journal of Medicine, 363*(22), 2124–2134.

Leape, L. L. (1994). Error in medicine. *Journal of the American Medical Association, 272*(23), 1851–1857.

Leape, L. L., Brennan, T. A., Laird, N., Lawthers, A. G., Localio, A. R., Barnes, B. A., . . . Hiatt, H. (1991). The nature of adverse events in hospitalized patients: Results of the Harvard Medical Practice Study II. *New England Journal of Medicine, 324*(6), 377–384.

Leapfrog Group. (2011a). *Homepage.* Retrieved November 7, 2011, from http://www.leapfroggroup.org/

Leapfrog Group. (2011b). *ICU physician staffing.* Retrieved November 6, 2011, from http://www.leapfroggroup.org/for_hospitals/leapfrog_hospital_survey_copy/leapfrog_safety_practices/icu_physician_staffing

Leapfrog Group. (2011c). *Computerized physician order entry.* Retrieved November 6, 2011, from http://www.leapfroggroup.org/for_hospitals/leapfrog_hospital_survey_copy/leapfrog_safety_practices/cpoe

Medical errors in the USA: Human or systemic. (2011). *The lancet.* Retrieved November 7, 2011, from http://www.thelancet.com/journals/lancet/article/PIIS0140-6736(11)60520-5/fulltext?rss=yes

National Association of Boards of Pharmacy. (2011). *Medication error reporting: CQI programs offer avenue to vital follow-up.* Retrieved November 7, 2011, from http://

www.nabp.net/news/medication-error-reporting-cqi-programs-offer-avenue-to-vital-follow-up/

National Coordinating Council for Medication Error Reporting and Prevention. (1998–2011). *About medication errors.* Retrieved October 2, 2011, from http://www.nccmerp.org/aboutMedErrors.html

National Patient Safety Foundation. (2011). *About us.* Retrieved October 2, 2011, from http://www.npsf.org/about-us/mission-and-vision/

National Quality Forum. (2008). *National priorities and goals.* Retrieved November 5, 2011, from http://www.nationalprioritiespartnership.org/uploadedFiles/NPP/About_NPP/ExecSum_no_ticks.pdf

National Quality Forum. (2011a). *Mission and vision.* Retrieved May 20, 2012, from http://www.qualityforum.org/About_NQF/Mission_and_Vision.aspx

National Quality Forum. (2011b). *NQF national priorities partnership.* Retrieved November 6, 2011, from http://www.qualityforum.org/Setting_Priorities/NPP/National_Priorities_Partnership.aspx

National Quality Forum. (2011c). *NQF releases updated serious reportable events.* Retrieved November 7, 2011, from http://www.qualityforum.org/News_And_Resources/Press_Releases/2011/NQF_Releases_Updated_Serious_Reportable_Events.aspx

Pay for Performance: An Overview. (2011). *Healthcare economist.* Retrieved November 6, 2011, from http://healthcare-economist.com/2011/01/20/pay-for-performance-an-overview/

Thomas, E. J., Studdert, D. M, Newhouse, J. P., Zbar, B. I. W., Howard, K. M., Williams, E. J., & Brennan, T. A. (1999). Costs of medical injuries in Colorado and Utah in 1992. *Inquiry, 36*(3), 255–264.

Van Den Bos, J., Rustagi, K., Gray, T., Halford, M., Ziemkiewicz, E., & Shreve, J. (2011). The $17.1 billion problem: The annual cost of measurable errors. *Health Affairs, 30*(4), 596–603.

Walker, E. P. (2011). *Medicaid (AND Medicare) to quit paying for preventable events.* Retrieved November 6, 2011, from http://www.freerepublic.com/focus/f-news/2728495/posts

WHO Collaborating Centre for Patient Safety Solutions. (2008). *Patient safety solutions.* Retrieved May 20, 2012, from http://www.ccforpatientsafety.org/Patient-Safety-Solutions/

## BIBLIOGRAPHY

Karamchedu, M., Muppalla, S., & Capobianco, R. (2011). Moving beyond Medicare's ACOs to accountable care. *American Health & Drug Benefits, 4*(4), 204–206.

Barker, L. M., & Nussbaum, M. A. (2011). Fatigue, performance and the work environment: A survey of registered nurses. *Journal of Advanced Nursing, 67*(6), 1370–1382.

Burns, J. (2011). Are we finally getting serious about medical errors? *Managed Care, 20*(5), 23–28.

Chen, Y. (2011). Why are health care report cards so bad (good)? *Journal of Health Economics, 30*(3), 575–590.

Clarke, C. M., & Persaud, D. (2011). Leading clinical handover improvement: A change strategy to implement best practices in the acute care setting. *Journal of Patient Safety, 7*(1), 11–18.

Dudas, R., Bundy, D., Miller, M., & Barone, M. (2011). Can teaching medical students to investigate medication errors change their attitudes towards patient safety? *BMJ Quality & Safety, 20*(4), 319–325.

Hannawa, A. (2011). Shedding light on the dark side of doctor–patient interactions: Verbal and nonverbal messages physicians communicate during error disclosures. *Patient Education & Counseling, 84*(3), 344–351.

Helmchen, L. A., Richards, M. R., & McDonald, T. B. (2011). Successful remediation of patient safety incidents: A tale of two medication errors. *Health Care Management Review, 36*(2), 114–123.

McKinney, M. (2011). Going beyond saying you're sorry: More hospitals using quick remediation strategies following medical errors. *Modern Healthcare, 41*(13), 32–33.

Mészáros, K., Lopes, I., Goldsmith, P., & Knapp, K. (2011). Interprofessional education: Cooperation among osteopathic medicine, pharmacy, and physician assistant students to recognize medical errors. *Journal of the American Osteopathic Association, 111*(4), 213–218.

Milton, C. L. (2011). An ethical exploration of quality and safety initiatives in nurse practice. *Nursing Science Quarterly, 24*(2), 107–110.

Piper, L. E. (2011). The ethical leadership challenge: Creating a culture of patient- and family-centered care in the hospital setting. *Health Care Manager, 30*(2), 125–132.

Pepe, J., & Cataldo, P. (2011). Manage risk, build a just culture. *Health Progress, 92*(4), 56–60.

Agency for Healthcare Research and Quality. (2011). Public report cards prompt nursing homes to spend more on clinical services. *AHRQ Research Activities, 365*(15), 16.

Quality, Safety, and Education for Nurses. (2011). *About QSEN*. Retrieved November 6, 2011, from http://www.qsen.org/about_qsen.php

Samra, H. A., McGrath, J. M., & Rollins, W. (2011). Patient safety in the NICU: A comprehensive review. *Journal of Perinatal & Neonatal Nursing, 25*(2), 123–132.

Wang, J., Hockenberry, J., Chou, S., & Yang, M. (2011). Do bad report cards have consequences? Impacts of publicly reported provider quality information on the CABG market in Pennsylvania. *Journal of Health Economics, 30*(2), 392–407.

# Unit 4

# Legal and Ethical Issues

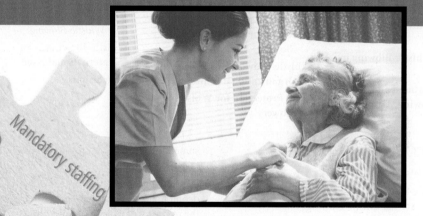

Mandatory staffing

Workplace violence

Entry into practice

## Chapter 16

# Whistle-Blowing in Nursing

Carol J. Huston

## ADDITIONAL RESOURCES

Visit thePoint for additional helpful resources
- eBook
- Journal Articles
- WebLinks

## LEARNING OBJECTIVES

*The learner will be able to:*

1. Define whistle-blowing and differentiate between internal and external whistle-blowing.

2. Identify conditions that should be met before whistle-blowing occurs, as well as situations in which whistle-blowing is clearly indicated.

3. Examine how cultural background may affect a nurse's willingness to blow the whistle on unsafe practices.

4. Identify risks and retaliatory consequences frequently experienced by whistle-blowers as a result of their actions.

5. Explore why reactions to whistle-blowers are often mixed and why the courage to speak out is something we honor more often in theory than in fact.

6. Differentiate among the consequentialist, deontological, and utilitarian viewpoints regarding the purposes of whistle-blowing.

7. Analyze how whistle-blowing could be considered a failure of organizational ethics.

8. Delineate strategies to create an organizational climate that both discourages the need for whistle-blowing and supports the whistle-blower when it is necessary for him or her to come forward.

9. Identify strategies that whistle-blowers should use to reduce the likelihood of retaliation and to reduce their legal liability.

10. Analyze existing and proposed federal and state legal protections for whistle-blowers.

11. Identify the process used by a whistle-blower to file a *qui tam* or whistle-blower lawsuit under the False Claims Act and the potential benefits of doing so.

12. Reflect on his or her willingness to assume the personal risks associated with whistle-blowing, should the need arise.

---

Watergate break-in...Enron and the artificial manipulation of energy prices...Martha Stewart and insider trading...WorldCom and accounting fraud...Bridgestone and Firestone tires...Dow Corning and silicone breast implants...Morgan Stanley and overcharging customers...fraudulent bank loans and artificial home price inflation. All of these high-profile cases, involving some degree of ethical malfeasance, have led the U.S. public to an increased sense of moral awareness about what is right and what is wrong. In addition, these cases have all come to the attention of the public as the result of *whistle-blowing*.

Lachman (2008) defines whistle-blowing in the nursing context as the "action taken by a nurse who goes outside the organization for the public's best interest when it is unresponsive to reporting the danger through the organization's proper channels" (p. 126). Similarly, the Free Online Dictionary (2011) defines a whistle-blower as "an informant who exposes wrongdoing within an organization in the hope of stopping it" (para. 2).

> **CONSIDER THIS** Virtually all definitions of whistle-blowing suggest the importance of advocating for others who may be harmed.

It is generally accepted that there are two types of whistle-blowing: internal and external. *Internal whistle-blowing* typically involves reporting concerns up the chain of command within an organization in the hope that whatever the problem is, it will be resolved. *External whistle-blowing* involves reporting concerns outside the organization and, in particular, to the media. In many cases, whistle-blowing becomes external only if inadequate action is taken at the organizational level to address the concerns of the whistle-blower. In some cases, however, whistle-blowing becomes external in an effort to embarrass an organization publicly or to seek financial redress.

> **DISCUSSION POINT**
>
> Is it ever appropriate to whistle-blow externally before attempting to resolve the problem internally?

In an era of managed care, declining reimbursements, and the ongoing pressure to remain fiscally solvent, the risk of fraud, misrepresentation, and ethical malfeasance in health care organizations has never been higher. As a result, the need for whistle-blowing has also likely never been greater.

This chapter explores the effect of "groupthink" on the likelihood that whistle-blowers will come forward. In addition, it presents select cases of whistle-blowing. Personal risks associated with whistle-blowing are described, as are the mixed feelings many individuals hold about whistle-blowing. Whistle-blowing is also explored as a failure of organizational ethics and strategies are identified to create an organizational climate that both discourages the need for whistle-blowing in the first place and supports the whistle-blower when it is necessary for him or her to come forward. Finally, legal protections for whistle-blowing are discussed.

> **CONSIDER THIS** "To see what is right, and not do it, is want of courage, or of principles."—Confucius

## GROUPTHINK AND WHISTLE-BLOWING

Being a whistle-blower takes great courage and self-conviction because it requires the whistle-blower to avoid *groupthink*—an inappropriate conformity to group norms. Going outside group norms often carries significant personal and professional risks. Unfortunately, these risks are more common than not, as whistle-blowers are more likely to be viewed as disloyal employees than courageous public servants (Boumil, Nariani, Boumil, & Berman, 2010).

For example, Colvin (2002) recounted how Sherron Watkins, an accountant, first blew the whistle on Enron's complex "special-purpose entities." She detailed them in a memo to Chief Executive Officer Ken Lay, her boss's boss's boss. She understood that something wrong was going on—something everyone else seemed to think was perfectly okay—and that public revelation would be disastrous.

What Colvin argued was most important in this scandal was that Watkins had access to the same facts as many other people inside Enron, yet somehow she was able to escape the groupthink that ensnared her colleagues. Soon after writing the memo, she identified herself as its author and met with Mr. Lay. When her memo eventually became public, the wrongness of what happened was apparent even internally (Colvin, 2002).

Colvin recounts a similar story at WorldCom, where Cynthia Cooper, another internal auditor, saw something that did not look right and took matters into her own hands. In this case, Cooper began investigating some of the company's capital expenditures and discovered bookkeeping entries that would eventually uncover what is likely the largest accounting fraud in U.S. history.

Faced with disturbing facts, Cooper discussed her findings with the company's controller and with Scott Sullivan, the chief financial officer. Sullivan tried to explain to her why costs that had previously been expensed were suddenly being capitalized. Then he asked her to stop the audit, which was being conducted early, and to put it off until the third quarter. She did not. Instead, she continued—and immediately went over her boss's head and called the chairman of the board's audit committee. He arranged to meet with her and the company's new auditor, KPMG. Two weeks later, WorldCom announced that it would restate earnings by US$3.9 billion—the largest restatement ever.

Again, Colvin (2002) suggested that the importance of Cooper's refusal to postpone her audit, as Sullivan had asked, is even greater than it may appear. Facts uncovered about the company, combined with the memo Sullivan wrote to the board in a last-ditch attempt to defend himself, show that if Cooper had "been a good soldier," the whole problem might have been concealed forever.

A similarly unsettling case was reported by Smith (2008), who profiled corporate whistle-blower Dana de Windt, a stockbroker at the financial services firm of Morgan Stanley. De Windt complained to government regulators that the company was cheating brokerage clients, having overcharged brokerage customers on 2,800 purchases of US$59 million of bonds. De Windt repeatedly confronted his bosses with "questions tucked inside a thick, three-ring binder" for more than 4 years, and management's response was simply for "him to get over it" (para 5). Finally, de Windt reported the situation to regulators, and in August 2007, Morgan Stanley settled the resulting complaint brought by the U.S. Securities and Exchange Commission (SEC) by paying a US$6.1-million fine.

Finally, Schulman (2007) presented the story of Leroy Smith, a safety manager at a federal prison in California, who exposed "hazardous conditions in a prison computer recycling program where inmates were smashing monitors with hammers, unleashing clouds of toxic metals" (para. 1), despite being threatened with termination and other types of retaliation. Although Smith eventually went on to be named "Public Servant of the Year" by the U.S. Office of Special Counsel (the federal agency charged with protecting government employees who expose waste, fraud, and abuse), his recognition ceremony was canceled at the last minute due to what Schulman called "ludicrous" reasons. In addition, things did not change at the prison as a result of the whistle-blowing. Smith concluded that his experience "was a beacon of false hope for public servants who are trying to correct wrongdoing," and Schulman agreed, noting that "given the current climate for whistle-blowers, false hope might be all the hope there is" (para. 3).

> CONSIDER THIS  Although the U.S. public wants corruption and unethical behavior to be unveiled, the individual reporting such behavior is often looked on with distrust and considered to be disloyal.

Indeed, Schulman (2007) alleged that "a series of court rulings, legal changes, and new security and secrecy policies have made it easier than at any time since the Nixon era to punish whistle-blowers" (para. 3). William Weaver, a professor of political science at the University of Texas-El Paso and a senior adviser to the National Security Whistle-blowers Coalition, agreed and stated that he now counsels federal employees against coming forward in any situation (Schulman, 2007). He said that he warns them that it will destroy their lives, cost them their families and friends, and squander their life savings on attorneys.

Perhaps the most frightening aspect of these four cases is that the responses by management at Enron, WorldCom, Morgan Stanley, and the California prison are not unique. Many organizations are aware of problem situations but choose to ignore them until a crisis occurs or the problem becomes public.

Some nurses take comfort in thinking that any moral professional would report substandard care. The reality, however, is often very different, and many professionals are torn between what they believe they should do and what they actually do. This is particularly disconcerting, and those who bear witness are required to overcome groupthink despite their moral distress. This is a primary reason why so many whistle-blowers delay in reporting their concerns outside the organization.

---

**DISCUSSION POINT**

Why is speaking out often honored more in theory than in fact?

---

**DISCUSSION POINT**

In the United States, there is some evidence that the events of September 11, 2011, have made people more public spirited and more inclined to blow the whistle. Do you think this inclination is driven more by fear or by a desire to promote public good?

---

## EXAMPLES OF WHISTLE-BLOWING IN NURSING

With the current nursing shortage, complaints about unsafe staffing and the use of unlicensed assistive personnel to perform nursing tasks outside their scope of practice are common. Worse yet, some nurses claim that they have been told to participate in illegal or unethical activities—things such as fraudulently altering medical records, falsifying insurance claims, and covering up the failure to meet mandated staffing ratios.

A review of the literature reveals multiple case studies of whistle-blowing by nurses. For example, in 2007, two nurses in Missouri blew the whistle on what they felt to be nursing home abuse and neglect of nursing home residents, which involved gross malpractice (McCranie, 2007). In addition, the nurses alleged that the nursing home operator was defrauding Medicare and Medicaid by providing essentially worthless care to the nursing home residents. According to the nurses, many of the patients suffered from "dehydration, weight loss, and preventable bed sores that eventually led to amputations," that "nursing home staffing was cut to unacceptable levels to save money" and that "other nurses misused patients' medicines, which were not locked securely" (McCranie, 2007, para. 2).

In a similarly disconcerting, high-profile whistle-blower case in New Mexico, six nurses at Memorial Medical Center in Las Cruces independently voiced concerns to their nurse managers over a 6-year period regarding inadequate and inappropriate care being given by an osteopathic physician on staff (Bitoun Blecher, 2001–2010). In addition, the nurses brought the alleged shortcomings of this particular doctor to the attention of other physicians. The doctor in this case was later accused of negligence and incompetence after one of her patients died from sepsis and another suffered a serious injury.

For reasons that are still unclear, however, the hospital failed to act on the nurses' complaints. Instead, the hospital challenged the nurses' actions and disciplined them, citing state regulations that forbid sharing patient information for any reason. The hospital also retaliated after the case was filed and the nurses agreed to testify against the doctor. One of the nurses retired and later heard that she had been blackballed by the institution, whereas a second nurse allegedly was offered a management position in the hospital after being identified as a potential witness for the hospital (Hook, 2001).

The American Nurses Association (ANA) responded by filing an *amicus curiae* ("friend of the court") brief on behalf of the nurses. This brief cited conflict and ambiguity in New Mexico law and urged the court to protect the nurses, who were exercising their ethical responsibility. The ANA argued that the application of the state regulation in question limited the ability of the nurse to report incompetent practice, which is a statutory mandate (Hook, 2001).

Tariman (2007) presented the story of Barry Adams, a registered nurse (RN) who blew the whistle on unsafe nurse staffing and its effect on patient care. Despite reporting his concerns to his supervisors and filing an official hazards report with the director of nursing at his institution, he received no response. He was then fired for an alleged insubordination. Fortunately, Adams had documented his actions, as well as the poor patient outcomes, including patient falls and medication errors. Adams was vindicated by the National Labor Relations Board when they ruled that he had been fired illegally for whistle-blowing (Tariman, 2007).

Similarly, Mason (2011) shared the recent story of two nurses, Anne Mitchell and Vicki Galle, who blew the whistle on a physician for a variety of charges including unprofessional conduct, via what they thought was a confidential report to the state board for medicine.

Instead of the physician being investigated, the nurses found themselves the target of unprofessional conduct charges brought by the local sheriff and county attorney, who were friends and business associates of the reported physician. In the end, the nurses who had a combined 47 years of experience at the hospital, were fired. The charges for Galle and Mitchell were eventually dropped and the sheriff, county attorney, and hospital administrator were indicted for retaliating against the whistle-blowers. Each faces six counts, including misuse of official information and retaliation, which are third-degree felonies (Sack, 2011). The nurses sued the county and settled for a shared US$750,000 (Sack, 2011).

Clearly, patient advocacy has a central role in nursing. So too does professional advocacy, through which nurses are committed to improving the practice of nursing and maintaining the integrity of the health care profession. Both advocacy roles suggest that the nurse is accountable for assuring that at least minimum standards are met. All of these cases depict nurses who believed that they were acting honorably in the role of patient advocate. Yet all suffered negative consequences, including job loss. Unfortunately, this is more common than not.

---

CONSIDER THIS   Advocacy is the foundation and essence of nursing, and nurses have a responsibility to promote human advocacy (Marquis & Huston, 2012).

---

It is important, however, to remember that whistle-blowing should never be considered the first solution to ethically troubling behavior. Indeed, it should be considered only after prescribed avenues of solving problems have been attempted. This is true, however, only if patients' lives are not at stake. In those cases, immediate action must be taken.

In addition, the employee should typically go up the chain of command in reporting his or her concerns. This process, however, must be modified when the immediate supervisor is the source of the problem (Lachman, 2008). In such a case, the employee might need to skip that level to see that the problem is addressed.

There are other general guidelines for blowing the whistle that should also be followed, including carefully documenting all attempts to address the problem and being sure to report facts and not personal interpretations. These guidelines, as well as others, are presented in Box 16.1.

## BOX 16.1   GUIDELINES FOR BLOWING THE WHISTLE

- Stay calm and think about the risks and outcomes before you act.

- Know your legal rights, because laws protecting whistle-blowers vary by state.

- First, make sure that there really is a problem. Check resources such as the medical library, the Internet, and institutional policy manuals to be sure.

- Seek validation from colleagues that there is a problem, but do not get swayed by groupthink into not doing anything if you should.

- Follow the chain of command in reporting your concerns, whenever possible.

- Confront those accused of the wrongdoing as a group whenever possible.

- Present just the evidence; leave the interpretation of facts to others. Remember that there may be an innocent or good explanation for what is occurring.

- Use internal mechanisms within your organization.

- If internal mechanisms do not work, use external mechanisms.

- Document carefully the problem that you have seen and the steps that you have taken to see that it is addressed.

- Do not expect thanks for your efforts.

*Source:* Bitoun Blecher, M. (2001–2010). *What color is your whistle?* Retrieved May 20, 2011, from http://www.minoritynurse.com/?q=workplace-issues/what-color-your-whistle; Myers, A. (2008b). How to blow the whistle safely? *Nursing Standard, 22*(25), 24.

## CULTURAL BACKGROUND AND WHISTLE-BLOWING

For some minority nurses, cultural issues further complicate whether a decision is made to blow the whistle and, if so, how it should be done. For example, "nurses with certain cultural backgrounds—for example, some Asians, Filipinos, and Africans—may be more reluctant to blow the whistle because they've been raised to respect a clear chain of command and hierarchy" (Bitoun Blecher, 2001–2010, para. 12). The same goes for nurses whose first language is not English. According to Winifred Carson, nurse practice counsel for the ANA, "They fear problems related to communication—whether they accurately communicate the magnitude of the problem and whether not speaking English as a first language would be used against them if they continue to challenge authority" (Bitoun Blecher, 2001–2010, para. 14).

Bitoun Blecher (2001–2010) suggested that "reporting incidents of wrongdoing in the workplace is always a risky business—but for minority nurses who blow the whistle, the stakes are even higher" (para. 1). Carson stated that minority nurses are more apt to be retaliated against, especially if they are working in nonminority settings (Bitoun Blecher, 2001–2010, para. 7).

## THE PERSONAL RISKS OF WHISTLE-BLOWING

Being a whistle-blower is not without risks. Indeed, it is filled with risks. Unfortunately, most whistle-blowers set out believing that their actions will be welcomed, only to discover that the problems raised go much deeper than they imagined and the personal consequences can be overwhelming. Such consequences include negative reactions from coworkers, losing one's job, and, in the extreme, legal retaliation. In many cases, whistle-blowers are fired from their jobs, especially those who are termed *at-will* employees.

Bitoun Blecher (2001–2010) concurs, noting an Australian survey of 95 nurses that suggested that there were severe repercussions for the 70 nurses who reported incidents of misconduct but few professional consequences for the 25 nurses who remained silent: "Fourteen percent of the whistle-blowers reported being treated as traitors, 16% received professional reprisals in the form of threats, 14% were rejected by peers, 11% were reprimanded, 9% were referred to a psychiatrist and 7% were pressured to resign" (para. 6).

CONSIDER THIS  Our culture still often labels whistle-blowers as "snitches," "moots," and "tattletales" (Hill, 2010, p. 8).

Peters et al.'s (2011) interviews with Australian nurses whose actions had been affirmed by whistle-blowers or who were whistle-blowers themselves also suggested that whistle-blowing brought about negative effects in virtually every aspect of their lives. The nurses shared such problems as tremendous and chronic distress, acute anxiety, flashbacks, nightmares, and disturbing thoughts. Peters et al. concluded that many nurse whistle-blowers were not prepared for the impact on their personal, emotional, physical, and professional welfare.

Research by Jackson et al. (2010) also revealed whistle-blowing to be highly stressful for nurses with whistle-blowers having to balance their need to act in accordance with a duty of care, the fear of repercussions, and the belief that no one would listen (See Research Study Fuels the Controversy 16.1).

In addition, Wilkes, Peters, Weaver, and Jackson (2011) noted that many whistle-blowers report negative impacts on their family life, including strained relationships with family members, dislocation of family life, and exposing family to public scrutiny. Wilkes et al. note that the harm caused to the nurses who blow the whistle is not restricted to one party but is echoed in family life as well.

Clearly, whistle-blowers should never assume that doing the right thing will protect them from retaliation. Instead, potential whistle-blowers should determine their legal duty for reporting and carefully research the specifics of their protection under the law. In addition, they should try to report anonymously when possible. Moreover, they must be prepared to defend their claims. In addition, prospective whistle-blowers should always at least try to solve problems internally before going public. When that is impossible and there is a clear indication of serious harm, they must document their actions and go public. They should also seek support and counsel before taking any steps.

It is clear, then, that whistle-blowers often face both social and work-related retaliation, and that at times this retaliation can be severe and life altering. Yet it must be noted that at least some self-satisfaction and pride must come with the recognition that unethical behavior has been exposed and that at least the potential for correction is possible because of the whistle-blower's actions. Box 16.2 summarizes some of the pros and cons of whistle-blowing.

## ETHICAL DIMENSIONS OF WHISTLE-BLOWING

Hook (2001) suggested that "although the average patient's immediate response to whistle-blowing would probably be a resounding 'hurrah!', whistle-blowing

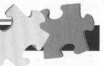

## RESEARCH STUDY FUELS THE CONTROVERSY 16.1

### THE EXPERIENCE OF WHISTLE-BLOWING

This research explored the reasons behind the decision to blow the whistle and provided insights into nurses' experiences of being whistle-blowers.

Jackson, D., Peter, K., Andrew, S., Edenbrough, M., Halcombe, E., Luck, L., . . . Wikles, L. (2010). Understanding whistleblowing: Qualitative insights from nurse whistleblowers. *Journal of Advanced Nursing, 66*(10), 2194–2201.

### STUDY FINDINGS

Using a qualitative narrative inquiry design, data were collected from 11 nurse whistle-blowers from a range of general and specialty clinical areas, using in-depth semistructured interviews. Participants reported whistle-blowing as highly stressful but believe they were acting in accordance with a duty of care. The findings were clustered into three main themes, namely, (1) reasons for whistle-blowing: *I just couldn't advocate*, (2) feeling silenced: *Nobody speaks out*, and (3) climate of fear: *You are just not safe.*

The researchers concluded that there is a need for greater clarity about the role nurses have as patient advocates. Furthermore, they suggested there is a need to develop clear guidelines that create opportunities for nurses to voice concerns and to ensure that health care systems respond in a timely and appropriate manner and a need to foster a safe environment in which to raise issues of concern.

### BOX 16.2    PROS AND CONS OF WHISTLE-BLOWING

**Pros**

- Protects patients
- Improves quality of care
- Meets professional expectations and standards
- Satisfies ethical duty
- Brings problems out into the open
- Provides validation of concerns and moral

**Cons**

- Poses personal and professional risks
- Casts doubt on motives
- Leads to possible job loss or employer retaliation
- Is typically a tiring, anxiety-producing, and often frustrating experience

can create considerable moral distress for nurses as they weigh the consequences of their actions against the duties of their profession" (para. 4). Clearly, nurses are bound to the role of patient advocacy by ethical codes of conduct and this requires them to safeguard patients from harm (Hill, 2010). The problem is that nurses also have professional commitments to their employer and to other health care professionals, and this loyalty to the employer can be misplaced when it leads to patient harm. The end result all too often then is a conflict between principles and duty. This tension between loyalty to employer and the need to protect patients is a major reason so many nurses delay in blowing the whistle.

Davis and Konishi (2007) discussed this moral conflict in their study of 24 Japanese nurses and viewed whistle-blowing as an act of the international nursing ethical ideal of advocacy, as well as in the larger context of professional responsibility. In this study, 10 of the nurses had previously reported another nurse and 12 had reported a physician for a wrongful act. Being direct and openly discussing sensitive topics is not valued in Japan because "such behavior disrupts the most fundamental value, harmony" (p. 194). In addition, whistle-blowing challenges long-held cultural values of group loyalty and "saving face." This requires Japanese nurses to make a professional judgment based on the perceived extent of potential harm to a patient and how the individual defines professional responsibility in the light of her or his advocacy function: "It could be considered irresponsible to report every witnessed act that could be viewed as wrong, just as it would be irresponsible not to report what is judged to be a serious wrongdoing" (p. 200).

Lachman (2008) suggested that the ethics of this divided loyalty can be viewed in relation to its moral purpose, whether that is to maximize the benefit and minimize the harm (a consequentialist view) or to fulfill a duty (a deontological Kantian view). If whistle-blowing is aimed at changing a situation for the better, the consequentialist moral framework becomes paramount. If whistle-blowing is viewed as the fulfillment of a duty to keep promises or protect patients, then the deontological framework becomes paramount. Hill (2010) agrees suggesting that Kantian (duty), virtue, and utilitarian ethical principles and theories justify whistle-blowing.

A strong argument can be made, however, for the precedence of the nurse's duty to the patient over his or her duty to the employer. Indeed, nurses must always remember that their primary professional responsibility is to their patients, not to their employers. As such, the need to uphold the rights of others, to promote fairness, and to provide for the greater good become paramount.

---

### DISCUSSION POINT

Can you think of a situation in which you have been involved in which *utilitarianism* (the greater good) would support not blowing the whistle on unethical behavior?

---

CONSIDER THIS   A whistle-blower must blow the whistle for the right reason for it to be a moral action.

---

The ANA *Code of Ethics for Nurses With Interpretive Statements* may also provide guidance for nurses who are considering becoming a whistle-blower. Provision 3 of the *Code of Ethics* states that the nurse "promotes, advocates for, and strives to protect the health, safety, and rights of the patient" (ANA, 2001, para. 25). In addition, Section 3.5 states:

> As an advocate for the patient, the nurse must be alert to and take appropriate action regarding any instances of incompetent, unethical, illegal, or impaired practice by a member of the health care team or the health care system, or any action on the part of others that places the rights or best interest of the patient in jeopardy. (para. 32)

Ethical codes of conduct from Canada, the United Kingdom, Australia, and Japan mandate similar action: "The Code of Ethics for nurses developed by the Japanese Nursing Association for both registered and licensed practical nurses notes: 'The nurse protects and safeguards individuals when their care is endangered or inhibited.' This can include whistle-blowing, although this word is not in the code" (Davis & Konishi, 2007, p. 195).

Such ethical codes bind nurses to the role of patient advocacy and compel them to take action when the rights or safety of patients are jeopardized. The bottom line is that although whistle-blowing can result in negative consequences for both the employing institution and the whistle-blower, nurses must uphold a professional standard and protect their patients. Perhaps that is why Lachman (2010) suggests that nurses who speak out against unethical, unlawful, or outdated practices must demonstrate moral courage.

## WHISTLE-BLOWING AS A FAILURE OF ORGANIZATIONAL ETHICS

Ethical organizations practice in such a way that patients and workers are protected from harm. Lachman (2008) argues then that whistle-blowing is indicative of ethical failure at the organizational level because the organization is failing to address accountability for the safety and welfare of the patients. The nurse or other employees feel compelled to take action against the wrongdoing in an effort to fulfill their professional obligations.

---

CONSIDER THIS   The motive of most whistle-blowers is advocacy, not troublemaking.

---

Myers (2008a) agreed, pointing out

*Every organization faces the risk that something can go seriously wrong, and whether this is caused by the rare case of deliberate malpractice or, as is more likely, because of substandard practice or a serious mistake, the people who are most likely to suspect it are those working in or for the relevant organization.* (p. 3)

It is imperative then that nurses working on the frontline be encouraged to speak up and that they be supported in their actions to do so. For example, nursing departments within hospitals should provide their nurses with an ethics committee chaired by a nurse with experience in bioethical issues (not one who has a vested interest in promoting administrative or hierarchical constraints). Nurse managers should promote the values inherent in patient advocacy, and the organization should openly support individuals who are willing to take the risk of being a whistle-blower. The reality is that if an employee is willing to go to the trouble and risk the repercussions of blowing the whistle, those concerns should be taken seriously and investigated.

General Secretary Peter Carter of the Royal College of Nursing agreed, suggesting that workplaces must strive to be more transparent so that nurses feel safe addressing problems. In addition, nurses should feel confident that all safety issues will be addressed immediately in a positive manner (Waters, 2008).

---

CONSIDER THIS   "One person can root out corruption and abuse of power. Once he understands this, he is redeemed and can break out of the trap of fear, and break free into the light of integrity and justice. That is the effect of seeing a brave whistle-blower stand up and win; it inspires the rest of us" (Scott Bloch, director of the Office of Special Counsel, as cited by Schulman, 2007, para. 1).

---

## LEGAL PROTECTION
## FOR WHISTLE-BLOWERS

There is no universal legal protection for whistle-blowers; however, under the 1st and 14th Amendments to the U.S. Constitution, state and local government officials are prohibited from retaliating against whistle-blowers. In addition,

*Although they do not fall under the category of "whistle-blower" protections, the laws protecting individual*

*employees from mistreatment in the workplace, such as Title VII of the Civil Rights Act or the Fair Labor Standards Act, also protect employees from retaliation for asserting their rights under those laws. For example, it is illegal to terminate an employee for reporting sexual harassment, or for challenging an employer's failure to pay overtime.* (Joseph and Herzfeld LLP, 2011, para. 13)

In addition, there is some whistle-blower protection at the state level. As of November 2011, however, only 21 states (Box 16.3) had passed some type of whistle-blower legislation, although a number of other states since that time, have at least introduced such legislation (ANA, 2011). The problem is that although some of these state laws prohibit retaliation, the standards for proving retaliation vary.

---

**BOX 16.3   STATES WITH WHISTLE-BLOWER PROTECTION AS OF NOVEMBER 2011**

Arizona (2003)
California (2003/2007)
Nevada (2002/2009)
Colorado (2007)
New Jersey (2006/2008)
Florida (2002)
New York (2002)
Georgia (2007)
Ohio (2001)
Hawaii (amended 2002)
Oregon (2001/2009)
Illinois (2003)
Texas (2007)
Indiana (2005)
Utah (2003)
Maine (2003/2007)
Vermont (2004/2008)
Maryland (2002)
Virginia (2003)
Michigan (2002)
West Virginia (2001)

*Source:* ANA (2011). *Whistle-blower protection.* Retrieved November 6, 2011, from http://ana. nursingworld.org/MainMenuCategories/ANA-PoliticalPower/State/StateLegislativeAgenda/ Whistleblower_1.aspx

For example, in Massachusetts,

*If an employee reports legitimate violations of policy or patient care standards, state law requires the employer to correct the violations and prohibits them from taking retaliatory action against the whistle-blower, including discharge, suspension, demotion, or denial of promotion. If these actions occur, the employee can report the employer to the attorney general's office, which may act on the public's behalf to protect the employee.* (Bitoun Blecher, 2001–2010, para. 53)

Joseph and Herzfeld LLP (2011) suggest, however, that employees in most states increase their likelihood of whistle-blower protection under general statutes or common law if they meet criteria similar to those established at the federal level: (1) They must be acting in good faith that the employer or its employees are breaking the law in some way, (2) they must complain about that violation either to the employer or to an outside agency, (3) they must refuse to be a party to the violation, and (4) they should be willing to assist in any official investigations of the violation.

---

### DISCUSSION POINT

What whistle-blowing protections, if any, exist in the state where you live? Is any legislation pending?

---

## The False Claims Act

Some whistle-blower legislation has been enacted at the federal level, however, to encourage people to report wrongdoings. One such piece of legislation is the False Claims Act (FCA), originally a Civil War statute, which encourages whistle-blowers to come forward regarding fraud committed against the federal government and to file a lawsuit seeking lost monies in the government's name.

The individual would file a *qui tam* or whistle-blower lawsuit and provide knowledge that a person defrauded the government (Hill, 2010). "In the United States qui tam whistle-blowers (also known as 'relators') are private citizens empowered with the right, as well as an economic incentive, to hire counsel and assume the position of law enforcement in matters involving alleged fraud against the government" (Boumil et al., 2010, p. 19). In the 7-year period following the revision of the

FCA in 1986, more than 1,000 qui tam lawsuits were filed, with settlements, verdicts, and fines totaling more than US$1 billion (Boumil et al., 2010).

For example, a whistle-blower may have knowledge of a colleague inappropriately billing Medicare or Medicaid. The FCA provides protection for government whistle-blowers, thereby prohibiting employers from punishing employees who report the fraud or assist in the investigation of the fraud. If the whistle-blower is dismissed or discriminated against in any way as a result of the lawsuit, the whistle-blower can file a claim against that employer for unlawful retaliation.

To have a case brought to trial under federal law, the whistle-blower must first exhaust his or her internal chain of command and then file a complaint with the Department of Health and Human Services (DHHS). If the DHHS decides that the complaint is valid, the government proceeds with litigation against the employer, and the whistle-blower receives a percentage of the damages awarded. The case discussed earlier in this chapter involving the two nurses in Missouri who alleged nursing home abuse and fraud was a False Claims Act *qui tam* lawsuit.

One of the best known cases involving the FCA involved four health care professionals who opened a home infusion company known as Ven-A-Care in the Florida Keys (Taylor, 2001). The company provided care to terminally ill patients who had acquired immunodeficiency syndrome (AIDS). A large national chain, National Medical Care (NMC) approached Ven-A-Care about becoming a partner. Ven-A-Care refused because they believed NMC was using fraudulent schemes as part of their business practices. As a result, NMC countered by offering allegedly illegal incentives to local physicians to refer their patients to its Key West clinic, and Ven-A-Care was forced out of business as a result (Taylor, 2001).

One of Ven-A-Care's owners contacted government regulators in 1991 about NMC's business practices, but no action was taken. In June 1994, Ven-A-Care filed a civil whistle-blower suit against NMC in Miami. The case was later transferred to the U.S. Attorney's office in Boston. The end result was that NMC was partly dismantled, sold, and absorbed by German dialysis giant Fresenius. Fresenius paid the U.S. Justice Department US$486 million in civil and criminal fines to settle Ven-A-Care's civil whistle-blower lawsuit. At least three top NMC executives pleaded guilty to criminal kickback and conspiracy charges and received prison sentences and fines, and three NMC divisions pleaded guilty to criminal fraud and kickback charges and were excluded from Medicare and Medicaid programs. None of the

Key West doctors ever faced charges for their role in the NMC scheme there. Under the federal FCA, Ven-A-Care and its partners were entitled to a US$40 million recovery (Taylor, 2001).

A different whistle-blower suit was brought by the four Ven-A-Care partners in 1995 in Miami federal court against more than 20 pharmaceutical companies (Taylor, 2001). This suit alleged that drug manufacturers manipulated the benchmark price Medicare uses to reimburse doctors for administering a relatively small number of drugs. That standard, known as the *average wholesale price*, is set and reported by the drug manufacturers and bears little resemblance to the average selling price of a drug.

The suit alleged that drug companies set an artificially high average wholesale price to encourage doctors who administer medications to patients with cancer, hemophilia, or AIDS to prescribe their drugs. Then physicians were encouraged to bill government health programs at 95% of average wholesale price, guaranteeing a huge built-in profit. Through that practice, called "marketing the spread," physicians stood to gain hundreds of dollars in profits per dose just for administering a drug, whereas the drug companies gained a captive market share and fat profits (Taylor, 2001).

The end result was a US$14 million settlement with New Haven, Connecticut–based drug giant Bayer Corporation. The suit rocked the pharmaceutical industry and further stirred outrage in Congress and among consumer groups about high prescription-drug prices and illegal marketing practices. It was the first of an expected 20 settlements, and it took more than 5 years from the time the suit was filed until the first drug company settled (Taylor, 2001).

A more recent case in which a *qui tam* lawsuit was filed occurred when a former employee at a nursing home in Tennessee filed a lawsuit after he was fired for pointing out instances of Medicare and Medicaid fraud at the nursing home (Rosenfeld, 2011). The employee alleged that the nursing home was double-billing for some patient services as well as billing Medicare and Medicaid for the care of unqualified patients. Vanguard denied any wrongdoing but did pay back US$2 million as compensation for the amount it allegedly overbilled the federal health care systems (Rosenfeld, 2011).

Because the FCA has been fairly effective in detecting fraud at the federal level, state versions of the FCA have also passed. Under these state laws, whistle-blowers can file lawsuits seeking lost monies in the state or local government's name and share in the proceeds.

Weaknesses in the federal law, however, have come to light. Zeller (2008) stated that the FCA does not apply to subcontractors, only to companies dealing directly with the government. This prompted two senior members of the House Judiciary Committee to introduce a companion bill in 2008 to add subcontractors to the legislation in an effort to modernize the law. Immediately, trade groups spoke up against making the change, arguing that this change would raise costs and discourage contractors from working with the government due to fears of unfounded claims by whistle-blowers. Sponsors of the bill argued that contractors only need to play by the rules to avoid penalties and that "some contractors have gotten a free ride when courts threw out cases involving subcontractors or barred testimony from whistle-blowers because they weren't privy to specific details of billing documentation" (Zeller, 2008, para. 7).

In contrast, a Supreme Court ruling in 2008 narrowed the application of the False Claims Act, limiting the liability of those who do not bill the government directly but go through another entity that contracts with the United States (Sorrel, 2008). "Justices clarified that the plaintiffs must show that the defendants intended to defraud the U.S. and not another entity, and that alleged false statements were relevant to the government's decision to pay the claim" (Sorrel, 2008, para. 5). In other words, it is not enough to show that government money was involved in fraud; plaintiffs must show there was fraud against the government to obtain government funds. Some legal experts say the decision could make it more difficult for whistle-blowers to prove certain cases using the false claims statute as opposed to other state or federal antifraud remedies (Sorrel, 2008).

## Other Federal Legislation Related to Whistle-Blowing

Another piece of legislation, the Whistleblower Protection Act of 1989, protects federal employees who disclose government fraud, abuse, and waste. The Whistleblower Protection Enhancement Act of 2007 extended the Whistleblower Protection Act of 1989 to federal employees who specialize in national security issues. In addition, the Paul Revere Freedom to Warn Act protects federal employee whistle-blowers who speak out about abuse, harassment, and unethical behavior in the workplace (Hill, 2010).

The National Labor Relations Act might protect employees in the private sector from retaliation when employees act as a group to modify working conditions or ask for better wages. The best protection for nongovernmental employees in the United States at this time, however, is likely the Sarbanes-Oxley Act of 2002. This act dramatically redesigned federal regulation of public company corporate governance and reporting obligations and provided some protection for whistle-blowers who report fraud in publicly traded companies to the proper authorities (Occupational Safety and Health Administration, 2006).

Employees in these companies who experience retaliation for whistle-blowing have 90 days to file a written complaint with OSHA: "If the evidence supports an employee's claim of retaliation and a settlement cannot be reached, OSHA will issue an order requiring the employer to reinstate the employee, pay back wages" (Occupational Safety and Health Administration, 2006, para. 11). After OSHA issues its final ruling, either party may request a full hearing before an administrative law judge of the Department of Labor. That decision can then be appealed to the Department's Administrative Review Board for final review.

## WHISTLE-BLOWING AS AN INTERNATIONAL ISSUE

Whistle-blowing cases involving nurses are not limited to the United States. Myers (2008a) recounted the story of significant failings in infection control (an outbreak of *Clostridium difficile*) that caused, or probably caused, at least 90 deaths at Maidstone and Tunbridge Wells NHS Trust, Kent, England. The 2007 investigation found that although clinical staff reportedly raised concerns about the spreading infection, no effective action was taken. In short, the nurses' concerns went unheeded.

Indeed, a recent survey of 752 nurses by *Nursing Standard* and the whistle-blowing charity Public Concern at Work revealed that the number one reason that nurses cited for not raising a patient safety concern was that nothing would be done (Waters, 2008). The frustrating part of this is that 68% of these nurses had serious concerns about patient safety during the last 3 years. Of these, 87% said that they had reported their concerns, usually to their line managers. Only 29% of respondents thought that their manager had handled their concerns well and that patient risks had been addressed or resolved properly; 47% thought that the issues were handled "badly" and that safety concerns were overlooked; and 23% of those who had reported safety issues thought that the risks they identified went on to harm patients (Waters, 2008).

Another report from England highlights not only the difficulty that whistle-blowers face in changing bad situations but also the personal consequences they often suffer as a result of their whistle-blowing. Scott (2008) told the story of Moi Ali, a nurse who exposed how pedophile nurses escaped punishment in the United Kingdom. As a result of her whistle-blowing, she was "pressured to quit" two top jobs, one as a board member of NHS Lothian and the second as vice president of the nurses' regulatory body—the Nursing and Midwifery Council (Scott, 2008, para. 3). Ali asserted that she was asked to leave both positions because her superiors felt that "her whistle-blowing had impacted her position." Her superiors responded that the decisions to resign were entirely her own.

A similar story comes from yet another country. In November 2002, four nurses in New South Wales, Australia, went public with their concerns about how clinical incidents were managed and patient safety at two hospitals (Johnstone, 2005). Eight months later, the same thing happened in Queensland, when "Toni Hoffman, the charge nurse of the intensive care unit at Bundaberg Base Hospital, raised serious concerns about the practices of a newly appointed surgeon, Dr Jayant Patel" (Johnstone, 2005, p. 8). She believed that the surgeon's practice was placing patients at unacceptable risk of preventable adverse events, including death. After 2 years of trying to address the problem within the hospital, she went public with her concerns: "What has since been described as a 'medical scandal' of unprecedented dimensions in Australia, suddenly emerged as front-page news here and around the world, again highlighting the role and responsibility of nurses as advocates for patient safety and quality care" (Johnstone, 2005, p. 8).

In both Australian cases, the nurses took their concerns about patient safety and quality of care repeatedly to management and were ignored. In addition, nurses in both cases reported high levels of intimidation after reporting their concerns to the appropriate authorities and were dissuaded from speaking freely at inquiries established to investigate the issues. Finally, in both cases, there was an apparent failure of whistle-blower laws to protect the nurses (Johnstone, 2005).

---

CONSIDER THIS   That nurses have had to resort to whistle-blowing "to try and remedy a serious wrong detected in the course of their work is a travesty, not only of the principles and practice of good clinical governance and clinical risk management, but also of justice" (Johnstone, 2005, p. 8).

The lack of protection for whistle-blowers then is a global problem. In fact, Company Law ("Company Law," 2010) notes that while whistle-blowing has gained advocates and acceptance as an organizational control strategy internationally, legislative bodies in other countries have taken a variety of approaches to whistle-blowing.

One approach has been the United Kingdom's Public Interest Disclosure Act, which passed in July 1998 and was fully implemented by 2001. Under this act, whistle-blower disclosures to employers, regulatory bodies, and the media are protected from retaliation. Employers who retaliate may be subject to unlimited compensation in fines. This is because whistle-blowers are viewed as witnesses acting in the public interest. The burden of proof, however, is on the employee to show that the disclosure was protected and that the disclosure was the reason for dismissal (Goldman & Lewis, 2007).

The law was tested in 2011 when Shanta Sangraula, president of the Nepalese Nurses Association UK, was dismissed by the owners of the Whitefriars Nursing Home in Southall after she raised concerns about abuse of elderly residents by colleagues and poor administration of medicines (Ford, 2011). An employment tribunal in Watford ruled that the care home's actions had been unreasonable and that Sangraula had raised her concerns in good faith. She was awarded £15,000 for unfair dismissal (Ford, 2011).

In addition, the Royal College of Nursing (RCN, 2009) launched a dedicated telephone line and website in 2009 to allow RCN members to share in confidence any serious and immediate worries they had regarding patient safety in their workplaces. This action was the result of a survey of more than 5,000 RCN members that showed that 78% of respondents said they would be concerned about victimization, personal reprisals, or a negative effect on their career if they were to report concerns to their employers. While "99% of registered nurses understood their professional responsibility to report worries about patient safety, fears about personal reprisals meant that only 43% would be confident to report concerns without thinking twice" (RCN, 2009, para. 6).

Boumil et al. (2010) suggest, however, that international adoption of legislation such as the False Claims Act or qui tam laws would do much to expose fraud and increase the protection for whistle-blowers from retaliation globally. Such legislation would, however,

> require a political and legal infrastructure that encourages and rewards individuals to come forward and perform as a surrogate police force to enforce a matter of great concern to the public's health. At present, some are closely scrutinizing the US False Claims Act, but so far there is little movement toward widespread embracing of its methodology. (p. 27)

Company Law ("Company Law," 2010) disagrees, suggesting that better whistle-blower legislation will do little to solve the problem since such laws are flawed through exemptions and built-in weaknesses. Company Law argues that such laws only give the illusion of protection since they generally come into play only after disclosures have been made and reprisals have begun. In addition, as a result of such legislation, whistle-blowers may put their trust in law rather than developing the skills they need to achieve their goals more directly.

---

### DISCUSSION POINT

Would international adoption of legislation similar to the False Claims Act increase the likelihood that whistle-blowers will both come forward and be protected from recrimination globally?

---

### CONCLUSIONS

Nurses as health care professionals have a responsibility to uncover, openly discuss, and condemn short-cuts that threaten the clients they serve. Clearly, however, there has been a collective silence in many such cases. The reality is that whistle-blowing offers no guarantee that the situation will change or the problem will improve, and the literature is replete with horror stories regarding negative consequences endured by whistle-blowers. The whistle-blower cannot even trust that other health care professionals with similar belief systems about advocacy will value their efforts because the public's feelings about whistle-blowers are so mixed. In addition, state laws vary and protections for the nongovernment employee whistle-blower are often limited.

For all these reasons, it takes tremendous courage to come forward as a whistle-blower. It also takes a tremendous sense of what is right and what is wrong, as well as a commitment to follow a problem through until an acceptable level of resolution is reached. Whistle-blowers are heroes and should be treated as such; their courage is nothing short of exceptional. How unfortunate that we frequently do not treat them that way.

# FOR ADDITIONAL DISCUSSION

**1.** Why do Americans have a "love–hate" relationship with whistle-blowers? Is this dichotomy prevalent in other countries as well?

**2.** Which is greater for you personally—your duty to your patients, your duty to your employer, or your duty to yourself? How do you sort out what you should do when these duties are in conflict?

**3.** Do you believe that most whistle-blowing must be external before appropriate action is taken?

**4.** Should whistle-blowers receive compensation under the False Claims Act?

**5.** Would you be willing to bear the risks of becoming a whistle-blower?

**6.** Do you believe that there is more, less, or the same amount of whistle-blowing in health care as in other types of industries?

**7.** Can you identify a whistle-blowing situation in which it might be appropriate to go outside the chain of command in reporting concerns about organizational practice?

# REFERENCES

American Nurses Association. (2001). *Code of ethics for nurses with interpretive statements*. Washington, DC: Author. Retrieved April 30, 2005, from http://www.nursingworld.org/ethics/code/protected_nwcoe303.htm

American Nurses Association. (2011). *Whistleblower protection*. Retrieved May 20, 2012, from http://ana.nursingworld.org/MainMenuCategories/ANAPoliticalPower/State/StateLegislativeAgenda/Whistleblower_1.aspx

Bitoun Blecher, M. (2001–2010). *What color is your whistle?* Minoritynurse.com. Retrieved November 7, 2011, from http://www.minoritynurse.com/features/nurse_emp/05-03-02c.html

Boumil, S., Nariani, A., Boumil, M., & Berman, H. (2010). Whistleblowing in the pharmaceutical industry in the United States, England, Canada, and Australia. *Journal of Public Health Policy, 31*(1), 17–29.

Colvin, G. (2002). Wonder women of whistleblowing. *Fortune, 146*(3). Retrieved May 20, 2012, from http://money.cnn.com/magazines/fortune/fortune_archive/2002/08/12/327047/index.htm

Company Law—Whistleblower concept in India with respect to US and UK Laws: A comparison. (2010, August 28). *Free law projects*. Retrieved November 14, 2011, from http://lawprojectsforfree.blogspot.com/2010/08/company-law-whistleblower-concept-in.html

Davis, A. E., & Konishi, E. (2007). Whistleblowing in Japan. *Nursing Ethics, 14*(2), 194–202.

Ford, S. (2011, October). Whistleblowing nurse wins £15,000 payout after unfair dismissal. *Nursingtimes.net*. Retrieved November 15, 2011, from http://www.nursingtimes.net/nursing-practice/clinical-specialisms/management/whistleblowing-nurse-wins-15000-payout-after-unfair-dismissal/5036046.article

The Free Online Dictionary. (2011). *Whistleblower* (Definition). Retrieved November 7, 2011, from http://www.thefreedictionary.com/whistleblower

Goldman, L., & Lewis, J. (2007). Blowing the whistle. *Occupational Health, 59*(11), 16–17.

Hill, T. (2010). Whistleblowing: The patient or the paycheck? *Kansas Nurse, 85*(2), 4–8.

Hook, K. (2001, Fall). Toward an ethical defense of whistleblowing. *American Nurses Association: Ethics and Human Rights Issues Update, 1*(2). Retrieved April 30, 2005, from http://www.ana.org/ethics/update/vol1no2a.htm

Jackson, D., Peters, K., Andrew, S., Edenbrough, M., Halcombe, E., Luck, L., ... Wikles, L. (2010, October). Understanding whistleblowing: Qualitative insights from nurse whistleblowers. *Journal of Advanced Nursing, 66*(10), 2194–2201.

Johnstone, M. J. (2005). Issues: Whistleblowing and accountability. *Australian Nursing Journal, 13*(5), 8.

Joseph and Herzfeld LLP. (2011). *Whistleblower and Sarbanes Oxley claims*. Retrieved November 7, 2011, from http://www.jhllp.com/lawyer-attorney-1324989.html

Lachman, V. D. (2008). Whistleblowers: Troublemakers or virtuous nurses? *Medsurg Nursing, 17*(2), 126–128, 134.

Lachman, V. D. (2010, September). Strategies necessary for moral courage. *Online Journal of Issues in Nursing, 15*(3). Retrieved November 16, 2011, from http://nursingworld.org/MainMenuCategories/AN-AMarketplace/ANAPeriodicals/OJIN/TableofContents/Vol152010/No3-Sept-2010/Strategies-and-Moral-Courage.html

Marquis, B., & Huston, C. (2012). *Leadership roles and management functions in nursing* (6th ed.). Philadelphia, PA: Lippincott Williams & Wilkins.

Mason, D. J. (2011). *Public officials indicted in RN whistleblowing case.* Retrieved November 6, 2011, from http://centerforhealthmediapolicy.com/2011/01/14/public-officials-indicted-in-rn-whistleblowing-case/

McCranie, F. (2007). *Nursing home abuse and fraud exposed by nurses in Qui Tam whistleblower case.* Retrieved November 14, 2011, from http://www.whistleblowerlawyerblog.com/2007/06/nursing_home_abuse_and_fraud_e.html

Myers, A. (2008a). Whistleblowing saves lives. *Nursing Management—UK, 15*(3), 3.

Myers, A. (2008b). How to blow the whistle safely. *Nursing Standard, 22*(25), 24.

Occupational Safety and Health Administration. (2006). *OSHA fact sheet: Filing whistleblower complaints under the Sarbanes-Oxley Act.* Retrieved November 14, 2011, from http://www.osha.gov/Publications/osha-factsheet-sox-act.pdf

Peters, K., Luck, L., Hutchinson, M., Wilkes, L., Andrew, S., & Jackson, D. (2011). The emotional sequelae of whistleblowing: Findings from a qualitative study. *Journal of Clinical Nursing, 20*(19/20), 2907–2914.

Rosenfeld, J. (2011, November 22). *Nursing home operator to reimburse government for double billing.* Retrieved May 20, 2012, from http://www.nursinghomesabuseblog.com/whistleblower-qui-tam-claims/nursing-home-operator-to-reimburse-government-for-double-billing/

Royal College of Nursing. (2009, May 11). *RCN launches phone line to support whistleblowing nurses.* Retrieved November 6, 2011, from https://www.rcn.org.uk/newsevents/news/article/uk/rcn_launches_phone_line_to_support_whistleblowing_nurses

Sack, K. (2011, January 14). Sheriff charged in Texas whistle-blowing case. *New York Times.* Retrieved November 7, 2011, from http://www.nytimes.com/2011/01/15/us/15nurses.html?_r=1

Schulman, D. (2007). Office of Special Counsel's war on whistleblowers. *Mother Jones.* Retrieved August 17, 2008, from http://www.motherjones.com/news/feature/2007/05/dont_whistle_while_you_work.html

Scott, M. (2008). *NHS whistleblower Moi Ali forced to quit over nurse row.* Retrieved August 17, 2008, from http://www.sundaymail.co.uk/news/newsfeed/2008/06/29/nhs-whistleblower-moi-ali-forced-to-quit-over-nurse-row-78057-20624687/

Smith, R. (2008, May 24). A Morgan Stanley crusader; Bond-pricing issues prompt one broker's inside investigation. *Wall Street Journal (Eastern edition),* p. B1. Retrieved May 20, 2012, from http://online.wsj.com/article/SB121158398445518845.html

Sorrel, A. L. (2008). *Supreme Court tightens scope of False Claims Act.* Retrieved August 21, 2008, from http://www.ama-assn.org/amednews/2008/07/28/gvsa0728.htm

Tariman, J. D. (2007). Straight talk: When should you blow the whistle for ethical reasons? *ONS Connect, 22*(2), 22–23.

Taylor, M. (2001). Four found whistleblowing the best revenge. *Modern Healthcare, 31*(24), 32–34.

Waters, A. (2008, June). Blowing the whistle. *Nursing Management—UK, 15*(3), 7.

Wilkes, L. M., Peters, K., Weaver, R., & Jackson, D. (2011). Nurses involved in whistleblowing incidents: Sequelae for their families. *Collegian, 18*(3), 101–106.

Zeller, S. (2008, June 30). Whistleblowing pay hike? Updating a Civil War law to help whistleblowers. *CQWeekly-Vantage Point,* p. 1746. Retrieved May 20, 2012, from http://library.cqpress.com/cqweekly/document.php?id=weeklyreport110-000002908705&%20type=toc&num=161&

## BIBLIOGRAPHY

Abbasi, K. (2011). A way forward for whistleblowing. *Journal of the Royal Society of Medicine, 104*(7), 275.

Bjorkelo, B., Einarsen, S., & Matthiesen, S. (2010). Predicting proactive behaviour at work: Exploring the role of personality as an antecedent of whistleblowing behaviour. *Journal of Occupational & Organizational Psychology, 83*(Part 2), 371–394.

Black, P. (2010). Breaking taboo: Dilemma of whistleblowing. *British Journal of Nursing (BJN), 19*(1), 5.

Bolsin, S., Pal, R., Wilmshurst, P., & Pena, M. (2011). Whistleblowing and patient safety: The patient's or the profession's interests at stake? *Journal of the Royal Society of Medicine, 104*(7), 278–282.

Braillon, A. (2010). Whistleblowing: Neither reward, nor protection. *Journal of Public Health Policy, 31*(2), 278–279.

Fagan, J. (2011). If whistleblowing was easy, it would happen. *Nursing Times, 107*(15–16), 9.

Gallagher, A. (2010). Whistleblowing: What influences nurses' decisions on whether to report poor practice? *Nursing Times, 106*(4), 22–25.

Grainger, M. (2011). Whistleblowing: Is it worth it? *British Journal of Nursing (BJN), 20*(12), 775.

Jackson, D., Peters, K., Andrew, S., Edenborough, M., Halcomb, E., Luck, L., . . . Wilkes, L. (2010). Trial and retribution: A qualitative study of whistleblowing and workplace relationships in nursing. *Contemporary Nurse: A Journal for the Australian Nursing Profession, 36*(1/2), 34–44.

Jane, D. (2011, November 5). *Undesirable effects of whistleblowing*. Retrieved November 6, 2011, from http://nursingcrib.com/news-blog/undesirable-effects-of-whistleblowing/

Mansbach, A., & Bachner, Y. (2010). Internal or external whistleblowing: Nurses' willingness to report wrongdoing. *Nursing Ethics, 17*(4), 483–490.

Moore, L., & McAuliffe, E. (2010). Is inadequate response to whistleblowing perpetuating a culture of silence in hospitals? *Clinical Governance: An International Journal, 15*(3), 166–178.

Qui tam changes may bring more fraud suits. (2010). *Healthcare Risk Management, 32*(1), 8–9.

Reid, J. (2010). The NHS must support staff to speak out against poor practice. *Nursing Times, 106*(43), 9.

Salcido, R. (2010). Qui tam: False Claims Act. *Advances in Skin & Wound Care, 23*(11), 487.

West, F. (2011). Whistleblowing at work. *Nursing in Practice: The Journal for Today's Primary Care Nurse, 61*, 18.

Whitehead, B., & Barker, D. (2010). Does the risk of reprisal prevent nurses blowing the whistle on bad practice? *Nursing Times, 106*(43), 12–15.

# Chapter 17

# Impaired Nursing Practice
## *What Are We Doing About It?*

Jennifer Lillibridge

## ADDITIONAL RESOURCES

Visit the Point for additional helpful resources
- eBook
- Journal Articles
- WebLinks

## CHAPTER OUTLINE

## LEARNING OBJECTIVES

*The learner will be able to:*

1. Examine the prevalence of substance abuse in the nursing profession and compare this prevalence with that in the other health care professions.

2. Reflect on possible reasons for the inadequacy of current empirical research studies examining chemical impairment in nursing.

3. Describe early risk factors that result in an increased risk for chemical addiction in the nursing profession.

4. Explore why the early identification of risk factors and substance misuse increases the likelihood of successful intervention and treatment of the impaired nurse.

5. Identify common behaviors and actions that might signify chemical impairment in an employee or colleague.

6. Analyze how personal feelings, values, and biases regarding chemical impairment might alter a colleague's or manager's ability to confront and/or help the chemically impaired employee.

7. Explore reasons why nurses with substance abuse problems often fail to receive the same caring attitude or approach from their peers that is extended to other individuals who misuse drugs and alcohol.

8. Identify State Board of Nursing reporting requirements for nurses suspected of chemical dependency or of diverting drugs for personal use.

9. Describe typical components of a state diversion program, as well as a "return to work" contract, for a chemically impaired nurse.

10. Identify the driving forces that compelled most State Boards of Nursing in the United States to move from mandatory disciplinary action for impaired nurses to diversion program treatment.

11. Reflect on personal feelings regarding the extent to which a State Board of Nursing has the right and/or responsibility to invade the impaired nurse's privacy to ensure recovery is ongoing.

"Helping the impaired nurse is difficult but not impossible. The choices for action are varied. The only choice that is clearly wrong is to do nothing" (National Council of State Boards of Nursing [NCSBN], 2001, p. iv). Definitions of impaired practice vary, but most include that professional judgment is impaired due to the use of drugs or alcohol (or mental illness) and this interferes with the ability of the health professional to provide quality, safe nursing care.

The problem of impaired nursing practice has plagued nursing for decades; however, it continues to remain both poorly researched and poorly understood. Several explanations for the lack of recent research and the continuation of the problem can be found: (1) nurses find it difficult to talk openly about and report a situation in which "one of their own" may be engaging in behavior that puts them and their patients at risk, (2) nurses are reluctant to self-disclose a substance abuse problem due to the stigma, and (3) there is a lack of federal funding to research impaired nursing practice. In addition, the NCSBN (Darbro, 2011) suggests that stigma and negative stereotyping leads to underreporting, as well as "the tendency to protect or ignore workplace indicators of problem behaviors" (p. 42).

A discussion about impaired nursing practice often raises more questions than it answers. Two key issues surround impaired nursing practice. The first is concern for patient safety. The second is concern for the health of the impaired nurse. With denial common, the problem can go without detection or treatment for years. When nurses divert drugs for personal use and make poor, often critical judgments while providing care to the vulnerable, the risk for harm to patients is high (Epstein, Burns, & Conlon, 2010; Talbert, 2009).

Without wanting to discount the individual nurse with a substance abuse problem, patient safety is at the forefront of national considerations about professional nursing practice and the future of nursing (Finkelman & Kenner, 2009; Quality & Safety in the Education of Nurses [QSEN], 2011). Given this agenda, it seems critical that preventing impaired practice and dealing with it when it does happen should be inclusive in all discussions about patient safety. Talbert (2009) emphasizes that "substance abuse among nurses is a problem that threatens the delivery of quality care and professional standards of nursing" (p. 17). Although a literature search revealed limited new research since 2009 on the topic of impaired nurses/health care professionals, summaries of the issue, discussion articles, anecdotal pieces, and evidence-based care sheets keep this topic alive and warranting our attention (Bettinardi-Angres & Bologeorges, 2011; Monroe & Kenaga, 2010; Pinto & Schub, 2010; Talbert, 2009).

## PREVALENCE OF THE PROBLEM

Estimates on the prevalence of chemical dependency in the nursing profession are varied; efforts to quantify the prevalence are fraught with problems. It has been suggested that the difficulty may be due in part to the fact that self-disclosure is reduced due to the stigma associated with substance abuse (Monroe & Kenaga, 2010). The NCSBN estimation of prevalence of nurses suffering from addiction to drugs and/or alcohol is 16% (NCSBN, 2010). Another estimate suggests that "between 10 and 20 percent of nurses will have a substance abuse problem at some point in their lives" ("I Think," 2011, p. 24). Pinto and Schub (2010) estimate the problem to be approximately 10% to 15% for health care professionals generally. However, there continues to be no recently published large-scale prevalence studies on substance abuse in the nursing profession and many of the estimations are based on substance abuse in the general population, then looking at women within that group as the profession is largely composed of women.

Previously, it has been suggested that prevalence is not as important as patterns of abuse among health professionals, such as physicians and nurses. Although patterns of abuse may still be important, current thinking in the profession is more along the lines of whether the nurse can practice safely ("I Think," 2011). With this perspective, the behavior of the nurse becomes the issue and whether the nurse is making safe, appropriate decisions in the provision of quality patient care.

CONSIDER THIS  If 10% to 15% of nurses have a substance use problem, every nurse will likely work with chemically impaired colleagues at some time during his or her nursing career.

## OVERVIEW OF THE LITERATURE

One of the problems in reviewing recent literature is that research about impaired nursing practice is lacking. Recent research-based literature on the topic is disappointing, and gaps about all issues related to impaired nursing practice exist. An extensive review yielded limited new material on this persistent problem. Most new articles are discussion pieces, and many are anecdotal accounts about individual nurses, but very few are research based. Burman and Dunphy (2011) also explored the barriers that exist with advanced practice nurses confronting a colleague in which they believed practice misconduct had occurred due to substance abuse. These authors recommended standardizing practices, discussing ethical obligations, and addressing institutional policies and procedures. An evidence-based care sheet was published in 2010 by Pinto and Schub that is a compilation of information on substance abuse and nurses that focuses on two areas: what we know and what we can do. Unlike other published pieces that use very dated information, this reference uses literature from 2007 to the present only, which is encouraging that more recent information is being published.

There is no consistent theme in recent literature on substance abuse among nurses, nursing students, and health care professionals generally. Monroe and others (Monroe, 2009; Monroe & Kenaga, 2010; Monroe & Pearson, 2009; Monroe, Pearson, & Kenaga, 2008) have researched and written about student nurses; Bettinardi-Angres and Bologeorges (2011) focused on the practices of confronting/reporting impaired work colleagues; and studies were found about impaired physicians and nurse anesthetists. With limited recent empirically based research, there is little to help the profession move closer toward management and resolution of the problem, if indeed resolution is even possible.

### DISCUSSION POINT

Why hasn't more nursing research been conducted that explores the experiences and perspectives of nurses who misuse substances?

## Identifying Early Risk Factors for Substance Abuse

The very nature of the work of nurses seems to be challenged when risk factors are considered. Nurses have constant access to narcotics, and fatigue seems to come with the job, no matter what shift is worked. It is difficult to avoid job strain in the current health care environment, which is in the middle of the worst nursing shortage ever reported. Despite the difficulties inherent in the practice setting today, many nurses do work hard to get experience and increase knowledge so they can become specialists, only to find this, too, can put them at higher risk of turning to drugs or alcohol when coping is difficult. These issues highlight the complexity of the problem for the profession, requiring that all nurses become more aware of how to prevent it from occurring.

### DISCUSSION POINT

Due to long work hours, overtime (often mandatory), and job strain, is the nursing shortage contributing to the prevalence of nurses who misuse substances?

One study addressed the issue of identification of early risk factors for the development of substance abuse problems in health care professionals. This study broadly looked at a variety of health care professionals including nurses. Kenna and Lewis (2008) used a sample of 697 dentists, nurses, pharmacists, and physicians that was limited to one state. The aim was to look at risk factors for alcohol and other drug use in health care professionals. All data were self-reported. Several findings are noteworthy when discussing risk factors for nurses. Younger practitioners were at higher risk than their older colleagues. This is consistent with the literature about drug use in the general population. General moderate use of alcohol was a predictor for any drug use, significant or not. Social contact was not considered a risk factor, which supports the belief that there is not a professional drug culture in the health care setting.

Several conclusions can be drawn from this study. The first is that it is imperative that new graduate and younger nurses be educated about impaired practice and their increased risk, in the hopes of facilitating positive coping strategies and increasing the focus on prevention. This means that education about impaired practice risks must start in the nursing education community. Second, alcohol should not be dismissed as a legal drug that carries less significance in the broader picture of impaired practice. Finally, impaired practitioners tend to isolate themselves from others and not seek help readily. This speaks to the issue of reporting an impaired colleague, which is discussed later in the chapter.

> CONSIDER THIS Nurses are praised and looked up to by clients, society, and other nurses. Yet a nurse with a substance abuse problem does not seem to receive that same caring attitude from his or her peers.

## National Nursing Organizations

For policies to be in place at the local level, it is imperative that the positions of leading national nursing organizations about impaired practice be clear (Box 17.1). The American Nurses Association's (ANA) policy about impaired practice can be found on its website. The basis for the policy is the ethical duty of the nurse to the patient, specifically Provision 3 of the ANA (2010) *Code of Ethics for Nurses*. The advocacy role all nurses have is clear; nurses must report an impaired colleague. The ANA supports treatment as opposed to discipline and a process that facilitates reentry of the recovered nurse back into practice (ANA, 2008).

The focus of the position about impaired nursing practice of the American Association of Colleges of Nursing (AACN) is on policy development in nursing education (AACN, 1998). Their policy was written in 1994 and updated in 1998. The AACN's policy can

## BOX 17.1 NURSING ORGANIZATION POSITION STATEMENTS ON IMPAIRED PRACTICE

- **ANA**—http://gm6.nursingworld. org/MainMenuCategories/Policy-Advocacy/Positions-and-Resolutions/ ANAPositionStatements/Position-Statements-Alphabetically/Abuse-of-Prescription-Drugs.html

- **AACN**—http://www.aacn.nche. edu/publications/position/ substance-abuse-policy-and-guidelines

- **NCSBN**—https://www.ncsbn.org/ SUDN_10.pdf

also be found on its website. The policy has guidelines for prevention and management of substance abuse in the nursing education community. There are specific features that address the issue for students, faculty, and staff. Critical to successful policy development is attention to confidentiality and legal perspectives. From the perspective of process and content, the necessary areas are identification, intervention, evaluation, treatment, and reentry into practice. The AACN is in agreement with the ANA regarding the importance of treatment over a reasonable timeframe and a process for successful reentry into practice.

The National Council of State Boards of Nursing (NCSBN) published *Substance Use Disorder in Nursing* in 2011 and that manual can be found on their website. The purpose of the *Substance Use Disorder in Nursing* manual "is to provide practical and evidence-based guidelines for evaluating, treating and managing nurses with a substance use disorder" (NCSBN, 2011, p. 16). As with the AACN and the ANA, the NCSBN also supports early detection and treatment of the impaired nurse with the goal of returning a recovered nurse to work. The manual serves a dual purpose: (1) to assist alternative to discipline programs and state boards of nursing with program content and delivery and (2) to provide "theoretical and practical guidelines for clinicians, educators, policymakers and public health professionals" (NCSBN, 2011, p. 16). In addition to the completion of the *Substance Use Disorder in Nursing* manual, the NCSBN also compiled model guidelines for alternative programs and discipline monitoring programs (Darbro, 2011). The purpose of the model is to provide best practice, evidence-based guidelines that could be used by state boards of nursing for "evaluating, treating, monitoring, and managing health-care professionals with substance use disorders" (Darbro, 2011, p. 43).

## Nurses Reporting an Impaired Colleague— Issues and Ethics

It is the responsibility of every nurse to be aware of reporting requirements when a colleague is suspected of chemical dependency or of diverting drugs for personal use. No uniform agreement exists among the states as to what those reporting requirements are. Information regarding reporting requirements can be found from each State Board of Nursing, which often can be easily accessed via its website. Before a nurse can be reported or referred to a treatment program, there must be recognition that the nurse needs help. Recognizing that a nurse is impaired might not be easy. Some common

**BOX 17.2    SIGNS AND BEHAVIORAL CHANGES SUGGESTING CHEMICAL IMPAIRMENT**

**COMMON SIGNS OF IMPAIRMENT**

- Nurse appearing to be a "workaholic," arriving early, staying late, offering to work extra shifts, and offering to cover for breaks

- Often working in areas that have a high volume of commonly abused drugs; examples include the oncology department, the emergency department, and the operating room

- Volunteering to care for patients who have diminished awareness

- Frequent reports from patients that their pain medication is ineffective; narcotic count errors are common

- Peers complaining about the quality and quantity of the nurse's work

- Nurse volunteering for overtime

**BEHAVIORAL CHANGES**

- Increased irritability with patients and colleagues, often followed by extreme calm

- Social isolation; the person eats alone and avoids unit social functions

- Extreme and rapid mood swings

- Unusually strong interest in narcotics or the narcotic cabinet

- Sudden dramatic change in personal grooming or any other personal habits

- Extreme defensiveness regarding medication errors

*Source:* Marquis, B. L., & Huston, C. J. (2012). *Leadership Roles and Management Functions in Nursing: Theory & Application* (7th ed.). Philadelphia, PA: Lippincott Williams & Wilkins; "I think my colleague has a problem. . ." (2011). *Canadian Nurse, 107*(3), 24–28.

signs or behavior changes of a chemically impaired nurse are shown in Box 17.2.

CONSIDER THIS Whistle-blowing usually carries a negative connotation. Consider how you would feel if someone labeled you a whistle-blower for reporting an impaired peer.

In theory, reporting an impaired nurse seems like a decision that would be easy to make. The position of the ANA and other nursing organizations is clear: It is the ethical and legal duty of a nurse to advocate for public safety, their colleagues, and the profession (Burman & Dunphy, 2011). This means simply that it is a nurse's job to protect the patient from harm; if that means reporting an impaired colleague that is what one must do. In practice, however, the situation is anything but

clear. New research conducted with both nurses and physicians suggests that although both groups of professionals understand the need for reporting an impaired colleague, most do not report (Bettinardi-Angres & Bologeorges, 2011; DesRoches et al., 2011). Previous literature suggests that there is a "code of silence" about impaired practice. However, these newer studies suggest that other reasons are responsible for a lack of peer reporting. In the DesRoches et al. (2011) study, the main reason physicians did not report seemed to be that they thought someone else was dealing with the problem. However, Bettinardi-Angres and Bologeorges (2011) found the reasons were more complex. These authors identified some barriers as lack of general knowledge of substance abuse in the workplace, lack of a clear protocol or process for reporting or intervening, and lack of compassion in the workplace for peers. They also found that the word *confrontation* itself was a barrier to reporting and that perhaps more compassionate terminology would help, such as assisting a nurse, addressing a problem, and so forth. Research Study Fuels the Controversy extrapolates some of these reasons.

---

### DISCUSSION POINT

You suspect that a coworker/friend is diverting drugs for personal use. You find yourself covering up for her because you know that she is depressed, exhausted, and having family problems. Your supervisor makes a casual comment with similar suspicions. Your first instinct is to make excuses for your friend; what would you do?

---

## Impaired Practice Policies in the Workplace

It is a difficult and often traumatic experience for a nurse to report an impaired peer. The important considerations are that patients are not harmed, the nurse is helped, and the provider is protected. It is imperative that every health care facility and educational institution have an *Impaired Practice Policy* in place that clearly sets out the process that is to be followed if impaired practice is suspected (Palmer & Hoffman, 2007). An important component of any policy is the commitment to a drug- and alcohol-free workplace, whether that is a health care setting (Saver, 2008) or an educational environment. Another important component of any policy should include "procedures for returning to work, which normally

## RESEARCH STUDY FUELS THE CONTROVERSY

### ADDRESSING CHEMICALLY DEPENDENT COLLEAGUES

This two-phased, mixed-method study is one of the few recently published studies on substance abuse in the nursing profession. Phase 1 sought to better understand the variables associated with chemical dependency in nurses. These variables included "drugs of choice, the question of IV use, and the percentage of nurses diverting drugs" (Bettinardi-Angres & Bologeorges, 2011, p. 11). The qualitative phase 2 will be discussed here.

Bettinardi-Angres, K., & Bologeorges, S. (2011). Addressing chemically dependent colleagues. *Journal of Nursing Regulation, 2*(2), 10–15.

---

### STUDY FINDINGS

Phase 2 of the research aimed to explore the perceptions and attitudes of nurses in practice about confronting a colleague suspected of abusing substances and to investigate the reasons why confrontation did not occur. A semistructured interview approach was used to gather data about the topic. All nurses were asked the same three questions that focused on addressing suspicion of substance abuse with a colleague, reporting that colleague, and the reasons that might prevent the nurse from reporting the colleague.

Fifty-seven percent of nurses in the study indicated that even if they were suspicious that a colleague was using drugs or alcohol, they would be reluctant to confront them directly. Reasons were mixed but included not trusting their own judgment that their suspicions were correct, fear that harm might come to them, not wanting to "tell" on a peer, and that someone else was probably better prepared to deal with the situation.

An interesting aspect of these findings is that most of the nurses who would be comfortable confronting a colleague were experienced nurses with many years of professional practice. The finding that most of the nurses would not confront a suspected drug-using colleague is distressing as peer reporting and referral are the main recommendations made in the literature for identifying impaired health care professionals.

These authors make several recommendations: (1) emphasize the importance of education on chemical dependency that begins in nursing school, (2) develop clear standards or protocols that allow for confidential reporting of substance abuse in the workplace, (3) "establish nurse's well being committees in the workplace" (p. 15), and (4) ensure there is a climate of compassion in the workplace for both nurses and patients.

included a signed contract, restrictions on handling of narcotics, and random urine testing for drugs" (Saver, 2008, p. 12).

A nurse who is suspected of impaired practice should not be confronted unless there is a plan in place, whether it is a referral to a person or program within the facility or a referral to the treatment program for that particular state board of nursing. Many professional associations and treatment programs have peer-assistance hotlines in place that can also provide a variety of resources (Palmer & Hoffman, 2007). The key is that the nurse suspecting impaired practice and the nurse whose practice is being challenged should not feel alone in the process. Help is available and should be used.

## Alternative to Discipline/Diversion Programs

The disciplinary approach was the normal response to chemical impairment in most states through the 1980s. Following the ANA resolution in 1982 to support treatment of chemically dependent nurses, many states began to look at treatment and rehabilitation options instead of discipline (ANA, 1984).

In 2009, the NCSBN conducted a survey about alternative to discipline programs in the United States. Their results showed that there are 59 licensing jurisdictions for nurses in this country and that 41 of those 59 currently have alternative to discipline programs in place. That still leaves 18 that do not (NCSBN, 2009).

> CONSIDER THIS   Most addiction specialists and the American Medical Association view addiction as a chronic medical illness and argue that it should be approached in an analogous way to, say, diabetes or asthma.

Although most states now offer treatment options, the types of programs vary. Some programs are completely voluntary, which means that there is no threat of the nurse being reported to disciplinary authorities. The first treatment program offered was the Intervention Project for Nurses (IPN) in Florida in 1983. The IPN has a comprehensive website offering information about the history of the program, including frequently asked questions and available services.

California also offers a diversion program; information is available from the California Board of Registered Nursing (CBRN). Established in 1985, its goal is to "protect the public by early identification of impaired registered nurses and by providing these nurses access

to appropriate intervention programs and treatment services" (CBRN, 2011, para. 2). Impaired nurses can be self-referred or can be referred by family, coworkers, or the board. All licensed registered nurses residing in California are eligible to enter the program, but they must agree to enter the program voluntarily. Since 1985, more than 1,200 nurses have successfully completed the diversion program in California. Requirements for completion include "a change in lifestyle that supports continuing recovery and [having] a minimum of 24 consecutive months of clean, random, body-fluid tests" (para. 14). Confidentiality of participants is protected by law, and nurses who successfully complete the program have their records regarding chemical impairment destroyed.

A different approach is followed in the Texas Peer Assistance Program (TNA) for Nurses. This program offers services to nurses suffering from chemical dependency, as well as from anxiety and other mental health disorders. It requires abstinence, maintains confidentiality, is strictly voluntary, and is independent of the state licensing board (Van Doren, 2010). Information from the TNA website includes how and when to make referrals, how the program works, and important links to services and organizations.

Despite these examples of positive programs in existence, Monroe and Pearson (2009) highlight that there is a substantial lack of information in general about how these alternative to discipline programs work in most states. They found limited, dated literature with no clear or consistent definition of what constituted an alternative program. Without extensive research into outcomes of the different programs, it is difficult to conclude what type of program works best and how that can become more standardized across states.

Little is said in the literature about nursing students and what needs to be done when impairment is suspected or found. Monroe (2009) suggests developing a prototype alternative to discipline policy for nursing students, which is consistent with most State Boards of Nursing in terms of offering treatment instead of discipline. This approach for students should lead to earlier intervention and treatment because the student would be removed from practice early in the process, thus ensuring patient safety while also helping the student recover (Monroe, 2009). In a similar article, Monroe and Pearson (2009) support the notion that nursing students be offered the same process as registered practitioners (in most states), that is, be offered alternative to dismissal programs rather than be treated using punitive measures.

CONSIDER THIS   Although most states lean toward treatment rather than discipline for chemical dependency, many nurses still attach a stigma and think that impaired nurses should be punished and not allowed to return to work.

## The Recovered Nurse: Reentry Into Practice

When a nurse has completed a treatment or rehabilitation program and is ready to return to work, he or she typically encounters a number of issues. These issues include whether the nurse's practice is limited or restricted in some way, how long the nursing board has a right to invade the nurse's privacy to ensure that recovery is ongoing, where organizational responsibility ends, who bears the cost if the nurse does not return to work at full capacity, and ensuring that confidentiality is maintained (Box 17.3).

Although many anecdotal or discussion articles were found on the topic of what constitutes a disciplinary or

---

**BOX 17.3   ISSUES TO CONSIDER WHEN THE RECOVERED NURSE RETURNS TO WORK**

- Should the nurse returning to work following rehabilitation have his or her practice limited or restricted in some way, such as no exposure to the drug of choice or no access to controlled substances for a period of time?

- How long does the board of nursing have a right to invade the privacy of a recovered nurse?

- Where does the organizational responsibility end?

- Who bears the cost if the recovered nurse is not able to return to work at full capacity?

- Can confidentiality be maintained?

- Should the nurse be allowed to work in stressful practice areas?

- Should the nurse initially be allowed to work full-time?

---

treatment approach to impaired practice, few recent articles could be found that addressed the concerns of reentry of the impaired nurse to the practice setting. Wilson and Compton (2009) reviewed the literature about reentry of addicted certified registered nurse anesthetists and, similar to the general literature about chemical dependency and reentry in nursing, found that literature to be dated, with little empirical work to support how successful existing programs are.

Despite this, there are some general considerations that should be taken into account when a recovered nurse returns to work. To protect patient safety, practice restrictions may be in place for a varying time, depending on the length of the program and whether it was treatment based or disciplinary action occurred. Recovering nurses need to be reassured that their records are confidential and that they are kept separate from general personnel records. It is also important that staff nurses realize the commitment of the recovering nurse to reestablish his or her career and continue in the profession.

Most Board of Registered Nursing websites offer little information about the reentry process. Instead, they focus primarily on what should be done if someone suspects an impaired colleague, how to report it, the treatment or disciplinary action once impairment is identified, and the specific aspects of each program. A question that is left unanswered is how long the board follows a recovered nurse in terms of random drug testing. Some hospitals or health care agencies already do random drug testing, so the question of invasion of privacy has in some instances already been dealt with.

Angres, Bettinardi-Angres, and Cross (2010) suggest what they refer to as a *last-chance agreement*, which is a contract between the nurse and employer stating that in lieu of termination, a contract will be instated as a good faith agreement that the nurse will follow all stipulations. This usually begins with the nurse successfully completing a treatment program before reentry and then being returned to a setting where there is no access to controlled substances.

This process benefits the organization as well as the returning nurse. It is less expensive than replacing a nurse and can potentially boost morale because it demonstrates to other team members that the organization supports its employees. The contract approach supports the earlier work of Saver (2008) who also suggested that a written contract is useful because it puts in writing the expectations for the nurse. Another suggestion is for the nurse to attend a support group for chemically dependent nurses.

## DISCUSSION POINT

You just came from a staff meeting at which the nurse-manager informed everyone that a recovered nurse would begin working on the unit in a few weeks. Some nurses had the attitude that the nurse not be allowed back to work because he or she could not be trusted. How would you respond to your colleagues?

## Research Dissemination—Is It Happening?

Although there are limited new research findings to disseminate, the question still needs to be asked: Are the profession and education community applying/using what findings are available? Issues have been raised about student substance abuse. If you work in an educational setting or interact with students in your workplace, do you know what policies are in place if a student is suspected of impaired practice? More important, what is being done in the educational community to address the issue of alcohol and substance use by students that might be affecting their performance in the clinical setting? As suggested by the AACN (1998), it is critical that policies regarding impaired practice be clear and in place in the educational community and that all faculty and students be aware of the content of the policy.

The literature clearly states that impaired practice policies should be in place in every health care setting. However, anecdotal evidence suggests that many nurses in clinical practice have no knowledge of such policies and would not know what to do if they suspected a colleague was impaired. Impaired practice policies should be introduced during hospital orientation for new employees and during annual renewal of hospital safety procedures. This would highlight the issue for everyone and put the problem clearly in the spotlight, especially if issues such as barriers to reporting an impaired colleague and prevalence of the problem were discussed. Nurses should be allowed to ask questions so that they are clear about the process of reporting and so that a nurse who is using substances irresponsibly knows where to go for help.

## HOW CAN WE STOP LOSING NURSES TO SUBSTANCE ABUSE?

Preventative health care is finally receiving much needed attention in the media and in practice. Insurance companies are increasingly paying for prevention and screening procedures, yet many areas of health care still lag behind what would be ideal for preventative practices. The issue of preventing substance abuse is no exception to this situation. How can nurses individually and as a profession help to prevent the cycle of nurse addiction from starting?

Some of the risk factors for substance abuse that have been identified are difficult to modify. Nurses will always have easy access to narcotics, do shift work, and suffer from fatigue. The ongoing stress that has worked its way into clinical settings due to the nursing shortage seems a long way from dissipating. What, then, can be done to diminish the effects of these factors so that nurses do not turn to substances as an inappropriate coping mechanism?

Perhaps one avenue is to more fully explore the experiences of nurses who do not turn to substances. Although much has been written about self-care to prevent burnout (Marquis & Huston, 2012), no evidence could be found that linked burnout to harmful coping strategies, such as substance abuse. Do nurses who use self-care strategies to prevent burnout also use those same strategies to avoid harmful substance use? Perhaps this information about how nurses cope with difficulties of the workplace when they do not turn to drugs or alcohol will contribute to prevention. Most research focuses on the nurse who abuses drugs, when a great deal could be learned about positive coping behaviors from nurses who manage stress without abusing drugs.

Where does the education about substance abuse begin? Student nurses need not only to be made aware of the risks of substance abuse but also to be self-aware about their attitudes and beliefs regarding those who do abuse substances, whether those people are patients or colleagues. Nursing school is an incredibly stressful time for students. Not only could appropriate education in nursing school help to prevent the onset of substance abuse, it might also allow students to explore their feelings and beliefs about impaired practice. This increased self-awareness might help students to have empathy toward impaired nurses and encourage them to take the appropriate steps to assist a nurse or fellow student in getting help.

Nursing is going through a very tumultuous time. The nursing shortage is never far from the minds of most nurses as they struggle on a daily basis with low staffing levels and a stressed work setting. How this stress is channeled can lead a nurse to have positive or negative coping strategies. What are hospitals doing to acknowledge and diffuse this stress? Are nurses too stressed to seek counsel from each other when they have a particularly bad day? Are nurses debriefing with each other or at home so they can let go of the often traumatic nature of work and move forward? Nurses and nurse-managers need to answer these questions for their particular work settings to know whether they are doing enough for themselves, their colleagues, and their staff.

## CONCLUSIONS

Losing one nurse to substance abuse is losing one nurse too many. We are a profession known for its caring nature toward others, yet often we fail to care for ourselves. The harmful coping strategies that lead to substance abuse can begin even before nursing school. Educating our students may help us to increase awareness about this ever-present problem. If new graduates can bring current information to their nursing practice and be self-aware about their attitudes, beliefs, and coping strategies, then perhaps they can come armed with more positive strategies to help them when times get tough.

Do we teach our students, new graduates, and seasoned nurses to ask for help when they need it, or do we expect them to "do it all"?

Nurses who suspect an impaired colleague need to take action as they have both an ethical and legal obligation in the interest of patient safety (Talbert, 2009). If all nurses are aware of the problem of chemical dependency and take the initiative to confront or intervene when they suspect a colleague of impaired practice, we are one step closer to decreasing the incidence of substance abuse in the nursing profession.

Finally, responsibility rests not just with individual nurses but also with employers to create a positive work environment, to know employees so that confrontation can occur early, to increase awareness about substance abuse so that nurses are not afraid to ask for help, to ensure that an impaired practice policy is in place, and finally to provide a process that facilitates reentry into practice following recovery.

## FOR ADDITIONAL DISCUSSION

1. Explore your attitudes and beliefs about impaired nursing practice. How would you treat a colleague suspected of diverting drugs for personal use? How would you treat a recovered nurse returning to work?

2. What kind of peer support exists in your work setting? How do staff debrief from stressful situations?

3. What do you think is the best approach to deal with impaired practice—treatment or discipline? Did moral values play a part in your decision?

4. Should recovered nurses who return to work have a limited practice? If so, for how long, and with what types of limitations? How does this affect the workload of other nurses?

5. What practices are in place in your work setting that could deter a nurse from diverting drugs for personal use?

6. Have you known a colleague who was caught stealing drugs from work? If so, how was it handled? Did the nurse seek treatment and return to work? Could it have been managed better?

7. You are a nurse-manager for an intensive care unit and have been asked to talk to student nurses about impaired practice. What key points would you make?

8. Does your workplace have an impaired practice policy in place? If so, have you read it, and was it discussed during your initial hospital orientation? Is it discussed annually? If not, what might you do to ensure that one is in place?

## REFERENCES

American Nurses Association. (1984). *Addiction and psychological dysfunctions in nursing.* Kansas City, MO: Author.

American Nurses Association. (2010). *Code of ethics for nurses with interpretive statements.* Washington, DC:

Author. Retrieved from http://nursingworld.org/MainMenuCategories/ThePracticeofProfessional-Nursing/EthicsStandards/CodeofEthics.aspx

American Nurses Association. (2008). *Impaired nurse resource center.* Retrieved from http://nursingworld.org/MainMenuCategories/WorkplaceSafety/Work-Environment/ImpairedNurse

American Association of Colleges of Nursing. (1998). *Policy and guidelines for prevention and management of substance abuse in the nursing education community.* Retrieved from http://www.aacn.nche.edu/publications/position/substance-abuse-policy-and-guidelines

Angres, D. H., Bettinardi-Angres, K., & Cross, W. (2010). Nurses with chemical dependency: Promoting successful treatment and reentry. *Journal of Nursing Regulation, 1*(1), 16–20.

Bettinardi-Angres, K., & Bologeorges, S. (2011). Addressing chemically dependent colleagues. *Journal of Nursing Regulation, 2*(2), 10–15.

Burman, M. E., & Dunphy, L. M. (2011) Reporting colleague misconduct in advanced practice nursing. *Journal of Nursing Regulation, 1*(4), 26–31.

California Board of Registered Nursing. (2011). *What is the BRN's diversion program?* Retrieved from http://www.rn.ca.gov/diversion/whatisdiv.shtml

Darbo, N. (2011). Model guidelines for alternative programs and discipline monitoring programs. *Journal of Nursing Regulation, 2*(1), 42–49.

DesRoches, C. M., Rao, S. R., Fromson, R. J., Iezzoni, L., Vogeli, C., & Campbell, E. G. (2011). Physicians' perceptions, preparedness for reporting, and experiences related to impaired and incompetent colleagues. *Journal of the American Medical Association, 304*(2), 187–193.

Epstein, P. M., Burns, C., & Conlon, H. A. (2010). Substance abuse among registered nurses. *AAOHN Journal, 58*(12), 513–516.

Finkelman, A., & Kenner, C. (2009). *Teaching IOM: Implications of the Institute of Medicine reports for nursing education* (2nd ed.). Silver Spring, MD: American Nurses Association.

"I think my colleague has a problem . . ." (2011). *Canadian Nurse, 107*(3), 24–28.

Kenna, G. A., & Lewis, D. C. (2008). Risk factors for alcohol and other drug use by healthcare professionals. *Substance Abuse Treatment, Prevention, and Policy, 3*(3). Retrieved from http://www.biomedcentral.com/content/pdf/1747-597X-3-3.pdf

Marquis, B. L., & Huston, C. J. (2012). *Leadership roles and management functions in nursing: Theory and application* (7th ed.). Philadelphia, PA: Lippincott Williams & Wilkins.

Monroe, T. (2009). Addressing substance abuse among nursing students: Development of a prototype alternative-to-dismissal policy. *Journal of Nursing Education, 48*(5), 272–278.

Monroe, T., & Kenaga, H. (2010). Don't ask don't tell: Substance abuse and addiction among nurses. *Journal of Clinical Nursing, 20*(3/4), 504–509.

Monroe, T., & Pearson, F. (2009). Treating nurses and student nurses with chemical dependency: Revising policy in the United States in the 21st century. *International Journal of Mental Health Addiction, 7*(4), 530–540.

Monroe, T., Pearson, F., & Kenaga, H. (2008). Procedures for handling cases of substance abuse among nurses: A comparison of disciplinary and alternative programs. *Journal of Addictions Nursing, 19*(3), 156–161.

National Council of State Boards of Nursing. (2001). *Chemical dependency handbook for nurse managers.* Retrieved from https://www.ncsbn.org/chem_dep_handbook_intro_ch1.pdf

National Council of State Boards of Nursing. (2010). *Breaking the habit: When your colleague is chemically dependent.* Retrieved from http://www.google.co.in/url?sa=t&rct=j&q=&esrc=s&source=web&cd=1&ved=0CEAQFjAA&url=http%3A%2F%2Fwww.reshealth.org%2Fpdfs%2Fsubsites%2Faddiction%2Faddressing_chemically_dependent_colleagues.pdf&ei=4OooUKGkMIrRrQeS74HADA&usg=AFQjCNGqfEf2VY7K9l2bF_zgWdYRqwZ7fQ&sig2=vLyboFMIuFuxYc6FjZvIg

National Council of State Boards of Nursing. (2011). *Substance use disorder in nursing.* Retrieved from https://www.ncsbn.org/SUDN_10.pdf

National Council of State Boards of Nursing. (2011). *Substance use disorder in nursing: A resource manual and guidelines for alternative and disciplinary monitoring programs.* Retrieved from https://www.ncsbn.org/2106.htm

Palmer, L., & Hoffman, L. A. (2007). Detecting and preventing substance abuse in health care professionals. *Critical Care Alert, 15*(1), 5–8.

Pinto, S., & Schub, T. (2010). *Substance abuse in healthcare professionals: Evidence-based care sheet.* Glendale, CA: CINAHL Information Systems.

Quality and Safety Education for Nurses. (2011). *Project overview.* Retrieved from http://www.qsen.org/overview.php

Saver, C. (2008). Substance abuse in the OR: Why managers should not ignore it. *OR Manager, 24*(5), 1, 11–12.

Talbert, J. J. (2009). Substance abuse among nurses. *Clinical Journal of Oncology Nursing, 13*(1), 17–19.

Van Doren, M. (2010). Self-assessment in substance abuse: The pain and the promise. *Texas Board of Nursing Bulletin, 41*(2), 6–7, 13.

Wilson, H., & Compton, M. (2009). Reentry of the addicted certified registered nurse anesthetist: A review of the literature. *Journal of Addictions Nursing, 20*(4), 177–184.

## BIBLIOGRAPHY

Burman, M. E., & Dunpy, L. M. (2011). Reporting colleague misconduct in advance practice nursing. *Journal of Nursing Regulation, 1*(4), 26–31.

DuPont, R. L., McLellan, A. T., Carr, G., Gendel, M., & Skipper, G. E. (2009). How are addicted physicians treated? A national survey of physician health programs. *Journal of Substance Abuse Treatment, 37*, 1–7.

Kincheloe, D. M., & Litzenburg, T. A. (2010). Impaired health care practitioners: Help the healer help himself. *ED Legal Letter, 21*(9), 97–101.

Mikos, C. A. (2008). Increased authority to discipline licenses of impaired practitioners. *Florida Nurse, 56*(2), 10.

Raistrick, D., Russell, D., Tober, G., & Tindale, A. (2008). A survey of substance use by health care professionals and their attitudes to substance misuse patients (NHS staff survey). *Journal of Substance Use, 13*(1), 57–69.

Ramer, L. M. (2008). Using servant leadership to facilitate healing after a drug diversion experience. *AORN Journal, 88*(2), 253–258.

Savor, C. (2009). Drug diversion in the OR: How can you keep it from happening? *OR Manager, 25*(12), 1, 6–11.

Thomas, C. M., & Siela, D. (2011). The impaired nurse: Would you know what to do if you suspected substance abuse? *American Nurse Today, 6*(8), 1–5.

Van Doren, M. (2010). Self-assessment in substance abuse: The pain and the promise. *Texas Board of Nursing Bulletin, 41*(2), 6–13.

# Chapter **18**

# Collective Bargaining and the Professional Nurse

Carol J. Huston

## ADDITIONAL RESOURCES

Visit thePoint for additional helpful resources
- eBook
- Journal Articles
- WebLinks

## CHAPTER OUTLINE

**Historical Perspective of Unionization in the United States**

**Historical Perspective of Unionization in Nursing**

Unions Representing Nurses

Motivation to Join Unions

Reasons Not to Join Unions

Eligibility for Union Membership

Organizing a Union and Seeking Representation

Labor–Management Relationships

American Nurses Association and Collective Bargaining

Nurses and Strikes

Conclusions

## LEARNING OBJECTIVES

*The learner will be able to:*

1. Explore possible motivations behind nurses' decisions to join or not join unions.

2. Identify major U.S. legislation that has affected the ability of nurses to unionize over time.

3. Describe the shifting balance of power between unions and management in the United States over the last century and analyze the power balance that currently exists between the two entities.

4. Identify the largest unions representing health care employees, and nurses in particular.

5. Investigate the current status of rulings by the National Labor Relations Board (NLRB) and the courts regarding the definition of "supervisor" in nursing and the effect those rulings have on the eligibility of nurses for protection under the National Labor Relations Act (NLRA).

6. Delineate common union organizing strategies as well as specific steps for starting a union.

7. Debate the potential conflicts inherent in having the American Nurses Association serve as both a professional association for all nurses and as a collective bargaining agent.

8. Explore the impact management has on creating a work environment that eliminates or reduces the need for unionization.

9. Reflect on whether going on strike can be viewed as an ethically appropriate action for professional nurses.

10. Explore his or her beliefs about whether belonging to unions, a practice historically reserved for blue-collar workers, undermines nursing's quest for increased recognition as a profession.

There is likely no greater dichotomy than stereotypical images of nurses dressed in white uniforms and caps acting as handmaidens to physicians and angry nurses in picket lines waving strike placards at passersby. Although both of these images are stereotypical, they are at the heart of the debate about whether nursing, long recognized as a caring and altruistic profession, should be a part of collective bargaining efforts to improve working conditions.

*Collective bargaining* involves activities occurring between organized labor and management that concern employee relationships. Such activities include negotiation of formal labor agreements and day-to-day interactions between unions and management. A *labor union* (hereafter referred to as a *union*) is an organization of workers, often in a trade or profession, formed to protect their rights and interests and improve their economic status and working conditions through collective bargaining with employers.

Many nurses have strong feelings about unions and collective bargaining activities. Often these feelings have to do with their exposure to unions while growing up. Many nurses from working-class families were raised in a cultural milieu that promoted unionization. Other nurses know little about unions and know only what they have seen portrayed in the media. Some nurses, however, have been actively involved in collective bargaining in their place of employment and have emerged from the experience with either positive or negative impressions or a combination thereof.

Despite this tension, collective bargaining and unions are very much a part of many nurses' experiences. Although union membership in the private sector has been slowly declining, steady increases have occurred in the number of nurses represented by collective bargaining agents. In fact, membership in hospital nursing unions in the United States has grown 18% in the last 3 years (Spetz, Ash, Seago, & Hererra, 2011). Still, depending on the source used, only 16% to 22% of all nurses belong to collective bargaining units (discrepancies have to do with how the numbers are calculated). The issues driving nurses to pursue unionization, however, continue to exist. Increased nursing workloads and a feeling that management does not care are significant factors encouraging increased union activity at the close of the first decade of the 21st century.

This chapter explores the historical development of unions in the United States, particularly in nursing. The motivations behind nurses' decisions to join or not join unions are explored, and the unions that represent the majority of nurses are described. Union organizing strategies are presented, as are specific steps for starting a union. Emphasis is given to the importance of management creating a work environment that eliminates or reduces the need for unionization in the first place. The chapter concludes with a discussion of the definition of "supervisor" in nursing, types of labor union–management relationships, and whether striking can be viewed as an ethically appropriate action for professional nurses.

## HISTORICAL PERSPECTIVE OF UNIONIZATION IN THE UNITED STATES

Unions have been present in the United States since the 1790s. Skilled craftsmen formed early unions to protect themselves from wage cuts during the highly competitive era of industrialization. Strikes were rare and when they did occur, they were short and peaceful. This changed in the early 1800s, with strike activity increasing during economic prosperity and declining during less prosperous economic times. By the mid- to late 1800s, the labor movement began to more closely resemble what we see today. Unions started negotiating with employers, addressing not only wages but also work rules, hours, and grievances, thus arbitrating contracts between employees and employers.

By the 1930s, and after 4 years of the Great Depression, repressive management was the norm, and tensions were high between workers and their employers. There were no legal protections for workers, no overtime compensation, no child labor laws, and no health or safety regulations. Workers attempted to form unions to improve working conditions, but business owners responded by blacklisting organizers and using force to prevent strikes (Franklin D. Roosevelt Presidential Library, 1935).

President Franklin Roosevelt attempted to intervene by promoting the National Industrial Recovery Act, but he was forced to make an even bolder stand alongside labor when the Supreme Court ruled that act unconstitutional. Roosevelt promoted the National Labor Relations Act (NLRA), also known as the Wagner Act after New York Senator Robert Wagner, which was enacted in 1935. This act gave workers the right to form unions and bargain collectively with their employers (Box 18.1). It also provided for the creation of the National Labor Relations Board (NLRB) to oversee union certification, arrange meetings with unions and employers, and investigate violations of the law (Franklin D. Roosevelt Presidential Library, 1935).

**BOX 18.1 UNFAIR MANAGEMENT PRACTICES IDENTIFIED IN THE WAGNER ACT (1935)**

1. To interfere with, restrain, or coerce employees in a manner that interferes with their rights as outlined under the act. Examples of these activities are spying on union gatherings, threatening employees with job loss, or threatening to close down a company if the union organizes

2. To interfere with the formation of any labor organization or to give financial assistance to a labor organization

3. To discriminate with regard to hiring, tenure, and so on to discourage union membership

4. To discharge or discriminate against an employee who filed charges or testified before the NLRB

5. To refuse to bargain in good faith

With this rapid shift in power from management to labor, labor–management relationships were turbulent throughout the 1930s and 1940s. History books are filled with battles, strikes, mass-picketing scenes, and brutal treatment by both management and employees. The balance of power, however, fell to labor unions.

Because of this, it was necessary to pass additional federal legislation to restore what was perceived to be a balance of power with management. Passed in 1947, the Taft–Hartley Labor Act, also known as the Labor–Management Relations Act, retained the provisions under the Wagner Act that guaranteed employees the right to collective bargaining but added the provision that employees had the right to refrain from taking part in unions ("closed shops" were illegal; Box 18.2). In addition, the act permitted the union shop only after a vote of a majority of the employees. It also forbade *jurisdictional strikes* ("an illegal strike about which trade union should have the right to represent a particular group of employees in an organization", Business Dictionary, 2011), secondary boycotts, and unions from contributing to political campaigns.

**DISCUSSION POINT**

The Taft–Hartley Labor Act also required union leaders to affirm they were not supporters of the Communist Party. Why was this requirement a part of the act, and how did it mesh with the culture of the time?

Eventually, federal legislation such as the Fair Labor Standards Act (1938), the Occupational Safety and Health Act (1970), and the Equal Employment Opportunity Act (1972) were passed, providing federal protection for workers. These acts were important in the history of unions because unions no longer had to be the primary source of security for workers. As a result, there has been little growth of unions in the private and blue-collar sectors since membership peaked in the 1950s.

To counteract these dwindling numbers, several major unions merged, and new affiliations were formed. In addition, new organizing tactics were developed. Nowhere is this turnaround more apparent than in the health care industry.

**BOX 18.2 UNFAIR LABOR UNION PRACTICES IDENTIFIED IN THE TAFT–HARTLEY AMENDMENT (1947)**

1. Requiring a self-employed person or an employer to join a union

2. Forcing an employer to cease doing business with another person. This placed a ban on secondary boycotts, which were then prevalent

3. Forcing an employer to bargain with one union when another union has already been certified as the bargaining agent

4. Forcing the employer to assign certain work to members of one union rather than another

5. Charging excessive or discriminatory initiation fees

6. Causing or attempting to cause an employer to pay for unnecessary services

# HISTORICAL PERSPECTIVE OF UNIONIZATION IN NURSING

Collective bargaining was slow in coming to the health care industry for many reasons. Until labor laws were amended, unionization of health care workers was illegal. In addition, nursing's long history as a service commodity further delayed labor organization in health care settings.

---

### DISCUSSION POINT

Is it appropriate for nurses to organize into collective bargaining units, something historically reserved for blue-collar workers?

---

Initial collective bargaining in nursing took place in government or public organizations as a result of Executive Order 10988 issued by President John Kennedy. This 1962 order lifted restrictions that prevented public employees from organizing. As a result, city, county, and district hospitals and health care agencies joined collective bargaining in the 1960s.

In 1974, Congress amended the Wagner Act, extending national labor laws to private nonprofit hospitals, nursing homes, health clinics, health maintenance organizations, and other health care institutions. These amendments opened the door to much union activity for professions and the public employee sector. Indeed, a review of union membership figures shows that since 1960, most collective bargaining activity in the United States has occurred in the public and professional sectors of industry, most notably among faculty at institutions of higher education, teachers at primary and secondary levels, and physicians.

---

### DISCUSSION POINT

Why is white-collar union membership growing when the private and blue-collar sectors are not? Have societal norms altered perceptions regarding the appropriateness of unionization in white-collar industries?

---

From 1962 through 1989, there were slow but steady increases in the numbers of nurses represented by collective bargaining agents. In 1989, the NLRB ruled that nurses could form separate bargaining units, and union activity increased. However, the American Hospital Association immediately sued the American Nurses Association (ANA), and the ruling was put on hold until 1991 when the Supreme Court upheld the 1989 decision by the NLRB. A summary of the legislation affecting the development of unionization in nursing is shown in Table 18.1.

# UNIONS REPRESENTING NURSES

Various unions represent nurses and other health care workers. The Service Employees International Union (SEIU) is the largest union in the health care industry, with more than 1.1 million health care worker members, including nurses, licensed practical nurses (LPNs)/licensed vocational nurses (LVNs), doctors, lab technicians, nursing home workers, and home care workers (SEIU, 2011a).

The largest union and professional association of registered nurses is the National Nurses United (NNU), which was formed in December 2009 when the California Nurses Association (CNA)/National Nurses Organizing Committee (NNOC) joined with two other unions representing nurses (United American Nurses and the Massachusetts Nurses Association) to create a new 150,000+ member advocacy association (New National Nurses, 2010). Although each union maintained its separate identity, the NNU was intended to give union-represented nurses a national voice and strength based on numbers. Since 2009, NNU added 6,500 RNs from Florida, Illinois, Iowa, Nevada, and Texas and has grown to more than 170,000 members, including members from every state (NNU, 2011).

Other unions that represent nurses include the American Nurses Association (ANA); the National Union of Hospital and Health Care Employees of Retail, Wholesale and Department Store Union; the American Federation of Labor–Congress of Industrial Organizations (AFL-CIO); the United Steelworkers of America (USWA); the American Federation of Government Employees, AFL-CIO; the American Federation of State, County, and Municipal Employees, AFL-CIO; the International Brotherhood of Teamsters; the American Federation of State, County, and Municipal Employees, which operates mostly in the public sector; and the United Auto Workers.

Union representation also varies by state. The states with the most union organizing for all industries, including health care, are New York, California, Pennsylvania, Michigan, and Illinois.

| TABLE 18.1 | Labor Legislation | |
|---|---|---|
| **Year** | **Legislation** | **Effect** |
| 1935 | National Labor Relations Act/Wagner Act | Gave unions many rights in organizing; resulted in rapid union growth |
| 1947 | Taft–Hartley Amendment | Returned some power to management; resulted in a more equal balance of power between unions and management |
| 1962 | Executive Order 10988 (President John Kennedy) | Amended the 1935 Wagner Act to allow public employees to join unions |
| 1974 | Amendments to the Wagner Act | Allowed workers in nonprofit organizations to join unions |
| 1989 | National Labor Relations Board ruling | Allowed nurses to form separate bargaining units |

---

### DISCUSSION POINT

Is it appropriate for RNs to be represented by non-nursing unions? Why would nurses seek out non-nursing unions for representation?

## MOTIVATION TO JOIN UNIONS

Knowing that human behavior is goal directed, it is important to examine what personal goals union membership fulfills. Nurse-managers often tell each other that health care institutions differ from other types of industrial organizations. This is really a myth because most nurses work in large and impersonal organizations, just like workers in other industries.

CONSIDER THIS  People are motivated to join or reject unions as a result of many needs and values.

Deciding whether to join a union is a personal and often complex decision because there are typically many influencing factors. Both choices can be justified, however, so both driving and restraining forces for union membership are presented here.

There are six primary motivations for joining a union (Box 18.3). The first is to increase the power of the individual. Employees know that singly they are much more dispensable. Because a large group of employees is generally less dispensable, nurses greatly increase their bargaining power and reduce their vulnerability by joining a union. This is a particularly strong motivating

### BOX 18.3  REASONS NURSES JOIN UNIONS

**1.** To increase the power of the individual

**2.** To achieve wage advantages

**3.** To increase their input into organizational decision making

**4.** To eliminate discrimination and favoritism

**5.** Because they are required to do so as part of employment (closed shop)

**6.** To satisfy a social need to be accepted

**7.** Because they believe it will improve patient outcomes and quality of care

force for nurses when jobs are scarce and nurses feel vulnerable. Indeed, during the massive downsizing and restructuring of the 1990s, collective bargaining priorities shifted from wages and benefits to job security.

CONSIDER THIS  Although historically, unions focused heavily on wage negotiations, current issues deemed just as or more important by nurses are nonmonetary, such as guidelines for staffing, float provisions, shared decision making, and scheduling.

Union activity also tends to change in response to workforce excesses and shortages. For decades, employment demand for nurses has increased and decreased periodically. High demand for nurses is tied directly to a healthy national economy, and, historically, this has been correlated with increased union activity. Similarly, when nursing vacancy rates are low, union membership and activity tend to decline.

A second reason for joining unions is economics. In some organizations, pay is neither fair nor competitive, and most economists agree that joining a union typically is an effective means of raising one's pay. Indeed, the median weekly earnings of union workers are 28% higher than nonunion workers (average yearly difference of US$10,400) and according to a January 2011 Bureau of Labor Statistics report, workers who belong to a union typically earn higher pay than nonunion workers doing the same kind of job (SEIU, 2011b). In addition, 92% of union employees in the United States had access to health care benefits in 2009, as compared to only 68% of non-union workers, and companies with 30% or more unionized workers were five times as likely to have their entire family health insurance premium paid for, in comparison to companies with no unionized workers (SEIU, 2011b).

Another reason nurses join unions is to communicate their aims, feelings, complaints, and ideas to others. The desire to have input into organizational decision making is a strong motivator for people to join unions. A feeling of powerlessness or the perception that administration does not care about employees is one of the most common reasons for seeking unionization.

CONSIDER THIS  The rapid downsizing and restructuring of the 1990s left many nurses feeling that management did not listen to them or care about their needs. This discontentment provides a fertile ground for union organizers because unions thrive in a climate that perceives the organizational philosophy to be insensitive to the worker.

In addition, nurses join unions because they want to eliminate discrimination and favoritism. Unions emphasize equality and fairness. This might be an especially strong motivator for members of groups that have experienced discrimination, such as women and minorities.

The fourth primary motivation for joining a union stems from the social need to be accepted. Sometimes, this social need results from family or peer pressure. Because many working-class families have a long history of strong union ties, children are frequently raised in a cultural milieu that promotes unionization.

Another reason nurses join unions is because the union contract dictates that all nurses belong to the union. This has been a big driving force among blue-collar workers. However, the *closed shop*, or requirement that all employees belong to a union, has never prevailed in the health care industry. Most health care unions have *open shops*, allowing nurses to choose whether they want to join the union.

Finally, some nurses join unions because they believe that patient outcomes are better in unionized organizations due to better staffing and supervised management practices. One study published in 2004 found an association between nurse unions and lower risk-adjusted heart attack mortality; however, it was unclear if unions were actually the cause of the improved outcomes (Spetz et al., 2011). Longitudinal study follow-up by Spetz et al. (2011) found little relationship between unionization and patient outcomes (see Research Study Fuels the Controversy 18.1).

## REASONS NOT TO JOIN UNIONS

Just as there are many reasons to join unions, there also are many reasons nurses reject unions, including societal and cultural factors (Box 18.4). Many people distrust unions because they believe that they promote the welfare state and oppose the U.S. system of free enterprise. Other individuals reject unions because they feel a need to demonstrate that they can get ahead on their own merits.

### BOX 18.4   REASONS NURSES DO NOT WANT TO JOIN UNIONS

1. The belief that unions promote the welfare state and oppose the U.S. system of free enterprise
2. The need to demonstrate individualism
3. The belief that unionization allows for mediocrity and substandard practice
4. The belief that professionals should not unionize
5. Identification with management's viewpoint
6. Fear of employer reprisal
7. Fear of lost income associated with a strike or walkout

## RESEARCH STUDY FUELS THE CONTROVERSY 18.1

### UNIONIZATION AND PATIENT OUTCOMES

This study examined the impact of unionization on nurse staffing and patient outcomes in California general acute care hospitals using a longitudinal data set (1995 to 2006). Union data were collected through review of public records and a telephone survey and merged with the California Office of Statewide Health Planning and Development (OSHPD) Annual Hospital Disclosure data, as well as patient outcomes calculated using AHRQ Inpatient Quality Indicators and Patient Safety Indicators software.

The researchers estimated the effect of unionization on patient outcomes by using fixed-effects Poisson regression, with the observed number of cases as the dependent variable and the expected number of cases as the offset. Explanatory variables include staffing, patient volumes, casemix, service mix, profit status, system affiliation, market concentration, and HMO penetration.

Spetz, J., Ash, M., Seago, J., & Hererra, C. (2011). *Presentation: The effect of hospital unions on nurse staffing and patient outcomes in California.* Retrieved December 31, 2011, from http://ihea2011.abstractsubmit.org/presentations/1858/

### STUDY FINDINGS

By 2006, about half of all California hospitals were unionized. Preliminary analyses suggested that unionized hospitals had higher staffing, however, hospitals unionized between 1996 and 2006 differed little in the number of staff, with any

advantage from unionization negated by the implementation of minimum nurse-to-patient staffing regulations in 2004. Patient outcomes for most nursing-sensitive indicators improved over time, but little relationship was found between unionization and patient outcomes.

---

In addition, some professional employees reject unions for reasons that deal with class and education. They argue that unions were appropriate for the blue-collar worker but not for the university professor, physician, or engineer. Nurses rejecting unions on this basis usually are driven by a need to demonstrate their individualism and social status.

Other employees identify with management and thus frequently adopt its viewpoint toward unions. These nurses, therefore, reject unions because their values more closely align with management than with workers.

In addition, although employees are protected under the NLRA, some nurses reject unions because of fears of employer reprisal. Nurses who reject unions on this basis could be said to be motivated most of all by a need for job security.

Finally, some employees reject unions because they fear losing income associated with a strike or walkout. Strikes and walkouts are a reality of unionization; however, they are heavily regulated by law (striking is discussed later in this chapter).

Once managers understand the needs and driving forces behind nurses' decisions to join or reject unions, they can begin to address them. Organizations with

unfair management policies are more likely to become unionized. It is certainly then within managerial power to eliminate some of the needs staff feel for joining unions.

Managers can encourage feelings of power by allowing subordinates to have input into decisions that will affect their work. Managers also can listen to ideas, complaints, and feelings and take steps to ensure that favoritism and discrimination are not part of their management style. In addition, managers can strengthen the drives and needs that make nurses reject unions. By building a team effort, sharing ideas and future plans from upper management with the staff, and encouraging individualism in employees, managers can facilitate identification of the worker with management.

When nurses begin showing signs of job dissatisfaction (frustration, stress, perceived powerlessness), they are sending a wake-up call to nursing management. Leaders must be alert to employment practices that are unfair or insensitive to employee needs and intervene appropriately before such issues lead to unionization. However, organizations offering liberal benefit packages and fair management practices may still experience union activity if certain social and cultural factors are present. If union activity does occur, managers must be aware of specific employee and management rights so that the NLRA is not violated by either managers or employees.

## ELIGIBILITY FOR UNION MEMBERSHIP

The NLRA defines a supervisor as

*any individual having authority, in the interest of the employer, to hire, transfer, suspend, lay off, recall, promote, discharge, assign, reward, or discipline other employees, or responsibly to direct them, or to adjust their grievances, or effectively to recommend such action, if in connection with the foregoing the exercise of such authority is not of a merely routine or clerical nature, but requires the use of independent judgment.* (Matthews, 2010, para. 12)

Up until two decades ago, only *supervisors* in nursing were considered managers, and, as such, they were prohibited from joining unions.

However, a 2006 NLRB ruling deemed that *charge nurses* might also be considered supervisors since they are responsible for the coordination and provision of patient care throughout a unit (Matthews, 2010). Even part-time charge nurses were so labeled. This finding has been contested legally since that time and several interpretations have occurred. Reinterpretations by the NLRB are expected in the future.

In addition, the definition of supervisor in nursing came into question with several administrative and court rulings in the early 1990s. These rulings came about as a result of a case involving four licensed practical nurses (LPNs/LVNs) employed at Heartland Nursing Home in Urbana, Ohio. During late 1988 and early 1989, these LPNs complained to management about what they thought were disparate enforcement of the absentee policy; short staffing; low wages for nurses' aides; an unreasonable switching of prescription business from one pharmacy to another, which increased the nurses' paperwork; and management's failure to communicate with employees (NLRB, n.d.-a). Despite assurances from the vice president for operations that they would not be harassed for bringing their concerns to headquarters' attention, three of the LPNs were terminated as a result of their actions.

In response to what they perceived to be illegal termination, the LPNs filed for protection under the NLRA. The NLRB ruled that because the LPNs had responsibility to ensure adequate staffing, to make daily work assignments, to monitor the aides' work to ensure

proper performance, to counsel and discipline aides, to resolve aides' problems and grievances, to evaluate aides' performances, and to report to management, they should be classified as "supervisors," thereby making them ineligible for protection under the NLRA.

On appeal, the administrative law judge (ALJ) disagreed, concluding that the nurses were not supervisors and that the nurses' supervisory work did not equate to responsibly directing the aides *in the interest of the employer*, noting that the nurses' focus is on the well-being of the residents rather than on the employer.

In another turnabout, the U.S. Court of Appeals for the Sixth Circuit then reversed the decision of the ALJ, arguing that the NLRB's test for determining the supervisory status of nurses was inconsistent with the statute and that the interest of the patient and the interest of the employer were not mutually exclusive. The court said that, in fact, the interests of the patient are the employer's business and argued that the welfare of the patient was no less the object and concern of the employer than it was of the nurses. The court also argued that the statutory dichotomy the NLRB first created was no more justified in the health care field than it would be in any other business in which supervisory duties are necessary to the production of goods or the provision of services (*NLRB v. Health Care & Retirement Corp.*, 1994).

The court further stated that it was up to Congress to carve out an exception for the health care field, including nurses, should Congress not wish for such nurses to be considered supervisors. The court reminded the NLRB that the courts, and not the board, bear the final responsibility for interpreting the law. After concluding that the board's test was inconsistent with the statute, the court found that the four licensed practical nurses involved in this case were indeed supervisors and ineligible for protection under the NLRA (*NLRB v. Health Care & Retirement Corp.*, 1994).

This same interpretation, at least for full-time charge nurses, was used in another landmark court case in September 2006 to determine whether charge nurses, both permanent and rotating, at Oakwood Healthcare Inc. were "supervisors" within the meaning of the NLRA, such that they should be excluded from a unit of nurses represented by a union (Rothgerber, Johnson, & Lyons LLP, 2006):

*Notably, to be a supervisor, the NLRB found that an individual must spend "a regular and substantial portion of his/her work time performing supervisory functions. Thus, individuals who sporadically fill in and perform supervisory functions on a substitute basis, such as rotating charge nurses, would not fit the definition of supervisor.* (para. 7)

This was not the case, however, for the full-time charge nurses. The NLRB determined that permanent charge nurses were supervisors but rotating charge nurses were not if this role was less than 10% to 15% of their work time.

Matthews (2010) notes that the Oakwood case has set precedence and figured in approximately 35 subsequent decisions in both health care and industrial settings, although there have been no further rulings addressing the charge nurse/supervisor status. Hence the Oakwood ruling is still in effect today, specifying that nurses, on average, with less than 10% to 15% (equal to about one shift per pay period) of their time as charge nurse are considered staff nurses, while nurses working more than 15% of their professional time as charge nurses are considered supervisors.

---

### DISCUSSION POINT

Would the NLRB's definition of *supervisor* affect charge nurses' eligibility for union membership at the facility in which you work?

---

## ORGANIZING A UNION AND SEEKING REPRESENTATION

Unions use a variety of different tactics when organizing health care workers (Box 18.5). The first step in seeking union representation is determining that adequate levels of desire for unionization exist. The NLRB requires that at least 30% of employees sign an interest card before an election for unionization can be held. Most collective bargaining agents, however, require 60% to 70% of the employees to sign interest cards before they begin an organizing campaign. Union representatives are generally careful to keep a campaign secret until they are ready to file a petition for election. They do this so that they can build momentum without interference from the employer.

However, legislation was introduced in the 2007 Congress called the Employee Free Choice Act (HR 800). Had it passed, unions would have been allowed to request representation from the NLRB by the use of signed cards only. This would have eliminated the need for a secret ballot election to determine union representation. This bill passed the House of Representatives but failed a cloture motion, preventing consideration of the bill in the Senate, by roll call vote (S. 1041: Employee

---

### BOX 18.5   UNION ORGANIZING STRATEGIES

1. Meetings (both group and one-on-one)
2. Leaflets and brochures
3. Pressure on the hospital corporation through media and community contacts
4. Political pressure of regional legislators and local lawmakers
5. Corporate campaign strategies
6. Activism of local employees
7. Using lawsuits
8. Bringing pressure from financiers
9. Technology

---

Free Choice Act of 2007, 2007). The bill was reintroduced unsuccessfully in the 111th Congress in 2009. In 2010, however, four states (Arizona, South Carolina, South Dakota, and Utah) passed constitutional amendments guaranteeing a secret ballot on union recognition.

After enough interest cards have been signed, the organization must hold an election. At that time, all employees of the same classification, such as RNs, vote on whether they desire unionization. A choice in every such election is *no representation*, which means that the voters do not want a union. During the election, 50% plus one of the petitioned units must vote before the union can be recognized. Unions can also be decertified by a process similar to that of certification. *Decertification* can occur when at least 30% of the eligible employees in the bargaining unit initiate a petition asking to no longer be represented by the union.

There are important differences, however, between organizing in a health care facility and in other types of organizations. Generally, the solicitation and distribution of union literature are banned entirely in immediate patient care areas. Managers should never, however, independently attempt to deal with union-organizing activity. They should always seek assistance and guidance from higher-level management and the personnel department.

The entire list of rights for management and labor during the organizing and establishment phases of unionization is beyond the scope of this book.

Throughout the years, Congress has amended various labor acts and laws in the attempt to balance power between management and labor. At times, the balance of power has shifted to management or labor, but Congress eventually enacts laws that attempt to restore what it judges to be the balance. The manager must ensure that the rights of management and employees are protected.

## LABOR–MANAGEMENT RELATIONSHIPS

In the last 30 years, employers and unions have substantially improved their relationships. Although evidence is growing that contemporary management has come to accept the reality that unions are here to stay, businesses in the United States are still less comfortable with unions than their counterparts in many other countries. Likewise, unions have come to accept the fact that there are times when organizations are not healthy enough to survive aggressive union demands.

> CONSIDER THIS    It is possible to create a climate in which labor and management can work together to accomplish mutual goals.

Once management is faced with dealing with a collective bargaining unit, it has a choice of either accepting or opposing the union. It may actively oppose the union by using various union-busting techniques, or it may more subtly oppose the union by attempting to discredit it and win employee trust. *Acceptance* also may run along a continuum. The company may accept the union with reluctance and suspicion. Although they know that the union has legitimate rights, managers often believe they must continually guard against the union encroaching further into traditional management territory.

There is also the type of union acceptance known as *accommodation*. Increasingly common, accommodation is characterized by management's full acceptance of the union, with both union and management showing mutual respect. When these conditions exist, labor and management can establish mutual goals, especially in the areas of safety, cost reduction, efficiency, eliminating waste, and improving working conditions. Such cooperation represents the most mature and advanced type of labor–management relationships.

The bottom line is that the attitudes and the philosophies of the leaders in management and the union determine what type of relationship develops between the two parties in any given organization. When dealing with unions, managers must be flexible. It is critical that they do not ignore issues or try to overwhelm others with power. The rational approach to problem solving must be used.

It is also important to remember that employees have a right to participate in union organizing under the NLRA, and managers must not interfere with this right. Prohibited managerial activities include threatening employees, interrogating employees, promising employees rewards for cessation of union activity, and spying on employees. However, if management picks up early clues of union activity, the organization may be able to take legitimate steps that will discourage unionization of its employees.

> ### DISCUSSION POINT
>
> When unions are present in the workplace, what should be the relationship between them and management? What is accomplished by having a competitive or hostile relationship?

## AMERICAN NURSES ASSOCIATION AND COLLECTIVE BARGAINING

One difficult union issue faced by nurse-managers is the dual role of their professional organization, the ANA. The NLRB recognizes the ANA, at most state levels, as a collective bargaining agent. The use of state associations as bargaining agents is divisive among U.S. nurses. Some nurse-managers believe that they have been disenfranchised by their professional organization. Other managers recognize the conflicts inherent in attempting to sit on both sides of the bargaining table. Even for members who feel that the issue presents no real dilemma, there appears to be some conflict in loyalty.

This conflict has manifested itself in recent splitting away of state nurses associations from the parent ANA organization. Since California RNs broke from the ANA, a number of other states have disaffiliated and declared their independence. There are no easy solutions to the dilemma created by the dual role held by the ANA.

**DISCUSSION POINT**

If you are a student, do you belong to the state student nurses association? If you are an RN, have you joined your state nurses association? Why or why not?

Perhaps the nursing profession should look at the experience of the American Association of University Professors (AAUP), which serves as both a professional association that promotes academic freedom and other professorial concerns and as a collective bargaining unit. In addition, there is a fundraising foundation arm. Wilson (2008) noted that their duality of mission had resulted in declining membership, budget deficits, and membership conflicts. As a result, in June 2008, AAUP leaders met to discuss restructuring the organization. The resultant plan divided the AAUP into three separate entities: a professional association that promotes academic freedom and other academic concerns, a collective bargaining unit, and a fund-raising arm called the AAUP Foundation (Wilson, 2008). This allowed AUP members to determine which part of the organization they wished to support with their membership dues.

CONSIDER THIS   The ANA acts as both a professional association for RNs and a collective bargaining agent. To some nurses, this dual purpose poses a conflict in loyalty.

**DISCUSSION POINT**

Should the ANA—the recognized professional association for nurses in the United States— also be a collective bargaining agent?

## NURSES AND STRIKES

The NLRA states in part that employees shall have the right to engage in "other concerted activities" for the purpose of collective bargaining or other mutual aid or protection (application of the National Labor Relations Board n.d.-b). The phrase "other concerted activities" refers to "the right to effectively communicate with one another regarding self-organization at the jobsite" (para. 8).

The law then gives union members time to work together to determine whether strikes are necessary to achieve desired goals. Such strikes, however, are not allowed without giving the employer and the Federal Mediation and Conciliation Service (FMCS) 10 days' notice of the intent to strike. In doing so, the facility should have a reasonable amount of time to stop admitting patients, transfer existing patients to other facilities, and reduce medical procedures that require nurse-intensive labor. Problems occur when management continues to admit new patients or maintains normal operations.

**DISCUSSION POINT**

Can strikes, walkouts, "blue flu epidemics," and picket lines be considered ethical actions if nurses believe that they are the only way in which they can improve working conditions or ensure safe patient care?

The controversy over whether nurses should strike is long-standing and is likely at the heart of why so many individuals fear union activity. Critics of nurses having the ability to strike suggest that it is unethical because it leaves patients without care providers. Unions argue that strikes must be supported because they are used only as a last resort and after careful consideration of every factor. The issue of striking then continues to divide the nursing profession. Ironically, both proponents and opponents of strikes in nursing argue that they aim for the same goal: safe patient care.

Indeed, the ANA has held consistently for 50+ years that nurses not only have a right to strike but also have a professional responsibility and ethical duty to do so if it means maintaining work conditions conducive to providing high-quality care.

In addition to the moral dilemmas related to the decision to strike, nurses must also determine how they feel about crossing the picket line, should a strike occur. Nurses do have a choice not to participate in strikes or to cross picket lines when strikes occur. They risk derision by their peers in doing so, however, because strikebreakers, commonly known as "scabs," are viewed as taking management's side on the issue and may never be fully accepted by their peers after the strike action has ended.

## CONCLUSIONS

The question of whether nurses should participate in collective bargaining has been around since legislation made such organization possible. Advocates on both sides of the issues present earnest, well-reasoned arguments to support their positions. Clearly, nurses working in unionized organizations appear to have some economic advantage, and their individual vulnerability to arbitrary action on the part of their employer is reduced.

Yet nurse's longstanding struggle to be recognized as a profession underscores concerns that the profession's involvement in collective bargaining associations, historically reserved for blue-collar industries, may undermine this goal. In addition, some nurses think that union activities draw attention away from patients and patient-related activities. Union advocates argue the opposite—that improving pay, benefits, and working conditions ultimately leads to improved patient care.

There are also issues related to who can belong to a union, what the definition of "supervisor" is in nursing, and whether strikes and walkouts are ethically justified for nursing professionals. In addition, the dual role of the ANA as both the national organization for nurses and a collective bargaining agent poses ethical dilemmas for many nurses. Even unionized nurses cannot agree on the intensity and direction their unions should take, resulting in state unions breaking off from the ANA.

Finally, the relationships health care organizations have developed with their collective bargaining agents vary from direct opposition to collaboration. The effect of that relationship on working conditions and quality of patient care cannot be overstated. Unionization, then, is likely to continue to be fraught with challenges and will be one of the most passionate issues nurses will debate for some time to come.

## ACKNOWLEDGMENT

This chapter is reproduced, in part, with permission from Marquis, B., & Huston, C. (2012). Understanding collective bargaining, unionization, and employment laws. In *Leadership roles and management functions in nursing* (7th ed., pp. 513–536). Philadelphia, PA: Lippincott Williams & Wilkins.

## FOR ADDITIONAL DISCUSSION

**1.** Does the presence of unions increase the likelihood that management will be fairer and more consistent with employers?

**2.** How do you feel about the AAUP dividing the organization into three distinctive parts with separate activities—collective bargaining, academic support, and fund raising? Would a similar model work for the ANA?

**3.** Can the need for unionization be eliminated simply by management being more attentive to worker needs and being willing to provide employees reasonable working conditions and a voice in decision making?

**4.** Would you be willing to cross a picket line to work during an authorized strike?

**5.** Are there other ways nurses can increase their group power other than by unions? If so, are they as effective?

**6.** Some state unions are choosing to break off from the ANA. Does this further fragment nursing's collective power in the political arena by diminishing group size, or does it increase the broad-based support of nursing issues?

**7.** Do you believe that the current nursing shortage will accelerate the rate of unionization in nursing?

**8.** How does a nursing shortage affect a union's power in negotiating wages, benefits, and working conditions?

## REFERENCES

Business Dictionary. (2011). *Jurisdictional strike* [Definition]. Retrieved December 30, 2011, from http://www.businessdictionary.com/definition/jurisdictional-strike.html

Franklin D. Roosevelt Presidential Library and Museum. (1935). *Our documents: National Labor Relations Act.* Retrieved December 30, 2011, from docs.fdrlibrary.marist.edu/odnlra.html

Matthews, J. (2010). When does delegating make you a supervisor? *Online Journal of Issues in Nursing, 15*(2). Retrieved December 30, 2011, from http://www.nursingworld.org/MainMenuCategories/ANAMarketplace/ANAPeriodicals/OJIN/TableofContents/Vol152010/No2May2010/Delegating-and-Supervisors.aspx

National Labor Relations Board. (n.d.-a). *Case 09-CA-026348.*Retrieved December 30, 2011, from http://www.nlrb.gov/search/simple/all/Case%2009-CA-%20026348

National Labor Relations Board (n.d.-b) National Labor Relations Act. Retrieved Oct. 9, 2012 from https://www.nlrb.gov/national-labor-relations-act

National Nurses United. (2011). *About the NNU.* Retrieved December 31, 2011, from http://www.nationalnursesunited.org/pages/about

"New national nurses' union a reality!" (2010). *Michigan Nurse, 83*(1), 2–4.

NLRB v. Health Care & Retirement Corp., 114 S. Ct. 1778 (May 23, 1994). Retrieved December 31, 2011, from http://www.law.cornell.edu/supct/html/92-1964.ZS.html

Rothgerber, Johnson, & Lyons LLP. (2006). *Critical NLRB decision clarifies who may be a "supervisor" under the NLRA.* Retrieved August 21, 2008, from http://www.rothgerber.com/files/3337_EmpLawUpdateWinter2006.pdf

S. 1041: Employee Free Choice Act of 2007. (2007). Retrieved December 31, 2011, from http://www.govtrack.us/congress/bill.xpd?bill=s110-1041

Service Employees International Union. (2011a). *About SEIU.* Retrieved December 31, 2011, from http://www.seiu.org/our-union/

Service Employees International Union. (2011b). *The union advantage: Facts and figures.* Retrieved December 30, 2011, from http://www.seiu.org/a/ourunion/research/union-advantage-facts-and-figures.php

Spetz, J., Ash, M., Seago, J., & Hererra, C. (2011). *Presentation: The effect of hospital unions on nurse staffing and patient outcomes in California.* Retrieved December 31, 2011, from http://ihea2011.abstractsubmit.org/presentations/1858/

Wilson, R. (2008). Can reorganization save the AAUP? *Chronicle of Higher Education, 54*(42), A4.

## BIBLIOGRAPHY

August, J., & Grimm, B. (2011). Changing together: Kaiser-union partnership gets results. *Modern Healthcare, 41*(38), 20.

Budd, J., Gollan, P., & Wilkinson, A. (2010). New approaches to employee voice and participation in organizations. *Human Relations, 63*(3), 303–310.

Clover, B., & Santry, C. (2010). One in four nurses would strike as job fears increase. *Nursing Times, 106*(29), 1–3.

Goldberg, C. B., Clark, M. A., & Henley, A. B. (2011). Speaking up: A conceptual model of voice responses following the unfair treatment of others in non-union settings. *Human Resource Management, 50*(1), 75–94.

Huntington, J. (2011). What would Florence do? *Washington Nurse, 41*(2), 24–26.

Lawson, L. D., Miles, K. S., Vallish, R. O., & Jenkins, S. A. (2011). Labor relations: Recognizing nursing professional growth and development in a collective bargaining environment. *Journal of Nursing Administration, 41*(5), 197–200.

Labor law: Nurse fired for criticizing staffing, court sees unfair labor practice by hospital. (2010). *Legal Eagle Eye Newsletter for the Nursing Profession, 18*(2), 8.

Nurses hold record number of actions calling for tax on Wall Street. (2011). *National Nurse, 107*(7), 4–6.

Porter, C. (2010). A nursing labor management partnership model. *Journal of Nursing Administration, 40*(6), 272–276.

Porter, C., Kolcaba, K., McNulty, S., & Fitzpatrick, J. (2010). The effect of a nursing labor management partnership on nurse turnover and satisfaction. *Journal of Nursing Administration, 40*(5), 205–210.

Seago, J., Spetz, J., Ash, M., Herrera, C., & Keane, D. (2011). Hospital RN job satisfaction and nurse unions. *Journal of Nursing Administration, 41*(3), 109–114.

Sister Doris, G. (2011). New ground rules make for smoother union relations. *Health Progress, 92*(4), 54–55.

Sojourner, A. J., Grabowski, D. C., Min, C., & Town, R. J. (2010). Trends in unionization of nursing homes. *Inquiry, 47*(4), 331–342.

Spetz, J., Ash, M., Konstantinidis, C., & Herrera, C. (2011). The effect of unions on the distribution of wages of hospital-employed registered nurses in the United States. *Journal of Clinical Nursing, 20*(1/2), 60–67.

Twarog, J. (2011). Unfair labor practices and the National Labor Relations Act. *Massachusetts Nurse Advocate, 82*(1), 9.

Unionized hospital RNs slightly less satisfied with work than non-unionized RNs. (2011). *AHRQ Research Activities, 372,* 17.

Vesely, R. (2011). Healthcare unions strike . . . at each other in Calif., fighting for members. *Modern Healthcare, 41*(25), 25–26.

Wolschleger, S. M., & Prochaska, K. (2011). Learning what National nurses united is all about. *Michigan Nurse, 84*(4), 8–12.

# Chapter 19

# Assuring Provider Competence Through Licensure, Continuing Education, and Certification

Carol J. Huston

## ADDITIONAL RESOURCES

Visit thePoint for additional helpful resources

- eBook
- Journal Articles
- WebLinks

## LEARNING OBJECTIVES

*The learner will be able to:*

1. Differentiate between *competence* and *continuing competence* in a profession.

2. Identify stakeholders who would be affected by a movement to mandate continuing competence in nursing.

3. Identify driving and restraining forces to implementing mandatory reexamination as a prerequisite for license renewal in nursing.

4. Compare support for mandatory reexamination for license renewal in nursing with that of other health professions such as medicine and pharmacy.

5. Identify arguments for and against mandated continuing education for license renewal.

6. Compare continuing education requirements for nurses with those of physicians, physician assistants, pharmacists, respiratory therapists, and other health care professionals.

7. Describe personal and professional benefits of professional certification.

8. Delineate the roles/responsibilities assumed by the American Board of Nursing Specialties as the accrediting body for nursing certification.

9. Identify the strengths and weaknesses of using professional certification as an indicator of entry-level competence in advanced practice nursing.

10. Describe how portfolios and self-assessment, as tools for reflective practice, can further the goal of professional competence.

11. Explore the roles and responsibilities of the individual, employers, the state board of nursing, and professional associations in assuring both the initial and continued competence of health care practitioners.

12. Reflect on his or her beliefs regarding the need for and efficacy of mandating reexamination for licensure, continuing education, and certification for nurses to assure continuing competence.

How can one determine whether a nurse is competent? Does licensure assure competence? Does clinical performance assure competence? Does competence require clinical practice recency? Is it assured by professional certification? Would nurse residencies increase the competency of the new graduate nurse?

Unfortunately, in many states, a practitioner is determined to be competent when initially licensed and thereafter unless proven otherwise. Yet, clearly, passing a licensing examination and continuing to work as a clinician does not assure competence throughout a career. Competence requires continual updates to knowledge and practice, and this is difficult in a health care environment characterized by rapidly emerging new technologies, chaotic change, and perpetual clinical advancements.

For example, a recent paper excerpted from the Institute of Medicine (IOM) report *The Future of Nursing* suggests that nursing graduates now need competency in a variety of areas including continuous improvement of the quality and safety of health care systems, informatics, evidence-based practice, a knowledge of complex systems, skills and methods for leadership and management of continual improvement, population health and population-based care management, and health policy knowledge, skills, and attitudes (Cronenwett, 2011). One must at least question how many nurses currently in practice would be able to demonstrate competency in these areas.

In 1995, the Task Force on Healthcare Workforce Regulations of the Pew Health Professions Commission recommended changing how health care professions, including nursing, were regulated and suggested that continued competence should be assured as a regulatory board function (North Carolina Board of Nursing [NCBN], 2011). The Citizens Advocacy Center, a public policy organization located in Washington, D.C., concurred, as did the 1999 IOM in its report *To Err Is Human*, which included a recommendation for professional licensing bodies to assume the responsibility for determining licensees' competence and knowledge.

There is little disagreement that the knowledge health care professionals' need must be current and appropriate to their area of practice and that their care should be competent at the minimum. The challenge lies, however, in determining how best to assure that competence and in determining who should be responsible for its oversight.

This chapter explores definitions of *competence* with particular attention given to that of *continuing competence*. Licensure, periodic relicensure, continuing education, and professional certification are examined as potential strategies for assuring provider competence. The chapter also discusses the limitations of each of these strategies for assessing both initial and continuing competence, as well as the difficulties inherent in standardizing continuing competence requirements in a health care system composed of varied stakeholders. Finally, the chapter concludes with an exploration of portfolio development and reflective practice; contemporary strategies that allow health care professionals to carry out a self-assessment of their practice and to develop a personal plan for maintaining competence.

## DEFINING COMPETENCE

*Competence* in nursing can be defined in many ways. In a 1996 position paper titled *Assuring Competence: A Regulatory Responsibility*, the National Council of State Boards of Nursing (NCSBN) defined continued competence as "the application of knowledge and the interpersonal, decision-making, and psychomotor skills expected for the nurse's practice role, within the context of public health, welfare and safety" (NCSBN, 2005, para. 3). Paganini and Egry (2011) suggest that competence is the skill to develop knowledge and ability that enhances professional practice in multiple ways. As such, it is tied to experience and context. Hence, professional competence can be defined as the capacity to handle events and challenges effectively.

In 1999, the American Nurses Association (ANA) convened an expert panel that defined three types of competence in nursing: *continuing competence, professional* nursing competence, and continuing professional nursing competence. Special attention was given, however, to continuing competence because so many assumptions exist regarding the rights and responsibilities of consumers, individual nurses, and employers to see that such competence is present and promulgated. Indeed, it is continuing competence that is a primary focus of this chapter, given that initial licensure suggests that at least minimum competence levels were met at that time.

In 2007, the ANA released a draft position statement on competence and competency for public review and comment. The purpose of this position paper was to define competence ("performing successfully at an expected level") and competency ("an expected level of performance that results from an integration of knowledge, skills, abilities, and judgment within the context of current and projected professional directions"). Key excerpts from the final document released in 2008 are shown in Box 19.1.

Continued competence also was a focus of the NCBN (2011), which defined it as "the ongoing application of knowledge and the decision-making, psychomotor, and interpersonal skills expected of the licensed nurse within a specific practice setting resulting in nursing care that contributes to the health and welfare of clients served" (para. 4).

Clearly, although there is some overlap among these definitions, there is also a lack of consensus around what competence is and how it should be measured. There also appears to be difficulty in relating the continuing competence of providers with the roles they are asked to assume in the clinical setting. For example, some nurses develop high levels of competence in specific areas of nursing practice as a result of work experience and specialization at the expense of staying current in other areas of practice. Yet employers, who espouse the support of continuing competence, often ask registered nurses (RNs) to provide care in areas of practice outside their area of expertise because the current nursing shortage encourages them to do so. In addition, many current competence assessments focus more on skills than they do on knowledge.

> CONSIDER THIS  Nurses are often asked to float to or work in areas where their competence may be in question because their license allows them to work in virtually any area of practice.

In addition, professional nursing organizations decline to implement continuing competence mandates because they fear membership repercussions. For example, the American Nurses Credentialing Center (ANCC) continues to offer certification examinations for registered nurses without baccalaureate degrees, despite the recognition that such certification suggests advanced rather than basic practice.

---

**BOX 19.1    EXCERPTS FROM THE AMERICAN NURSES ASSOCIATION (ANA) DRAFT STATEMENT ON PROFESSIONAL ROLE COMPETENCE (APPROVED 5/28/2008)**

The ANA supports the following principles in regard to competence in the nursing profession:

• The public has a right to expect nurses to demonstrate competence throughout their careers.

• Nurses are individually responsible and accountable for maintaining competence.

• The nursing profession must shape and guide any process assuring nurse competence.

• Regulatory bodies define minimal standards for regulation of practice to protect the public.

• Employers are responsible and accountable to provide an environment conducive to competent practice.

• Assurance of competence is the shared responsibility of the profession, individual nurses, regulatory bodies, employers, and other key stakeholders.

Source: American Nurses Association. (2011). ANA position statement: Professional role competence. Retrieved November 19, 2011, from http://gm6.nursingworld.org/MainMenu Categories/Policy-Advocacy/Positions-and-Resolutions/ANAPositionStatements/Position-Statements-Alphabetically/Professional-Role-Competence.html

The ANA advocates that states defer competence monitoring to the professional association, without governmental involvement in the process, partly because of concern about misconduct charges if state regulators are involved and partly because memberships and revenues are likely to increase if the association monitors competence. Clearly, then, stakeholders and politics continue to influence how continuing competence is defined, used, and promulgated.

The issue is also complicated by the fact that there are no national standards for defining, measuring, or requiring continuing competence in nursing. In addition, specialty nursing organizations, state nurses associations, state boards of nursing, and professional nursing organizations have not reached consensus about what continuing competence is and how to measure it, although there is little debate that it is needed. The reality is that given the multiplicity and variations of the definition of continuing competence and the number of stakeholders affected by its promulgation, identifying and mandating strategies that assure the continuing competence of health care providers will be very difficult.

CONSIDER THIS There is no consensus about how to define or objectively measure competence in nursing practice.

## PROFESSIONAL LICENSURE

Licensure can be defined as

*the granting of permission by a competent authority (usually a government agency) to an organization or individual to engage in a practice or activity that would otherwise be illegal. Licensure is usually granted on the basis of education and examination rather than performance. It is usually permanent, but a periodic fee, demonstration of competence, or continuing education may be required.* (The Free Dictionary by Farlex, 2011, para. 1)

Most health care professionals must be licensed, and this license is assumed to provide at least some assurance that the practitioner is competent in his or her field at the time of initial licensure.

## Licensure Processes in Nursing

One of the most important purposes of the NCSBN and its 60 state boards of nursing (one in each of 46 states, 2 in 4 states, 1 in the District of Columbia, and 1 in each of 5 U.S. territories) is to protect the health, safety, and welfare of the public (Boards of Nursing, 2010; NCBSN, 2011a). This is done by having a regulatory role in the accreditation of nursing education programs, through licensure, and by implementing and enforcing the Nurse Practice Act. In addition, the NCSBN has created and disseminated numerous nursing practice and regulation resources on nursing practice and education and maintains a database on nursing disciplinary actions taken across the nation.

It is for the licensing examinations for RNs and licensed practical nurses/vocational nurses (LPNs/LVNs), however, that the NCSBN and its state boards of nursing are probably best known. The NCSBN has developed two licensure examinations to test the entry-level nursing competence of candidates for licensure as registered nurses and as LPNs/LVNs. These examinations, the National Council Licensure Examinations (NCLEX-RN and NCLEXPN), are administered with the contractual assistance of a national test service (NCSBN, 2011b) and test integrated nursing content. Passage of the NCLEX suggests that the individual has been deemed by the state to have met minimal competence standards for entry into practice; however, this does reflect or measure the many higher level competencies achieved in different types of education programs for nurses.

Despite this flaw, licensure by examination continues to be a highly regarded strategy for assuring competence levels of health care professionals such as nurses. Indeed, some professional organizations and regulatory bodies suggest that RNs should be required to repeat the NCLEX periodically or that nurses should be required to take examinations similar in scope to the NCLEX for license renewal.

Efforts to implement mandatory reexamination as a prerequisite for license renewal in nursing, however, have met with minimal success. This is because there is little agreement about what such an examination should look like, how it would be administered, and how often it should be required. Nonetheless, multiple states have introduced legislation with varying approaches from retesting to requiring a provider to demonstrate competence in the workplace, but resistance is high, and there is little hope that periodic reexaminations to assess competence will be a part of nursing's immediate future.

In addition, 23 states currently participate in the Nurse Licensure Compact (NLC), which allows a nurse to have a license in one state and to practice in other states, as long as that nurse is subject to each state's practice laws and discipline. Such a compact further reduces the likelihood that a nurse would require NCLEX reexamination during his or her career, despite crossing state lines where the initial nursing license was obtained.

## Licensure Processes in Medicine

In contrast to the NCLEX, U.S. medical licensure examinations are developed using a competence-based process that requires examinees to be cognizant of practice changes, the evidence required for practice, and the knowledge necessary to be competent into the future. In addition, to achieve full authority to practice independently, physicians are required to pass three licensure examinations (U.S. Medical Licensing Examination, 1996–2011). Furthermore, a clinical skills examination was implemented in 2004.

In addition, although periodic reexamination was recommended in 1967 by the Bureau of Health Manpower of the U.S. Department of Health for licensure of physicians as of 1971, the decision regarding whether to do so has been left to the discretion of individual states. In most states, this is simply a matter of completing mandatory continuing education requirements and having no disciplinary actions filed against their license.

As a result, a committee of the Federation of State Medical Boards (FSMB) recommended in 2007 that

*boards require doctors applying for relicensure to participate in self-evaluation and practice assessment, show continued competence in areas such as patient care and medical knowledge, and complete an exam in their practice areas. The process, committee members said, would be similar to maintenance of certification, a voluntary program used by specialty boards to ensure lifelong learning as a part of board certification. Members said most medical boards likely would accept recertification as meeting the maintenance of licensure requirements.* (Adams, 2007, para. 3–4).

## Licensure Processes in Pharmacy

Pharmacists have also been reluctant to embrace the IOM's *To Err Is Human* recommendation that periodic reexamination of key providers is critical to resolving health care quality problems, especially medical errors. Pharmacists take a licensing exam on graduation, known as the North American Pharmacist Licensure Examination (NAPLEX). The NAPLEX is a computer-adaptive examination that consists of 185 multiple-choice test questions. The NAPLEX is just one component of the licensure process and is used by the boards of pharmacy as part of their assessment of a candidate's competence to practice as a pharmacist (National Association of Boards of Pharmacy [NABP], 2011a).

In addition, 48 jurisdictions require a Multistate Pharmacy Jurisprudence Examination (MPJE), which combines federal- and state-specific questions to test the pharmacy jurisprudence knowledge of prospective pharmacists. Arkansas, California, Guam, Puerto Rico, Virginia, and the Virgin Islands do not participate (NABP, 2011b). The MPJE consists of 90 multiple-choice test questions. Reciprocity is then granted between states by an electronic licensure transfer program. At present, pharmacists are not required to retake the NAPLEX at any point for license renewal.

---

### DISCUSSION POINT

Why are professional health care organizations reluctant to support reexamination as a means of assuring continuing competence? Who are the stakeholders involved? What are some ramifications of adopting such a mandate?

## CONTINUING EDUCATION

Instead of requiring health care providers to periodically repeat their initial licensure examinations, many professional associations and states have mandated continuing education (CE) for license renewal. This has been done in an attempt to promote continued competence and is less controversial than periodic reexamination for licensure.

### Continuing Education in Nursing

A majority of the states in the United States have some kind of requirements for CE for professional nurse license renewal. These requirements typically vary from a few hours to 30 hours, every 2 years (Box 19.2). There is no requirement for continuing education for registered nurses in Arizona, Colorado, Connecticut, Georgia, Hawaii, Idaho, Illinois, Maine, Maryland, Mississippi, Missouri, Montana, New York, Oklahoma, South Dakota, Tennessee, Vermont, Virginia, Washington, and Wisconsin ("What Continuing Education", 1999–2011). Every other state has some sort of requirement for registered nurses.

Some states—Colorado, for example—required CE at one time but removed that requirement because it felt that CE did not guarantee competence. Similarly, Hawaii discontinued CE requirements for many professions, including nursing and physical therapy, because of high costs of these courses to the individual practitioner, considerable costs to the state to administer the legislation, and the inability to demonstrate positive outcomes.

---

### BOX 19.2 SAMPLE STATE CONTINUING EDUCATION (CE) REQUIREMENTS FOR NURSES

- *Arkansas:* 15 practice focused contact hours every 2 years, or certification or recertification during the renewal period by a national certifying body or completion of 1 college credit hour course in nursing with a grade of C or better during licensure period (Arkansas Board of Registered Nursing, 2011).

- *California:* 30 hours every 2 years (California Board of Registered Nursing, 2011).

- *Florida:* 24 hours every 2 years with 2 hours dedicated to prevention of medical errors. In addition, HIV/AIDS is now a one-time, 1-hour CE requirement to be completed prior to the first renewal and Domestic Violence CE is now a 2-hour requirement every third renewal (Florida Board of Registered Nursing, 2011).

- *Iowa:* 36 hours for a 3-year license and 24 hours for licenses less than 3 years (Iowa Board of Nursing, 2007).

- *Michigan:* Not less than 25 hours of continuing education, with at least 1 hour in pain and symptom management (Michigan Nurses Association, 2009).

- *New Jersey:* 30 hours every 2 years (Continuing Education Requirements, 2011).

- *New York:* 3 contact hours infection control every 4 years and 2 contact hours child abuse (one time; Continuing Education Requirements, 2011).

- *North Dakota:* 12 contact hours every 2 years (Continuing Education Requirements, 2011).

- *Ohio:* 24 hours every 2 years including a minimum of 1 contact hour related to the law (ORC 4723) and the rules (OAC 4723 1–23) governing nursing practice in Ohio (Continuing Education Requirements, 2011).

- *Oregon:* One-time, 7-hour course on pain management (Continuing Education Requirements, 2011).

- *Texas:* 20 hours every 2 years (Texas Board of Nursing, 2011).

## Continuing Education in Medicine

Forty-four states plus Guam, Puerto Rico, and the Virgin Islands require some form of continuing medical education (CME) for relicensure of medical doctors (MDs) and for doctors of osteopathy (DOs), although the requirements frequently differ for the two groups (Medscape Education, 2011).

The number of required hours also varies dramatically by state. For example, Montana, Colorado, Indiana, New York, Oregon, South Dakota, and Vermont require no CME hours for either MDs or DOs. North Carolina and Illinois require 150 hours every 3 years, whereas Wisconsin requires only 30 hours every 2 years and Arkansas requires only 20 hours each year (Medscape Education, 2011). It should be noted, however, that some medical specialty societies, specialty boards, hospital medical staffs, the Joint Commission, and insurance groups require physicians to demonstrate continuing education, even if the state does not require this for relicensure.

In addition, many states have laws that direct the format of the CME. Miller et al. (2008) stated that 17 of the 68 medical and osteopathic licensing boards "require physicians to participate in legislatively mandated topics that may have little to do with the types of patients seen by the applicant physician" (p. 95). Required topics include pain management, AIDS, and domestic violence. Other states require that physicians renewing their licenses must receive instruction on ethics and professional responsibility.

Furthermore, unlike nursing CE, which is typically monitored by the state boards of nursing, there is no central repository of CME. Instead, accredited CME providers are required to keep records of *CE credits* awarded to physicians who participate in their activities for 6 years, and physicians are responsible for maintaining a record of their CME credits from all sources.

Miller et al. (2008) argued that using CME to ensure continued competence is flawed and that CME for physicians must evolve from counting hours of course time to recognizing physician achievement in knowledge, competence, and performance. In addition, Miller et al. advocated that "state medical boards should require valid and reliable assessment of physicians' learning needs" and that "CME planners should create learning activities on the basis of the assessed practice needs of physicians" (p. 97), rather than having a CME system that encourages coursework based on interest alone.

## Continuing Education in Other Health Care Professions

Almost all states require CE for pharmacists, and most require the CE be from approved sources such as the American Council on Pharmacy Education. Sometimes carryover of hours or units is allowed, and sometimes the type is proscribed.

In addition, many states require acupuncturists, audiologists, and occupational therapists to have CE for license renewal. Physician Assistants (PAs) must log 100 hours of continuing medical education every 2 years and sit for a recertification every 6 years to maintain their national certification (American Academy of Physician Assistants, 2011).

In addition, 48 states (Colorado and Wyoming do not) and the District of Columbia mandate CE for relicensure for dentists, with a range of 12 to 25 hours per year with some states requiring annual CE completion and others requiring a sum total every 2 or 3 years (DDS Training, 2011).

## Does Requiring Continuing Education Ensure Competence?

The CE approach to continuing competence continues to be very controversial because there is limited research demonstrating correlation among CE, continuing competence, and improved patient outcomes. In addition, many professional organizations have expressed concern about the quality of mandated CE courses and the lack of courses for experts and specialists. Likewise, there is no agreement on the optimal number of annual credits needed to ensure competence. Until consensus can be reached regarding how CE should be provided and how much is needed, and until research findings show an empirical link between CE and provider competence, it is difficult to tout CE as a valid and reliable measure of continuing competence. Taft and Sparks (2008) summarized the pros and cons of mandating continuing education for nurses (Box 19.3).

## CERTIFICATION

As defined by the American Board of Nursing Specialties (ABNS, 2005), certification is "the formal recognition of the specialized knowledge, skills, and experience demonstrated by the achievement of standards identified by a nursing specialty to promote optimal health outcomes" (para. 1).

Certification does not, however, include a legal scope of practice. The ANCC suggested, however, that it "does protect the public by enabling anyone to identify competent people more readily; aids the profession by encouraging and recognizing professional achievement; recognizes specialization, enhances professionalism and, in some cases, serves as a criterion for financial reimbursement" (ANCC, 2011a, para. 1). Organizations offering specialty certifications for nurses include the ACCN, the American Association of Critical Care

---

### BOX 19.3 PROS AND CONS OF CONTINUING EDUCATION REQUIREMENTS FOR NURSES

**Pros**

- Demonstrates professionalism

- Demonstrates commitment to maintaining competence

- Demonstrates attention to patient safety and a reduction in medical errors

- Motivates employers to support continuing education needs of RN employees

- Raises the standard for continuing education for all nurses

- Research supports the conclusion that continuing education positively affects nursing practice

**Cons**

- Seat time does not guarantee learning

- Difficult to agree on competence standards

- Administrative and monitoring costs

- Concerns about the cost, access, quality, and relevance of continuing education offerings

- Research is inconclusive about the benefits of mandatory continuing education over voluntary continuing education

- Difficult to measure outcomes of mandatory continuing education on patient care due to the many variables that influence patient outcomes, including the individual nurse, the choice of the continuing education program, the continuing education program itself, learning styles, professionalism, and accountability

*Source:* Taft, L., & Sparks, R. K. (2008). Mandatory continuing education for nurses. *Nursing Matters, 19*(3), 4.

Nursing, the American Association of Nurse Anesthetists, the American College of Nurse Midwives, the Board of Certification for Emergency Nursing, and the Rehabilitation Nursing Certification Board.

## Becoming Certified

To achieve professional certification, nurses must meet eligibility criteria that may include years and types of work experience, as well as minimum educational levels, active nursing licenses, and successful completion of a nationally administered examination. Certifications normally last 5 years.

## The American Board of Nursing Specialties

In addition to the large numbers of certified nurses, there are many different types of nursing certification credentials, and certification programs often have very different standards. This makes it difficult for providers and consumers to determine the value of a particular nursing certification. For this reason, the ABNS was created in 1991 to create uniformity in nursing certification, advocate for consumer protection by establishing specialty nursing certification, and increase public awareness of the value of quality certification to health care.

The ABNS is composed of nurse-certifying organizations from around the world. As the only accrediting body specifically for nursing certification, the Accreditation Council provides a peer-review process for accrediting nursing certification programs that demonstrate compliance with ABNS standards.

## The American Nurses Credentialing Center

The ANCC calls itself "the largest and most prestigious nurse credentialing organization in the United States" (ANCC, 2011b, para. 4). The ANA established the ANA Certification Program in 1973 to provide tangible recognition of professional achievement in a defined functional or clinical area of nursing. The ANCC, a subsidiary of the ANA, became its own corporation in 1991, and since then has certified more than a quarter million nurses and approximately 75,000 advanced practice nurses (ANCC, 2011a). The ANCC administers more than 20 specialty and advanced practice certification examinations each year at authorized testing agencies across the country.

## Certification and the Advanced Practice Nurse

Advanced practice nurses were the first nurses to use professional certification as a means of documenting advanced knowledge in practice. In 1946, the American Association of Nurse Anesthetists began certifying nurse anesthetists. The American College of Nurse Midwives soon followed. Most states now use certification as an indicator of entry-level competence in advanced practice nursing, which includes clinical nurse specialists (CNS) and nurse practitioners (NPs).

Even the NCSBN, which originally proposed second licensure for NPs, now recognizes the certification examination as the regulatory mechanism for advanced nursing practice. A master's degree is required to take the certification examinations for advanced practice nurses. Certification, then, in the case of the advanced practice nurse is not really voluntary; it is required to ensure public safety and enhance public health.

---

**DISCUSSION POINT**

The ANCC currently does not allow educational waivers for the CSN- or NP-certifying examination (all applicants must have at least a master's degree). Do you support this decision to not "grandfather" advanced practice nurses who completed their educations through certifying programs (no master's degree) and who are currently practicing in an advanced role? Why or why not?

---

**DISCUSSION POINT**

Physician Assistants must pass a national certification examination for licensure. Why is this not also required for nurse practitioners?

---

## The Effect of Professional Certification

A great deal of research has been completed the last decade regarding the use of certification to ensure competence and its inherent value. Most of these studies suggest that certification does have an effect on both improved patient outcomes and the creation of a positive work environment.

A recent study by Kendall-Gallagher, Aiken, Sloane, and Cimiotti (2011) found that nurse specialty certification was associated with better patient outcomes; however, certification had no impact on mortality and failure to rescue when the nurse did not have a baccalaureate degree. The researchers suggested then that since certification was not a substitute for education, employers might want to invest in improving nursing education levels for staff without BSN degrees, rather than investing in specialty certification for these nurses.

Research done by Krapohl, Manojlovich, Redman, and Zhang (2010) found no correlation between the proportion of certified nurses on an intensive care unit and three nursing sensitive patient outcomes, although educational levels of the nurses were not considered. The association between nurses' perception of overall workplace empowerment and certification, however, was positive.

Krischke (2010) agrees, suggesting that nurses who achieve specialty certification have more credibility to their professionalism and that this external validation of a specialized knowledge basis is one of the most important reasons most individuals seek certification. Krischke also notes that certification adds to both income and hiring potential. Indeed, a 2011 salary survey found an increase in salaries for nurses when they achieved higher academic degrees and when they achieved certification in a specialty area (Nurses Earn More, 2011).

Research by Haskins, Hnatiuk, and Yoder (2011) also found that certification validated nurses' qualifications and expertise, provided for increased career opportunities and enhanced professional autonomy. The impact on salary, however, was unclear (see Research Study Fuels the Controversy 19.1). Box 19.4 provides a summary of some of the personal benefits associated with specialty certification.

## Creating Work Environments That Value Certification

It is middle- and top-level nurse managers who play the most significant role in creating work environments that value and reward certification. For example, nurse managers can grant tuition reimbursement or salary incentives to workers who seek certification. This is critical because the greatest barrier to nurses obtaining specialty certification in a recent study was the cost of the examination and the greatest barrier to recertification was the fee for renewal (Haskins et al., 2011). Managers can also show their support for professional certification by giving employees paid time off to take the certification exam and by publicly recognizing employees who have achieved specialty certification.

Managers should also encourage certified nurses to promote their achievements by introducing themselves as certified medical-surgical nurses to patients, wearing

### BOX 19.4 PERSONAL BENEFITS OF PROFESSIONAL CERTIFICATION

**Professional certification**

- Provides a sense of accomplishment and achievement
- Validation of specialty knowledge and competence to peers and patients
- Increased credibility
- Increased self-confidence
- Promotes greater autonomy of practice
- Provides for increased career opportunities and greater competitiveness in the job market
- May result in salary incentives

their certification pins, and publicly displaying their credentials (Haskins et al., 2011). In doing so, the certified nurse acts as a role model to other nurses considering specialty certification.

Altman (2011) notes that many nurses do not seek certification due to a fear of test taking or failure, and she suggests that nurse leaders can play a pivotal role in supporting employees to overcome these fears. It may be as simple as providing study resources, granting time off to study, supporting nurses verbally during their certification journey, and rewarding and recognizing staff who do become certified.

### DISCUSSION POINT

Do most employers value professional certification? Do nurses value it? Does the general public value it? On what criteria do you base your answer?

### REFLECTIVE PRACTICE

Kinsella (2010) suggests that *reflective practice*, a term coined by Donald Schon, is one of the most popular theories of professional knowledge in the last 20 years. Reflective practice is defined by the NCBN (2011) as "a process for the assessment of one's own practice to identify and seek learning opportunities to promote

## RESEARCH STUDY FUELS THE CONTROVERSY 19.1

### PERCEIVED VALUE OF CERTIFICATION

Haskins, Hnatiuk, and Yoder (2011) distributed the 18-item Perceived Value of Certification Tool, developed by the Competency and Credentialing Institute, electronically to 6,775 medical/surgical nurses. The response rate was 26% (1,748 responded with 1,659 completed surveys, 89 partial responses, and 481 emails returned).

Haskins, M., Hnatiuk, C., & Yoder, L. H. (2011). *Medical-surgical nurses' perceived value of certification study.* *MEDSURG Nursing, 20*(2), 71–93.

### STUDY FINDINGS

Data indicated certified medical-surgical nurses had a positive perception of the value of certification. Responses by both certified and noncertified nurses to survey statements indicated a high level of agreement with the value statements about certified practice, although a higher percentage of certified nurses reported agreement with the value statements than non-certified nurses. The one statement that received a low level of agreement by both groups of respondents was "Certification increases salary."

More than 98% of respondents reported enhanced feelings of personal accomplishment as a result of certification. More than 97% reported personal satisfaction with having attained specialty certification, and the same percentage reported feeling validated about their specialized knowledge. All of this led to enhanced professional credibility and new professional challenges.

The researchers concluded that while nursing licensure is intended to ensure minimal competency of professional nurses, certification demonstrates nurses' achievement of a high level of competence or expertise in a particular area or specialty.

---

continued competence" (para. 7). Inherent in the process is the evaluation and incorporation of this learning into one's practice. Such self-assessment is gaining popularity as a way to promote professional practice and maintain competence. Perhaps that is why nursing is moving away from a continuing education model to a reflective practice/professional portfolio model for competence assessment (O'Malley, 2008).

For example, North Carolina now requires RNs to use a reflective practice approach to carry out a self-assessment of her or his practice and develop a plan for maintaining competence (NCBN, 2011). This assessment is individualized to the licensed nurse's area of practice. RNs seeking license renewal or reinstatement must attest to having completed the learning activities required for continuing competence and be prepared to submit evidence of completion if requested by the board on random audit (NCBN, 2011).

Similarly, the Nurses Association of New Brunswick (NANB) developed a mandatory continuing competence program for implementation in 2008 that requires registered nurses to demonstrate on an annual basis how they have maintained their competence and enhanced

their practice (NANB, 2011). The three steps of the NANB mandatory Continuing Competence Program (CCP) are as follows:

1. Self-assessment of nursing practice to determine learning needs
2. Development and implementation of a learning plan to meet the identified learning needs
3. Evaluation of the effect of learning activities.

> CONSIDER THIS Competence is continually maintained and acquired through reflective practice, lifelong learning, and integration of learning into nursing practice (NANB, 2011).

The College of Registered Nurses of British Columbia (CRNBC) also has a mandatory CCP in place. This program was created in 2000 in response to the Health Professions Act, which required the establishment and maintenance of a CCP to promote high practice standards among registered nurses. In the year before license renewal, registrants are expected to

> complete a self assessment using CRNBC's Professional Standards for Registered Nurses and Nurse Practitioners, and where relevant, review the practice standards and the Scope of Practice Standards to identify learning needs; obtain peer feedback; develop and implement a learning plan based on their self assessment and peer feedback; and evaluate the impact of last year's learning on their practice. (Winslow, 2008, p. 17)

Of the just more than 2,900 CRNBC registered nurses audited in 2008, only 177 received "conditions" on their licensure for noncompliance with the continuing competence requirements (Winslow, 2008). Registrants are allowed to practice only for an additional 3 months before requirements must be met.

## Portfolios and Self-Assessment

Portfolio development is another strategy the individual RN can use to be reflective about his or her practice and/or to assess or demonstrate competence: Sherrod (2007) suggests the professional portfolio typically contains a number of core components, such as biographical information; educational background; certifications achieved; employment history; a one- to two-page resume; a competence record or checklist; personal and professional goals; professional development experiences, presentations, consultations, and publications; professional and community activities; honors and awards; and letters of thanks from patients, families, peers, organizations, and others.

O'Malley (2008) suggested that the portfolio should not, however, just be a collection of certificates nor a diary or logbook. Instead, she suggested that it be a "living document" that demonstrates critical thinking, values, skills, and, perhaps most important, reflection. O'Malley suggested that the writer and the reader of the portfolio should experience a nursing career journey with diverse sources of evident and written reflections.

McColgan (2008) agreed, suggesting that portfolios allow nurses to assess their competence, complete work-based reflection, pursue lifelong learning, create career paths, and pursue professional development. McColgan concluded that for portfolios to work effectively, nurses and their employers must have a working partnership and jointly appreciate the value and the opportunities that exist through personal portfolio development.

> CONSIDER THIS   All nurses should maintain a portfolio to reflect their professional growth throughout their career.

## WHO IS RESPONSIBLE FOR COMPETENCE ASSESSMENT IN NURSING?

Who, then, has the responsibility for competence assessment in nursing? Should it be the individual, the employer, the regulatory board, or the certifying agency? Is it a shared responsibility? If so, are these entities willing to work together to create an integrated and systematic approach to promoting continuing competence in nursing?

Certainly, an individual responsibility for maintaining competence is suggested by the *ANA Code of Ethics for Nurses With Interpretive Statements* in its assertion that nurses are obligated to provide adequate and competent nursing care (ANA, 2001). State nurse practice acts also hold nurses accountable for being reasonable and prudent in their practice. Both standards require the nurse to have at least some personal responsibility for continually assessing his or her professional competence through reflective practice.

> CONSIDER THIS   The individual registered nurse has a professional obligation to maintain competence.

The role of the professional association also lacks clarity. Although professional associations develop and promote standards, there is no oversight function of either initial or continuing competence.

Employers also play a role in assuring competence of employees by performing periodic performance appraisals and by carrying out the requirements of the accrediting bodies to ensure the ongoing competencies of employees. Yet employers are often among the first to argue that "a nurse is a nurse is a nurse" when it comes to meeting mandatory staffing or licensure requirements.

Regulatory boards, such as the state boards of nursing, regulate initial licensure, monitor compliance with requirements for license renewal, and take action when professional standards are breached. Yet, clearly, licensure and relicensure per se do not guarantee competence, particularly in a discipline as broad in scope and practice as nursing.

Finally, certifying organizations do help to identify those individuals who have an expertise in a specific area of practice; however, knowledge expertise does not always translate into practice expertise. A lack of professional certification does not necessarily mean that the nurse lacks continuing competence. Recertification does not ensure continued expertise because recertification is usually a product of meeting CE requirements rather than reexamination.

## CONCLUSIONS

The challenge in assuring competence in nursing is that nursing practice is dynamic, and thus best practice must be continually redefined as a result of new discoveries. Licensure, continuing education, and professional certification can only ensure provider competence if they reflect the latest thinking, research, and clinical practice needs. In addition, each of these three strategies is limited in its effectiveness as a competence assessment strategy.

Clearly, the NCLEX, as it currently exists, assures only minimum entry-level competence for professional nursing practice. Given that NCLEX content derives from a retrospective model and that technological changes and the rate of knowledge acquisition are increasing exponentially in the 21st century, the knowledge base of the newly licensed nurse has a great likelihood of being dated even before examinations are scored. In addition, as long as a single NCLEX exists and there are multiple levels of educational entry into practice, the examination will continue to have to meet educational content directed at the lowest educational level of entry.

In addition, health care professionals, professional organizations, and regulatory bodies are reluctant to implement mandatory reexamination for licensure. One must at least question whether this is because of the fear that many providers would be unable to demonstrate the continuing competence necessary for relicensure.

CE has similar limitations for assuring provider competence. Some states do not require nurses to complete CE. Those that do demonstrate wide variation in how much CE is required, what content can be included, and how that CE can be provided. In addition, there is no guarantee that completing CE courses results in a change in the provider's knowledge level or practice or even that the content provided in the CE course is current and relevant.

Finally, professional certification does ensure that the nurse has some specialized area of knowledge and practice expertise. The reality, however, is that many nurses perform outside of the area of their certification expertise each and every day in their jobs, particularly if their area of specialty certification expertise is narrow. In addition, there are multiple certifying bodies and numerous types of certification. Determining the exact value of that certification in terms of improving patient care has not completely been ascertained.

How best to ensure provider competence cannot yet be answered. Efforts that address the need to do so are under way, but these efforts have not been coordinated or integrated by the professional associations, regulatory bodies, and stakeholders that are affected. In addition, most professional entities involved in ensuring continuing competence are reluctant to mandate interventions for fear of alienating stakeholders. Individual practitioners also seem reluctant to embrace reflective practice or to put the thought and effort into creating portfolios that identify continuing competence in concrete and measurable ways. Until the focus rests solely on the need to protect patients and improve the quality of health care, mandated interventions for continuing competence are likely never to occur and provider competence will not be assured.

## FOR ADDITIONAL DISCUSSION

**1.** Who should be responsible for the cost of ensuring provider competence—the provider, the employer, the clients that are served, or some other entity?

**2.** How likely is it that states, professional organizations, professional certifying organizations, and employers will be willing to agree on standardized measures for assessing professional competence?

**3.** Would most RNs support mandatory development of a portfolio? Are most RNs actively engaged in reflective practice in an effort to assess their ongoing competence?

**4.** Why should the entry-level examination for nursing be broad and general in scope, whereas continuing competence is arguably demonstrated by professional certification in specialty areas?

**5.** Are cost and access deterrents to professional certification? If so, how can these barriers be overcome?

**6.** Do most nurses view continuing education coursework as a reliable and valid tool for increasing provider competence?

**7.** Should nurses be required to complete mandated continuing education hours in the area of nursing practice in which they work?

**8.** Are there core competencies all licensed nurses must achieve regardless of the setting in which they practice?

## REFERENCES

Adams, D. (2007). *Stricter requirements sought for relicensure as medical boards draft proposal.* Retrieved August 22, 2008, from http://www.ama-assn.org/amednews/2007/12/24/prl21224.htm

Altman, M. (2011). Let's get certified: Best practices for nurse leaders to create a culture of certification. *AACN Advanced Critical Care, 22*(1), 68–75.

American Academy of Physician Assistants. (2011). *Information about PAs and the PA profession.* Retrieved November 19, 2011, from http://www.orthocarolina.com/uploads/news/Information%20About%20PAs%20and%20the%20PA%20Profession.pdf

American Board of Nursing Specialties. (2005). *Promoting excellence in nursing certification: A position statement on the value of specialty nursing certification.* Retrieved November 2011, from http://nursingcertification.org/pdf/value_certification.pdf

American Nurses Association. (2001). *Code of ethics for nurses with interpretive statements.* Washington, DC: Author.

American Nurses Association. (2011). *ANA position statement: Professional role competence.* Retrieved November 19, 2011, from http://gm6.nursingworld.org/MainMenuCategories/Policy-Advocacy/Positions-and-Resolutions/ANAPositionStatements/Position-Statements-Alphabetically/Professional-Role-Competence.html

American Nurses Credentialing Center. (2011a). *Certification FAQs.* Retrieved November 19, 2011, from http://www.nursecredentialing.org/FunctionalCategory/FAQs/CertiticationFAQs.aspx

American Nurses Credentialing Center. (2011b). *About ANCC.* Retrieved November 19, 2011, from http://www.nursecredentialing.org/FunctionalCategory/AboutANCC.aspx

Arkansas Board of Registered Nursing. (2011). *Continuing Education.* Retrieved November 19, 2011, from http://www.arsbn.arkansas.gov/education/Pages/continuingEducation.aspx

Boards of nursing in the United States state-by-state web links. (2010). Retrieved November 19, 2011, from http://www.medscape.com/viewarticle/482270

California Board of Registered Nursing. (2011). *Continuing education for license renewal.* Retrieved November 18, 2011, from http://www.rn.ca.gov/licensees/ce-renewal.shtml

Continuing education requirements by state: New Hampshire-Oregon. (2011). *Advance for Nurses.* Retrieved November 19, 2011, from http://nursing.advanceweb.com/Article/Continuing-Education-Requirements-by-State.aspx

Cronenwett, L. R. (2011). *The future of nursing education.* Retrieved November 23, 2011, from http://www.iom.edu/~/media/Files/Activity%20Files/Workforce/Nursing/Future%20of%20Nursing%20Education.pdf

DDS training. (2011). Retrieved November 19, 2011, from http://www.ddstraining.com/dental-ce-by-state

Florida Board of Registered Nursing. (2011). *Continuing education requirements.* Retrieved November 19, 2011, from http://www.health-first.org/internal_access/education/fbn_con_ed_requirements_feb17.pdf

The Free Dictionary by Farlex. (2011). *Licensure* [Definition]. Retrieved November 19, 2011, from http://medical-dictionary.thefreedictionary.com/licensure

Haskins, M., Hnatiuk, C., & Yoder, L. H. (2011). Medical-surgical nurses' perceived value of certification study. *MEDSURG Nursing, 20*(2), 71–93.

Iowa Board of Nursing. (2007). *Continuing education: The basic requirements.* Retrieved November 18, 2011, from http://www.iowa.gov/nursing//continuing_ed/basic_requirement.html

Kendall-Gallagher, D., Aiken, L. H., Sloane, D. M., & Cimiotti, J. P. (2011). Nurse specialty certification, inpatient mortality, and failure to rescue. *Journal of Nursing Scholarship, 43*(2), 188–194.

Kinsella, E. (2010). Professional knowledge and the epistemology of reflective practice. *Nursing Philosophy, 11*(1), 3–14.

Krapohl, G., Manojlovich, M., Redman, R., & Zhang, L. (2010). Nursing specialty certification and nursing-sensitive patient outcomes in the intensive care unit. *American Journal of Critical Care, 19*(6), 490–499.

Krischke, M. M. (2010). *The benefits of nursing specialty certification.* Retrieved November 19, 2011, from http://www.nursezone.com/Nursing-News-Events/more-features/The-Benefits-of-Nursing-Specialty-Certification_34206.aspx

McColgan, K. (2008). The value of portfolio building and the registered nurse: A review of the literature. *Journal of Perioperative Practice, 18*(2), 64–69.

Medscape Education. (2011). *State CME requirements.* Retrieved November 19, 2011, from http://www.medscape.org/public/staterequirements

Michigan Nurses Association. (2009). *Continuing education requirements for Michigan nurses.* Retrieved November 18, 2011, from http://www.michigan.gov/documents/lara/LARA_Nursing_CE_Brochure_5-11_376431_7.pdf

Miller, S., Thompson, J., Mazmanian, P., Aparicio, A., Davis, D., Spivey, B. E., & Kahn, N. B. (2008). Continuing medical education, professional development, and requirements for medical licensure: A white paper of the Conjoint Committee on continuing medical education. *Journal of Continuing Education in the Health Professions, 28*(2), 95–98.

National Association of Boards of Pharmacy. (2011a). *North American Pharmacist Licensure Examination (NAPLEX).* Retrieved November 19, 2011, from http://www.nabp.net/programs/examination/naplex/index.php

National Association of Boards of Pharmacy. (2011b). *MPJE.* Retrieved November 19, 2011, from http://www.nabp.net/programs/examination/mpje/

National Council State Boards of Nursing. (2005). *Fast facts about the continued competence practice analysis.* Retrieved November 19, 2011, from https://www.ncsbn.org/pdfs/07_25_05_continued_comprtencyt_faq.pdf

National Council State Boards of Nursing. (2011a). *About NCSBN.* Retrieved November 18, 2011, from https://www.ncsbn.org/about.htm

National Council State Boards of Nursing. (2011b). *NCLEX examinations.* Retrieved November 19, 2011, from https://www.ncsbn.org/nclex.htmAc

North Carolina Board of Nursing. (2011). *Continuing competence.* Retrieved November 18, 2011, from http://www.ncbon.com/content.aspx?id=664

Nurses Association of New Brunswick. (2011). *Continuing competence program.* Retrieved November 21, 2011, from http://www.nanb.nb.ca/index.php/practice/ccp

Nurses earn more with specialty certification. (2011). *AACN Bold Voices, 3*(9), 5.

O'Malley, P. A. (2008). Profile of a professional. *Nursing Management, 39*(6), 24–27, 48.

Paganini, M. C., & Egry, E. Y. (2011). The ethical component of professional competence in nursing: An analysis. *Nursing Ethics, 18*(4), 571–582.

Sherrod, D. (2007). Professional portfolio: A snapshot of your career. *Nursing, 37*(Suppl. 1), 18.

Taft, L., & Sparks, R. K. (2008). Mandatory continuing education for nurses. *Nursing Matters, 19*(3), 4.

Texas Board of Nursing. (2011). *Continuing competency: Lifelong learning. Understanding and complying with the continuing competency requirements, including continuing education, for nurses in Texas.* Retrieved November 19, 2011, from http://www.bon.state.tx.us/nursingeducation/ceu.html

U.S. Medical Licensing Exam. (1996–2011). *Overview: Introduction.* Retrieved November 19, 2011, from http://www.usmle.org/bulletin/overview/

What continuing education does a nurse need. (1999–2011). Retrieved November 18, 2011, from http://www.ehow.com/facts_4969045_continuing-education-does-nurse-need.html

Winslow, W. (2008). Personal practice review inspires RNs to be lifelong learners. *Nursing BC/College of Registered Nurses of British Columbia, 40*(3), 16–19.

## BIBLIOGRAPHY

Bolden, L., Cuevas, N., Raia, L., Meredith, E., & Prince, T. (2011). The use of reflective practice in new graduate registered nurses residency program. *Nursing Administration Quarterly, 35*(2), 134–139.

Chambers, S., Brosnan, C., & Hassell, A. (2011). Introducing medical students to reflective practice. *Education for Primary Care, 22*(2), 100–105.

Chang, M., Chang, Y., Kuo, S., Yang, Y., & Chou, F. (2011). Relationships between critical thinking ability and nursing competence in clinical nurses. *Journal of Clinical Nursing, 20*(21/22), 3224–3232.

Dobson, C., & Hess, R. R. (2010). Pursuing competence through continuing education. *Journal of Nursing Regulation, 1*(2), 8–13.

Fahy, A., Tuohy, D., McNamara, M. C., Butler, M., Cassidy, I., & Bradshaw, C. (2011). Evaluating clinical competence assessment. *Nursing Standard, 25*(50), 42–48.

Green, T., Dickerson, C., & Blass, E. (2010). Using competences and competence tools in workforce development. *British Journal of Nursing, 19*(20), 1293–1298.

Kaplow, R. (2011). Symposium introduction: Creating a culture to promote nursing specialty certification. *AACN Advanced Critical Care, 22*(1), 23–24.

Lenburg, C. B., Abdur-Rahman, V. Z., Spencer, T. S., Boyer, S. A., & Klein, C. J. (2011). Implementing the COPA model in nursing education and practice settings: Promoting competence, quality care, and patient safety. *Nursing Education Perspectives, 32*(5), 290–296.

Ryan, M. (2011). Evaluating portfolio use as a tool for assessment and professional development in graduate nursing education. *Journal of Professional Nursing, 27*(2), 84–91.

Smith, L. S. (2011). Showcase your talents with a career portfolio. *Nursing, 41*(7), 54–56.

Sulosaari, V., Suhonen, R., & Leino-Kilpi, H. (2011). An integrative review of the literature on registered nurses' medication competence. *Journal of Clinical Nursing, 20*(3/4), 464–478.

Sturmberg, J., & Hinchy, J. (2010). Borderline competence—From a complexity perspective: Conceptualization and implementation for certifying examinations. *Journal of Evaluation in Clinical Practice, 16*(4), 867–872.

Vernon, R., Chiarella, M., & Papps, E. (2011). Confidence in competence: Legislation and nursing in New Zealand. *International Nursing Review, 58*, 103–108.

Wilkerson, B. (2011). Specialty nurse certification effects patient outcomes. *Plastic Surgical Nursing, 31*(2), 57–59.

XiaoJing, H., Dan, Z., & MinHua, Z. (2011). Clinical nursing faculty competence inventory—Development and psychometric testing. *Journal of Advanced Nursing, 67*(5), 1109–1117.

# Unit 5

# Professional Power

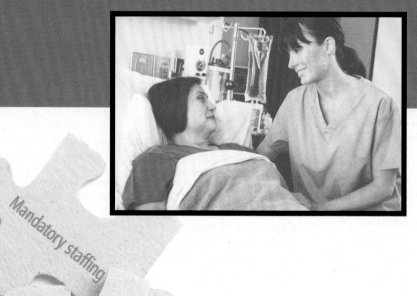

Mandatory staffing

Workplace violence

Entry into practice

# Chapter 20

# The Nursing Profession's Historic Struggle to Increase Its Power Base

Carol J. Huston

## ADDITIONAL RESOURCES

Visit thePoint for additional helpful resources
- eBook
- Journal Articles
- WebLinks

## CHAPTER OUTLINE

**Factors Contributing to Powerlessness in Nursing**
*Oppression of Nurses as a Group*
*Failure to Align Fully With the Feminist Movement*
*Limited Collective Representation of Nurses*
*Socialization of Women to View Power and Politics Negatively*
*Inadequate Recognition of Nursing as an Educated Profession With Evidence-Based Practice*

*The Nursing Profession's History of Being Reactive in National Policy Setting*

**Driving Forces to Increase Nursing's Power Base**
*Timing Is Right*
*Size of the Nursing Profession and Diversity of Our Practice*
*Nursing's Referent Power*
*An Increasing Knowledge Base and Education for Nurses*
*Nursing's Unique Perspective*
*Consumers and Providers Want Change*

**Action Plan for the Future**
*Place More Nurses in Positions of Influence*
*Stop Acting Like Victims*
*Become Better Informed About All Health Care Policy Efforts*
*Build Coalitions Inside and Outside of Nursing*
*Conduct More Research to Strengthen Evidence-Based Practice*
*Support Nursing Leaders*
*Mentor Future Nurse Leaders and Plan for Leadership Succession*

**Conclusions**

## LEARNING OBJECTIVES

*The learner will be able to:*

1. Explore factors that historically led to nursing's limited power as a profession.

2. Examine characteristics of oppressed groups and analyze whether the nursing profession displays those characteristics.

3. Examine factors that led to the divergence of the nursing profession and feminism in the 1960s and 1970s and subsequently to their convergence in the mid-1980s as part of second-wave feminism.

4. Analyze the influence of gender in how many nurses view policy and politics, the willingness of nurses to work together collectively to achieve common goals, and the mentoring opportunities available to the profession's future leaders.

5. Identify driving forces in place to increase the nursing profession's power base.

6. Identify potential partners/external stakeholders/alliances which could strengthen the nursing profession's power in national and global policy arenas.

7. Identify nurses currently holding elected office in Congress and state legislatures, as well as the significant committees they serve on or positions they hold.

8. Identify issues currently being debated in the legislature that affect nursing and health care.

9. Explore individual, organizational, and professional responsibilities for succession planning to ensure that an adequate number of highly qualified nursing leaders exist in the future.

10. Reflect on whether the need to be politically competent should be internalized by nurses as a moral and professional obligation.

Power is an elusive concept. The word *power* is derived from the Latin verb *potere*, meaning "to be able," thus, power may be appropriately defined as that which enables an individual or a group to accomplish goals. Power can also be defined as the capacity to act or the strength and potency to accomplish something (Marquis & Huston, 2012). Having power then gives an individual or a group the potential to change the attitudes and behaviors of others.

How individuals view power, however, varies greatly. Indeed, power may be feared, worshipped, or mistrusted, and it is frequently misunderstood (Marquis & Huston, 2012). Many women (and thus nurses) have historically demonstrated ambivalence toward the concept of power and some have even eschewed the pursuit of power.

This likely occurred as a result of how many women were socialized to view power, believing that women do not inherently possess power (formal or informal) or authority. In addition, rather than feeling capable of achieving and managing power, many women feel that power manages them. These gender-based perceptions are changing, yet women still have much ground to make up in terms of learning to use power as a tool for personal and professional success.

Similarly, the nursing profession has not historically been the powerful force it could be in dealing with issues directly affecting health care and the profession itself. In a recent Gallup poll of more than 1,500 thought leaders from insurance, corporate, health services, government and industry, as well as university faculty, the majority felt that nurses should have more influence in many areas of the health care system, including reducing medical errors, increasing the quality of care, promoting wellness, improving efficiency, and reducing costs (Robert Wood Johnson Foundation [RWJF], 2011a). In addition, these thought leaders said that "nurses should have more influence than they do now on health policy, planning, and management. But when asked how much influence various professions and groups are likely to have in health reform, opinion leaders put nurses behind government, insurance, and pharmaceutical executives, and many others—and they see real barriers to nursing leadership" (RWJF, 2011a, para. 2).

Indeed nurses are often thought of as an apolitical group. As a result, nursing has more often than not been reactive (rather than proactive) in the policy arena, addressing proposed legislation after its introduction rather than drafting or sponsoring legislation that reflects nursing's agenda. As a result, external forces (typically male dominated and medically focused) have often controlled nursing.

All of these factors have contributed to the nursing profession having a relatively small power base in the political arena and some invisibility as a force in health care decision making. This chapter explores factors that have led to this relative powerlessness as a profession. Driving forces are identified that are in place to increase nursing's professional power. The chapter concludes with an action plan to increase nursing's power base so that the profession is recognized as an increasingly significant force in health care decision making in the 21st century.

## DISCUSSION POINT

Why is it that nurses, the largest group of health professionals, with perhaps the greatest firsthand knowledge of the health care problems faced by consumers, have not historically been an integral part of health care policy decision making?

## FACTORS CONTRIBUTING TO POWERLESSNESS IN NURSING

Many factors have contributed to the nursing profession's relative powerlessness in health care policy setting. Six factors are discussed in this chapter (Box 20.1).

**BOX 20.1    FACTORS CONTRIBUTING TO POWERLESSNESS IN NURSING**

1. The oppression of nurses as a group
2. Nursing's failure to fully align with the feminist movement
3. Limited collective action by nurses
4. The socialization of women to view power and politics negatively
5. The inadequate recognition of nursing as an educated profession with evidence-based practice
6. The nursing profession's history of being reactive (rather than proactive) in national policy setting

## Oppression of Nurses as a Group

Dong and Temple (2011) note that "oppression requires a set of norms that are determined by a dominant group and a belief of the inferiority of those outside the dominant group" (p. 169). The attributes of oppression then are unjust treatment, the denial of rights, and the dehumanizing of individuals. As such, Dong and Temple suggest that nurses and the nursing profession both work with oppressed groups and are themselves an oppressed group.

Indeed, nursing historically has been controlled by outside forces with greater prestige, power, and status. Generally, these forces were patriarchal and male dominated, such as medicine and hospital administration. For example, in the early 1900s, physicians attempted to exclude women from knowledge emerging from the basic sciences and their refusal to let nurses use new instrumentation sustained women's subordination in nursing, although many nurses continually and actively sought greater scientific knowledge and techniques and incorporated these into their education.

Even as of late 2011, some physicians were openly suggesting that they should be the only health care professional qualified to directly treat patients, despite the fact that many of the health care professions, including nurses, now hold advanced degrees including doctorates (Harris, 2011). Indeed, some physicians and their allies are currently pushing legislative efforts to restrict the right to use the title of "doctor." Dr. Roland Goertz, the board chairman of the American Academy of Family Physicians, suggests that physicians are worried about "losing control" of the term *doctor* because it has defined the medical profession for centuries. Indeed, he argued

that patients could be confused about the roles of various health professionals if other professions are able to call themselves doctor.

One must question whether this elitism is more an effort to control money, power, and prestige than it is a concern about whether patients will be confused. Harris (2011) notes that research evidence exists to show that advanced practice nurses can achieve similar, if not better, outcomes than many primary care physicians. In this respect then, the battle over the title "doctor" is likely a proxy for a larger struggle related to dominance and status.

The research suggests that when a group is oppressed, it tends to have value confusion and low self-esteem. This occurs because the dominant groups identify their norms and values as the "right ones" and use their initial power to enforce them as the status quo. Oppressed groups accept these norms, at least externally, in an effort to gain some power and control. For example, nursing's oppressors have not always held the same values as nursing (i.e., caring, nurturance, and advocacy). This has led to confusion for some nurses and even, at times, contempt for their own profession and what it represents.

For example, Brann (2010) suggests that a predominance of task orientation, horizontal violence, and a lack of engagement exemplify how nurses have lost a sense of profession through oppression. She concludes that increased recognition of nurses' work; greater awareness of what nurses say about each other; and involvement in decision-making processes will help to reduce oppression in nursing. "Nursing leaders owe it to the staff, their facilities, and patients to begin the process of nurse empowerment and leave the history of oppression where it belongs—in the past" (Brann, 2010, p. 18).

> **CONSIDER THIS** Badmouthing one's own profession may be a sign of oppression and values confusion.

## Failure to Align Fully With the Feminist Movement

A second factor contributing to nursing's relative powerlessness is the profession's failure to align fully with the feminist movement. Although both nurses and women have improved their status in the last four decades, nursing has not kept pace with the progress women have made in other areas. This has occurred, because, at least in part, nurses have not been fully engaged in the feminist movement.

This occurred for several reasons. One was that many feminists in the 1960s and 1970s were influenced by a more radical feminist perspective and, as a result, spoke out against women becoming nurses because it suggested that female nurses were in subordinate, caregiving roles. In addition, many nurses feared public identification with feminism.

The reality, however, is that nursing continues to be a profession composed of approximately 94% women, and this figure has changed very little over time. This is noteworthy, given that there have been major gender shifts in virtually all of the other traditionally female-dominated professions (such as social workers, librarians, K-to-12 teachers) since the 1970s.

> ## DISCUSSION POINT
>
> Many nursing leaders in the early 1900s were political activists, actively involved in social issues such as women's suffrage and public health. At what point did nursing diverge from a sociopolitical agenda and why?

Although having female dominance in the profession may have some benefits, it also poses some liabilities. Indeed, some nursing leaders have suggested that nursing will never attain greater status and power until more men join the ranks (see Chapter 9). Others think that adding men to nursing's ranks is not the answer. Instead, nurses need to accept the responsibility for addressing the problems that have historically plagued the profession and take whatever steps are necessary to proactively build a power base that does not depend on gender.

CONSIDER THIS   Being a female professional in a male-dominated health care system brings to mind the "Ginger Rogers syndrome." Both Ginger Rogers and her dancing partner, Fred Astaire, were known as wonderful dancers, but Fred Astaire's name always came first, and he always received the greater recognition. In reality, Ginger Rogers danced the same steps as Fred Astaire, but she did them backward and in high heels. So, who deserved the greater recognition?

Susan Malka (as cited in Irvine, 2008) suggested, however, that nursing's divergence from feminism has changed. She noted that in the mid-1960s through the mid-1980s, the nursing profession was focused on

defining the profession and was out of step with the feminist movement. From the mid-1980s to the present, however, nursing became more compatible with *second-wave feminism*, in that the profession began actively lobbying for greater rights and recognition, more men joined the profession, and women became nurses by choice, not because it was one of the few career choices open to them. Feminist issues such as pay equity and equal opportunities for advancement are now widely espoused by nurses.

Jagger (as cited by Thompson, 2011) agrees, suggesting that feminism is now more of a continuing cluster of social and political ideals that evolve and change. As such, it merges with larger social values, such as freedom, justice, equality, and democracy and aims to uncover inequality in areas as diverse as class, religion, and sexuality.

In addition, recognition that assertive, independent nurses cannot exist if they have been socialized to be dependent women is growing. Similarly, it is improbable, if not impossible, for female nurses to implement expanded roles in advanced practice if they are unaware of or unwilling to recognize the social constraints imposed on them because they are women. Clearly, the battles between the American Medical Association (AMA) and advanced practice nurses about scope of practice, reimbursement, and the need for medical oversight are likely related as much to gender as they are to competition over patients (see Chapter 22).

Nurses need then to continue to examine the progress women have made in other professions and work with them inside and outside of nursing to strengthen power for women everywhere. This holds true for the men in nursing as well because the relative powerlessness of the profession transfers to them too, despite gender differences. Both male and female nurses must solve problems, work to advance the science of nursing, network to increase nursing's knowledge base and power, and provide mutual support.

## Limited Collective Representation of Nurses

A third factor limiting the development of the nursing profession's power base is the inadequate collective representation of nurses by groups, such as collective bargaining agents and professional nursing organizations. Only about 15% of the 3.1 million nurses in the United States belong to collective bargaining units (Marquis & Huston, 2012). Less than 3% of nurses (approx. 175,000) belong to the American Nurses Association (ANA), the nationally recognized professional organization for all registered nurses, whose mission is to advance and protect the profession (Union Facts, 2011). These relatively small membership numbers directly reflect the money that is available for lobbyists to represent nursing in the political arena. In contrast, the American Medical Association (AMA) has one of the most powerful lobbying organizations in the United States.

> CONSIDER THIS  Nurses must be represented in mass before they will be able to significantly affect the decisions that directly influence their profession.

There are many reasons for the small representation of nurses in the ANA. The dual and often conflicting role of the ANA as both a professional organization for nurses and a collective bargaining agent is certainly one reason (see Chapter 18). In addition, some nurses think that state nurses associations have been burdened with the task of collective bargaining under the federation model of the ANA and that other programs have suffered as a result of funds being used for collective bargaining. Other nurses have expressed concerns about the cost of membership in the ANA or argued that the ANA is not responsive enough to the needs of the nurse at the bedside. Other nurses look on nursing as a job and not as a career and have little interest in professional issues outside of their immediate work environment.

> ### DISCUSSION POINT
>
> Do you belong to a professional nursing organization? Why or why not? Do contemporary nursing leaders espouse this as a value? Is it encouraged in the workplace and in the academic world?

Whether these issues are valid is almost immaterial. The reality is that as long as such a small percentage of nurses belong to the ANA, the economic power of the ANA will be limited, as will its ability to significantly influence policy setting and legislation. Perhaps even more importantly, until nurses are willing to work together collectively in some form, they will be unlikely to increase either their personal or their professional power.

> CONSIDER THIS  At times, nurses have lacked pride in their collective groups and have viewed alignment with other nurses as alignment with other powerless persons, something that does little to advance an individual's professional power.

Unfortunately, more often than not, nurses in this country have not acted cohesively, whether at the local level, fighting for wage increases, or at the national level, attempting to influence health policy. Even the various professional nursing organizations to which nurses belong have not historically worked together cooperatively. The reality is that nurses continue to be widely divided on basic issues such as entry into practice, mandatory staffing ratios, and collective bargaining. Strategies to promote greater nurse unity are shown in Box 20.2.

### BOX 20.2  STRATEGIES FOR PROMOTING UNITY WITHIN THE NURSING PROFESSION

1. Nurses must respect each other's specialties and work toward enriching each other's job and work environments.

2. Nurses must acknowledge the different expertise that will help promote the quality care expected of them.

3. Nurses need to be self-aware regarding their behaviors that lead to disunity.

4. Nurses need to examine and learn from the nursing legacy that has negatively affected their behavior individually and collectively.

5. Accommodation of new vibrant views should be encouraged. This could be done through proper mentoring of the newly graduated nurses.

6. Collaboration among nursing organizations and working collectively, as in a union, would strengthen nursing.

*Source:* Thupayagale-Tshweneagae, G., & Dithole, K. (2007). Unity among nurses: An evasive concept. *Nursing Forum, 42*(3), 143–146.

> CONSIDER THIS  A metaphor for increasing nursing's power base through collective action would be a snowball. Individual snowflakes are fragile, but when they stick together, they become a powerful force.

## Socialization of Women to View Power and Politics Negatively

A fourth factor contributing to powerlessness in the nursing profession has been the socialization of women to view power and politics negatively. Politics is the art of using legitimate power wisely, and it requires clear decision making, assertiveness, accountability, and the willingness to express one's views (Marquis & Huston, 2012). It also requires being proactive rather than reactive and demands decisiveness.

Fuller (2011) suggests that politics is difficult for nurses because nurses tend to be direct, honest, and forthright and because nurses often stand on principle and speak out on what they believe. She notes, however, that this is not always the best strategy in politics. Nurses must, however, recognize that power and politics provide opportunities for change—the chance to make things better for both nurses and clients. Therefore, all nurses should seek skill in being able to appropriately intervene in political processes.

> CONSIDER THIS  Changing nurses' view of both power and politics is perhaps the most significant key to proactive rather than reactive participation in policy setting.

Nurses must perceive a need not only to be more knowledgeable about power, negotiation, and politics but also to be more involved in broad social and political issues. This requires becoming politically astute. Nurses need to understand what politics means, and they need to become experts in using politics to help nursing achieve both its professional goals and the needs of their clients.

## Inadequate Recognition of Nursing as an Educated Profession With Evidence-Based Practice

A fifth factor contributing to the nursing profession's relative powerlessness is the inadequate recognition of nursing as a profession driven by research and the pursuit of higher education. Although nurses should value

highly the caring, intuitive, nurturing part of nursing practice, the nursing profession has been negligent about equally emphasizing their extensive scientific knowledge base and the high level of critical thinking and analysis professional nurses use every day in their clinical practice.

Both the art and the science of nursing require highly developed skills and a well-developed knowledge base. The nurse of the 21st century has an extensive knowledge base in the sciences as well as in the arts. In addition, nurses must be expert critical thinkers, as they are required to continually look for and analyze subtle clues in their client data, make independent nursing diagnoses, and create plans of care. Constant assessment and adjustment to the plan of care are almost always necessary, so nurses must be highly organized and know how to set priorities. In addition, nurses must have highly refined communication skills, well-developed psychomotor skills, and sophisticated leadership and management skills. This is the image nurses must promote to the public.

> ### DISCUSSION POINT
>
> If the public was asked to list five adjectives to describe nursing, what would they be? Would the art or the science of nursing be recognized more? Would nurses use different adjectives?

## The Nursing Profession's History of Being Reactive in National Policy Setting

The last factor discussed here as contributing to a relative lack of professional power in nursing is the profession's history of being reactive rather than proactive in national policy setting regarding nursing practice. *Reactive* means waiting until there is a problem and then trying to fix it. *Proactive* is more anticipatory; it means developing appropriate policy before taking action or a problem occurs.

Unfortunately, the nursing profession has been far from proactive in shaping its own course or that of the health care system. In the 1990s, health care became big business. Managed care proliferated, and gatekeepers, not providers and consumers, began deciding who needed care and how much care was needed. Hospitals lost their place as the center of the health care universe as client care shifted from inpatient hospital stays to outpatient and ambulatory health care settings. Physicians lost much of their autonomy to practice medicine as they saw fit as insurers increasingly placed restrictions not only on which physicians patients could see but also on what services the physician was authorized to prescribe.

Patients found themselves with limited choices of providers, longer wait times for care, more rules to follow, and more confusion about what would and would not be a covered expense. At the same time, registered nurses (RNs) in record numbers, for the first time in history, were downsized, restructured, and often replaced by a cheaper counterpart in an effort to reduce costs.

Many nurses felt both overwhelmed and helpless with this degree of change. However, these changes did not happen overnight. Many of them were incremental and insidious, and the health care system changes occurred with little concerted effort by nurses to stop them.

There is a brief parable that Peter Senge (1990) wrote about in *The Fifth Discipline* that nurses should keep front and foremost when they think about the need to be proactive, even with incremental change. It's called "The parable of the boiled frog" and it goes like this:

> *If you place a frog in a pot of boiling water, it will immediately try to scramble out. But if you place the frog in room temperature water, and don't scare him, he'll stay put. Now, if the pot sits on a heat source, and if you gradually turn up the temperature, something very interesting happens. As the temperature rises from 70 to 80 degrees Fahrenheit, the frog will do nothing. In fact, he will show every sign of enjoying himself. As the temperature gradually increases, the frog will become groggier and groggier, until he is unable to crawl out of the pot. Though there is nothing restraining him, the frog will sit there and boil. He will boil to death, oblivious to what is happening to him.*

CONSIDER THIS Gradual but constant change may be even more dangerous than cataclysmic change because resistance is less organized.

Clearly, nursing can no longer afford to be reactive in the policy arena. Instead, the profession must determine its priorities and then create a plan for action which is strategic and timely relative to the debates taking place at the national and global levels.

# DRIVING FORCES TO INCREASE NURSING'S POWER BASE

So what is the likelihood that the nursing profession will ever be a powerful force in health care decision making and the political arena? The answer is unclear, although the likelihood of this happening is increasing because of several driving forces in place. This chapter discusses six of these forces (Box 20.3).

## Timing Is Right

Timing is everything. The political ferment regarding the need for further health care reform continues to escalate, and issues of cost and access are paramount in this country. For 2012, the United States will spend more than US$1 trillion on health care annually, an amount equal to 18% of the gross domestic product (GDP; U.S. Government Spending, 2011). In fact, the United States spends more than any other industrialized country in the world (two to three times that of many industrialized countries). In addition, the country spends nearly three times as much on hospital care and almost five times as much on administration compared with all other OECD countries for which there are data (Matthews, 2011). Yet its rankings in terms of life span, infant mortality, and teenage pregnancy are much lower than many countries that spend significantly less on health care.

In addition, there are more than 45 million uninsured individuals in the United States and likely tens of millions more who are underinsured. While recently enacted health care reform laws will provide many of the currently uninsured at least some basic level of coverage, these laws will not take effect until 2014.

In addition, Singhal, Stueland, and Ungerman (2011) point out that reform provisions will fundamentally

---

**BOX 20.3 DRIVING FORCES TO INCREASE NURSING'S POWER BASE**

1. The timing is right.
2. The size of the nursing profession and the diversity of our practice
3. Nursing's referent power
4. The increasing knowledge base and education for nurses
5. Nursing's unique perspective
6. The desire for change among consumers and providers

alter the social contract inherent in employer-sponsored medical benefits and how employees value health insurance as a form of compensation. Thus, while the new laws guarantee at least some right to health insurance regardless of an individual's medical status, they "minimize the moral obligation employers may feel to cover the sickest employees, who would otherwise be denied coverage in today's individual health insurance market" (Singhal et al., 2011, para. 9). Singhal et al. suggest that most employers will seek value-creating options and even those employers that intend to provide benefits similar to those they currently offer, will likely take no-regrets moves, like tailoring plans to maximize what their employees will value most about employer-sponsored insurance. This radical restructuring of employer-sponsored health benefits alone should draw a crowd of interested parties to the policy table.

Furthermore, as a result of publications like *To Err Is Human*, consumers, health care providers, and legislators are more aware than ever of the shortcomings of the current health care system, and the clamor for action has never been louder (see Chapter 15). Clearly, the public wants a better health care system and nurses want to be able to provide high-quality nursing care. Both are powerful elements for change, and new nurses are entering the profession at a time when their energy and expertise will be more valued than ever.

## Size of the Nursing Profession and Diversity of Our Practice

The second driving force for increasing nursing's professional power base is the size of the profession and the diversity of nursing practice. Numbers are the lifeblood of politics. McNeal (2011) notes, however, that candidates seeking office are typically only interested in those constituents who regularly engage in voting activities and who make their influence and issues known. If nurses do not vote as a block then, their political voice becomes diluted. The nursing profession's size then is perhaps its greatest asset, and its potential for a collective voting block should increasingly be recognized as a force to deal with.

> CONSIDER THIS   Collective involvement of only a fraction of the nation's 3.1 million registered nurses in health care policy would produce a significant voting block.

> **DISCUSSION POINT**
>
> Have nurses ever made a concerted effort to vote collectively? What positions have professional organizations such as the ANA taken on recent election issues or candidates for office? Have endorsements by professional nursing organizations influenced how you vote?

In addition, the diversity of the settings within which nurses practice creates a foundation of strength since it allows them to take evidence from a wide variety of sources, develop arguments based on the data discovered, and demonstrate that nurses' power comes not only from their work at the bedside but also from their role as actors in larger social and political arenas (D'Antonio et al. 2010).

## Nursing's Referent Power

A third driving force for increasing the power of the profession is the referent power nurses hold. *Referent power* is the power one has when others identify with you or what you symbolize; therefore, you have their admiration or respect (Marquis & Huston, 2012). Nurses have a high degree of referent power because of the trust and credibility given to them by the public. Donelan, Buerhaus, DesRoches, and Burke (2010) agree, noting that "the public trusts nurses' honesty and integrity and values the profession and that places nurses in a position to be a critical void for the patient in the public sphere" (p. 179).

## An Increasing Knowledge Base and Education for Nurses

A fourth driving force for increasing the power of the profession is nursing's increasing knowledge base. Indeed, the Institute of Medicine (2011) in *The Future of Nursing: Focus on Education* notes that

> *transforming the health care system to provide safe, quality, patient-centered, accessible, and affordable care will require a comprehensive rethinking of the roles of many health care professionals, nurses chief among them. To realize this vision, nursing education must be fundamentally improved both before and after nurses receive their licenses.* (para. 1)

Fortunately, more nurses are being prepared at the master's and doctoral level than ever before. However, while 13% of nurses hold a graduate degree, less than 1% have a doctoral degree (IOM, 2011). "Nurses with doctorates are needed to teach future generations of nurses and to conduct research that becomes the basis for improvements in nursing science and practice" (IOM, 2011, para. 11). The report recommended doubling the number of nurses with a doctorate by 2020.

Furthermore, leadership, management, and political theory are increasingly a part of baccalaureate nursing education, although the majority of nurses still do not hold baccalaureate degrees. These are learned skills, and, collectively, the nursing profession's knowledge of leadership, politics, negotiation, and finance is increasing. This can only increase the nursing profession's influence outside the field.

## Nursing's Unique Perspective

A fifth driving force for increasing the nursing profession's power base is the unique philosophical perspective nursing brings to the health care arena. Nursing's perspective is unique as a result of its blending of art and science—a blending of "caring" and "curing," so to speak. The caring part of the nursing role is better known and better understood by the public. It is what historically has defined nursing. It is important that nurses not forget or underappreciate the unique values nursing represents because these are the values that make the profession different from all the others. These same values will make nursing irreplaceable in the current health care system.

The "science" part of nursing is less understood by the public. Nursing has an extensive scientific knowledge base, and the high level of critical thinking and analysis professional nurses use every day in their clinical practice is enormous. Nursing practice is increasingly becoming *evidence based*, meaning that nursing practice reflects what the literature says is "best practice." That is, the practice of nursing is research based and scientifically driven (see Chapter 2). Unfortunately, consumers, legislators, and sometimes even other health care professionals fail to recognize this. Nursing then must do a better job of explaining and emphasizing both the art and the science of its practice.

## Consumers and Providers Want Change

Finally, health care restructuring and health care reform are resulting in unrest for health care consumers, as well as providers. Limited consumer choice, hospital restructuring, the downsizing of registered nursing, and the Institute of Medicine (IOM) medical errors reports were the sparks needed to mobilize nurses, as well as consumers, to take action. Nurses began speaking out about how downsizing and restructuring were affecting the care they were providing and the public began demanding accountability. The public does care who is caring for them and how that affects the quality of their care. The good news, then, is that the flaws of the health care system are no longer secret and nursing has the opportunity to use its expertise and influence to help create a better health care system for the future.

## ACTION PLAN FOR THE FUTURE

Based on these driving forces, an action plan can be created to increase the power of the nursing profession in the 21st century. This chapter identifies seven possible strategies to achieve this goal (Box 20.4).

## Place More Nurses in Positions of Influence

The IOM (2011) suggested that for health care reform to work, that nurses must be a part of decision-making processes in the health care system. This is true even at the organizational level. For example, although nurses typically represent the greatest percentage of the

---

**BOX 20.4    ACTION PLAN FOR INCREASING THE POWER OF THE NURSING PROFESSION**

1. More nurses must be placed in positions of influence.
2. Nurses must stop acting like victims.
3. Nurses must become better informed about all health care policy efforts.
4. Coalition building must occur within and outside of nursing.
5. More research must be done to strengthen evidence-based practice.
6. Nursing leaders must be supported.
7. Attention must be paid to mentoring future nurse leaders and leadership succession.

workforce in hospitals, few nurses serve on hospitals boards or hold positions of significant power.

For this reason, the Honor Society of Nursing, Sigma Theta Tau International (STTI; 2011) has created a number of resources for nurses interested in gaining the skill set necessary to serve on the boards of health care institutions. One resource is a 2-year *Board Leadership Development* program which focuses on increasing knowledge and skills in the areas of strategic thinking and planning, fiduciary oversight, board and staff partnerships, and generative governance. Online educational resources are also available for nurses interested in learning how to be knowledgeable, contributing leaders on national and international not-for-profit boards.

In addition, nurses must be placed in national positions that influence public policy. For example, a significant effort began in 2005 to establish an *Office of the National Nurse* in the United States, who would serve as an assistant to the surgeon general. A National Nursing Network Organization was formed, and legislation has repeatedly been introduced in Congress since 2006 to achieve this goal.

Most recently, Texas Congresswoman Eddie Bernice Johnson introduced HR 3679, The National Nurse Act of 2011 on December 15, 2011 (The National Nurse for Public Health, 2011). This legislation, co-led by Congressman Peter King (NY-3) would create a National Nurse for Public Health by designating the existing position of the chief nurse officer of the U.S. Public Health Service to serve in that capacity. This bill elevates this nurse into a full-time leadership position to focus on the critical work needed to address national priorities of health promotion and disease prevention. Major efforts would be directed at improving health literacy and decreasing health disparities in America (The National Nurse for Public Health, 2011). Proponents of the idea suggest that such a position would raise the profile of nursing and assist in a nationwide cultural shift to prevention and health promotion. Opponents suggest that this might not be the best way to effect change both within nursing and in the health care system.

Not all positions that influence public policy, however, occur at the national level. Indeed, few leaders burst on to the national scene directly. Instead, they assume leadership roles in entities such as medical centers, community hospitals, government agencies, and insurance companies.

Running for and holding elected office is, however, the ultimate in political activism and involvement. A total of seven nurses held office in the 112th Congress (Four New Nurses to Join 112th Congress in January, 2010). Many more nurses hold elected office in state legislatures.

In fact, nurses are uniquely qualified to hold public office because they have the greatest firsthand experience of problems faced by patients in the health care system, as well as an ability to translate the health care experience to the general public. As a result, more nurses must seek out this role. In addition, because the public respects and trusts nurses, nurses who choose to run for public office are often elected. The problem then is not that nurses are not being elected . . . the problem is that not enough nurses are running for office.

## Stop Acting Like Victims

A second part of the action plan to increase the power of the nursing profession in the 21st century is that nurses must stop acting like victims. This is not to say that some nurses have not been victimized. The reality, however, is that nursing, like any other profession, has positive and negative attributes. Whining and acting like a victim never fixes problems. Nurses unhappy with their career choice either need to fix what is wrong or leave and find a job that fulfills their expectations.

In addition, it is critical that each nurse never lose sight of his or her potential to make a difference. Some legislators and nursing employers have argued that "a nurse is a nurse is a nurse." This is wrong. Nurses can be whatever they want to be in nursing, and they can achieve that goal at whatever level of quality they choose. The bottom line, however, is that the profession will only be as smart, as motivated, and as directed as its weakest link. If the nursing profession is to be the powerful force it can be, it needs to be filled with bright, highly motivated people who want to make a difference in the lives of the clients with whom they work, as well as in the health care system itself.

---

CONSIDER THIS   Individuals may be born average, but staying average is a choice.

---

Nurses also must realize that part of the reason nursing has been invisible or portrayed inappropriately in the media is that nurses have not assumed the spokesperson roles they could have or should have for their profession. Donelan et al. (2010) note that nurses and nursing associations need well-honed messages and they need to master the tools of communication—news media, research publications, surveys, and advertising. The IOM report provides a "window of opportunity to put nursing issues on the national agenda and national stage," but it will be "critically important that nurses follow the release of that report with research, new strategies for change, and further inquiry" (Donelan et al., 2010, p. 179).

## Become Better Informed About All Health Care Policy Efforts

The third step of the action plan is that nurses must become better informed about all health care policy efforts—especially those that influence their profession. This is difficult because no one can do this but nurses. This means grassroots knowledge building and involvement. Nurses need to be better-informed consumers and providers of health care.

> CONSIDER THIS   Nurses who do not understand the legislative process will not be able to influence the policy-making process.

Indeed, although nurses are held in high esteem by the public, physicians are more visible than nurses in media coverage, public policy, and political spheres (Donelan et al., 2010). The result is that nursing issues may be overshadowed by other health priorities. Research undertaken by Donelan et al. (2010) found that while nursing issues are considered at the policy table, all too often they do not include effective policy solutions (see Research Study Fuels the Controversy 20.1).

One effort to increase the number of nurses who are well prepared to influence health policy at the local, state, and national levels was the launch of the American Nurses Advocacy Institute (ANAI) in 2009 (Trossman, 2011). ANAI fellows attend a 2+ day seminar in Washington, D.C. to strengthen their competence in the political arena and participate in a yearlong formal mentoring program. The institute covers content such as the advocacy process, criteria and methods for conducting political environment scans, effective strategies for creating and sustaining policy change, and coalition building (Trossman, 2011).

Another program which helps nurses acquire the leadership skills to shape health care locally and nationally is the *Robert Wood Johnson Foundation Executive*

## RESEARCH STUDY FUELS THE CONTROVERSY 20.1

### NURSING'S VISIBILITY IN THE POLICY ARENA

The purpose of this research was to understand the visibility and salience of the health workforce in general, to gain an understanding about the effectiveness of messages concerning the nursing workforce in particular, and to understand why nursing workforce issues do not appear to have gained more traction in national health care policy making. To answer these questions, the researchers administered a national survey to 301 nursing thought leaders via mail, telephone, and online. One hundred twenty-three respondents completed questionnaires for a response rate of 41%.

Donelan, K., Buerhaus, P., DesRoches, C., & Burke, S. (2010). Health policy thoughtleaders' views of the health workforce in an era of health reform. *Nursing Outlook, 58*(4), 175–180.

### STUDY FINDINGS

Thought leaders agreed that nurses were critical to the quality and safety of our health care system, that there are current nursing shortages, and that nursing shortages will be intensified by health reform. Thought leaders reported, however, that while they do hear about nursing issues frequently, they do not view most sources of information as proposing effective policy solutions. For example, while the thought leaders suggested that nursing organization support was important to the passage of health care reform, only 7% said these organizations were "very effective" in proposing solutions. The researchers concluded that while nursing has achieved certain successes in the recent health care reform debate, that this study highlighted a critical gap in effective policy advocacy and leadership to advance nurse workforce issues higher on the national health agenda.

*Nurse Fellows* program (RFJF, 2011b). This three-year program allows Fellows to "strengthen their leadership capacity and improve their abilities to lead teams and organizations in improving health and health care. The program targets 20 leadership competencies focused on leading oneself, leading others, leading the organization, and leading in health care."

Not all nurses, however, need to or want to be this involved in politics and policy setting. Determining how directly or indirectly one should be involved is a personal decision. Fortunately, nurses are in the enviable position of having great credibility with legislators and the public. For nurses who choose to be directly involved in politics and policy setting, they can seek public office or become more involved in lobbying legislators about issues pertinent to health care and nursing. Such lobbying can be done either in person or by writing, and there are many good sources on how to do both (see Chapter 23). The legislator needs to understand why this is an issue that is critical to not only the nursing profession but also to his or her constituents. It is important, then, to create a need for the legislator to listen to what is being said.

Nurses can also give freely of their time and money to support nursing's position in the legislative arena. This can be done indirectly by contributing to professional associations such as the ANA, which have lobbyists in the legislative arena to protect nursing's interests, or by giving money directly to a political campaign. In this case, nurses should try to give early and to make as large a contribution as possible. It is the early and significant contributions that are remembered most.

Nurses interested in a more indirect contribution to policy development may work to influence and educate the public about nursing and the nursing agenda to reform health care. Either role is helpful—at least the nurse will have made a conscious decision to be involved. Other strategies for effecting change through political involvement are noted in Box 20.5.

## Build Coalitions Inside and Outside of Nursing

The fourth step of the action plan to increase professional power in the 21st century is for the nursing profession to look within itself as well as beyond its organizations for coalition building. For example, in September 2011, National Nurses United (the largest union of and professional association of registered nurses in the United States with more than 150,000 members), coordinated

more than 10,000 registered nurses across the nation as they "staged 61 actions in 21 states to call for a tax on Wall State in order to raise revenue for healing Main Street America." This protest was likely the biggest series of events ever hosted by nurses in U.S. history (Nurses Hold Record Number, 2011).

Belonging to professional nursing organizations is another way in which nurses can network for coalition building. Coalitions have been formed within nursing groups as well. The Tri-Council for Nursing is an alliance of four autonomous nursing organizations: the AACN, the ANA, the AONE, and the NLN. The Tri-Council focuses on leadership for education, practice, and research.

The Council for the Advancement of Nursing Science (CANS) is another example of coalition building among nursing groups. The Council is composed of representatives from the four major regional research societies, STTI, the American Academy of Nursing; and the National Institute of Nursing Research (CANS, 2011).

Similarly, the National Federation for Specialty Nursing Organizations and the Nursing Organizations Liaison Forum, an entity of the ANA, merged in 2001 to become the Nursing Organizations Alliance (NOA), also known as The Alliance. The Alliance "provides a forum for identification, education, and collaboration building on issues of common interest to advance the nursing profession" (The Alliance, 2011, para. 1).

> **CONSIDER THIS** More collaboration among nursing organizations would increase the power of the nursing profession.

### DISCUSSION POINT

All too frequently, the AMA and the ANA stand in opposition to each other in the legislative arena. Are there health care issues on which they could partner? Are there issues on which the ANA and the American Hospital Association could partner?

Nurses have not done as well, however, in building political coalitions with other interdisciplinary professionals with similar challenges. Nurses have also not

## BOX 20.5 POLITICAL ACTIVITIES TO EFFECT CHANGE

1. Campaigning
   a. Know the issues associated with pending or potential legislation and formulate a view related to that legislation.
   b. Organize a "call to action" by urging nursing health professionals to contact a legislator and identifying a legislator's position on an issue.
   c. Work for a political candidate.
   d. Attend political meetings.
   e. Make a campaign contribution.
   f. Provide links to a candidate's website.

2. Communicating
   a. Join organizations and assist in the development and wide dissemination of policy statements.
   b. Write letters to the editors of well-known lay newspapers and professional health care journals.
   c. Contact legislators.
   d. Present congressional testimony.
   e. Become a consultant to political candidates, help write their campaign message, and prepare policy briefings.
   f. Use social network media to get the message out to broader audiences.
   g. All television networks are required to provide free advertising space for public service announcements (PSAs). Volunteer to write the script for those PSAs.

3. Voting
   a. Register to vote and take the lead in organizing voter registration activities.
   b. Public universities are mandated to ensure that all college students are made aware of the process for registering to vote. Ensure that nursing students are aware of the process and engage them in debating the issues.
   c. Promote the appointment of qualified nurses of key governmental positions.

4. Protesting
   a. Participate in a boycott.
   b. Support an action to strike.
   c. Organize a march.
   d. Oppose legislation.

*Source:* McNeal, G. J. (2011). Politicization: The power of influence. *ABNF Journal, 22*(3), 51–52.

done well in building political coalitions with legislators. Most legislators have a great deal of respect for nurses but know little about their qualifications to speak with authority about the health care system. Nurses need to become experts at political networking, making tradeoffs, negotiating, and coalition building. They also need to see the bigger picture of health care. This is not to say that nurses should lose sight of client needs but that they must do a better job of seeing the bigger picture and of building and strengthening alliances with others before they will be seen as powerful and capable.

Finally, Donelan et al. (2010) note that nurses have done well in building alliances with many organizations that care for and about safety and quality health care. They suggest, however, that more attention must be given to building alliances with hospitals and physicians.

## Conduct More Research to Strengthen Evidence-Based Practice

Another critical strategy for increasing nursing's power base is to continue to develop and promote evidence-based practice in nursing. Great strides have been made in researching what it is that nurses do that makes a difference in patient outcomes (research on *nursing sensitive outcomes*), but more needs to be done. Nursing practice must reflect what research has identified as best practices, and a better understanding of the relationship between nursing practice and patient outcomes is still needed.

> CONSIDER THIS   Only relatively recently has research been able to prove that patients get better because of nurses and not in spite of them.

Building and sustaining evidence-based practice in nursing will require far greater numbers of master's and doctorally prepared nurse researchers, as well as entry into practice at an educational level similar to that of other professions. Social work, physical therapy, and occupational therapy all now have the master's or doctoral degree as the entry level into practice. Nursing cannot afford to continue debating whether a bachelor's degree is necessary as the minimum entry level into professional practice (see Chapter 1).

## Support Nursing Leaders

Another part of the action plan to increase the profession's power is that nurses must support their nursing leaders and recognize the challenges they face as visionary change agents. Nurses have often viewed their leaders as rule breakers, and this has often occurred at a high personal cost to innovators.

In addition, nurses often resist change and new ideas from their leaders and instead look to leaders in medicine and other health-related disciplines. Some of this occurs as a result of nurse leaders being discounted, at least in part, because of their female majority, and also in part to the low value placed on nursing expertise. "Nursing needs a more coordinated strategic effort that puts the profession in the public eye as a value and participating part of the leadership of the profession and the care team of the patient" (Donelan et al., 2010, p. 179).

It is important to remember that, typically, it is not outsiders who divide nursing followers from nursing leaders. Instead, the division of nursing's strength often comes from within. Nursing leaders must be perceived as the profession's best advocates. Differing viewpoints should not only be acknowledged but also be encouraged. There is a proper arena for conflict and argument, but the outward force presented must be one of unity and direction.

## Mentor Future Nurse Leaders and Plan for Leadership Succession

Finally, and perhaps most important, before nursing can become a powerful profession, nurses must actively plan for leadership succession and care for younger members by providing mentoring opportunities. It is the future leaders who face the task of increasing nursing's power base in the 21st century.

Female-dominated professions have a history of exemplifying what is known as the *queen bee syndrome*. The queen bee is a woman who, after great personal struggle, becomes successful in her career. Her attitude, however, is that because she had to make it on her own with so little help, other novices should have to do the same. Thus, there has been inadequate empowering of young nurse leaders by older, more established nurse leaders. It is the young who hold not only the keys to the present but also the hope for the future. The nursing profession is responsible for ensuring leadership succession and is morally bound to do it with the brightest, most highly qualified individuals.

> ### DISCUSSION POINT
>
> Is the nursing profession proactive in planning its leadership succession, or is it a change that occurs by drift?

## CONCLUSIONS

D'Antonio et al. (2010) suggest that while marginalization, invisibility, and gender issues have been and continue to be a part of nursing's history, there is also evidence of strength, purpose, and successful political action. Still, there is little doubt that nursing, as a female-dominated profession, will face more challenges than male-dominated professions in having a strong voice in health care policy. Nursing lobbyists in the nation's capitol are influencing legislation on quality, access to care, patient and health worker safety, health care restructuring, reimbursement for advanced practice nurses, and funding for nursing education. Representatives of professional nursing organizations regularly attend and provide testimony at government agency meetings to be sure that the "nursing perspective" is heard on health policy issues.

Yet, clearly, nurses, as health care professionals, need to have greater input into and control over how the health care system evolves in this country. We need a health care system that will guarantee basic, affordable health care coverage for all citizens and in which all the members of the multidisciplinary health care team work together to create policy and provide care based on what is best for the patient. We also need a health care system that is accountable for its outcomes—that recognizes that individuality, autonomy, quality, and basic human dignity are essential components of health care services and that the bottom line is not always a number.

The nursing profession must be held accountable for being an integral force in shaping such a health care system. Indeed, nursing has a moral and professional obligation to do so. McNeal (2011) perhaps says it best:

*For too long the discipline of nursing has quietly watched as other disciplines have slowly taken over many duties that were once only within the purview of the nursing profession. Pharmacy chains now conduct blood pressure screening and provide immunizations; retail stores have opened convenience clinics throughout the nation staffed by family nurse practitioners; and, social workers perform case management activities. At no other time in the history of this profession has the Office of the President recognized the value of nursing by creating ample provisions within the Healthcare Reform Act to facilitate nursing's ability to take the lead. This is our time, this is our moment. Let's not permit this time to pass us by.* (p. 52)

## FOR ADDITIONAL DISCUSSION

1. Should the nursing profession target the recruitment of men into nursing in an effort to increase professional power?

2. What partners/external stakeholders should the nursing profession seek in terms of alliances or coalitions to strengthen its position in the policy arena?

3. What are the priority issues the nursing profession should identify in creating a proactive legislative agenda?

4. Will nursing ever be able to increase its power base if it does not increase its educational entry level to a level similar to that of other health care professions?

5. Do nursing schools provide enough content on politics, policy, and leadership for nurses to develop some degree of political competence? If not, what is missing?

6. Do most nurses internalize the need to be politically competent as a moral and professional obligation?

7. What legislative issues being debated have the greatest potential effect on nursing and health care?

# REFERENCES

The Alliance. (2011). *Home page.* Retrieved December 28, 2011, from http://www.nursing-alliance.org/content.cfm/id/about_us

Brann, M. (2010). Leading nursing from its dark side of history: Oppression. *Nevada RN Formation, 19*(4), 6.

Council for the Advancement of Nursing Science. (2011). *Home page.* Retrieved December 28, 2011, from http://www.nursingscience.org/

D'Antonio, P., Connolly, C., Wall, B., Whelan, J., & Fairman, J. (2010). Histories of nursing: The power and the possibilities. *Nursing Outlook, 58*(4), 207–213.

Donelan, K., Buerhaus, P., DesRoches, C., & Burke, S. (2010). Health policy thoughtleaders' views of the health workforce in an era of health reform. *Nursing Outlook, 58*(4), 175–180.

Dong, D., & Temple, B. (2011). Oppression: A concept analysis and implications for nurses and nursing. *Nursing Forum, 46*(3), 169–176.

Four New Nurses to Join 112th Congress in January. (2010). Retrieved December 29, 2011, from http://www.capitolupdate.org/index.php/2010/12/four-new-nurses-to-join-112th-congress-in-january/

Fuller, W. (2011). What can you do for us? *Florida Nurse, 59*(3), 2–6.

Harris, G. (2011). *When the nurse wants to be called "doctor."* Retrieved December 29, 2011, from http://www.nytimes.com/2011/10/02/health/policy/02docs.html?_r=1&adxnnl=1&pagewanted=all&adxnnlx=1325141350-1L247LFAkXoylKPfw5Kmxw

Institute of Medicine. (2011). *The future of nursing: Focus on education.* Retrieved December 29, 2011, from http://www.iom.edu/Reports/2010/The-Future-of-Nursing-Leading-Change-Advancing-Health/Report-Brief-Education.aspx

Irvine, H. (2008, February 17). Review: *Daring to care: American nursing and Second-Wave feminism* [by Susan Gelfand Malka]. *Feminist Review.* Retrieved August 29, 2008, from http://feministreview.blogspot.com/2008/02/daring-to-care-american-nursing-and.html

Marquis, B., & Huston, C. (2012). *Leadership roles and management functions in nursing* (7th ed.). Philadelphia, PA: Lippincott Williams & Wilkins.

Matthews, D. (2011). Research desk: Where does the U.S. spend more on health care? [Erza Klein's Wonkblog]. *Washington Post.* Retrieved December 28, 2011, from http://www.washingtonpost.com/blogs/ezra-klein/post/research-desk-where-does-the-us-spend-more-on-health-care/2011/08/01/gIQA40CPnI_blog.html

McNeal, G. J. (2011). Politicization: The power of influence. *ABNF Journal, 22*(3), 51–52.

The National Nurse for Public Health. (2011). *Special interest: HR 3679.* Retrieved December 28, 2011, from http://www.nationalnurse.blogspot.com/

Nurses hold record number of actions calling for tax on Wall Street. (2011). *National Nurse, 107*(7), 4–6.

Robert Wood Johnson Foundation. (2011a). *Nursing leadership from bedside to boardroom: Opinion leaders' perceptions.* Retrieved December 29, 2011, from http://www.rwjf.org/pr/product.jsp?id=54350

Robert Wood Johnson Foundation. (2011b). *Robert Wood Johnson Foundation Executive Nurse Fellows.* Retrieved December 28, 2011, from http://www.rwjfleaders.org/programs/robert-wood-johnson-foundation-executive-nurse-fellows-programe

Senge, P. (1990). *The fifth discipline.* New York, NY: Doubleday/Currency.

Sigma Theta Tau International Honor Society of Nursing. (2011). *Board leadership development program.* Retrieved December 27, 2011, from http://www.nursingsociety.org/LeadershipInstitute/Omada/Pages/omada_main.aspx

Singhal, S., Stueland, J., & Ungerman, D. (2011). How US health care reform will affect employee benefits. *McKinsey Quarterly.* Retrieved December 29, 2011, from http://www.mckinseyquarterly.com/How_US_health_care_reform_will_affect_employee_benefits_2813

Thompson. C. (2011). *Role of feminist theory in nursing.* Retrieved December 28, 2011, from http://www.ehow.com/about_6589371_role-feminist-theory-nursing.html

Thupayagale-Tshweneagae, G., & Dithole, K. (2007). Unity among nurses: An evasive concept. *Nursing Forum, 42*(3), 143–146.

Trossman, S. (2011). Political advocacy, anyone? *American Nurse, 43*(3), 1–7.

Union Facts. (2011). *American Nurses Association (ANA).* Retrieved December 30, 2011, from http://www.unionfacts.com/union/American_Nurses_Association

U.S. Government Spending. (2011). *Total budgeted government spending expenditure GDP—CHARTS—Deficit debt.* Retrieved December 29, 2011, from http://www.usgovernmentspending.com/

## BIBLIOGRAPHY

Brody, A., Barnes, K., Ruble, C., & Sakowski, J. (2012). Evidence-based practice councils potential path to staff nurse empowerment and leadership growth. *Journal of Nursing Administration, 42*(1), 28–33.

Burke, J. (2011a). Talking politics. *Registered Nurse Journal, 23*(2), 18–20.

Burke, J. (2011b). With involvement comes influence. *Registered Nurse Journal, 23*(4), 20–22.

Dolinar, D., & Weisbrich, M. (2012). Connecting the dots: Nursing practice and legislation. *Nursing Voice, 17*(1), 7.

Falter, E. (2012). Nursing leadership... From the board room to the bedside. *Nursing Administration Quarterly, 36*(1), 17–23.

Gambardella, L. C. (2011). Nursing and politics: Strange bedfellows or compatible partners in practice? Building a passion for political action (Reprinted with permission from *The DNR Reporter*, November–January, 2011). *Nursing News, 35*(2), 13.

Habel, M. (2011). The power of change: Nurses make the difference. *Nurse.Com (DC/Maryland/Virginia), 21*(15), 36–41.

Harmer, R. (2011). Politics is an issue for us all. *Nursing Children & Young People, 23*(7), 12.

Hassmiller, S., & Combes, J. (2012). Nurse leaders in the boardroom: A fitting choice. *Journal of Healthcare Management, 57*(1), 8–11.

Hicks, B. (2011). Gender, politics, and regionalism: Factors in the evolution of registered psychiatric nursing in Manitoba, 1920–1960. *Nursing History Review, 19*, 103–126.

Kramer, M., Maguire, P., Halfer, D., Budin, W., Hall, D., Goodloe, L.,... Lemke, J. (2012). The organizational transformative power of nurse residency programs. *Nursing Administration Quarterly, 36*(2), 155–168.

Lyttle, B. (2011). Politics: A natural next step for nurses. *New Jersey Nurse, 41*(3), 6.

Manning, M., & Grosso, D. (2011). Doctor of nursing practice students advocating for health care access, quality, and reform: From the virtual classroom to Capitol Hill. *Journal of Nursing Education, 50*(1), 14–20.

McCarthy, M., & Unberhagen, K. (2012). Nurse empowerment... Powerful nurses can create change. *Nurse. Com (DC/Maryland/Virginia), 22*(4), 8.

MacPhee, M., Skelton-Green, J., Bouthillette, F., & Suryaprakash, N. (2012). An empowerment framework for nursing leadership development: Supporting evidence. *Journal of Advanced Nursing, 68*(1), 159–169.

McSherry, R., Pearce, P., Grimwood, K., & Mcsherry, W. (2012). The pivotal role of nurse managers, leaders and educators in enabling excellence in nursing care. *Journal of Nursing Management, 20*(1), 7–19.

Rudge, T., Holmes, D., & Perron, A. (2011). The rise of practice development with/in reformed bureaucracy: Discourse, power and the government of nursing. *Journal of Nursing Management, 19*(7), 837–844.

Sanchez, L., & Cralle, L. (2012). Attaining employee empowerment. *Nurse Leader, 10*(2), 38–40.

Seenandan-Sookdeo, K. I. (2012). The influence of power in the Canadian healthcare system. *Clinical Nurse Specialist: The Journal for Advanced Nursing Practice, 26*(2), 107–112.

Sieloff, C. L., & Bularzik, A. M. (2011). Group power through the lens of the 21st century and beyond: Further validation of the Sieloff-King Assessment of group power within organizations. *Journal of Nursing Management, 19*(8), 1020–1027.

Vandenberg, H. E. R., & Hall, W. A. (2011). Critical ethnography: Extending attention to bias and reinforcement of dominant power relations. *Nurse Researcher, 18*(3), 25–30.

# Chapter 21

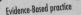

# Professional Identity and Image

Carol J. Huston

Visit thePoint for additional helpful resources
- eBook
- Journal Articles
- WebLinks

## LEARNING OBJECTIVES

*The learner will be able to:*

1. Explore the roots and prevalence of historical and contemporary nursing stereotypes, including nurse as angel of mercy, love interest (particularly to physicians), sex bombshell/naughty nurse, handmaiden to the physician, and battle-axe, as well as the stereotype of the male nurse as being gay, effeminate, or sexually predatory.

2. Identify common public portrayals or descriptions of nurses in terms of gender, dress, and role responsibilities.

3. Examine the role that organizations such as the Center for Nursing Advocacy and Truth About Nursing have assumed in addressing inaccurate or negative portrayals of nursing in the media and the process they use to raise public and professional awareness of the issues surrounding nursing's public image.

4. Analyze the effect of inaccurate nursing stereotypes on the profession's ability to recruit the best and brightest students to nursing, as well as on the collective identity and self-esteem of all nurses.

5. Name well-known fictional nurse characters depicted in contemporary media (television and movies) and identify the nursing stereotypes they best represent.

*continued*

6. Discuss the challenges inherent in attempting to change deeply ingrained stereotypes about nursing that are likely instilled very early in childhood.

7. Analyze how a lack of uniformity in dress and the way in which nurses introduce themselves to patients have contributed to the public's confusion about who is a nurse.

8. Explore the roles and responsibilities that individual nurses, employers, professional associations, and the media have to see that nurses are portrayed accurately and positively to the public.

9. Assess the effect of strategies undertaken by professional coalitions and corporations such as Johnson & Johnson to improve recruitment and retention in nursing.

10. Reflect on the premise that every nurse controls the image of nursing.

11. Reflect on what image he or she would like the public to have of the nursing profession.

An *image* can be defined as a reproduction or an imitation of something or as a mental picture or impression of something (Merriam Webster Online Dictionary, 2011). In other words, an image is often an unknown reality because it depends on the subjective perception of others. Perhaps that is why the public image of the nursing profession is typically one dimensional and inaccurate.

If asked to describe a nurse, most of the public would use such terms as *nice*, *hardworking*, or *caring*. They would also use the terms *ethical* and *honest*. There is little question that the public trusts and respects nurses. In fact, since they were added to the list in 1999, nurses have ranked number one on every Gallup poll on honesty and ethics with the exception of 2001 (Jones, 2010). Few people, however, would use the terms *highly educated*, *bright*, *powerful*, *professional*, or *independent thinker* to describe a nurse. Even fewer would call the nursing profession *prestigious*.

### DISCUSSION POINT

If the nursing profession is so well thought of and so highly recommended, why do many of the brightest students look to medicine rather than nursing? Why are there such significant differences in terms of occupational prestige and status between medicine and nursing?

Many people would, however, describe a nurse as a caring young woman, dressed in a white uniform dress, cap, and shoes, altruistically devoted to caring for the ill ("angel of mercy"), under the supervision of a physician. Common job functions would be identified as making beds, passing out pills, emptying bedpans, giving shots,

and helping doctors. Some people, however, would allude, at least subtly, to a lustier image of sexy young females dressed in provocative attire and seeking sexual gratification from both patients and physicians. Still others might depict stern, aged "battle-axe" females thrusting hypodermic needles into recalcitrant patients and seemingly enjoying the discomfort they cause and the power that they hold.

What do these portrayals have in common? Almost nothing and yet everything. All are part of the convoluted, often conflicting stereotypical images of nurses. In addition, all of these images demean the true nature and complexity of nursing, and most are based almost entirely in fiction. Yet these stereotypes are pervasive, and efforts to change them have yielded only limited progress.

Clearly, public perceptions about the nursing profession are mixed and even contradictory at times. The public trusts and admires nurses, but this does not necessarily equate to respect. Nor does the public consider the profession prestigious or understand what nursing is all about.

The result of this public image confusion is that old stereotypes of nurses as overbearing, brainless, sexually promiscuous, and incompetent women are perpetuated, as are images of nurses as caring, hardworking, altruistic, and selfless. This image conflict is an enduring issue for nursing, and the profession's efforts to address the problem have been fragmented and largely unsuccessful. Indeed, many nurses believe nursing's image to be one of the most important and enduring issues they face as a profession.

This chapter explores common historical and contemporary nursing stereotypes. The effect of these inaccurate stereotypes on recruitment into the profession and the collective self-esteem and identity of nurses is examined. In addition, strategies for improving the

BOX 21.1    **COMMON NURSING STEREOTYPES**

- Angel of mercy
- Love interest (particularly to physicians)
- Sex bombshell/naughty nurse
- Handmaiden to the physician
- Battle-axe
- Male nurses as homosexual, effeminate, or sexually predatory

public image of nursing are presented, as are the challenges inherent in trying to change stereotypes that are ingrained in the profession's history and even in how nurses view themselves.

## NURSING STEREOTYPES

Of the many nursing stereotypes, the most common ones are shown in Box 21.1: the nurse as an angel of mercy; the nurse as a love interest (particularly to physicians); the nurse as a sex bombshell or "naughty nurse"; the nurse as a handmaiden to physicians; the nurse as a battle-axe; and the male nurse as gay, effeminate, or sexually predatory. All of these stereotypes are profiled in this chapter. In addition, contemporary nursing images as depicted in movies and on television are profiled in an effort to better identify what images of nursing are before the public, especially the young people who represent the potential future nursing workforce.

### Angel of Mercy

One of the oldest and most common nursing stereotypes is that of the nurse as an angel of mercy. Some individuals suggest that the image of the nurse as an angel with wings actually comes from the capes nurses historically wore as part of their uniforms. When most people think of nurses as angels of mercy, the saintly image of Florence Nightingale bringing comfort to maimed soldiers during the Crimean War comes to mind. Clearly, Florence Nightingale's legacy of caring is beyond remarkable; however, few individuals outside of nursing would recognize Nightingale as a politically astute, assertive change agent who used her knowledge of epidemiology and statistics to document the effectiveness of nursing interventions. Both images are equally important parts of her legacy.

The nurse "angel of mercy" stereotype continues to persist today, more than 100 years after Florence Nightingale's death. Indeed, a book published by Harlequin in 2008 titled *Single Dad, Nurse Bride* details the fictional life of an orthopedic doctor, Dr. Dane Hendricks, "who is every nurse's dream—handsome and a take charge kind of guy when it comes to medicine but also warm and humorous" (Amazon.com, 2008, para. 2). He is also wealthy. Rikki Johansen, "a conscientious nurse, taking to heart all the lessons she learned in nursing school,... always puts others before herself and as a result, she must drive a car that doesn't always start right away" (para. 4). "When Dane's brother is diagnosed with cancer and Rikki turns out to be the only bone marrow match, there is never any doubt what her choice will be" (para. 8).

Even contemporary health care organizations may unwittingly be perpetuating the stereotype. In May 2011, a major managed health care group (Kaiser Permanente) sponsored a 60-second radio ad as part of the Nurses Week celebration. While the ad was meant to honor nurses, the message perpetuated the angel of mercy stereotype suggesting that nurses are "noble" and "selfless," that they have a "colossal capacity to care," that their sympathy is "superhuman," and that nurses are self-effacing caregivers who endure exhausting, disgusting jobs (with frequent exposure to various "bodily fluids") without complaint (Truth About Nursing, 2011b). The ad even suggests that nurses have "gargantuan hearts which are all squishy with compassion, thumping away."

The Center for Nursing Advocacy (n.d.) has suggested that such images of the nurse as an "angel" or "saint" are generally unhelpful to the profession because they "fail to convey the college-level knowledge base, critical thinking skills, and hard work required to be a nurse. They also suggest that nurses are supernatural beings who do not require decent working conditions,

## BOX 21.2 THE NIGHTINGALE PLEDGE

I solemnly pledge myself before God and in the presence of this assembly, to pass my life in purity and to practice my profession faithfully. I will abstain from whatever is deleterious and mischievous, and will not take or knowingly administer any harmful drug. I will do all in my power to maintain and elevate the standard of my profession, and will hold in confidence all personal matters committed to my keeping and all family affairs coming to my knowledge in the practice of my calling. With loyalty will I endeavor to aid the physician, in his work, and devote myself to the welfare of those committed to my care.

*Source:* Florence Nightingale. The "Nightingale Pledge." (n.d.). Retrieved December 3, 2011, from http://www.countryjoe.com/nightingale/pledge.htm

adequate staffing, or a significant role in health care decision-making or policy" (para. 1).

Some individuals argue that the angel of mercy stereotype is unconsciously promoted by nurses even today—in the Nightingale pledge, for instance (Box 21.2). When one looks closely at the pledge, which originated in 1893 but is still cited frequently in nursing graduation ceremonies, it speaks of nurses forgoing their personal wants and needs for the good of others. Being giving and caring in nature is a wonderful thing, but to suggest that it should be done to the extent of self-neglect is likely not the desired message.

It is important to remember, however, that being an angel of mercy is not all bad. It does encompass behaviors that many nurses typify, such as caring and dedication. Unfortunately, the angel of mercy image all too often also carries with it the idea that pay is never an issue and that suffering must be a part of the nurse's life if the role is to have value. This intrapersonal conflict between the values of altruism and pay befitting a professional is still experienced by many nurses.

### Love Interest (Particularly to Physicians)

Another historical stereotype of nurses is that of a love interest, particularly to physicians. Doctor/nurse romance novels first appeared in the 1930s and 1940s, when becoming a nurse was one of the few career opportunities available to women besides secretarial work, teaching, and child care (Ryan, 2009–2011). Nurses in these novels were cast as intelligent, strong women who felt fulfilled in their careers until they met the physician who would eventually become their husband. Then their career would end, and the nurses would live happily ever after, caring for their spouse and children.

With the women's rights movement of the 1970s, women's career opportunities expanded and fewer books were devoted to women as nurses. In addition, readers' interest in medical romances dwindled. This is not to say that there are not still doctor/nurse romance novels. There are, but the characters typically are different from what they were in decades past. The female character in contemporary books is often now a determined but compassionate physician or at least a charge nurse of a critical care unit in a large, urban medical center, who is beautiful. The male character, however, almost always continues to be a physician, coping with a tragedy in his past, who is "brilliant, tall, and muscular" and "with chiseled features, working in emergency medicine" ("Lovesick Doctors," 2007).

Romantic relationships between nurses and doctors abound on contemporary television shows as well, such as *ER, Scrubs, House,* and *Gray's Anatomy.* It could be argued, however, that most of these relationships are not so much love interests as sexual liaisons.

### Sex Bombshell/Naughty Nurse

Another common nursing stereotype is that of the nurse as a sex bombshell or "naughty nurse." Use of the word *naughty* probably is not powerful enough, however, given that the depiction of nurses in the sex and pornography industry is even more rampant that the general sexual stereotyping of nurses in the media. In fact, for at least 40 years, nurses have been portrayed as sex objects both on television and in the movies. Indeed, movies in the 1960s, 1970s, and 1980s were filled with images of nurses garbed in miniskirts, sleazy, low-cut tops, and high heels, who spent all of their time fulfilling sexual fantasies and virtually no time providing care to patients.

One of the most famous portrayals of a lusty nurse during the 1970s was the character "Hot Lips" Houlihan in the movie M \* A \* S \* H (1970). Hot Lips was, at least at times, a positive role model for nursing, although her sexual proclivities were highlighted at least as much as her skills as a nurse. Hot Lips was also a key character in the television series (1972–1983); however, her sexual exploits were less of an issue.

One decade later, in the spring of 2004, a 10-week series titled *No Angels* depicting the lives of four young nurses appeared on television in the United Kingdom. Three nurses who reviewed the show said the characters were "all smoking, all drinking, sexed up independent women, sashaying through the wards en route to another wild night of clubbing or a steamy clinch in the linen cupboard" (Allen, 2004, para. 2). In fact, the press release for the show stated that *No Angels* was about the life, death, and lunacy inherent in nursing and the antics that nurses indulge in when they want to let off steam (Allen, 2004).

Nurses are even depicted as sex objects in television commercials. In 2003, Clairol Herbal Essences shampoo launched a commercial that showed a nurse abandoning her patient to wash her hair in his bathroom and then tossing her hair sensually at the patient as she left the room. Many nurses and nursing organizations, including the Center for Nursing Advocacy, condemned the unprofessional stereotype perpetuated in the ad and asked sponsor Procter & Gamble to discontinue it (Procter & Gamble Pulls Offending Ad, 2003). Procter & Gamble did issue an apology to nurses and pull the ad, stating that the company "holds the nursing profession in the highest esteem" (p. 35).

### DISCUSSION POINT

Do you think that the public truly believes that a nurse would abandon patient care duties to wash her hair in a patient's bathroom and then sensually shake her hair at the patient? If not, does the commercial still cause harm?

Another commercial sexualizing nurses was launched in September 2007 by Cadbury Schweppes Canada for Dentyne gum (Truth About Nursing, 2007). The Cadbury Schweppes ads showed female nurses being lured into bed with male patients the instant the male patients popped Dentyne into their mouths. The tag line for the commercial was "Get Fresh" and the message was that when hospitalized patients used Dentyne products, there would be an instant, erotic reaction from the "always available" bedside nurse.

More than 1,000 protest letters were sent from the website of the Registered Nurses Association of Ontario (RNAO) in response to the Cadbury Schweppes commercial (Truth About Nursing, 2007). Another 500 supporters from the Center for Nursing Advocacy wrote letters to top Cadbury Schweppes executives, leaving long messages explaining that such imagery reinforces a stereotype of workplace sexual availability that contributes to the global nursing crisis.

Initially, the company responded that its ads were causing no harm. On October 6, 2007, however, the company told the Center and RNAO that it would pull the ads and consult nurses in creating future U.S. and Canadian ads that involved nurses.

Another recent example of the perpetuation of the naughty nurse stereotype became apparent when the Heart Attack Grill, a theme restaurant in Arizona, began dressing their waitresses in naughty nurse uniforms, which included micro miniskirts, fishnet stockings, and high heels. Because nurses are already a highly sexually fantasized profession, the Center for Nursing Advocacy asked the Heart Attack Grill to reconsider their uniform choice when the restaurant opened in 2006. The Grill's owner, Jon Basso, who calls himself "Dr. Jon" and works in a medical lab coat, refused. In November 2011, a chapter of Truth About Nursing held a peaceful rally in front of the restaurant to protest the image of nursing being presented (Truth About Nursing, 2011a). Rally supporters argue that the Heart Attack Grill is reinforcing stereotypes that discourage practicing and potential nurses (especially men), fostering sexual violence in the workplace, and contributing to a general atmosphere of disrespect that weakens nurses' claims to adequate resources.

In addition, the State Board of Nursing filed a complaint with the Arizona Attorney General's office that Basso was illegally using the term *nurse* in advertising for his restaurant (Arizona Statute A.R.S. 32–1636 states only someone who has a valid nursing license can use the title "nurse"). The Attorney General sent Basso a letter informing him that he was illegally using the word "nurse" at his restaurant and on his website. Basso's response was a refusal to remove the word "nurse" from his website, but he did agree to insert an asterisk next to every nurse reference and to include a disclaimer that none of the women pictured on the website actually had any medical training or provide any real medical services.

## Handmaiden to the Physician

Perhaps the most pervasive stereotype of nurses is that of handmaiden to physicians. In the handmaiden role, the nurse simply serves as an adoring backdrop to the omnipotent physician, demonstrating little, if any, independent thought or action.

> **CONSIDER THIS** Nursing care is frequently perceived by the public as simple and unskilled.

This same view of nurses as a handmaiden to physicians in the 1950s and 1960s was reported in classic research by Philip and Beatrice Kalisch, who pioneered studies of nursing images in the 1970s. Indeed, during the 1970s, nurses generally had no substantial role in television stories and were a part of the hospital background in programs that focused on physician characters. When nurses were the focus of a program, the storyline frequently involved the nurse's personal problems rather than his or her role as a nurse and attributes such as obedience, permissiveness, conformity, flexibility, and serenity were emphasized.

Many of the commercial representations of nurses today continue to represent the stereotype of nurse as a handmaiden. For example, in spring 2008, the Angela Moore jewelry catalog featured "Nurse Nancy" bracelets and necklaces. According to Truth About Nursing (2008), the jewelry was composed of four different types of balls; one ball featured a smiling, rosy-cheeked nurse in white uniform and cap giving a balloon to a girl; the second ball had a ladybug next to a stethoscope; the third ball featured a nurse's cap with a thermometer; and the fourth ball had a stuffed bear holding flowers next to a lollipop. The text in the catalog "asked readers to buy the Nurse Nancy jewelry to celebrate the ladies who give lollipops and band aids a whole new meaning" (para. 1).

In response to letters of concern from nurses, the jewelry maker did agree to modify the description of the jewelry. According to Truth About Nursing (2008), however, what they changed it to was "Here's a special theme to celebrate the wonderful women who promote health and make us feel so much better. Talented, terrific and leaders to love!" (para. 3). Truth About Nursing suggested that "while this was probably an improvement over lollipops and band aids" (para. 4), it was still problematic in that it suggested that only women are nurses. In addition, they argued that "statements such as 'makes us feel so much better,' 'leaders to love,' and 'wonderful women' sound like adoration for someone's loving mom who makes them feel so much better by making them soup or tea" (para. 5), not that nurses are highly trained health care professionals who use both science and art to make a difference in their patient's outcomes.

## Battle-Axe

Few stereotypes in nursing are as dark or demented, however, as that of the nurse as a battle-axe. The battle-axe stereotype often depicts an overbearing, unhappy, mean senior nurse who intimidates both patients and staff. The movie *One Flew Over the Cuckoo's Nest* (1975) provides a perfect example of the battle-axe nurse (Nursing Stereotypes, n.d.). Nurse Ratched, a nurse in a mental hospital, fits the description of a battle-axe in almost every way. She craves power and control over others and forces patients to obey her every whim or suffer the repercussions.

Nurse Diesel, in the movie *High Anxiety* (1978), was another stereotypical battle-axe nurse, with the addition of enormous prosthetic breasts. As an overbearing, evil-charge nurse, Nurse Diesel continually displayed a dark sneer and a love of domination. Finally, Annie Wilkes from the novel and movie *Misery* gave new meaning to the sociopathic battle-axe nurse as she kidnapped, maimed, and held hostage a writer she admired and wanted to be close to.

Battle-axe stereotypes of nurses have always existed; however, they seemed to hit their peak in the 1970s and 1980s. There are, however, still multiple images of battle-axe nurses available on the Internet. It is also of interest that the battle-axe counterpart of male physicians in medicine is viewed less negatively. For example, the television show *House* stars a drug-addicted, rule-breaking, rude, and crude male physician whose bad behavior is excused by his brilliance and ability to often cure patients when all hope is lost.

## The Male Nurse: Gay, Effeminate, and Sexually Predatory

Female nurses are not the only ones who are stereotyped. Male nurse stereotypes are at least as prevalent as those for females, and the stereotypes for male nurses are virtually all negative, which only adds to the difficulty of recruiting men to the profession.

Male nurses are frequently stereotyped as being homosexual (or at least effeminate). In a December 2011 episode of the TV show *Desperate Housewives*, "major character Gaby tried to get past access restrictions at the rehabilitation facility where her husband was a resident by flirting with a male nurse, but she failed when the man simply pointed to his chest and said, 'male nurse'—meaning that he was of course gay and so not interested in Gaby" (Truth About Nursing, 2011f, para. 1).

Male nurses may even be stereotyped as being hypersexual and, as a result, the intent of their actions may be questioned as being either sexual in nature or, in some cases, even sexually predatory. This makes it very difficult for male nurses to demonstrate the caring, therapeutic interactions that are such an important part of nursing.

> CONSIDER THIS   Many male nurses live in fear of how their caring actions might be interpreted.

Another popular stereotype for male nurses is that they are nonachievers for going into nursing rather than more traditionally male occupations. This was certainly the case in the 2000 movie *Meet the Parents*. Unfortunately, despite the protestations of Greg Focker, the male registered nurse (RN) in the movie, that he loves nursing and became a nurse by choice, his future in-laws and other relatives constantly questioned his sexual orientation and manliness. They also clearly implied that Greg must have become a nurse because his test scores were not high enough for him to qualify for medical school.

Unfortunately, recent research by Bartfay, Bartfay, Clow, and Wu (2010) found a general perception in Canadian society that nursing is a more suitable career choice for women than men. Moreover, societal perceptions and stereotypes of male nurses (e.g., they are gay, effeminate, less compassionate and caring than female nurses) prevail, which may negatively contribute to their recruitment and retention in nursing programs. The researchers concluded that greater efforts are needed to recruit positive male role models in clinical practice and academia and that recruitment ads for nursing should make greater efforts to portray a positive male presence in the profession. These strategies will help to address in part the current national and global shortages for nurses and also help to encourage diversity in the profession (Bartfay et al., 2010).

## CONTEMPORARY NURSING STEREOTYPES ON TELEVISION

Television medical dramas currently provide the greatest number of visual images of nurses at work. In fact, a study by Donelan, Buerhaus, Desroches, Dittus, and Dutwin (2008) revealed that 60% of the general public watched television shows and news stories the prior year that included nurses or had seen advertisements about nursing. Although most suggested that fictional television shows made no difference in their level of respect for registered nurses, some respondents stated that such depictions increased their respect for nurses and others reported less as a result.

There is little doubt, however, that television medical dramas build on traditional stereotypes of nurses, as well as suggest new ones. One of the best known medical dramas in the past two decades, with strong nurse figures, was *ER* (1994–2009). This medical drama focused on the lives and events of the emergency department staff at County General Hospital in Chicago, a level I trauma center.

The character Carol Hathaway was perhaps the best known nurse on *ER*. After surviving the September 1994 pilot episode in which she tried to commit suicide, Hathaway became the charge nurse of the emergency department. She went on to have a sexual relationship with a physician and bore twins out of wedlock. Nurse Hathaway left the show in 1999—to join her physician love interest in another state.

Even with the departure of Nurse Hathaway, *ER* continued to provide probably the most influential portrayals of nurses on television. One of the highest profile nurses remaining on the show was Abby Lockhart, an alcoholic, former obstetrical nurse from a family afflicted with bipolar disorder. She started on the show as a medical student, dropped out of medical school, worked as a nurse, and then became a doctor. Abby had sexual relationships with several doctors on the show and eventually married one of them.

In addition, Samantha Taggart, a nurse who joined the *ER* cast in 2003, was a tough, free-spirited, single mother of an emotionally troubled child, who almost immediately entered into a sexual relationship with one of the physicians. In her introductory scene, "Sam" (who had come to the hospital inquiring about employment), grabbed a syringe and leaped to sedate an unruly patient through a central vessel in his neck. This behavior earned her not only a job but also the respect of her soon-to-be coworkers.

One newer TV show to stir nurses to action, however, is *Grey's Anatomy* (2005–present). Physician characters on this show provide all of the direct patient care as well as the emotional support of the patient and family. Nurses hold only trivial roles. Even more distressing is the fact that one of the most visible nurses on the show was the one who gave sexually transmitted diseases to the male physicians. Truth About Nursing (2011c) notes that a few episodes in season 7 did feature handsome male nurse (Eli), who "displayed a little skill and briefly stood up to the physicians, but by season's end, he was mainly a love interest for attending surgeon Miranda Bailey and no longer did any nursing work onscreen" (para. 8).

One of the most alarming contemporary visualizations of a nurse on TV, however, is *Nurse Jackie*, a series that premiered in 2009. The title character Jackie Peyton is a drug-addicted nurse who works in the emergency ward at All Saints' Hospital in New York City. Jackie often makes unethical and illegal decisions for the "good" of her patients, such as forging organ donor authorizations. In addition, although married, she has sex with the pharmacist at the hospital in exchange for drugs. In season 2, her drug addiction led her to falsify an MRI to get a phony prescription and to rip off a local drug dealer who embarked on revenge. In the most recent season, Jackie's addictions deepened to the point that she stole drugs from the oncology unit. When her theft was discovered, she was placed on probation by her employer and a sympathetic colleague in the lab perpetuated her employment by discarding her next contaminated urine drug test.

Perhaps what is most disturbing about Nurse Jackie is the attention this utterly dislikable nurse character receives solely as a result of her independent and strong-willed thinking. The reality is that this is a drug-addicted nurse who has little regard for any codes of ethics or the patients she is charged to care for. Her primary mission in life and at work is to attain the drugs she needs to fuel an ever-increasing addiction.

## THE IMAGE OF NURSING ON THE INTERNET

The Internet is also filled with images of nurses, some accurate and some very stereotypical. A recent review of nurse images on Google found thousands of inappropriate images of nurses. Many were sexually suggestive, as well as demeaning. Some were in caricature, but many were of young women dressed in cleavage-baring uniforms and wearing fishnet stockings, high heels, and garter belts.

Unprofessional images of nurses on the Internet do not always come from external sources, however. Sometimes, they come from health care professionals. Lagu, Kaufman, Asch, and Armstrong (2008) looked at how health care professionals (physicians and nurses) communicated through blogs on the Internet. In the 271 medical blogs reviewed, patients were described in 114 blogs (42.1%), and 45 blogs (16.6%) included sufficient information that patients would be able to identify their doctors or themselves. Three blogs showed recognizable photographic images of patients. The researchers concluded that whereas the Internet offers health care professionals the opportunity to share their narratives, revealing confidential information reflects poorly on blog authors and their professions.

In another review of 144 websites in 2001 and 152 websites in 2004, Kalisch, Begeny, and Neumann (2007) found that 70% of the Internet sites showed nurses as intelligent and educated and 60% as respected, accountable, committed, competent, and trustworthy. Nurses were also shown as having specialized knowledge and skills in 70% (2001) and 62% (2004) of the websites. However, images of the nurse as sexually promiscuous increased between 2001 and 2004, whereas images of the nurse as a committed, attractive/well-groomed, and authoritative professional decreased during the same time period. The researchers concluded that the Internet provides important opportunities for improving the image of the nurse.

Finally, a recent review of 40 comprehensive care center websites found that only two included broad representation of oncology nursing as part of the website (Boyle, 2010). The researcher concluded that the absence of nursing in lay-oriented media devalued oncology nurses' highly specialized knowledge and skill and suggested to the public that nurses are not integral members of the multidisciplinary team.

## HOW INGRAINED ARE NURSING STEREOTYPES?

Increasingly, researchers are concluding that inaccurate and negative stereotypes of nurses are not only well ingrained but also instilled early in life. Indeed, gender stereotyping about career opportunities begins at a very early age. By 3 years, most children already have firmly rooted gender-based ideas about the roles they can and should hold when they grow up.

This was borne out in research by Teig and Susskind (2008) of first graders (aged 6 to 8), who had already identified nursing as a high-status feminine occupation. This research suggested that boys attend to both gender roles and status when considering occupations, but that boys are willing to consider high-status "feminine" occupations as much as the low-status "masculine" jobs. Girls, however, focused primarily on the gender role of occupations and only attended to status within the less desirable masculine occupations. Teig and Susskind concluded that "if the social status of nurses is promoted during elementary school, it may enhance young boys' perceptions of the profession," and "if boys do not

eliminate nursing from future consideration during childhood, the percentage of men entering these vocations may increase" (p. 861).

The reality, then, is that by the end of middle school, most students report having their minds made up about desirable and undesirable careers. An unpublished study by Huston (see Research Study Fuels the Controversy 21.1) suggested that basic beliefs and stereotypes about professions such as nursing may be ingrained at a far

## RESEARCH STUDY FUELS THE CONTROVERSY 21.1

### SECOND-GRADERS' IMAGE OF NURSES

This unpublished study examined stereotypes held by 25 second-graders regarding "important" nursing roles and functions. In an effort to introduce students to nonhospital nursing roles, which students stated they already knew, a 30-minute slide show and discussion was held showing nurses actively engaged in less traditional nursing roles such as cardiac rehabilitation, primary care, flight nursing, education,

management, and public health. In addition, nurse practitioners were introduced as primary care providers. Students were shown photos of nurses in all types of garb, except for white uniforms. Efforts were made to assure ethnic and gender diversity in all presentation materials. At the conclusion of the presentation, students were asked to draw a picture of what they thought was the most exciting role that had been presented for nurses.

Huston, C. (n.d.). *Nursing stereotypes ingrained by second grade.* Unpublished manuscript.

### STUDY FINDINGS

The caption on the first drawing was "the nurse is doing surgery on a real important disease." In the second, the nurse, with a red cross on her white uniform, was noted to be "rushing" into the hospital. In the third, the nurse, in her white starched cap, was making up a hospital bed.

In the fourth drawing, the nurse was giving a hospitalized patient a backrub. In another, a dour nurse, as denoted by a capital N on her starched white cap with red cross on it, was entering a hospital nursery. In the sixth, a patient in a bed was hooked up to an intravenous line, expressing pain. The smiling nurse was walking away from him.

In the seventh drawing, the nurse was helping the child in the hospital bed, and it included a caption that the "nurse is in a rush." In another drawing, nurses were scurrying to patients in their hospital beds. Rushing, for nurses, seemed to be a recurrent theme.

In the eighth drawing, the most exciting role for a nurse was noted as transporting a cot from room to room. Similarly, another student noted that the most important thing a nurse did was to transport people to the operating room, and yet another

student noted that transporting patients in wheelchairs to their car was the most important thing that nurses did.

Several drawings included stern nurses in white uniforms and caps and with red crosses on their chests making patients take medicine that tasted bad. Others depicted nurses working in nurseries or teaching mothers how to care for a crying baby. Another depicted a flight nurse taking an injured patient to the hospital, and yet another showed a nurse, in a white uniform with a red cross on her chest and wearing a cap, taking blood pressures.

All of the nurses in the drawings were female and white. The overwhelming majority wore white uniforms and caps and had red crosses on their chests. All but one drawing depicted nurses in hospital settings. Many associated the nurse with pain or an unpleasant experience. Despite the educational intervention, these second-graders already held deeply ingrained stereotypes about nursing and nursing roles, which were resistant to change. This suggests that if stereotypes are this difficult to modify in second-graders, the challenges in changing the image of nursing with the greater public will likely be very difficult.

younger age and that waiting until fifth, sixth, or even seventh grade to address inaccurate or negative images of nursing might be too late. Clearly, an early positive image for students is important if this is the population group the profession hopes will solve the current shortage.

A similar study, published in 2011, examined the influence of a career education program on children's interest in nursing as a career choice, especially related to gender in fifth-grade students (Turner, 2011). Both male and female students expressed increased interest in nursing as a career after the education program, underscoring the positive effect career education can have on career choice, especially in stimulating interest in nursing (see Research Study Fuels the Controversy 21.2).

## THE CENTER FOR NURSING ADVOCACY AND TRUTH ABOUT NURSING

Most nurses are upset about their depiction in contemporary media, but their efforts to respond to and change the situation have been fragmented. A more unified voice became possible with the creation of the Center for Nursing Advocacy in 2001. The center was created when Sandy Summers and seven other graduate nursing students at the Johns Hopkins University in Baltimore joined forces to address the media's disrespectful portrayal of nursing.

In 2009, the center was dissolved as a result of legal wrangling around record keeping and allegations of unpaid taxes (Center for Nursing Advocacy Ceases Operation, 2009). Sandy Summers then set up a new organization, called Truth About Nursing, a 501(c)(3) nonprofit organization that seeks to increase public understanding of the central, frontline role nurses play in modern health care, to promote more accurate, balanced and frequent media portrayals of nurses, and increase the media's use of nurses as expert sources (Truth About Nursing, 2011e). "The Truth About Nursing's ultimate goal is to foster growth in the size and diversity of the nursing profession at a time of critical shortage, strengthen nursing practice, teaching and research, and improve the health care system" (Truth About Nursing, 2011e, para. 1).

## CONSEQUENCES OF INACCURATE OR NEGATIVE IMAGES

Inaccurate or negative public images of nursing have many consequences, particularly because these images influence the attitudes of patients, other health care providers, policy makers, and politicians. They even influence how nurses think about themselves. Sridevy and Baby (2010) note that nurses internalize their professional self-image based in part on the images of nursing held by society. Perhaps even more critical, given

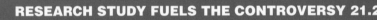

## RESEARCH STUDY FUELS THE CONTROVERSY 21.2

### FIFTH-GRADERS' IMAGE OF NURSES

This within-subjects study design compared interest in nursing as a career with 70 fifth-grade students before and after implementation of a 4-week career education program (four sessions of 2.5 hours each) about nursing. Research questions included (but were not limited to) what are the effects of race, having a family member who is a nurse, and knowing someone who is a nurse other than a family member on the students' interest in nursing as a career choice.

Turner, P. L. (2011). Enhancing nursing as a career choice with fifth-grade students. *Nursing Economics, 29*(3), 136–153.

### STUDY FINDINGS

There was a 61% ($p < 0.001$) increase of students expressing they would consider nursing as a career after participating in the career education program. This increased interest was seen in both male and female students. In terms of race, non-Black students showed a statistically significant increase in interest in nursing as a career choice while Black students did not, even though the percent increase of positive responses for Black students was greater than the increase of positive responses for non-Black students. Increased interest was most apparent in students who did not have a family member who was a nurse, although knowing a nurse other than a family member did not have a significant influence on students' expressed consideration of nursing as a career choice. The researcher concluded that exposing young students to practicing nurses is an important strategy for recruiting the next generation of nurses and that this responsibility falls to all nurses.

the current nursing shortage, is that negative attitudes about nursing might discourage capable prospective nurses who will instead choose another career that offers greater appeal in stature, status, and salary.

> CONSIDER THIS  Many nurses hold stereotypes about the profession to be true, just as the general public does.

## Recruitment Challenges

One significant consequence of the public not understanding both the scope of practice and the skill level required to be a nurse is that it may limit the profession's ability to recruit the best and brightest students. As with other predominantly female professions, the literature suggests that many clients and their families undervalue nursing and do not understand what it is that nurses do that makes a difference in patient outcomes. Indeed, many nurses will honestly admit that they had little factual basis for what nursing would be like when they chose it as a profession. Instead, what drove them to become a nurse were actually images that emphasized the caring, nurturing, and personal rewards associated with the profession.

Still, newer research is encouraging. Donelan et al. (2008) found that nursing, along with several other health/science careers, was viewed positively as a career choice by 70% of the public. Women were more likely than men to give nursing a positive rating (74% vs. 64%), as were those already employed in health care versus those who were not (80% vs. 68%). Finally, Donelan et al.'s research revealed that one in four Americans had personally considered a career in nursing, although only 15% identified it as a serious consideration.

In an effort to recruit young people into the profession, the drug company Johnson & Johnson (J&J) began a series of television advertisements in 2002 as a part of its Campaign for Nursing's Future. Three new 30-second ads were released in 2005 and 2007, highlighting different aspects of nursing practice and promoting diversity in nursing. New ads were released in 2011. While J&J's efforts have without doubt been the most organized and visible organizational effort to promote nursing in the past decade, some critics suggest that the ads have been too focused on the caring side of nursing and that more emphasis needs to be given to the expertise and science behind the decision making that saves patients' lives (Truth About Nursing, 2011d).

## CHANGING NURSING'S IMAGE IN THE PUBLIC EYE

Changing nursing's image in the public eye will not be easy. Nor will there be a silver bullet. Instead, multiple strategies are needed, including active interaction with the media and restriction of the term *nurse* to licensed nurses. In addition, nurses must increase their efforts to publicly praise and value nursing in addition to emphasizing how nursing uniquely contributes to patients achieving their desired health outcomes. Finally, nurses will need to become even more involved in the political processes that shape their profession.

Accomplishing this will take time and resources, including the time, energy, and funding of coalitions, foundations, and professional nursing organizations. Perhaps most important, it will take a concerted effort by individual nurses that will come only by first recognizing that there is a need to take action and then by doing what is necessary to achieve that goal.

### Finding a Voice in the Press

One of the most important strategies needed to change nursing's image is to change the image of nursing in the mind of the image makers. That means proactively seeking positive and accurate media exposure of what nursing really is and what nurses really do. This job cannot be left to professional nursing organizations or to the image makers. Nursing's contributions need to be recognized and proclaimed. Unfortunately, many nurses feel ill prepared or lack the self-confidence to interact with the media. Knowing how to interact with the media is not intuitive for most nurses. Media training should always be provided to give nurses the skills and self-confidence to be effective in this role. Tips for interacting with the media are shown in Box 21.3.

> CONSIDER THIS  Far too few nurses are both willing and appropriately trained to interact with the media.

Burke (2011) suggests that instead of being fearful of the media, nurses should view the desired relationship between the two as symbiotic. Nursing can use the media in order to expose the difficulties being encountered in the profession, and the media can provide more accurate stories about what nurses do and the difference nurses make in the lives of the populations they serve.

Nurse are uniquely qualified to speak with editors, reporters, and media producers on topics related to

## BOX 21.3   TIPS FOR INTERACTING WITH THE MEDIA

1. Be well informed about the topic.
2. Decide ahead of time what 2 to 3 key points you want to make and stay on track with the message.
3. Keep answers short, clear, and concise.
4. Stick to what you know and don't be pressured to answer questions you lack expertise in.
5. Talk in lay terms so that the public you want to reach understands your message.
6. Do not overestimate the reporter's expertise on the topic; be prepared to offer background information if necessary.
7. Remember that nothing is "off the record."
8. Be honest and friendly.
9. Respond immediately to media inquiries for interview since reporters are typically on short deadlines.
10. Be confident that you as a nurse are an expert on many issues consumers need and want to know.

health care because they have a view from the frontlines and are able to localize national health care issues. Nurses are also well qualified to simplify medical gibberish, explain the latest health care research, and identify current trends. Nurses, then, must be taught the basic skills necessary to self-confidently interact with the media. Nurses must also never pass up the opportunity to work with the media and should always view the media as playing a critical role in changing nursing's image.

> CONSIDER THIS  Nurses are experts in health care. Their invisibility in the media is likely a result of nurses lacking the basic skills and self-confidence to get involved, not that the media does not want to talk to nurses.

Finally, nurses should recognize that media stereotypes are not limited to nonprofessional sources. Even advertisements in medical and nursing journals often include stereotypical and demeaning nursing images, with frequent depictions of nurses as dependent, passive minor figures on the health care scene. If nurses are not depicted accurately in their own trade publications, how can they expect representation in other types of media to be better?

## Reclaiming the Title of "Nurse"

Another strategy needed to improve the image of nursing is to assure that use of the term *nurse* is limited to licensed nurses. The International Council of Nurses (ICN) stated in 2004 that the term "nurse" "should be protected by

law and applied to and used only by those legally authorized to practice the full scope of nursing" (ICN, 2004, para. 1). In addition, all state boards of nursing have passed legislation restricting unlicensed personnel from using the title of "nurse." Unfortunately, on a regular basis, nursing aides and attendants either intentionally or unintentionally misrepresent themselves as nurses.

With the increased use of unlicensed assistive personnel and cross-training in the 1990s, a blurring of titles, roles, and responsibilities occurred among RNs, licensed vocational nurses, and unlicensed support staff. Nametags increasingly recognized all staff as "care partners" or "associates," and some hospitals went so far as to prohibit the listing of RN on a name tag. At the same time, a loss of differentiated uniforms further added to the public's confusion about who truly was caring for them. In addition, the media frequently perpetuates the misappropriate use of the term "nurse" by referring to all nurse's aides, volunteers who do health-related work, and medical assistants as "nurses."

In addition, RNs often contribute to the confusion by how they introduce themselves to patients. Nurses are often very casual when introducing themselves to patients, rarely identifying their specific role as the leader of the health care team. Nor do they explain how the roles of other members of the health care team differ. This may be due in part to typical female role socialization, which encourages women not to promote themselves, or it may be part of a team-building effort. Either way, patients end up confused about who the leader of the team is or how their roles differ.

Jacobs-Summers and Jacobs-Summers (2011) urge nurses to project a professional image in all interactions. They suggest that when nurses meet patients, they introduce themselves as a nurse and include their surname as professionals do. This introduction should not be perceived as cold or formal; instead it demonstrates respect and pride in the profession.

Jacobs-Summers and Jacobs-Summers (2011) also encourage "nursing out loud." "This means describing more of what you're thinking while you're providing care, consistent with patient confidentiality and sensitivity. If you do, then patients, families, physician colleagues and others will get a better sense of your education and skill" (para. 5).

## Dressing Like Professionals

Nurses in this country began shedding their white uniforms in the 1960s as part of the anticonformist movement. As a result, the identity of the RN has blurred. Whereas nursing caps and white starched uniforms were often impractical in caring for acutely ill patients, 30 years ago the public knew who the nurse was by the uniform he or she wore. Today, many patients are unable to tell the members of the health care team apart, a problem that has become worse as the result of widespread adoption of scrubs as work uniforms.

Some nurse leaders have suggested that a return to white uniforms would restore the public's perception of nursing's professionalism. However, nurses are split on the issue of whether uniforms are essential to maintaining professionalism in nursing. They argue that comfort and uniformity of dress are equally important and that uniforms are not a requirement for professional trust and respect.

### DISCUSSION POINT

Is it the white uniform that makes the professional, or is it the actions nurses take that define what a nurse is?

Still, the Democratic Nursing Organization of South Africa (DENOSA), a large trade union in South Africa, argues that "nursing apparel will go a long way in restoring and upholding the professional image of nursing" (Sam, 2011, para. 1). DENOSA suggests that a professional image of nursing promotes nursing as a career choice and that complete and professional nursing apparel reassures patients and reinforces the professional role.

## Positive Talk by Nurses About Nursing

Another strategy for improving the image of nursing is to change how nurses talk about nursing to others. Some nurses bad-mouth the profession and discourage young adults from considering nursing as a profession, yet go on to bemoan the current nurse shortage. The effect of these comments by nurses to the general public should not be underestimated in terms of their effect on the recruitment of young people into the profession.

Donelan et al.'s (2008) research found that the public is significantly more likely to recommend a career in either nursing or medicine than are either doctors or nurses. In fact, Donelan et al. found that one in three Americans have discussed nursing as a career choice with a family member or friend, and so how nurses talk about nursing affects the perception of nursing by the general public.

The reality is that every nurse controls the image of nursing. Nursing, like any other profession, has strengths and weaknesses. It is important, however, that nurses enjoy their work, whatever it might be. Nurses should not stay in jobs that make them unhappy because it demoralizes everyone around them. Whining and acting like a victim does little to improve the situation.

The bottom line is that nurses must be ambassadors for the profession and tell the public that nursing is an essential service with equal worth to other professions; that it can provide many services better than other health care disciplines; and that nursing is often more cost-effective than other disciplines. The public's demand for nursing likely rests on the demand nursing creates for itself in the public's eye.

## Emphasizing the Uniqueness of Nursing

Another tactic nurses can use to improve nursing's image is not only to emphasize the profession's unique combination of "caring" and "curing" but also to underscore the depth and breadth of the scientific perspective that underlies its practice. Evidence-based practice and the application of best practice principles are an expectation for contemporary professional nursing practice. Nurses, then, must emphasize how clinical research and the use of current best evidence affect their decision making and the care they provide.

In addition, newer research on nursing sensitivity and nursing outcomes is able to clarify what it is that nurses do that makes a difference in patient outcomes; there is increasing recognition that patients get better as a result of nursing interventions, not despite them.

Generally speaking, however, the public knows very little about the research base that drives high-quality, evidence-based practice, and it is nurses who are in the best position to tell them about it.

## Participating in the Political Arena

The political process can influence nearly everything nurses do and every problem they confront each day. In addition, public opinion is often based on inaccurate images, and nursing is no exception. Participating in the political arena, then, becomes a powerful strategy for changing the public's image of nursing.

The reality, however, is that although the nursing profession has some strong professional organizations, of the approximately 3.1 million RNs in the United States, only a small percentage are members of national nursing organizations. This limits the profession's ability to be a force in the political arena. In addition, many nurses know little about the political process or feel too overwhelmed by the daily demands of their job to become involved in addressing larger professional issues in the political arena. Some nurses just assume that the best interests of the profession are being guarded by some unknown force out there. Legislators wonder whether inactivity means simply not caring or not having an opinion. The result is that nurses are inadequately represented in the political arena, and another

opportunity for nurses to be represented as knowledgeable, active participants in the health care system is lost.

Because the underlying causes of the profession's political inactivity are numerous, just as the strategies needed to address this issue are complex, it is only discussed briefly here. Instead, a separate chapter has been dedicated to more fully discuss the issue (see Chapter 23).

## CONCLUSIONS

Public identity and image have been a struggle for nurses for at least two hundred years. From a sociological perspective, conflicting stereotypes of nursing have not served the nursing profession well, and a disconnect continues to exist between reality and public image. The greater public clearly does not understand what professional nursing is all about, and the nursing profession has done a poor job of correcting long-standing, historically inaccurate stereotypes.

The responsibility for changing nursing's image lies squarely on the shoulders of those who claim nursing as their profession. Until such time as nurses are able to agree on the desired collective image and are willing to do what is necessary to both tell and show the public what that image is, little will change. Derogatory stereotypes are likely to continue to undermine public confidence in and respect for the professional nurse.

## FOR ADDITIONAL DISCUSSION

1. Historically, images of physicians in the media have been more positive than those of nurses. Why? What factors have led to this difference?

2. Some nurses feel that no longer wearing white uniforms and caps has reduced the professionalism of nursing. Is how nurses dress an important part of public image? Would reverting to more traditional nursing attire improve nursing's public image?

3. Would you want your son or daughter to be a nurse? What have you told them about nursing that would either encourage or discourage them from doing so?

4. Who are the best known nurses currently depicted in the media (radio, television, movies) you access on a regular basis? Do their characters represent nursing stereotypes that have been discussed in this chapter?

5. What do you believe to be the greatest restraining forces that discourage nurses from interacting with the media? Is media training the answer?

6. The contributions of J&J to improve the image of nursing and increase recruitment into the nursing profession are unparalleled. Why would a corporation such as J&J be interested in this pursuit? Why did such an initiative not originate with a professional nursing organization?

7. Are nurses confused about what shared image they want the public to have of their profession?

## REFERENCES

Allen, D. (2004). No holds barred. *Nursing Standard, 18*(24), 24–26.

Amazon.com. (2008). *Single dad, nurse bride* (Reader reviews). Retrieved May 20, 2012, from http://www.amazon.com/Single-Nurse-Harlequin-Medical-Romance/dp/037319904X

Bartfay, W., Bartfay, E., Clow, K., & Wu, T. (2010). Attitudes and perceptions towards men in nursing education. *Internet Journal of Allied Health Sciences & Practice, 8*(2).

Boyle, D. (2010). The invisibility of nursing: Implications from an analysis of National Cancer Institute-designated comprehensive cancer center websites. *Oncology Nursing Forum, 37*(2), E75–E83.

Burke, A. (2011). Dealing with the media. *World of Irish Nursing & Midwifery, 19*(4), 23.

Center for Nursing Advocacy. (n.d.). *Are nurses angels of mercy?* Retrieved September 3, 2008, from http://www.nursingadvocacy.org/faq/nf/are_nurses_angels.html

Donelan, K., Buerhaus, P., Desroches, C., Dittus, R., & Dutwin, D. (2008). Public perceptions of nursing careers: The influence of the media and nursing shortages. *Nursing Economics, 26*(3), 143–150, 165.

Florence Nightingale. "The Nightingale Pledge." (n.d.). Retrieved December 3, 2011, from http://www.countryjoe.com/nightingale/pledge.htm

Huston, C. (n.d.). *Nursing stereotypes ingrained by second grade.* Unpublished manuscript.

International Council of Nurses. (2004). *Position statement: Protection of the title "nurse."* Retrieved September 5, 2008, from http://www.icn.ch/images/stories/documents/publications/position_statements/B06_Protection_Title_Nurse.pdf

Jacobs-Summers, H., & Jacobs-Summers, S. (2011). *The image of nursing: It's in your hands.* Retrieved December 4, 2011, from http://www.nursingtimes.net/nursing-practice/clinical-specialisms/educators/the-image-of-nursing-its-in-your-hands/5024815.article

Jones, J. M. (2010). *Nurses top honesty and ethics list for 11th year.* Retrieved December 3, 2011, from http://www.gallup.com/poll/145043/nurses-top-honesty-ethics-list-11-year.aspx

Kalisch, B. J., Begeny, S., & Neumann, S. (2007). The image of the nurse on the Internet. *Nursing Outlook, 55*(4), 182–188.

Kennedy, S. (2009). Center for nursing advocacy ceases operation. *American Journal of Nursing, 109*(4), 14.

Lagu, T., Kaufman, E., Asch, D., & Armstrong, K. (2008). Content of weblogs written by health professionals. *Journal of General Internal Medicine, 23*(7). Retrieved May 20, 2012, from http://www.pharmalot.com/wp-content/uploads/2008/07/medical-blogs.pdf

Lovesick doctors and lovelorn nurses. (2007). *Nurse Ratched's Place.* Retrieved December 3, 2011, from http://nurse-ratcheds.blogspot.com/2007/11/lovesick-doctors-and-lovelorn-nurses.html

Merriam-Webster Online Dictionary. (2011). *Image* (Definition). Retrieved December 3, 2011, from http://www.merriam-webster.com/dictionary/image

*Nursing stereotypes: Images that underestimate the profession.* (n.d.). Retrieved December 3, 2011, from http://www.english.iup.edu/eaware/nursing/INDEX.htm

Procter & Gamble pulls offending ad. (2003). *Nursing, 33*(8), 35.

Ryan, K. (2009–2011). *Doctors and nurses.* Retrieved December 3, 2011, from http://www.rtbookreviews.com/content/theme-doctors-and-nurses

Sam, H. (2011). A clean, professional image. *Nursing Update, 35*(8), 28.

Sridevy, S., & Baby, P. (2010). Public verses self image of nurses. *International Journal of Nursing Education, 2*(1), 50–54.

Teig, S., & Susskind, J. (2008). Truck driver or nurse? The impact of gender roles and occupational status on children's occupational preferences. *Sex Roles, 58*(11/12), 848–863.

Truth About Nursing. (2007). *Getting fresher.* Retrieved December 5, 2011, from http://www.truthaboutnursing.org/news/2007/oct/06_dentyne.html

Truth About Nursing. (2008). *Let's "celebrate the ladies who give lollipops and band aids" with a Nurse Nancy bracelet!* Retrieved December 5, 2011, from http://www.truthaboutnursing.org/news/2008/mar/18_angela_moore.html

Truth About Nursing. (2011a). News on nursing in the media. *Heart Attack Grill: Successful protest in Las Vegas November 12!* Retrieved December 4, 2011, from http://truthaboutnursing.org/

Truth About Nursing. (2011b, May). News on nursing in the media: Take action! *That gargantuan heart all squishy with compassion thumping away!* Retrieved December 4, 2011, from http://truthaboutnursing.org/archives/2011/apr_may_jun.html#apr

Truth About Nursing. (2011c). *News on nursing in the media: Understaffed Fall 2011 TV review.* Retrieved December 4, 2011, from http://truthaboutnursing.org/archives/2011/jul_aug_sep.html#jul

Truth About Nursing. (2011d). *News on nursing in the media: Lucky charms.* Retrieved December 4, 2011, from http://truthaboutnursing.org/archives/2011/apr_may_jun.html

Truth About Nursing. (2011e). *Mission statement.* Retrieved December 4, 2011, from http://truthaboutnursing.org/about_us/mission_statement.html

Truth About Nursing. (2011f). *"Seriously? Male nurse."* Retrived December 31, 2011, from http://www.truthaboutnursing.org/news/2011/dec/04_desperate.html

Turner, P. L. (2011). Enhancing nursing as a career choice with fifth-grade students. *Nursing Economics, 29*(3), 136–153.

## BIBLIOGRAPHY

American College of Emergency Physicians. (2011). *Effective media interview techniques.* Retrieved December 4, 2011, from http://www.acep.org/content.aspx?id=21778

Ateah, C., Snow, W., Wener, P., MacDonald, L., Metge, C., Davis, P.,... Anderson, J. (2011). Stereotyping as a barrier to collaboration: Does interprofessional education make a difference? *Nurse Education Today, 31*(2), 208–213.

Boerner, H., & Hwang, L. (2010). Losing our voice. *National Nurse, 106*(8), 20–24.

Cabaniss, R. (2011). Educating nurses to impact change in nursing's image. *Teaching & Learning in Nursing, 6*(3), 112–118.

Dumont, C., & Tagnesi, K. (2011). Research corner. Nursing image: What research tells us about patients' opinions. *Nursing, 41*(1), 9–11.

Eley, D., & Eley, R. (2011). Personality traits of Australian nurses and doctors: Challenging stereotypes? *International Journal of Nursing Practice, 17*(4), 380–387.

Fehr, L. (2011). Colorado Nurses Association President... The invisible staff nurse. *Colorado Nurse, 111*(3), 2.

Help clean up the image of nursing. (2010). *Nursing Update, 35*(1), 40–41.

McMurry, T. (2011). The image of male nurses and nursing leadership mobility. *Nursing Forum, 46*(1), 22–28.

Morris-Thompson, T., Shepherd, J., Plata, R., & Marks-Maran, D. (2011). Diversity, fulfillment and privilege: The image of nursing. *Journal of Nursing Management, 19*(5), 683-92.

Nemeth, L. (2011). Nurse Jackie and nurse ethics: How TV and the media influence our public image. *Beginnings, 31*(2), 8–10.

Protection of the title "nurse" brief and talking points. (2010). *Wyoming Nurse, 23*(3), 12.

Toren, O., Kerzman, H., & Kagan, I. (2011). The difference between professional image and job satisfaction of nurses who studied in a post-basic education program and nurses with generic education: A questionnaire survey. *Journal of Professional Nursing, 27*(1), 28–34.

Wittmann-Price, R., Celia, L., Conners, C., Dunn, R., & Chabot, J. (2011). Exploring perceptions of nursing image in an inner-city hospital. *Nursing, 41*(9), 23–27.

# Chapter 22

## Advanced Practice Nursing
### *The Latest Issues and Trends*

Margaret Rowberg

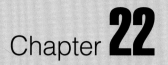

## ADDITIONAL RESOURCES

Visit thePoint for additional helpful resources
- eBook
- Journal Articles
- WebLinks

## LEARNING OBJECTIVES

*The learner will be able to:*

1. Differentiate between the definition of, educational preparation for, and roles commonly assumed by certified nurse-midwives (CNMs), clinical nurse specialists (CNSs), nurse practitioners (NPs), and certified registered nurse anesthetists (CRNAs).

2. Explore reasons why so few nurses seek doctoral education preparation, particularly the PhD.

3. Describe the impetus for and controversies associated with the granting of the doctor of nursing practice (DNP) degree.

4. Describe the driving and restraining forces for increasing the entry educational level for advanced practice nursing to that of a practice doctorate.

5. Identify the educational preparation and common role expectations of the clinical nurse leader (CNL).

6. Reflect on his or her interest in exploring advanced practice nursing as a career choice.

According to the American Association of Colleges of Nursing (AACN, 2010), "The health system's increasing demand for front-line primary care, and the accelerating drive toward managed care, prevention, and cost-efficiency are driving a need for nurses with advanced practice skills in this country" (para. 16). Although advanced practice registered nurses (APRNs) are skilled clinical practitioners, many do not have the knowledge and expertise needed to address the persistent professional issues which arise in the health care system.

In 2002, the AACN, in its landmark work, requested that a group of nurse leaders begin an evolving discussion about developing a clinical or practice doctorate. Several nursing schools had existing practice doctorate programs, and many more were assessing whether to develop such a program. The AACN (2007) thought it would be appropriate to develop a position about this degree because it believed that nursing had the "unparalleled opportunity and capability to address the critical issues that face the nation's current health care system" (p. 3). They also believed that nursing "has the answer to the predominant health care dilemmas of the future" (p. 3) and that "each of the prevailing health problems is suited to the nursing paradigm. Their amelioration is what nursing students are educated to do" (p. 4). Consequently, the AACN, upon task force recommendation, proposed furthering the development of both a clinical practice doctoral degree and the clinical nurse leader role.

Much has been written and published regarding the recommendations of the AACN task forces. This chapter discusses the development of the doctor of nursing practice (DNP) and the clinical nurse leader (CNL) and offers some insight into the current trends, issues, and concerns surrounding these evolving new roles.

## ROLE DEFINITION

According to the 2008 National Sample Survey of Registered Nurses, there are more than 254,000 APRNs in the United States (U.S. Department of Health and Human Services, Health Resources and Services Administration [HRSA], 2010, p. 19). Four categories of nurses are considered to be APRNs: nurse practitioners (NPs), clinical nurse specialists (CNSs), certified nurse midwives (CNMs), and certified registered nurse anesthetists (CRNAs).

More than 150,000 of the APRNs in the United States are NPs, including 19,000 who are both NPs and CNSs or NPs and CNMs. More than 59,000 are CNSs, 18,000 are CNMs, and 34,000 are CRNAs (HRSA, 2010, p. 19).

These numbers represent a 4.2% increase overall since 2004, when the previous survey was completed. The numbers also represent a 12.1% increase in NPs, an amazing 35.1% increase in CNMs and a 7.1% increase in CRNAs during this 4-year period. There was a 22.4% decline in the number of clinical nurse specialists during this time period (HRSA, 2010, p. 19). Although all advanced practice roles require specialization of knowledge and a high degree of practice autonomy, the roles and their associated scope of practice differ greatly.

## Nurse Practitioners

According to the American College of Nurse Practitioners (ACNP, n.d.),

> *Nurse practitioners (NPs) are registered professional nurses who are prepared, through advanced graduate education and clinical training, to provide a wide range of health care services, including the diagnosis and management of common, as well as complex, medical conditions to individuals of all ages.* (para. 1)

## Clinical Nurse Specialists

The National Association of Clinical Nurse Specialists (NACNS, n.d.) defines CNSs as

> *licensed registered nurses who have graduate preparation (Master's or Doctorate) in nursing as a Clinical Nurse Specialist. Clinical Nurse Specialists are expert clinicians in a specialized area of nursing practice, be it a population or setting, disease or medical subspecialty, a type of care or problem. Clinical Nurse Specialists practice in a wide variety of health care settings. In addition to providing direct patient care, Clinical Nurse Specialists influence care outcomes by providing expert consultation for nursing staffs and by implementing improvements in health care delivery systems. Clinical Nurse Specialist practice integrates nursing practice, which focuses on assisting patients in the prevention or resolution of illness, with medical diagnosis and treatment of disease, injury and disability.* (para. 1)

## Certified Nurse-Midwives

The American College of Nurse-Midwives (ACNM, 2010b) states,

> *Midwifery as practiced by Certified Nurse-Midwives (CNMs) and Certified Midwives (CMs) encompasses primary care for women across the lifespan from*

*adolescence to beyond menopause, with a special emphasis on pregnancy, childbirth, and gynecologic and reproductive health. Midwives perform comprehensive physical exams, prescribe medications including contraceptive methods, order laboratory and other diagnostic tests, and provide health and wellness education and counseling. The scope of practice for CNMs and CMs also includes treatment of male partners for sexually transmitted infections, and care of the normal newborn during the first 28 days of life.* (para. 1)

Certified nurse-midwives are registered nurses who have graduated from a nurse-midwifery education program accredited by the Accreditation Commission for Midwifery Education (ACME) and have passed a national certification examination to receive the professional designation of certified nurse-midwife. Nurse-midwives have been practicing in the United States since the 1920s (ACNM, 2010a).

*Certified midwives are individuals who have or receive a background in a health related field other than nursing and graduate from a midwifery education program accredited by ACME. Graduates of an ACME-accredited midwifery education program take the same national certification examination as CNMs but receive the professional designation of certified midwife.* (para. 2)

### Certified Registered Nurse Anesthetists

According to the American Association of Nurse Anesthetists (AANA, 2011),

*The practice of anesthesia is a recognized specialty within the profession of nursing. As one of the first nursing specialty groups, CRNAs have a longstanding commitment to high standards in a demanding field. As independently licensed health professionals, CRNAs are responsible and accountable for their practice.* (para. 1)

*A Nurse Anesthetist, or Certified Registered Nurse Anesthetist (CRNA), is a licensed professional nurse who provides the same anesthesia services as an anesthesiologist (MD).* (Allnursingschools.com, 2011, para. 1)

*CRNAs administer anesthesia and anesthesia-related care in four general categories: (1) pre-anesthetic preparation and evaluation; (2) anesthesia induction, maintenance and emergence; (3) post-anesthesia care; and (4) perianesthetic and clinical support functions.* (AANA, 2011, para. 12)

## BACKGROUND OF ADVANCED PRACTICE NURSING IN THE UNITED STATES

Advanced practice registered nurses have been making significant contributions to the health of the nation and around the world for almost 50 years, but they function in a health care system in the United States that is in need of change. In 1999, the Institute of Medicine (IOM; 1999) published its sentinel report *To Err is Human: Building a Safer Health System* that stated that as many as 98,000 people die each year due to errors that occur while receiving health care. The IOM (2001) further reported that "research on quality of care reveals a health care system that frequently falls short in its ability to translate knowledge into practice, and to apply new technology safely and appropriately" (p. 3).

Although these reports have been in existence for more than a decade, an unacceptable high number of errors continue to be reported. New safeguards have been put in place in most institutions, but nursing can and should be a key profession in leading the way to significant change to the health care system. According to the latest IOM (2011) report, *The Future of Nursing: Leading Change, Advancing Health,*

*The nursing profession has the potential capacity to implement wide-reaching changes in the health care system… By virtue of their regular, close proximity to patients and their scientific understandings of care processes across the continuum of care, nurses have a considerable opportunity to act as full partners with other health care professionals and to lead in the improvement and redesign of the health care system and its practice environment.* (p. 23)

One of the problems in achieving the goal of a patient-centered, cost-effective, and safe health care system is that nursing has so few nurses with doctoral degrees. According to the HRSA (2010), of more than 3 million nurses, only slightly more than 28,000 nurses in the United States obtained a doctorate after becoming a nurse (pp. 4–5). There has, however, been a significant increase in the number of nurses who have a master's degree or higher. This number has increased from 275,000 in 2000 to more than 400,000 in 2008 (HRSA, 2010, p. 5). The recent IOM (2011) report recognizes the need for more nurses who have higher degrees and has recommended that the number of nurses who have doctorates should be doubled by 2020, a date which will challenge schools, funders, and administrators alike.

The movement to increase the number of nurses who have doctorates may be having some impact. According to the National Science Foundation (NSF, 2010), almost 2,100 individuals were awarded doctorates in a health-related field in 2009, a number which shows a 48.8% increase over 1999 when only 1,400 doctorates were awarded in health (para. 6). At the same time, the NSF data show that more than three times as many individuals were awarded doctorates in engineering and more than 10 times as many doctorates in science than in a health-related field during this period (para. 1).

---

### DISCUSSION POINT

Why do you think so few nurses are willing to pursue a doctoral degree? Why is nursing not keeping the same pace as other professions such as engineering?

---

Why do not more nurses pursue advanced degrees? One reason is because salaries for people with these degrees, many of whom are in academic settings, have not kept pace with salaries in the clinical setting. The most recent statistics from the Bureau of Labor Statistics (May 2010) show nurses who are teaching as getting higher salaries than nurses who work in hospitals (US$74,180 vs. US$68,610 mean salary), but it is not unusual for nurses with 10 or more years of experience in the clinical setting to be making US$80,000 to 100,000/year. In fact, a recent salary survey by Pronsati and Gerchufsky (2011) revealed that nurse practitioners (NPs) who work in academe earn slightly more than US$80,000, while NPs in all settings averaged US$90,770 in 2010 (para. 3). AACN (2005b) found similar results and states, "Potential students calculate whether it profits them to seek doctoral study and enter academia when they can earn better salaries in non-academic master's-level positions" (para. 14).

Another reason is the length of time it takes to achieve a bachelor's or higher degree. It can take an associate degree nurse up to 5 years to achieve a master's degree. Obtaining a doctorate, particularly a PhD or DNS, may take another 5 to 6 years and for some, it can take even longer.

A third reason nurses do not pursue higher degrees is the costs related to returning to school. Although some organizations do offer tuition reimbursement, many nurses who obtain a master's or doctoral degree must personally pay for tuition and books or take out huge loans, which take years to pay back. The IOM (2011) suggests that ". . . nurses at all levels have few incentives to pursue further education" (p. 31).

These issues have contributed to a lack of appropriately prepared nurses who are willing to accept the challenges of the health care system and work toward effecting the needed changes. Research by PhD-prepared nurses is essential, but clinically active professionals who have a background in policy, leadership, and organizational behavior are vital to making needed changes. The National Academy of Sciences recommended in its celebrated work that nursing should "develop a new nonresearch clinical doctorate, similar to M.D. and Pharm.D. in medicine and pharmacy respectively" to help fill the need for practitioners and faculty (National Research Council, 2005, p. 74).

About the same time this report was released, landmark reports from the American Hospital Association Commission on Workforce for Hospitals and Health Systems (2002), the Joint Commission on Accreditation of Healthcare Organizations (JCAHO, 2002), and the Robert Wood Johnson Foundation (Kimball & O'Neill, 2002) were published which discussed the issues surrounding the nursing shortage and the need for health professionals to be educated with an emphasis on evidence-based practice. The United States faces several major problems: a health care system in need of reform, an increasing nursing shortage, and an insufficient number of practicing nurses who are educationally prepared to address these problems. The question becomes how nursing can address these issues.

---

### DISCUSSION POINT

How can nursing address the need for nurses who are educated with an emphasis on evidence-based practice?

---

In response to these questions, the AACN initiated several task forces to assess these issues. In 2002, one expert group was asked "to examine the current status of clinical or practice doctoral programs, compare various models, and make recommendations regarding future development" (AACN, 2004, p. 1). The group was to determine whether a practice doctorate would be an appropriate degree for advanced practice registered nurses. Another task force was asked to assess how nursing could provide the kind of leadership needed in light of the issues in the health care system and the ever-increasing nursing shortage. Ultimately, the board of the AACN proposed to its members that the DNP degree and the CNL role be developed.

## THE DOCTOR OF NURSING PRACTICE

It is important to start the discussion of the DNP with the exact words from AACN to clarify why it recommended that this new degree be developed. In its classic position statement, the AACN (2004) stated,

> Doctoral programs in nursing and other practice disciplines can be categorized into two distinct types: research-focused and practice-focused. The term practice, specifically nursing practice, as conceptualized in this document refers to any form of nursing intervention that influences health care outcomes for individuals or populations, including the direct care of individual patients, management of care for individuals and populations, administration of nursing and health care organizations, and the development and implementation of health policy. Preparation at the practice doctorate level includes advanced preparation in nursing, based on nursing science, and is at the highest level of nursing practice.
>
> What distinguishes this definition of practice from others is that it includes both direct care provided to patients by individual clinicians as well as direct care policies, programs and protocols that are organized, monitored, and continuously improved upon by expert nurse clinicians. (p. 3)

---

CONSIDER THIS   The definition of practice has been expanded to include policy and program development with ongoing continuous quality-improvement strategies.

---

It is frustrating for APRNs to learn that despite the fact that the master's degree required many clinical hours and course credits, it often does not provide an education in areas such as leadership, health policy, practice management, information technology, process and outcomes evaluation, and similar topics that are vital to health care. Further, the IOM (2011) has recommended that nurses must "demonstrate new competencies in systems thinking, quality improvement, and care management and a basic understanding of health policy and research" (p. 31). APRNs are finding that they must take continuing education courses to help fill the gap. Schools of nursing have struggled to keep up with the increasing demand for this knowledge while maintaining a reasonable length to their master's degree programs. Consequently, the AACN responded to proactively move forward to develop the practice or clinical doctorate.

It is important to realize that doctoral programs are not new to nursing. Hawkins and Nezat (2009) reported that the first doctoral programs in nursing were offered in the 1920s at Columbia University, which awarded a doctor of education degree, and the first PhD in nursing program was established at New York University (p. 92). When the first doctor of nursing science (DNS/DNSc) programs were begun, schools stated that these degrees were "different" from a PhD, but it soon became clear that most of these programs were research-focused much like the PhD and not practice based.

Practice-based doctorates are also not new to nursing. The first program began at Case Western Reserve University [CWRU; 2010a] in 1979 as a doctor of nursing (ND) degree. This degree was converted to the doctor of nursing practice (DNP), but the focus has always been to "prepare nurses to serve as leaders in nursing practice" (CWRU, 2010b, para. 3).

There is some confusion, however, regarding the differences between a research doctorate (PhD or DNS/DNSc) and a practice doctorate (DNP or ND). The AACN (2006) provided an excellent explanation in its introduction to the DNP Essentials document:

> Doctoral programs in nursing fall into two principal types: research-focused and practice-focused. Most research-focused programs grant the Doctor of Philosophy degree (PhD), while a small percentage offers the Doctor of Nursing Science degree (DNS, DSN, or DNSc). Designed to prepare nurse scientists and scholars, these programs focus heavily on scientific content and research methodology; and all require an original research project and the completion and defense of a dissertation or linked research papers. Practice-focused doctoral programs are designed to prepare experts in specialized advanced nursing practice. They focus heavily on practice that is innovative and evidence-based, reflecting the application of credible research findings. The two types of doctoral programs differ in their goals and the competencies of their graduates. They represent complementary, alternative approaches to the highest level of educational preparation in nursing. (p. 3)

One of the major issues that supported the move to the practice doctorate was the need for many APRN programs to increase the "number of didactic and clinical clock hours far beyond the requirements of master's education in virtually any other field.... Many NP master's programs now exceed 60 credits and cannot be completed in less than three years" (AACN, 2004a, para. 20). As a result, AACN (2004a) suggested,

*In response to changes in health care delivery and emerging health care needs, additional knowledge or content areas have been identified by practicing nurses. In addition, the knowledge required to provide leadership in the discipline of nursing is so complex and rapidly changing, that additional or doctoral level education is needed.* (para. 22)

Based on the work of the task force, the AACN (2004a) endorsed the position statement on the practice doctorate in nursing recommending that all advanced practice nursing education change from graduating APRNs with master's degrees to doctoral degrees by 2015. AACN (2006) then continued its work in this area and approved a document titled *The Essentials of Doctoral Education for Advanced Practice Nursing*. These essentials are similar in focus to the *Essentials of Baccalaureate Education for Professional Nursing Practice* (AACN, 2008). This DNP document provided schools of nursing with the key content areas that should be included in the DNP curriculum. It was not intended to be prescriptive of actual courses but to provide guidelines and standards around which faculty can develop

the courses that they feel are appropriate to their DNP degree. These essentials are shown in Box 22.1, as well as on the AACN website.

---

### DISCUSSION POINT

As the 2015 deadline approaches, how difficult do you believe it will be for APRN programs to achieve the recommendations of the AACN?

---

In the years since these documents have been published, many changes have occurred. It is interesting to note that schools adopted the recommendations with less resistance than previously seen in nursing. In October 2012, 190 schools were listed on the AACN website as offering DNP programs, with another 100 stating to the AACN that would have a program in the near future (AACN, 2012a). Nurse practitioner programs are the ones most quickly moving to the DNP.

The American Nurses Association (ANA, 2010) issued its first position statement on the DNP in 2010 and recommends that the DNP be "recognized as the terminal practice-focused degree in the nursing profession" but also "supports both master's and doctoral level of preparation as entry into APRN practice through a period of transition" (ANA, 2010, pp. 8–9).

---

### BOX 22.1   THE ESSENTIALS OF DOCTORAL EDUCATION FOR ADVANCED PRACTICE NURSING

1. Scientific underpinnings for practice
2. Organizational and systems leadership for quality improvement and systems thinking
3. Clinical scholarship and analytical methods for evidence-based practice
4. Information systems/technology and patient care technology for the improvement and transformation of health care
5. Health care policy for advocacy in health care
6. Interprofessional collaboration for improving patient and population health outcomes
7. Clinical prevention and population health for improving the nation's health
8. Advanced nursing practice

*Source:* American Association of Colleges of Nursing. (2006). *The essentials for doctoral education for advanced practice nursing.* Retrieved from http://www.aacn.nche.edu/DNP/pdf/Essentials.pdf

Though the change to the DNP by schools of nursing has occurred with little controversy, some nursing leaders continue to debate its necessity (Chase & Pruitt, 2006; Cronenwett et al., 2011; Dreher, 2011; Fontaine & Langston, 2011; Fulton & Lyon, 2005; Gilliss & Hill, 2011; Malone, 2011; Meleis & Dracup, 2005; Milton, 2005). Nursing historically has been unwilling to accept innovation in a timely manner. It has been more than 50 years, and yet nursing still cannot agree on the appropriate degree for entry into practice. Now the argument has become whether to adopt the DNP as entry into practice for APRNs. The acceptance of the DNP has occurred in a fairly short time period and may be reflective of a better understanding by nursing leaders that, due to the persistent health care system issues, nursing must finally be one of the leaders in change.

## What Do the APRN Organizations Think?

Some of the APRN organizations were quick to respond to the recommendation to adopt the DNP degree as the entry into practice for APRNs by 2015. The National Organization of Nurse Practitioner Faculties (NONPF) began work on the practice doctorate in 2001. In April 2011, it released its final document on the core competencies for nurse practitioner education and practice at the doctoral level. In the end, the NONPF decided that it could not support the 2015 deadline for NP programs to prepare graduates at the doctoral level (Fitzpatrick & Wallace, 2009; NONPF, 2011) but acknowledged that the DNP is a worthwhile goal for NP programs to attain and recommended that programs transition at a pace that would continue to ensure quality.

---

### DISCUSSION POINT

Should the NONPF establish a new deadline for making the change to doctoral-level education of nurse practitioners?

---

The other three advanced practice specialties (CNS, CNM, and CRNA) have taken a more conservative approach to the DNP recommendation. Their representative associations have published position statements that offer different views on the topic.

The National Association of Clinical Nurse Specialists (NACNS, 2009) decided to remain neutral about the recommendation and has requested ongoing dialogue to tackle lingering concerns. The association did state that the "NACNS supports CNS education at the master's or the doctoral level, including programs that offer the practice doctorate, providing that established, validated CNS competencies and education program standards are met" (para. 2).

The nurse-midwives stated that though they see the DNP as an option, it "should not be a requirement for entry into midwifery practice" (American College of Nurse Midwives [ACNM], 2009a, para. 1). One must keep in mind though that this group also resisted master's-level preparation as entry into midwifery practice and only began enforcing that mandate in 2010 (ACNM, 2009b). The ACNM believes that midwives, for decades, "regardless of terminal degree, are safe, cost-effective providers of maternity and women's health care" (para. 3).

In an effort to thoroughly examine the issues and arrive at a logical decision, AANA commissioned a task force that did an extensive study of the issue and published support for mandating the DNP but decided that the timeline should be extended to 2025 based on the outcomes of the study (American Association of Nurse Anesthetists [AANA], 2007, p. 9).

---

CONSIDER THIS  All advanced practice nursing organizations have established their own guidelines for changing to doctoral education.

---

## Issues and Concerns—Where We Are Now

With the release of the AACN position statement, the need for the DNP was challenged and important questions were raised (Fulton & Lyon, 2005; Meleis & Dracup, 2005; Milton, 2005). Much of the initial concern over the DNP was resolved with AACN's clarification of the role and its ultimate release of the DNP Essentials document. However, some issues persist. These concerns include the timing of the recommendation; questions over the DNP not including adequate theory; the effect of the DNP on nursing education, particularly PhD programs; concern that DNP graduates who become faculty members may not be able to attain tenure; and apprehension about DNP programs having the same degree of rigor as other doctoral programs. It is, however, unclear why nurses feel compelled to argue over a practice doctorate when the IOM is demanding that nursing develop a degree that focuses on practice and the clinical setting.

## Timing

Meleis and Dracup (2005) initially argued that the timing for introduction of the DNP was inappropriate because this recommendation was "detracting from other pressing matters related to quality and safe care" (para. 20). This author would argue that statement alone is an argument for the DNP because nursing's focus on health promotion and disease prevention is fundamental to effecting the needed changes in the health care system. Having nurses prepared at the doctoral level is vital for that change to occur because DNP coursework includes topics such as policy, evaluation, and leadership, areas which may not previously have been covered at the master's level. Nurses prepared in these new content areas are more knowledgeable when sitting in policy meetings and will be agents for system changes.

Cronenwett et al. (2011) argue that the timing may have been right when AACN originally introduced the DNP but due to changes in the economy, it is no longer appropriate to introduce new programs. To the contrary, now is an appropriate time as nursing programs are looking at ways to strengthen its education at all levels in an effort to ensure inclusion of the IOM competencies into curriculum. The economic downturn is forcing schools to focus on quality and safety while at the same time being more efficient in their financial resources.

This author believes that having only a research-focused doctoral degree in nursing limits the dissemination of the important outcomes nursing has achieved. The main focus of PhD programs is the development of research, which does not always include implementation of that research. DNP graduates have the coursework and clinical practice preparation to use the work of the PhD or DNS nurse through implementation of the research to effect change and improve care.

It is interesting to note that concerns about timing are continuing. Cronenwett et al. (2011) recently

recommended that APRN education remain at the master's level and the DNP be awarded only as a post-master's degree. Much commentary occurred because of these recommendations. Malone (2011) agreed, stating that "we (the National League for Nursing) have long held that to exclude nurses from a variety of entry points... is short-sighted" (p. 117). This author would argue that the data are clear that schools cannot continue to educate APRNs at the master's level and be able to keep the program at a reasonable length. As previously stated, the health care system desperately needs nurses with the knowledge of policy, practice management, informatics, and other topics which cannot be included in the current master's curriculum.

Gilliss and Hill (2011) also agreed with Cronenwett et al. (2011) and "look forward to the authors' future thinking" (p. 120). Fontaine and Langston (2011) further supported Cronenwett et al. and presented a doomsday response when they remarked that "the 2015 date has served to confuse the profession and the public, create anxiety in faculty and current master's students and leads to yet another division of the nursing profession" (p. 121). The public does get confused about nursing and its role because there is no clear designation as to which individuals are registered nurses in the clinical setting, but having a deadline for implementation of a practice doctorate does not contribute to that confusion. One could agree that faculty may indeed be anxious, but their greatest concern is the need to squeeze the required content into a master's degree. This discussion then appears to perpetuate the never-ending turmoil within the nursing profession and prevents its leaders from focusing on the more important issues in the health care system.

Instead of embracing change as supported by the IOM, these nursing leaders are insisting on continuing along the same path in which nursing has been trapped for decades. As Benner, Sutphen, Leonard, and Day (2010) discuss in the Carnegie report *Educating Nurses: A Call for Radical Transformation*, the major goal in education should be to "focus on changes in teaching and learning that will unburden overloaded curricula" (p. 8). To accomplish this, they recommend "approaches to teaching and student learning that will best prepare both today's and tomorrow's nurses" (p. 8). Though these authors are speaking mainly about baccalaureate education, these same words can and should be applied to master's education of the APRN and provide the logic for the need to move to the DNP.

Though Cronenwett et al. (2011) present their argument for the DNP as only a post-master's degree, they are expressing the usual nursing clash over innovative ideas. As Dreher (2011) suggests, the argument against the DNP is the same resistance that nursing leaders have presented over the BSN as entry into practice and the master's degree as the level needed for APRN certification (p. 126). In this author's opinion, nursing cannot afford, in light of the IOM recommendations, to drag its feet in implementing this change.

Dreher (2011) suggests that though Cronenwett et al. (2011) support the PhD, they "disdain the need to establish practice doctorates to place the profession in equal status among other practice doctorates, e.g., pharmacy, medicine, dentistry, clinical psychology, podiatry, optometry, physical therapy" (p. 126).

Potempa (2011) adds to the discussion in her assertion that

> Compelling arguments can be made that students and the profession are better served by programs that move baccalaureate graduates seamlessly into DNP programs without a break in their studies. Using this model, students may indeed progress more quickly to the terminal degree and incur fewer educational expenses than students who complete a master's program and then return to school years later to complete a doctorate. (p. 124)

Though the discussions may continue, the evidence is clear that schools of nursing are adopting the DNP at record speed and nurses are flocking to these programs to obtain this degree.

## Effect of the DNP on Nursing Education

Important questions have been raised over the effect of the DNP on nursing education. One such concern is how schools that do not offer doctorates will approach the DNP recommendation. An example of this issue occurs in the state of California where there is a two-tiered classification of higher education—the University of California (UC) system and the California State University (CSU) system. The CSU system by design was not meant to award doctoral degrees because this role was designated for the UC system. There has been extensive discussion about the DNP at the chancellor's level for both systems. The doctoral barrier was previously broken when a bill was passed that allowed a school within the CSU system to award educational doctorates (EdD) (Goulette, 2008, p. 8). This law provided the impetus for allowing the DNP in the CSU. In 2010, Assembly Bill 867 (Nava) California State University: Doctor of Nursing Practice Degree passed the California legislature

and was signed into law. This bill now allows the CSU to offer three pilot DNP programs in the state. What schools will be selected as pilot programs, what will happen to the remaining NP programs which will stay at the master's level, and how the state will actually implement this law in light of its horrific financial problems will be interesting to watch.

Another concern expressed about the effect of the DNP on nursing education relates to the actual content of each DNP program. During the many early discussions (Fulton & Lyon, 2005; Meleis & Dracup, 2005; Milton, 2005), comments were made that there were great differences in program content among DNP programs. One could also argue that there is considerable variance in content in PhD programs, but it should be expected that content in either degree will vary depending on its focus.

The literature has been questioning the DNP since the beginning. Meleis and Dracup (2005) began some of the discussion when they stated that "all doctoral education must be designed to help define, generate, develop, translate and test the substantive base of knowledge in nursing" (para. 12). This statement implies that practice doctorates will not contribute to this knowledge base. Edwardson (2010) agrees, arguing that

> The scholarship (of the DNP) focuses on integration, application, and teaching of knowledge. The scholarship of the DNP graduate may add to the store of generalizable knowledge, but in most cases will be more local and practical in nature than that developed by the PhD-prepared nurse. They will be able to exploit the evidence base to strengthen evidence-based practice. (p. 138)

The DNP Essentials document describes the requirements of DNP student final project, which may focus on "manuscripts submitted for publication, systematic review, research utilization project, practice topic dissemination, substantive involvement in a larger endeavor, or other practice project" (AACN, 2006, p. 20). A review of some outstanding DNP projects found that they met and exceeded these criteria. These projects have been defining, translating, and testing the research. An excellent example is A. Matos-Pagan (personal communication, March 19, 2011), who developed a coalition of nurses who were trained to respond to disasters on the island of Puerto Rico. Her work has continued and is now expanding to other islands in the Caribbean. Examples of other DNP student projects can be found at a website dedicated to the doctor of nursing practice (Doctors of Nursing Practice, 2009–2010).

CONSIDER THIS    Student DNP projects are using research and translating them into positive outcomes in practice.

Nursing should be focusing on what the public needs to improve its health instead of arguing over the necessity of a new degree. In fact, Weisbrod et al. found that some nurse leaders feel that PhDs "may have been too focused on research while neglecting faculty and nonacademic responsibilities" (AANA, 2007, p. 106). It is unclear what is meant by "nonacademic responsibilities," but it might be interpreted as meaning that many PhD nurses do not work in a clinical practice. By not being clinically active, these nurses are teaching students with no real understanding of current practice issues. The initiation of a doctorate that focuses on clinical practice provides a needed balance and should aid in improving the profession and the lives of patients.

There has also been concern that the practice doctorate or DNP will detract from nurses applying to PhD programs. Quite to the contrary, the DNP ensures that the PhD will remain focused on research. As there were no other options, nurses pursued that degree but having both degrees now offers nurses the choice which will best meet their needs. Based on conversations with several directors of DNP programs, nurses, particularly APRNs, had not considered pursuing a doctorate because their only option was research-based PhD degrees. The rapid growth of DNP programs nationwide reflects that nurses would indeed like to obtain doctoral degrees but want them to be relevant to their clinical practice. As suggested by Fitzpatrick and Wallace (2009), "The strength of the Doctor of Nursing Practice movement as we know it today is evidence that the nursing education and professional practice communities were ready for the change" (p. xv).

CONSIDER THIS    Many nurses never pursued doctoral degrees because the PhD degree was their only option.

Some nurse leaders have expressed concern, however, that the DNP will not increase the number of nursing faculty because there are no teaching courses included in the curriculum (Chase & Pruitt, 2006;

Malone, 2011; National League of Nursing, 2007). The AACN (2009), in fact, stated that the DNP graduates, as well as PhD graduates, would need additional education if their intent was to teach at the collegiate level (p. 13). Previously, Chase and Pruitt admitted, "Unfortunately, PhD programs also fail to prepare educators who understand curriculum development and evaluation" (p. 159). Consequently, all persons who wish to be educators need to understand that neither of these nursing doctorates will prepare them to teach at the collegiate level, and they must pursue additional coursework that focuses on teaching. The unfortunate outcome for California since the passing of AB 867 is that the DNP programs must "focus on the preparation of clinical faculty to teach in postsecondary nursing education programs and may also train nurses for advanced nursing practice or nurse leadership, or both" (p. 2). Knowing that teaching is not the focus of the DNP, it will be interesting to see how this part of the law will be implemented.

## Concern That DNP Graduates Who Become Faculty May Not Attain Tenure

Another common concern that arises about DNP graduates is that they may not be able to obtain tenure and equal status with PhDs in academia. The AACN (2009) states on its website,

*Though primarily an institutional decision, AACN is confident that a DNP faculty member will compete favorably with other practice doctorates in tenure and promotion decisions, as is the case in law, education, audiology, physical therapy, pharmacy, criminal justice, public policy and administration, public health, and other disciplines.* (para. 11)

It goes on to say that "AACN data from 2009 show that doctoral students who also teach are just as likely to have a DNP as a PhD. This indicates that graduates of both types of doctoral programs are finding teaching positions" (para. 11).

A small survey of DNP directors by this author found though that there would, in fact, be some challenges for DNP-educated faculty in obtaining tenure. O'Dell (2010), cofounder of Doctors of Nursing Practice, LLC, did state,

*Many colleges of nursing are not offering tenure to DNP-prepared graduates. Some say that tenure should be reserved for researchers that generate new nursing*

*knowledge, and that a DNP does not have the education or even the expectation to produce original scholarly work.* (para. 3)

He not only went on to say that the lack of being offered tenure is creating issues on some campuses but also felt that some universities "are entrenched in very old traditions" (para. 5) and obtaining tenure for DNPs may take some time.

This author, however, did not find any barriers to her appointment as a tenure track faculty and found through a web search that most nursing faculty career opportunities stated that the applicant needed to have a master's in nursing and an undefined doctorate in nursing or related field with some universities actively seeking applicants who have the DNP (HigherEdJobs, 2011a, 2011b).

---

CONSIDER THIS  Resistance to hiring nursing faculty with DNP degrees for tenure track positions in universities may be decreasing.

---

## Do DNP Programs Have the Same Amount of Rigor as Other Doctoral Programs?

Milton (2005), in her classic article on ethics and the DNP, commented that because there is no recommended theory and research in the curriculum, DNP graduates would not be able to make decisions based on evidence and best practices and could not "provide optimal nursing services" (p. 115). She cited Sigma Theta Tau International's (STTI, 2005) statement on evidence-based practice, which discusses having "access to the most recent research" (para. 4). This comment by Milton implied that DNPs cannot understand the need for an evidence-based focus in their practice when, in fact, evidence-based practice is listed third in the DNP Essentials document (AACN, 2006). She then contradicted her own comments and actually provided support for the DNP noting, "The past, present and future are cocreated [sic] a new all-at-once as novel activities and projects in education, research, and practice are offered for advancement and enhancement of the discipline" (p. 155). The AACN-recommended design of all DNP projects is to improve practice and/or provide better patient outcomes (AACN, 2006) that would meet Milton's description of "novel activities and projects." In

addition, the NONPF (2007) released a paper on the criteria for scholarly projects with most programs having written guidelines and requirements of a quality DNP project, which should dispel this apprehension.

One must question whether the concern about rigor should even be part of the discussion because there are distinct differences between research-based and practice-based degrees but both are completed in universities which must meet the standards of the professional accrediting bodies. The notion that DNPs would not be able to make decisions based on evidence is not supported by any data. Edwardson (2010) discusses the concern over rigor between the DNP and PhD but emphasizes that these degrees have different purposes and thus should not include the same content. She states, "The PhD degree has as its express purpose the preparation of scholars to articulate and generate knowledge for the discipline" (p. 137). She further suggests,

*The purpose of the DNP, on the other hand, is to prepare practitioners to take the knowledge created by researchers and theoretical scholars and use it in the delivery of services and advancement of policies that support high-quality health care. This is not to say that the DNP-prepared nurse does not engage in scholarship. Rather, the scholarship focuses on integration, application, and teaching of knowledge. The scholarship of the DNP graduate may add to the store of generalizable knowledge, but in most cases will be more local and practical in nature than that developed by the PhD-prepared nurse. They will be able to exploit the evidence base to strengthen evidence-based practice.* (p. 138)

---

CONSIDER THIS  DNP graduates base their practice on the latest evidence as defined in the third item of the DNP Essentials document.

---

In addition, the Commission on Collegiate Nursing Education (CCNE), the independent accrediting agency for the AACN, released a press report stating, "In a move consistent with other health professions,…[CCNE] has decided that only practice doctoral degrees with the Doctor of Nursing Practice (DNP) title will be eligible for CCNE accreditation" (AACN, 2005a, para. 1). This support by the CCNE reinforces that these programs do indeed meet the rigor of any doctoral degree.

Finally, with the development of the DNP Essentials, the AACN (2006) laid the groundwork for a strong and rigorous curricular model. The suggestion that the PhD is the only worthwhile doctoral program and that the DNP could not be as rigorous or as valuable to the profession is discourteous to the many outstanding institutions that have initiated DNP programs. Edwardson (2010) supports this belief when she states, "This is a real concern only if schools of nursing fail to insist on comparable rigor in the two programs" (p. 138) and suggests that "DNP preparation will deliberately prepare clinicians who base their practices in quality evidence and fill an important gap in practice such as being the principal providers of primary care" (p. 138).

## Concern That the DNP Curriculum Does not Include Theory

When the discussion on the DNP began, Whall (2005) and Milton (2005) questioned the lack of theory in DNP programs. Algase (2010) in her recent editorial supports this premise. She goes so far as to suggest that theory must be part of DNP education; otherwise DNPs will be "less equipped than those with research-focused doctorates" (p. 93). While these authors imply that DNP graduates have lesser knowledge, they miss the point that theories are often integrated throughout a curriculum depending on the particular course and topic. The fact that these theories may not be nursing theories may be an issue for some, but nursing in the 21st century does not practice in a vacuum. The profession must consider that nurses are working as part of an interdisciplinary team and need to understand many types of theories. The inability to understand nonnursing theories has been one of the major barriers to nurses effecting significant change. In addition, because the BSN curriculum includes courses that discuss a number of theories, professional nurses have the needed theoretical background.

Business, leadership, and organizational theories, not just nursing theories, are crucial for nurse leaders working to transform the health care system, making acquisition of this knowledge vital for the DNP. Leaders require knowledge of all conceptual theories if they are to be successful in their attempts at change.

> CONSIDER THIS The nursing profession must understand theories from all disciplines if it is to effect change in the health care system.

## Recent Developments

Some recent, very disconcerting developments have occurred regarding the DNP. In June 2008, at the American Medical Association (AMA) House of Delegates (HOD) meeting, physicians passed two resolutions about the DNP: "Citing patient safety concerns, members of the AMA House of Delegates protested the unregulated expansion of doctors of nursing practice and urged organized medicine to ensure transparency on and supervision of their role in medical care" (Sorrel, 2008, p. 25). Although this resolution is only a policy statement and not legally binding, it does demonstrate a continued effort by medicine to attempt to control nursing. It is not in the purview of physicians to dictate the role of nursing and its right to practice. Medicine frequently comments about patient safety issues but in this situation has no evidence to support its position. A review of the 1999 IOM report should remind physicians that they have more issues surrounding patient safety than do APRNs.

Another resolution, number 214, was also passed and states, "RESOLVED, That our AMA adopt policy that Doctors of Nursing Practice must practice as part of a medical team under the supervision of a licensed physician who has final authority and responsibility for the patient" (Sorrel, 2008, p. 19). Many nursing organizations submitted comments or testified against this resolution to no avail.

A more recent document was published in 2009 by the American College of Physicians (ACP, 2009). In this document, the ACP takes the position that physicians are the "most appropriate health care professionals for many patients" (p. 1). It further suggests that the reason nursing decided to move to the DNP was "to improve the quality of NP education" (p. 5). There has never been a question about the quality of NP education. One of the main reasons programs are moving to the doctoral level is to finally award a degree that reflects the number of units taken by students. As stated in the AACN (2004) position statement on the practice doctorate in nursing,

> *The growing complexity of health care, burgeoning growth in scientific knowledge, and increasing sophistication of technology have necessitated master's degree programs that prepare APNs to expand the number of didactic and clinical clock hours far beyond the requirements of master's education in virtually any other field.* (para. 22)

It further states,

> *In response to changes in health care delivery and emerging health care needs, additional knowledge or*

*content areas have been identified by practicing nurses. In addition, the knowledge required to provide leadership in the discipline of nursing is so complex and rapidly changing that additional or doctoral level education is needed.* (para. 23)

The ACP (2009) also states that the education of physicians and NPs are not equivalent and feels that NPs cannot function in the same capacity as physicians because physicians have so much more education than NPs. The document states,

*Training of physicians involves 50 years of premedical college education, 50 years of medical school that includes 50 years of clinical rotations, 50 years or more of clinical residency training with up to 80-hour workweeks, additional fellowship subspecialty training, and continuing medical education.* (p. 9)

This statement notes that NPs do not spend an equivalent amount of time in their education and suggests they cannot function at the expected level needed for their chosen area of practice. NPs do, however, spend 4 years in the baccalaureate nursing education, and 2 to 3 additional years obtaining a master's degree while typically working as a registered nurse and gaining needed clinical experience. The question must be asked whether NPs need 13 years of education and advanced clinical training to perform the role.

Most NPs programs require at least 1 year of clinical experience as a registered nurse before applying to the NP program and candidates must have received a bachelor's degree in nursing. In this author's experience as an NP program coordinator, most NP students have 5 to 50 years of experience as a nurse. In the end, it is not unusual for an NP to have 7 to 9 or more years of collegiate education and many more years practicing as a registered nurse before taking on the APRN role.

At the same time, there has never been the suggestion that NPs and physicians practice the same but it also does not mean that one practices better or more safely than the other. Physicians practice from a medical model while nursing practices from the nursing model. The main difference between these models is that nurses emphasize health promotion and disease prevention—a key component of NP practice and one that many patients value. It is interesting to note that in recent years medical schools are now talking about the importance of health promotion and disease prevention, partially in response to the quality and safety movement.

The ACP (2009) document does encourage collaboration. As stated in the IOM report, *Health Professions Education: A Bridge to Quality* (2003), health care professionals "work in interdisciplinary teams—cooperate, collaborate, communicate and integrate care in teams to ensure that care is continuous and reliable" (p. 45). NPs have always advocated that all health care providers, including physicians, NPs, physical therapists, pharmacists, and respiratory therapists among others, work together to provide the highest quality of care, but it does not mean that the physician is or should be the lead/main provider.

It is unfortunate that many physicians continue to believe that the health care system is a pyramid and that they are at the pinnacle with the right to direct all other health care professionals. Physicians have no legal right to attempt to regulate advanced practice registered nurses or to state that NPs must function under the direct supervision of a physician. Boards of nursing are the legal bodies that regulate nursing and monitor its practice. State nurse practice acts clarify the role and function of a nurse. One can only imagine the backlash if nursing tried to tell physicians how to practice. Unfortunately, the medical community seems determined to continue its long history of trying to defend what it believes is its turf.

> **CONSIDER THIS** The medical community has no legal right to attempt to regulate advanced practice registered nurses or to state that they must function under the direct supervision of a physician.

The goal instead should be to work in collaboration and as a team, given that all health care professionals make significant contributions to the health of the patient. One would think that the medical profession would focus on the more important issue of providing safe and high-quality care instead of wasting time and energy trying to regulate other providers who have extensive documentation of their worth. Any concern over the quality of care provided by NPs has been eliminated in multiple studies. The most recent one by Newhouse et al. (2011) reviewed the literature from 1990 to 2008 on care provided by APRNs in comparison with physician care.

*The results indicate APRNs provide effective and high-quality patient care, have an important role in improving quality of patient care in the United States, and could help to address the concerns about whether care provided by APRNs can safely augment the physician supply to support reform efforts aimed at expanding access to care.* (p. 1)

Another recent development was the AMA resolution (Sorrel, 2008), which called for limitations on the use of the term *doctor* and suggested that it be restricted to physicians, dentists, and podiatrists. After much discussion, however, the terminology was changed to say that all professionals must clearly identify their qualifications and credentials to patients. A floor amendment was approved that AMA will support legislation to "make it a felony for non-physician health care professionals to misrepresent themselves as physicians" (Sorrel, 2008, p. 25).

Why some physicians believed it was necessary to make such an amendment is unclear, given that it has always been illegal to misrepresent oneself as a licensed health care professional. Unfortunately, the ACP (2009) also felt compelled to discuss this issue in its monograph and suggests that the use of the term "doctor" by NPs could lead to confusion by the public. Patients are highly informed today and are more than capable of distinguishing among the many health care providers. It is unclear why physicians have such great concern about NPs with doctorates when so many health care providers today also have doctoral degrees. Most NPs clearly emphasize to their patients that they are nurse practitioners and not physicians.

Nursing must continue to be vigilant about these attempts to encroach on its right to practice. The IOM (2011) is recommending that all levels of nursing should be allowed and encouraged to perform to the full scope of their practice. Nurses must be strong advocates for the profession by joining and being actively involved in professional associations that focus on monitoring practice issues and voting for legislators who will support the role. Legislators must be kept informed of nursing practice and its meaning and provide documentation of its outstanding patient outcomes. Nursing must define nursing before others take away the freedom to practice.

*needs of society, this is not just a matter of increasing the volume of the nursing workforce. The nursing profession must produce quality graduates who:*

- *Are prepared for clinical leadership in all health care settings;*
- *Are prepared to implement outcomes-based practice and quality improvement strategies;*
- *Will remain in and contribute to the profession, practicing at their full scope of education and ability; and*
- *Will create and manage microsystems of care that will be responsive to the health care needs of individuals and families. (Batalden et al., as cited in AACN, 2007)*

The document states that

*. . . unless nursing is able to create a professional role that will attract the highest-quality women and men into nursing, it will not be able to fulfill its covenant with the public. The CNL addresses this call for change.* (AACN, 2007, p. 5)

The many advances in science and technology over the last century have put increased pressure on nursing education to produce graduates who have the educational preparation and expertise to meet the challenges in health care in the 21st century. This effort must occur through collaboration of education and practice. For too many years, nursing education has functioned somewhat in a vacuum without input from the practice setting as to its needs. "Change cannot occur in isolation. Nursing education must collaborate and work in tandem with the health care delivery system to design and test models for education and practice that are truly client-centered, generate quality outcomes and are cost-effective" (AACN, 2007, p. 6).

---

CONSIDER THIS   Nursing must continue to be vigilant about these attempts to encroach on its right to practice.

---

CONSIDER THIS   Nursing education must collaborate and work in tandem with the health care delivery system to design and test models for education and practice that are truly client centered, generate quality outcomes, and are cost-effective.

---

## THE CLINICAL NURSE LEADER

The AACN (2007) released its original white paper on the CNL with the following critical statement:

*While there is ample evidence for the need to produce many more nurses to meet the pressing health care*

According to Tornabeni and Miller (2008), "Central and key to the process of developing this role had been a commitment to engage multiple stakeholders in the process" (p. 609). Tornabeni and Miller reported on a task force that monitored the implementation of pilot projects in which schools of nursing joined with practice partners to initiate the CNL role (p. 609). The projects were able to demonstrate that just adding a CNL did not effect the changes anticipated: "Practice sites needed to redesign their patient care delivery models to center the care around the expertise the CNL would bring to patient care" (p. 609). It was also decided that the "skills and competencies required in this role" (p. 610) necessitated recommending that the CNL be educated through a master's degree curriculum.

"The CNL is a leader in the health care delivery system across all settings… functions within a microsystem and assumes accountability for healthcare outcomes for a specific group of clients" (AACN, 2007, p. 6). In addition, the CNL applies the best evidence to practice and provides or manages at the point of care. He or she designs, implements, and evaluates care by coordinating, delegating, and supervising the care provided by the health care team (p. 6).

Porter-O'Grady, Clark, and Wiggins (2010) make the important point,

> As medical care and clinical services have bcome more complex, narrowly defined, and increasingly technologically based, the requisites for specialization, depth of knowledge, and advancing clinical competence have created both the requisite for highly skilled practice and increasing dependence on the centrality of the nurse's role in correlating, integrating, and facilitating the continuum of care. (p. 38)

In developing this new role for nursing, the AACN (2007) made 10 assumptions for preparation of the CNL. These assumptions are shown in Box 22.2 and can be viewed on the AACN website. At first glance, these assumptions seem intuitive to nursing practice, but unfortunately not all are being integrated into the practice of each individual nurse. By making these declarative statements, the AACN is helping to clarify the role of the CNL.

A key area of focus of the CNL is integrating the care of all health care providers. As Tornabeni and Miller (2008) noted, "The goal is to develop strong communication between health professionals through patient-centered care and to create synergy, collaboration, and value for the contributions each discipline brings to patient care" (pp. 610–611).

It is expected that the CNL will

1. provide and manage care, including the delegation of tasks and supervision and evaluation of personnel and care outcomes

2. critically evaluate and anticipate risks to client safety

3. profile patterns of need and tailor interventions using an evidence-based approach

4. advocate for clients and community and assume accountability for delivery of high-quality care

5. assume the role of educator

---

## BOX 22.2   ASSUMPTIONS FOR PREPARING CLINICAL NURSE LEADERS

1. Practice is at a microsystems level.
2. Client care outcomes are the measure of quality practice.
3. Practice guidelines are based on evidence.
4. Client-centered practice is intra- and interdisciplinary.
5. Information will maximize self-care and client decision making.
6. Nursing assessment is the basis for theory and knowledge development.
7. Good fiscal stewardship is a condition of quality care.
8. Social justice is an essential nursing value.
9. Communication technology will facilitate the continuity and comprehensiveness of care.
10. The clinical nurse leader must assume guardianship for the nursing profession.

*Source:* American Association of Colleges of Nursing. (2007). *White paper on the education and role of the clinical nurse leader.* Retrieved from http://www.aacn.nche.edu/Publications/WhitePapers/ClinicalNurse-Leader07.pdf

6. be responsible for the provision and management of care in and across all environments

7. be a member and leader of the health care team (AACN, 2007, pp. 11–12).

The AACN finalized its vision of the CNL by recommending core competencies and a framework of the potential curriculum. Porter-O'Grady et al. (2010) state,

> *The coursework provides theoretical and clinical experiences that result in competencies that prepare the CNL to be a strong leader and clinician in today's healthcare setting. Skills and competencies include systems thinking, risk analysis, techniques in quality improvement at the micro- and mesosystem level, use of evidence-based practices, and the ability to laterally integrate care over the healthcare continuum for vulnerable and complex patients.* (p. 39)

The CNL role is being accepted across the country with positive outcomes. As of February 2011, there were more than 2,000 nurses certified as a CNL (AACN, 2012b) with more than 100 schools offering the CNL curriculum (AACN, 2012c).

Unfortunately, controversy usually accompanies any innovation and change. The clinical nurse specialists believe that the CNL functions in a manner similar to their practice. The NACNS declared that the "educational level of the CNL has been increased to a master's level preparation creating even further overlap with the competencies of the CNS" (NACNS, 2005, para. 2). The position statement further stated that "the similarity in the described roles, the resulting role confusion, and issues regarding a clear use of educational and institutional resources for duplicative efforts at a time when resources are scarce" (NACNS, 2005, para. 6) continues to be a concern.

---

### DISCUSSION POINT

Does the CNL role overlap with the role of the CNS?

---

The CNS concern revolved around their belief that the CNL and CNS have overlapping roles and competencies. The NACNS questioned how, in light of limited resources, this role could be added when CNSs, case managers, and nurse managers already function in parallel roles: "We believe that the roles that can accomplish

the bridging of the chasm already exist in the system" (NACNS, 2005, para. 8), and they requested that the nursing profession continue to "support CNS education and practice" (para. 8). As there is no information to be found on the NACNS website since these papers were published more than 6 years ago, it must be presumed that the association has given up its protest against the CNL.

Support for the CNS role is actually coming from nurses who have become CNLs: "The CNL is a master's prepared advanced generalist nurse. This differs from, but compliments, the role of the clinical nurse specialist (CNS), who is a master's prepared APN with a specialty focus" (Poulin-Tabor et al., 2008, p. 624). An example of the collaboration and interdisciplinary approach of the clinical nurse leader is the following:

> *I consulted the diabetic clinical nurse specialist as well as the heart failure CNS for the best approach for in-hospital and outpatient goals for this patient. As a result of working with the patient, physician assistants, doctors, social worker, dietician and clinical nurse specialists... the patient was discharged safely home without readmission.* (Poulin-Tabor et al., 2008, p. 627)

Although the concern of the NACNS can be appreciated, the CNL is definitely providing a new approach and focus. As the NACNS states in its documents, the clinical nurse specialist helps to improve nursing practice, but the CNL is patient focused, providing care across the care continuum. Patients are followed prior to hospital admission, during their stay, and after discharge. Although it is agreed that case managers work in a similar fashion, the point of the CNL role is that *all* patients receive this special attention, not just ones with certain diagnosis.

Sherman, Clark, and Maloney (2008) made specific note that "what surfaced in the discussion was the need for a consistent figure to act as a point person for staff, physicians, patients, and families" (p. 56). Poulin-Tabor et al. (2008) stated, "We focus on the patients as a whole rather than as a sum of their parts. As this has not been the traditional approach in medicine, it has been a noticeable difference to the patients and families that we touch" (p. 628).

---

CONSIDER THIS    The CNL acts as a point person for staff, physicians, patients, and families.

Too many stories have been told by patients and their families about the disorganization of and lack of caring by health care professionals. Sitting for an hour after the scheduled time for an outpatient procedure is unfortunately the norm. Discharges get delayed because no planning occurred. Cancellation of procedures wastes staff time and ties up operating/procedure rooms unnecessarily. The cost savings to the health care delivery system can be seen within months of initiating the CNL role. Although there is the added expense of the CNL salary and benefits, the overall cost savings can be significant (Harris & Ott, 2008). Harris and Ott (2008) further suggest that it is necessary to "move nursing practice from process to synthesis, from enumerating function to delineating value, from focus on the action of work to the product of that work, from the emphasis on effort to the determination of value" (p. 38).

However, before the CNL is employed, the rationale for hiring someone for this role should be made clear. Specific objectives that clarify the expected outcomes should be written. Reasons for and against the initiation of the CNL, as well as the probable costs and benefits, should be identified. Finally, alternatives and consequences should be assessed. All stakeholders need to be aware of "the possibilities to address any issue(s) and any future opportunities" (Harris & Ott, 2008, p. 27).

Porter-O'Grady et al. (2010) suggest that it is:

> . . . up to the CNO to serve as the leader in crafting the landscape and translating it to other stakeholders, creating an environment that allows the CNL to lead in that change and advance the nursing role for 21st century practice. (p. 41)

Indeed, nursing at the veteran affairs (VA) is being transformed through the use of the CNL. The Office of Nursing Services (ONS, 2011) awarded 15 innovation awards to CNL groups across the country in 2011 related to the theme of Strategies for Implementing and Sustaining the Clinical Nurse leader (CNL) Role. Most VA medical centers have implemented the role. Kennedy (2011), editor-in-chief of the *American Journal of Nursing,* reported that other health systems are looking at the CNL role and made the point that a recruiter from a Texas hospital system intended to hire more than 50 CNLs in the coming year (para. 5).

The nurses who are functioning as CNLs best state the case for the role:

> *We humanize and personalize the health care experience and in doing this, have rediscovered the art of nursing. . . . We believe that the role of the CNL will be instrumental as a coordinator and change agent to meet not only the demands of today but to anticipate the demands of tomorrow.* (Poulin-Tabor et al., 2008, p. 628)

The role of the CNL will continue to be assessed in the coming years, but it appears that these nurses are making a difference in the lives of their patients. As stated by Harris (2009), "The journey for CNLs has begun and is a promising dimension of health care quality and performance as care is coordinated and less fragmented" (p. 118). Documentation of CNL outcomes is provided in Research Study Fuels the Controversy 22.1.

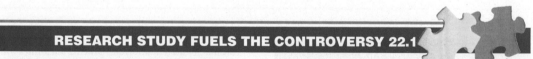

## RESEARCH STUDY FUELS THE CONTROVERSY 22.1

### EFFECT OF THE CLINICAL NURSE LEADER

Two case studies were discussed that examined the role of the clinical nurse leader (CNL) and its effect on improving quality and patient safety. One study focused on quality of care by assessing rates of patient falls, the percentage of patients who reported that their pain had been well managed, and the percentage of patients who reported "excellent" to the nurse response to calls and overall care. A final area of evaluation looked at length of stay.

Stanley, J. M., et al. (2008). The clinical nurse leader: A catalyst for improving quality and patient safety. *Journal of Nursing Management, 16,* 614–622.

### STUDY FINDINGS

Pain management satisfaction went from 82% prior to the residency by the CNL student to 96% during her time on site. This rate fell to baseline rates after her departure (p. 617). Satisfaction with care and response to calls rose from 87% and 58%, respectively, to 99% and 96% (p. 617). Fall rates and injury due to those falls more than doubled during the student CNL's clinical experience: "One reason, supported by the student's journal

*continued*

entries, is that in the process of frequent rounding, patients were found to have fallen" (p. 618).

The other study had some difficulty in assessing the true effect of the implementation of the CNL because data collection was poor prior to initiation of the role. Since that time, "the unit reports no nosocomial pressure ulcer development, 100%

compliance with pneumonia and flu vaccine administration, and the implementation of heart failure patient education and smoking cessation counseling" (p. 618). It was also found that the length of stay decreased by almost 1 day on the oncology unit.

## CONCLUSIONS

The controversy over the clinical practice doctorate will probably continue for many years, but advanced practice registered nursing must consider what level of education is needed to adequately care for patients in today's health care system. Of equal importance is that individual APRNs must learn from the lessons of the past and develop the skills needed to survive as a vital constituent of the health care system in the 21st century. The movement to the DNP is a crucial part of that process.

In addition, the CNL role provides exciting new opportunities for nursing and the health care system. As the number of nurses with this specialty increases, the public will become more aware of the positive outcomes these individuals bring to their care. There is little doubt that advanced practice nursing makes valuable contributions to the health care system. Doctors of nursing practice and clinical nurse leaders will have a significant impact on the health care of tomorrow.

## FOR ADDITIONAL DISCUSSION

1. Can the public appropriately distinguish between the many doctoral degrees offered by universities?

2. Will offering the DNP decrease the number of PhD candidates?

3. Is it necessary for DNP graduates to have coursework in nursing theory?

4. Should the medical profession be allowed to dictate the scope of practice for DNPs or other nurses?

5. Does the CNL function differently than a CNS

## REFERENCES

Algase, D. (2010). Essentials of scholarship for the DNP: Are we clear yet? [Editorial]. *Research and Theory for Nursing Practice: An International Journal, 24*(2), 91–93.

All Nursing Schools. (2011). *Certified nurse anesthetist (CRNA) career overview.* Retrieved from http://www.allnursingschools.com/nursing-careers/nurse-anesthetist/registered-nurse-anesthetist

American Association of Colleges of Nursing. (2004). *Position statement of the practice doctorate in nursing.* Retrieved from http://www.aacn.nche.edu/DNP/pdf/DNP.pdf

American Association of Colleges of Nursing. (2005a). *Commission on collegiate nursing education moves to* consider *for accreditation only practice doctorates with the DNP degree title.* Retrieved from http://www.aacn.nche.edu/news/articles/2005/commission-on-collegiate-nursing-education-moves-to-consider-for-accreditation-only-practice-doctorates-with-the-dnp-degree-title

American Association of Colleges of Nursing. (2005b). *Faculty shortages in baccalaureate and graduate nursing programs: Scope of the problem and strategies for expanding the supply.* Retrieved from http://www.aacn.nche.edu/publications/whitepapers/faculty-shortages.htm

American Association of Colleges of Nursing. (2006). *The essentials for doctoral education for advanced practice nursing.* Retrieved from http://www.aacn.nche.edu/DNP/pdf/Essentials.pdf

American Association of Colleges of Nursing. (2007). *White paper on the role of the clinical nurse leader.* Retrieved from http://www.aacn.nche.edu/publications/white-papers/cnl

American Association of Colleges of Nursing. (2008). *The essentials of baccalaureate education for professional nursing practice.* Retrieved from http://www.aacn.nche.edu/education/pdf/BaccEssentials08.pdf

American Association of Colleges of Nursing. (2009). *Frequently asked questions: AACN position statement on the practice doctorate in nursing.* Washington, DC: Author. Retrieved from http://www.aacn.nche.edu/DNP/DNPFAQ.htm

American Association of Colleges of Nursing. (2010). *Your nursing career: A look at the facts.* Washington, DC: Author. Retrieved from http://www.aacn.nche.edu/students/your-nursing-career/facts

American Association of Colleges of Nursing. (2012c). *CNL programs.* Retrieved from http://www.aacn.nche.edu/cnl/about/cnl-programs

American Association of Colleges of Nursing. (2012b). *CNL directory.* Retrieved from http://www.aacn.nche.edu/cnl/cnl-connect

American Association of Colleges of Nursing. (2012a). *Doctor of Nursing Practice (DNP) programs.* Washington, DC: Author. Retrieved from https://www.aacn.nche.edu/dnp/program-schools

American Association of Nurse Anesthetists. (2007). *Report of AANA task force on doctoral preparation of nurse anesthetists.* Park Ridge, IL: Author.

American Association of Nurse Anesthetists. (2011). *Qualifications and capabilities of the certified nurse anesthetist.* Retrieved from http://www.aana.com/ceandeducation/becomeacrna/Pages/Qualifications-and-Capabilities-of-the-Certified-Registered-Nurse-Anesthetist-.aspx

American College of Nurse-Midwives. (2009a). *Mandatory degree requirements for entry into midwifery practice.* Retrieved from http://www.midwife.org/ACNM/files/ACNMLibraryData/UPLOADFILENAME/000000000076/Mandatory_Degree_Req_for_Entry_Midwifery_Practice_7_09.pdf

American College of Nurse-Midwives. (2009b). *Midwifery education and the doctor of nursing practice (DNP).* Retrieved from http://www.midwife.org/ACNM/files/ACNMLibraryData/UPLOADFILENAME/000000000079/Midwifery%20Ed%20and%20DNP%207.09.pdf

American College of Nurse-Midwives. (2010a). *Our credentials.* Retrieved from http://www.midwife.org/Our-Credentials

American College of Nurse-Midwives. (2010b). *Our scope of practice.* Retrieved from http://www.midwife.org/Our-Scope-of-Practice

American College of Nurse Practitioners. (n.d.). *What is a nurse practitioner?* Retrieved from http://www.acnpweb.org/files/public/What_is_a_Nurse_Practitioner.pdf

American College of Physicians. (2009). *Nurse practitioners in primary care* [Policy monograph]. Philadelphia, PA: Author.

American Hospital Association Commission on Workforce for Hospitals and Health Systems. (2002). *In our hands, how hospital leaders can build a thriving workforce.* Chicago, IL: Author. Retrieved from http://www.aha.org/advocacy-issues/workforce/inourhands2001.shtml

American Nurses Association. (2010). *Position statement. The doctor of nursing practice: Advancing the nursing profession.* Retrieved from http://www.doctorsofnursingpractice.org/cmsAdmin/uploads/ANA_Position_Statement_on_DNP_as_a_Terminal_Degree_6_14_2010.pdf

Benner, P., Sutphen, M., Leonard, V., & Day, L. (2010). *Educating nurses: A call for radical transformation* (The Carnegie Foundation for the Advancement of Teaching). San Francisco, CA: Jossey-Bass.

Bureau of Labor Statistics. (2010). *Occupational employment and wages, May 2010.* Retrieved from http://www.bls.gov/oes/current/oes291111.htm

Case Western Reserve University. (2010a). *History of the DNP at FPB.* Retrieved from http://fpb.case.edu/DNP/history.shtm

Case Western Reserve University. (2010b). *Pathways to the DNP.* Retrieved from http://fpb.case.edu/GradEntry/pathways.shtm#dnp

Chase, S. K., & Pruitt, R. H. (2006). *The practice doctorate: Innovation or disruption?* Retrieved from http://www.doctorsofnursingpractice.org/cmsAdmin/uploads/Chase2006.pdf

Cronenwett, L., Dracup, K., Grey, M., McCauley, L., Meleis, A., & Salmon, M. (2011). The doctor of nursing practice: A national workforce perspective. *Nursing Outlook, 59*(3), 9–17. doi:10.1016/j.outlook.2010.11.003

Doctors of Nursing Practice. (2009–2010). DNP *scholarly projects: Archived and searchable.* Retrieved from http://www.doctorsofnursingpractice.org/studentprojects.php

Dreher, M. (2011). The doctor of nursing practice: A national workforce perspective—A response. *Nursing Outlook, 59*(3), 126–127. doi:10.1016/j.outlook.2011.03.013

Edwardson, S. (2010). Doctor of philosophy and doctor of nursing practice as complementary degrees. *Journal of Professional Nursing, 26*(3), 137–140. doi:0.1016/j.profnurs.2009.08.004

Fitzpatrick, J., & Wallace, M. (2009). *The doctor of nursing practice and clinical nurse leader: Essentials of program development and implementation for clinical practice.* New York, NY: Springer.

Fontaine, D., & Langston, N. (2011). The master's is not broken: Commentary on *The Doctor of Nursing Practice: A Workforce Perspective. Nursing Outlook, 59*(3), 121–122. doi:10.1016/j.outlook.2011.03.003

Fulton, J., & Lyon, B. (2005). The need for some sense making: Doctor of nursing practice. *Online Journal of Issues in Nursing, 10*(3). Retrieved from http://nursingworld.org/MainMenuCategories/ANAMarketplace/ANAPeriodicals/OJIN/TableofContents/Volume102005/No3Sept05/tpc28_316027.html

Gilliss, C., & Hill, M. (2011). Commentary: The doctor of nursing practice: A national workforce perspective. *Nursing Outlook, 59*(3), 119–120. doi:10.1016/j.outlook.2011.03.014

Goulette, C. (2008). *A look at current state legislation and government-related issues: Doctor nurse.* Retrieved from http://nursing.advanceweb.com/Article/From-the-Hill-4.aspx

Harris, J. L. (2009). Clinical nurse leader (CNL) experiences. In J. J. Fitzpatrick & M. Wallace (Eds.), *The doctor of nursing practice and clinical nurse leader* (pp. 107–118). New York, NY: Springer.

Harris, J. L., & Ott, K. (2008). Building the business case for the clinical nurse leader role. *Nurse Leader, 6*(4), 25–28, 37.

Hawkins, R., & Nezat, G. (2009). *Doctoral education: Which degree to pursue.* Retrieved from http://www.doctorsofnursingpractice.org/cmsAdmin/uploads/Hawkins2009.pdf

HigherEdJobs. (2011a). *Faculty Doctor of Nursing Practice.* Retrieved from http://www.higheredjobs.com/faculty/details.cfm?JobCode=175319154

HigherEdJobs. (2011b). *Faculty–nursing–Dallas.* Retrieved from http://www.higheredjobs.com/faculty/details.cfm?JobCode=175527811&Title=Faculty%20-%20Nursing%20-%20Dallas%20-%20 11NU02

Institute of Medicine of the National Academies. (1999). *To err is human: Building a safer health system.* Washington, DC: National Academies Press.

Institute of Medicine of the National Academies. (2001). *Crossing the quality chasm.* Washington, DC: National Academies Press.

Institute of Medicine of the National Academies. (2011). *The future of nursing: Leading change, advancing health.* Washington, DC: National Academies Press.

Joint Commission on Accreditation of Healthcare Organizations. (2002). *Health care at the crossroads: Strategies for addressing the evolving nursing crisis.* Chicago, IL: Author. Retrieved from http://www.jointcommission.org/assets/1/18/health_care_at_the_crossroads.pdf

Kennedy, M. (2011). True believers at the 2011 clinical nurse leader summit. *American Journal of Nursing, 5*(16). Retrieved from http://ajnoffthecharts.com/2011/01/26/true-believers-at-the-2011-clinical-nurse-leader-summit/

Kimball, B., & O'Neill, E. (2002). *Health care's human crisis: The American nursing shortage.* Princeton, NJ: The Robert Wood Johnson Foundation. Retrieved from http://www.rwjf.org/files/publications/other/NursingReport.pdf

Malone, B. (2011). Commentary on *The Doctor of Nursing Practice: A National Workforce Perspective. Nursing Outlook, 59*(3), 117–118. doi:10.1016/j.outlook.2011.03.002

Meleis, A. I., & Dracup, K. (2005). The case against the DNP: History, timing, substance, and marginalization. *Online Journal of Issues in Nursing, 10*(3). Retrieved from http://www.nursingworld.org/MainMenuCategories/ANAMarketplace/ANAPeriodicals/OJIN/TableofContents/Volume102005/No3Sept05/tpc28_216026.aspx

Milton, C. L. (2005). Scholarship in nursing: Ethics of a practice doctorate. *Nursing Science Quarterly, 18*(2), 113–116.

National Association of Clinical Nurse Specialists. (2005). *NACNS Update on the Clinical Nurse Leader (CNL).* Retrieved from http://www.nacns.org/docs/PositionOnCNL.pdf

National Association of Clinical Nurse Specialists. (n.d.). *What is a clinical nurse specialist?* Retrieved from http://www.nacns.org/html/cns-faqs1.php

National Association of Clinical Nurse Specialists. (2009). *Position statement on the nursing practice doctorate.* Retrieved from http://www.nacns.org/docs/PositionOnNursingPracticeDoctorate.pdf

National League of Nursing. (2007). *Reflections and dialogue: Doctor of nursing practice (DNP).* Retrieved from http://www.nln.org/aboutnln/reflection_dialogue/refl_dial_1.htm

National Organization of Nurse Practitioner Faculties. (2007). *NONPF recommended criteria for NP scholarly projects in the practice doctorate program.*

Retrieved from http://www.nonpf.com/associations/10789/files/ScholarlyProjectCriteria.pdf

National Organization of Nurse Practitioner Faculties. (2011). *Nurse practitioner core competencies.* Retrieved from http://www.nonpf.com/associations/10789/files/IntegratedNPCoreCompsFINAL-April2011.pdf

National Research Council. (2005). *Advancing the nation's health needs: NIH research training programs.* Retrieved from http://books.nap.edu/openbook.php?record_id=11275&page=74

National Science Foundation. (2010). *Number of doctorates awarded continue to grow in 2009.* Retrieved from http://www.nsf.gov/statistics/infbrief/nsf11305/

Newhouse, R., Stanik-Hutt, J., White, K., Johantgen, M., Bass, E., Zangaro, G.,... Weiner, J. (2011). *Advance practice nurse outcomes 1990–2008: A systematic review.* Advance online publication. Retrieved from https://www.nursingeconomics.net/ce/2013/article3001021.pdf

Office of Nursing Services. (2011). *2010 Award winners.* Retrieved from http://www.va.gov/NURSING/nationalawards.asp

O'Dell, D. (2010). *DNP answers: Tenure for DNP graduates* (Web log comment). Retrieved from http://community.advanceweb.com/blogs/np_7/archive/2010/06/26/tenure-for-dnp-graduates.aspx

Porter-O'Grady, T., Clark, J., & Wiggins, M. (2010). The case for clinical nurse leaders: Guiding nursing practice into the 21st century. *Nurse Leader, 8*(1), 37–41. doi:10.1016/j.mnl.2009.11.002

Potempa, K. (2011). The DNP serves the public good. *Nursing Outlook, 59*(3), 123–125. doi:10.1016/j.outlook.2011.03.001

Poulin-Tabor, D., Quirk, R. L., Wilson, L., Orff, S., Gallant, P., Swan, N., & Manchester, N. (2008). Pioneering a new role: The beginning, current practice and future of the clinical nurse leader. *Journal of Nursing Management, 16,* 623–628.

Pronsati, M., & Gerchufsky, M. (2011). National salary report 2010. *Advance for NPs & PAs.* Retrieved from http://nurse-practitioners-and-physician-assistants.advanceweb.com/Features/Articles/National-Salary-Report-2010.aspx

Sherman, R., Clark, J. S., & Maloney, J. (2008). Developing the clinical nurse leader role in the twelve bed hospital model: An education/service partnership. *Nurse Leader, 6*(3), 54–58.

Sigma Theta Tau International. (2005). *Evidenced based nursing position statement.* Retrieved from http://www.nursingsociety.org/aboutus/PositionPapers/Pages/EBN_positionpaper.aspx

Sorrel, A. L. (2008). *Physicians demand greater oversight of doctors of nursing.* Retrieved from http://www.ama-assn.org/amednews/2008/07/07/prsd0707.htm

Stanley, J. M., Gannon, J., Gabuat, J., Hartranft, S., Adams, N., Mayes, C.,... Burch, D. (2008). The clinical nurse leader: A catalyst for improving quality and patient safety. *Journal of Nursing Management, 16*(5), 614–622.

Tornabeni, J., & Miller, J. F. (2008). The power of partnership to shape the future of nursing: The evolution of the clinical nurse leader. *Journal of Nursing Management, 16*(5), 608–613.

U.S. Department of Health and Human Services, Health Resources and Services Administration. (2010). *The registered nurse population: Initial findings from the 2008 National Sample Survey of Registered Nurses.* Retrieved from http://bhpr.hrsa.gov/healthworkforce/rnsurveys/rnsurveyinitial2008.pdf

Whall, A. (2005). "Lest we forget": An issue concerning the Doctorate in Nursing Practice (DNP). *Nursing Outlook, 53*(1), 1.

## BIBLIOGRAPHY

Boland, B., & O'Sullivan, A. (2010). *Climb to new educational heights.* Retrieved from http://www.doctorsofnursingpractice.org/cmsAdmin/uploads/Boland2010.pdf

Chism, L. (2009). *Understanding the DNP.* Retrieved from http://www.doctorsofnursingpractice.org/cmsAdmin/uploads/Chism2009.pdf

Clark, R. C. (2011). The doctor of nursing practice graduate in practice. *Clinical Scholars Review, 4*(2), 71–77.

Drayton-Brooks, S. M., Barksdale, D. J., & Werner, K. E. (2011). An alternative view of the doctor of nursing practice. *Nursing Outlook, 59*(3), 115–116. doi:10.1016/j.outlook.2011.03.004

Florczak, K. (2010). *Research and the doctor of nursing practice: A cause for consternation.* Retrieved from http://www.doctorsofnursingpractice.org/cmsAdmin/uploads/Florczak2010.pdf

Institute of Medicine of the National Academies. (2003). *Health professions education: A bridge to quality.* Washington, DC: National Academies Press.

Retrieved from http://books.nap.edu/openbook.php?record_id=10681&page=45

Kelly, K. (2010). Is the DNP the answer to the nursing faculty shortage? Not likely! *Nursing Forum, 45*(4), 266–270. doi:10.1111/j.1744-6198.2010.00197.x

National League of Nursing. (2007). *Reflections and dialogue: Doctor of nursing practice (DNP).* Retrieved from http://www.nln.org/aboutnln/reflection_dialogue/refl_dial_1.htm

O'Sullivan, A. L., Carter, M., Marion, L., Pohl, J. M., & Werner, K. E. (2005). Moving forward together: The practice doctorate in nursing. *Online Journal of Issues in Nursing, 10*(3). Retrieved

from http://www.paeaonline.org/index.php?ht=a/GetDocumentAction/i/69226

Spear, H. (2006). Letter to the editor on "Doctor of Nursing Practice." *Online Journal of Issues in Nursing.* Retrieved from http://www.nursingworld.org/MainMenuCategories/ANAMarketplace/ANAPeriodicals/OJIN/LetterstotheEditor/JoanRosenBlochLetter.aspx

Vincent, D., Johnson, C., Velasquez, D., & Rigney, T. (2011). *DNP-prepared nurses as practitioner-researchers: Closing the gap between research and practice.* Retrieved from http://www.doctorsofnursingpractice.org/cmsAdmin/uploads/Vincet_et_al.pdf

## Chapter 23

# Nursing, Policy, and Politics
## Understanding the Connection and Importance of Getting Involved

Donna M. Nickitas

## ADDITIONAL RESOURCES

Visit thePoint for additional helpful resources
- eBook
- Journal Articles
- WebLinks

## CHAPTER OUTLINE

## LEARNING OBJECTIVES

*The learner will be able to:*

1. Define the terms *politics* and *policy* and explore their relationship.

2. Differentiate among the problem stream, the political stream, and the policy stream in John Kingdon's three-stream model of policy development.

3. Identify nursing leaders who were pioneers in public policy and describe their contributions in effecting social change.

4. Explore the relationships among social inequity, health disparities, and access to health care.

5. Cite examples of actions nurses might take to increase their political influence in public policy.

6. Investigate the most significant nursing issues being debated in the policy arena and predict the next "great" policy issues for debate.

7. Lobby a legislator, either in writing or face-to-face, about an issue related to nursing education, research, practice, or health care.

## INTRODUCTION

One important way for nurses to assume leadership roles and advance the nation's health is through involvement in the policy-making process (Institute of Medicine [IOM], 2011). Nurses play an essential role in supporting and realizing a vision for health care that is affordable, accessible, and of high quality. When nurses are full partners in the policy-making process, they achieve substantial improvements at the state, local, and national levels in both care delivery and health policy. In order to influence health policy, the nursing profession must stand ready to use the necessary knowledge and evidence needed to transform policy at all levels of the profession: practice, education, research, and leadership.

Policy issues affect all aspects of the nursing profession, including issues such as safety and quality, educational capacity and student diversity, nursing workforce shortages, mandatory overtime, nurse-staffing, workplace bullying and violence, whistle blowing, and the treatment of chemically impaired nurses. All have been shaped and/or influenced by the profession and the public at large. Indeed, nurses have long been involved in shaping health and public policy through the ages. For example, many of the early nursing leaders and activists, including Florence Nightingale, Lillian Wald, and Lavina Dock, embraced the social issues of the day within the profession. It was assumed that nurses had a key role in sharing "with society the responsibility for initiating and supporting action to meet the health and social needs of the public, in particular those of vulnerable populations" (International Council of Nurses [ICN], 2006, p. 2).

Professional advocacy and activism also created some of the earliest policy debates within nursing, including the requirements around the "training and education" of nurses. Subsequent debates continue to this day on the need for nurses to achieve higher levels of education and training to ensure the delivery of safe, patient-centered care across setting. The landmark report of the IOM and the Robert Wood Johnson Foundation, *The Future of Nursing, Leading Change, Advancing Health* (2011), calls for nurses to be better prepared with requisite competencies, such as leadership, health policy, system improvements, research, evidence-based practice, and collaboration, to deliver high-quality care, as well as competency in specific content areas including community, public health, and geriatrics. For nurses to practice to their fullest extent of their education and training, they must have both regulatory and legislative endorsement for entry into practice, licensure, and appropriate scope of practice activities.

State legislatures are responsible for the adoption of licensure laws relating to the practice of nurses and the protection of the public. Today, these laws continue to define the scope of nursing practice and licensure as distinctly separate from medicine and inclusive of responsibilities independent of medicine (National Council of State Boards of Nursing [NCSBN], 2009). To ensure the public continues to benefit from the care they receive, the NCSBN has launched an innovative, multistate study to evaluate safety and quality in nurse transition to practice programs. The mission of the NCSBN is to provide education, service, and research through collaborative leadership to promote regulatory excellence for patient safety and public protection (NCSBN, 2011).

---

CONSIDER THIS Nursing's involvement in policy and politics has resulted in state nurse practice acts that regulate nursing practice for patient safety and public protection. The NCSBN is a nonprofit organization whose members include the boards of nursing in the 50 states, the District of Columbia and four U.S. territories—American Samoa, Guam, Northern Mariana Islands, and the Virgin Islands.

---

In this chapter, nursing, policy, and politics are examined from the underlying assumption that nursing is a public good. In fact, society calls upon the profession to play a critical role in the advancement of the health of the public. It is this commitment to societal well-being and promise that nursing has made to meet the demands for health services for all citizens. Therefore, nurses at all levels of the profession—education, practice, and research must understand and appreciate how they make crucial contributions to society. This enduring commitment in fulfilling the social contract for care with society (Crigger, 2008; ICN, 2006; Kelley, Connor, Kun, & Salmon, 2008) is part of nursing's "overwhelming society responsibility of improving the health of the public" (Fry, 1983, p. 63). By improving the public's health and providing health care services, nursing seeks to protect, promote, and optimize health and well-being; prevent illness and injury; alleviate suffering through the diagnosis and treatment of human response; and advocate for the care of individuals, families, communities, and populations (American Nurses Association [ANA], 2010).

> CONSIDER THIS   Nursing's involvement in policy and politics has resulted in state nurse practice acts that allow such laws as the regulation of minimum staffing ratios, use of mandatory overtime, autonomy of practice, and scope of practice and reimbursement for advanced practice nurses (APNs).

The importance of nurse's role in health care delivery as well as in developing, promoting, or redesigning health and other related public policies cannot be overstated (Leavitt, 2009). Donna E. Shalala, chair of the Robert Wood Johnson Foundation (RWJF) Initiative of the Future of Nursing at the Institute of Medicine, recently stated that ". . . we cannot improve the quality of health care in our country without a central role for Nursing. The context has to be improving health care quality and value. This is about the patients. No one knows this better than the nursing profession" (Nickitas, 2011a, p. 23). An example that illustrates nursing's central role is in the 2010 *Affordable Care Act*. It calls for an expanded role for nurses in the design of more efficient and cost-effective models of health care delivery (Daley, 2011a). Participating in shaping health and public policy is an essential part of the professional nursing role because policy shapes the environment in which nurses provide care and determines the scope of their responsibilities.

"Nurses' political involvement is an important professional activity that advances the nursing profession while also improving the public's health" (Hall-Long, 2009, p. 78). This chapter defines policy, explains the policy process and the role of nurses in that policy process, and demonstrates how policy and politics are inextricably linked. John Kingdon's three-streams of policy development, as well as a continuum of political engagement activities, are discussed. The relationship between politics and policy are examined to demonstrate how nurses can participate in both.

In addition, this chapter identifies nursing leaders who were pioneers in public policy, traces nursing's involvement in key policy/political debates throughout the 20th century and early 21st century, and includes contemporary issues being debated today in the political arena such as health care reform and the need to prepare and enable nurses to lead change to advance health

(IOM, 2011). Finally, because politics is part of every organization and a part of government at every level, the political skills necessary for nurses to protect their practice, their profession, and the patients entrusted to their care are identified. The chapter includes a toolkit or a working model of how to "do" political advocacy and action so that nurses can increase their influence in policy and make sure the contributions of nurses are visible (Nickitas, 2011d).

> CONSIDER THIS   Nurses have a professional obligation to articulate how intellectually demanding and complex nursing care is and to demonstrate the ways in which they have developed and implemented innovative models of care that promote health reform: expanding access, improving quality and safety, and reducing costs (Nickitas, 2011b, p. 95).

## DEFINING POLITICS AND POLICY

It is critical to describe and define the meaning of the terms *policy* and *politics* well as to clarify the relationship between them. Policy, in this chapter is used to refer to government programs. The word *policy* is Greek in origin and is linked to citizenship (Online Dictionary of Social Sciences, n.d.). In government, it comes from the relationship of citizens to one another in public (Aries, 2011). Government policy and programs often intervene within organizations and delivery of health care services to assure greater equality in the distribution of goods and services. Policy represents the manifestations of ideology or belief systems about how the world should work (Rushefsky, 2008). Therefore, *public policy* is a term used that describes government actions and is divided into three areas: foreign policy, economic policy, and social policy (Lowi & Ginsberg, 1998). Foreign policy acts to defend our national sovereignty. Economic policy promotes and regulates markets. Social policy seeks to improve the conditions of American society and achieve greater social equity.

Policy is enacted through government systems in the legislative, executive, or judicial branches of government that have authoritative capacity decision made to direct or influence the actions, behaviors, or decisions of others (Block, 2008). Each branch of government plays a vital role in the formulation and regulation of health policy.

**DISCUSSION POINT**

How does health policy connect to how care and treatment are provided at the institutional level and at the governmental level? What factors must be considered before policy development begins at both levels?

**CONSIDER THIS** Policy always has a moral dimension because it relates to decisions about how to act toward others. "It involves the choices that a society or organization makes to reach a desired action and reflects the values and beliefs of those who develop the policies" (Leavitt, 2009, p. 73).

## FEDERAL POLICY

At the federal level, the U.S. Congress and the President make policy in three major areas: defense, domestic, and foreign. Health-related policies can be found in all three areas. Health-related *defense* policies include what kinds of health care the military and their families will receive and whether United States engages war to protect the homeland. *Domestic* policy refers to policies such as the recent reenactment of the 2010 Affordable Care Act, a comprehensive law aimed to protect consumers, increase access to care, promote health, improve and refocus the health care delivery system, and control costs.

Health is also a major part of *foreign* policy. Congress decides whether to assist other nations with preventing HIV/AIDS or in providing family planning and nutrition assistance to developing countries.

**CONSIDER THIS** Nurses serving in the military are affected by *defense* policy, nurses working to improve global health in developing countries are affected by *foreign* policy, and nurses working within the health care system anywhere in the United States are affected by *domestic* policy. The President and the Congress decide how tax dollars are allocated and spent on defense, foreign aid, and domestic health care. If more money is spent to fund one policy initiative over another, then less is available for others, unless taxes are increased.

## POLICIES AND VALUES

Policy involves the setting of goals and priorities by a society or an organization and the decisions about how and what resources should be used to achieve those goals. Thus, policies expressed as goals, programs, proposals, laws, and regulations that reflect the values and beliefs of those who develop the policies (Milstead, 2011).

Frequently, female policy makers, regardless of their political party, have tended to promote policies that address social issues such as family medical leave, child care, and domestic violence (Freeman, 2008). Mason, Leavitt, and Chafee (2012) suggest that women who became involved in political activism were likely to focus on community, collective responsibility, and connectedness, in contrast to men, who focused on individual rights. Similarly, policies developed by nurses have frequently shown a strong belief in the importance of assisting people to care for themselves despite their illness or disability, and this belief has distinguished nursing from other professions. Caring, whether it is for families, for patients, or for the environment, is a value central to nursing. Watson (2008) suggests that to help the current health care system retain its most precious resource, competent caring professional nurses, a new generation of health professionals must ensure care and healing for the public, while learning about the value of serving others.

Unfortunately, caring is not a value that receives much attention from institutions and government policy makers. Nurses have had some success at the state and federal levels at moving such a policy agenda forward; however, if nurses want policies that reflect nursing's values, then nurses must get involved in the policy process that makes decisions on which policies to adopt, and that requires involvement in politics.

**DISCUSSION POINT**

What values are reflected in state nurse practice acts that address the scope of nursing practice for registered nurses (RNs) and advanced practice nurses? Similarly, what values are reflected in state policies that allow chemically impaired nurses to participate in diversion programs rather than face disciplinary proceedings?

## Politics

Definitions of *politics* stem from the original Greek meaning, which referred to the government of the city-state; the actions of a government, politician, or political party; the process by which communities make decisions and govern; or the managing of a state or government. In addition, politics is the process of influencing the allocation of scarce resources required for policy goals to be achieved (Chaffee, Mason, & Leavitt, 2012). It involves power and influence for key decision making and requires significant investment in social capital. Politics is often described as the process of who gets to decide what will be done and when it will be done (Milstead, 2011).

In governing, politics is an activity that is central to developing policy that protects the well-being of society. Although this chapter focuses on policy and politics as they relate to government, many of the principles are applicable to nongovernmental institutions and organizations as well. Therefore, nurses must understand how politics drives policy decisions and have the necessary skills and competencies to care for society, regardless of their institution or organizational affiliation.

---

CONSIDER THIS   To lead change and be successful, nurses must understand the values and political issues at hand. Nurses who assume the role of politician advocates will seek to

1. believe that they have the power and expertise to convince others for the need to change,

2. adapt themselves to handle the broader political value issues, and

3. learn to effectively mobilize their expert power and muscle to influence key stakeholders for the needed change. (Robertson & Middaugh, 2011)

---

Indeed, politics is part of all organized human activity; any group of two or more individuals has to establish how to make decisions that require common action and how to resolve conflicts. In fact, Kraft and Furlong (2010) suggest that politics involves how conflicts in society are identified and resolved in favor of set of priorities or values over another. Because resources (money, time, and personnel) are limited or finite, choices must be made regarding their use. There is no perfect process for selecting optimum choices because whenever one

valuable option is chosen, usually some other option must be left out. The challenge for policy analysts and political action is to understand how these choices are organized and which ones have the most influence and why.

For nurses to have the ability to advocate for others and effectively shape policy, they must have the necessary political skill. This requires the ability to understand another's values and position and to use that understanding to influence others to act. Ferris, Davidson, and Perrewe (2005) have identified four essential components to mastering the necessary political skill:

1. *Social astuteness:* The ability to assess one's own behavior and the behavior of others; including the ability to address social situations.

2. *Interpersonal influences:* The ability to use oneself to influence others so as to be productive in behavior and action regardless of the situation.

3. *Networking ability:* The ability to use a variety of networks of individuals and organizations to position oneself to respond to opportunities and situations as they arise.

4. *Apparent sincerity:* The ability to demonstrate meaningful gratitude, authenticity, and integrity.

Just as nurses have learned to effectively use the nursing process to manage patient care, so too must they learn to use the political process. The skills that govern nursing practice can be artfully shaped and directed toward political advocacy and action.

## CONCEPTUALIZING POLITICS AND POLICY DEVELOPMENT

Although there are many models for conceptualizing politics and policy development, the Kingdon's streams of policy development (Sabatier, 1999) provides a broad and comprehensive framework for assessing policy development and a continuum for political engagement.

### Kingdon's Three Streams of Policy Development

Kingdon posited that there are *three streams* that determine why some problems are chosen over others for policy development (Sabatier, 1999; Box 23.1). The three streams are the *problem stream*, the *policy stream*, and the *political stream*. These three streams often flow endlessly without converging, but when the streams come together, a window of opportunity opens to move an agenda, to legislate, or to regulate policy solutions to problems.

## BOX 23.1 THE THREE STREAMS OF JOHN KINGDON'S STREAMS

1. *Problem:* embodies the process of problem recognition
2. *Policy:* embodies the formulation and refining of policy proposals as responses to problem recognition
3. *Politics:* considers the associated benefits and costs to subgroups of the population and the degree of external pressure the legislator feels to take action

## BOX 23.2 TEN UNIVERSAL COMMANDMENTS OF POLITICS FOR NURSES

1. The personal is political. Each of us is just one personal or social injustice away from being involved in politics.
2. Friends come and go, but enemies accumulate.
3. Politics is the art of the possible, and majority rules.
4. Be polite, be persistent, be persuasive.
5. Ignore your mother's rule: Do talk to strangers.
6. Money is the mother's milk of politics.
7. Negotiate visibility. Take credit, take control.
8. Politics has a "chit economy." So keep track.
9. Reputations are permanent.
10. Don't let 'em get to ya.

*Source:* Dodd, C. (2008). Play to win: Know the rules. In C. Harrington & C. Estes (Eds.), *Health policy: Crisis and reform in the U.S. health care delivery system* (pp. 15–26). Sudbury, MA: Jones & Bartlett.

The *problem stream* includes what are defined as problems, indicators of a problem, and the social construction of problems. It also includes how problems come to the attention of policy makers, such as in the form of causal stories or personal experiences. For example, U.S. Representative Caroline McCarthy, a licensed practical nurse, ran for Congress after her husband and son were shot on the Long Island Railroad in New York and she wanted to pass gun control legislation.

Another example of the problem stream coming to the attention of the general public and legislators is the current nursing shortage. The Johnson & Johnson Campaign for Nursing's Future (2011) has established and invested in a US$50-million national initiative designed to enhance the image of the nursing profession, recruit new nurses and nurse faculty, and help retain nurses currently in the profession. This campaign has garnished much attention surrounding the nursing shortage and the need to support expanding funding for scholarship and training to make the nursing workforce more diverse, particularly in the areas of gender and race/ethnicity.

In 2010, approximately 27% of prelicensure RN students were members of a minority group, compared with almost 37% of the U.S. population to whom they will eventually provide care. Males represent 13% of prelicensure programs, up from a low of 10% in 2003 (IOM, 2011). Again, the message here is that nursing needs to expand both its diversity and numbers of the U.S. workforce. Dodd (2008) reminds us in her Ten Universal Commandments of Politics for Nurses (Box 23.2) that the personal is political and that each of us is just one personal or social injustice away from being involved in politics (p. 16) when it comes to the significance of the problem stream.

Kingdon's second stream is the *policy stream*. Ideas that are potential policy solutions are considered based on their "technical feasibility and value acceptability" (Sabatier, 1999, p. 76). The reality is that policy makers are presented with many problems, and it is impossible to address all of them. Policy makers, then, must set an agenda that reflects their values and select problems on which to focus legislation or regulatory action that fits their priorities. Because policy makers want to be successful (for reelection and job security), most avoid introducing legislative or regulatory proposals that are unlikely to pass and/or to be implemented.

For example, Rep. McCarthy's failure to ban guns occurred because Americans value the "right to bear arms" as protected by the Second Amendment of the U.S. Constitution. She was successful, however, in leading the fight to at least pass a temporary ban on assault weapons (the legislation passed in 1993 and was made effective for 10 years, expiring in September 2004) because

Americans value their safety. Banning assault weapons provided safety and protected the guarantees of the Second Amendment.

> ## DISCUSSION POINT
>
> California is the only state that has enacted minimum licensed staff-to-patient ratios in acute care hospitals, and this passed only after vigorous opposition from the state hospital association. Is this an issue most state legislators would be eager to take on? Is such an issue "technically feasible and value acceptable"?

*The political stream* is the third and final stream. Politics, according to Kingdon, describes an environment that includes (1) the national mood—what the public sentiment is on issues, (2) support or opposition of *interest groups*, and (3) legislative or executive branch turnover accompanied by a change in political ideology and values (Sabatier, 1999). In other words, the political stream looks at associated benefits and costs to subgroups of the population and the degree of external pressure the legislator feels to take action.

An example of a strong *political stream* occurred when support from the public, professional nursing, and consumer and hospital organizations came together to help fund the Nursing Education Act. In contrast, the ban on assault weapons met with opposition because of the change of national mood, the turnover of Congress and the White House to Republican rule, and the powerful interest group of the National Rifle Association.

The significance of *interest groups* as part of the political stream cannot be overestimated. Indeed, throughout history, ideological interest groups have shaped social change. Interest groups provide politicians with one of three resources essential for their success (i.e., reelection). The first, and sometimes seemingly most important, is money; the second is the ability to mobilize voters; and the third is image. It is this image enhancement that may be most significant for nurses in terms of legislative interest. Clearly, having the support of nurses improves a candidate's image.

Historically, nurses have ranked high in public opinion polls, and the public believes that the endorsement of nurses demonstrates a candidate's integrity.

> CONSIDER THIS Nurses continue to outrank other professions in Gallup's annual Honesty and Ethics survey. Eighty-one percent of Americans say nurses have "very high" or "high" honesty and ethical standards, a significantly greater percentage than for the next highest rated professions, military officers and pharmacists. Americans rate car salespeople, lobbyists, and members of Congress as having the lowest honesty and ethics, with the last two getting a majority of "low" or "very low" ratings (Gallop Poll, 2011).

Nursing is a profession of more than 3 million members nationally. When divided by 435 congressional districts nationally, there are approximately 5,000 RNs per congressional district who can and have mobilized voters. The power of the "nursing numbers" converts to votes that can make the difference in electing officials who support and endorse nursing's core values and positions.

A strong political stream, however, is not enough. Convergence of the three streams is required. Nursing and the professional organizations that represent nursing (interest groups) in the legislature at the state and federal levels, then, have repeatedly worked to achieve this degree of stream convergence in public policy decisions related to health care. For example, the robust body of evidence by Mary Naylor, PhD, RN, professor at the University of Pennsylvania School of Nursing, proposed that transitional care can improve health outcomes and reduce hospital readmissions as well as provide range of solutions to reduce avoidable hospitalizations and health care costs (Naylor et al., 2004). Specifically, Naylor's research shows that the use of nurses, often master's prepared, who work with patients, family caregivers, and health teams can prevent medical errors and assure continuity of care as patients navigate a very fragmented health care system (Naylor et al., 1999; Naylor et al., 1994).

Transitional care—short-term services that bridge gaps between hospital and home—focuses on identifying and addressing patients' and family caregivers' goals, as well as their needs for education and support, such as access to community services, to prevent poor outcomes. Naylor's evidence provides those responsible for implementing community-based care transitions programs, Accountable Care Organizations, and other innovative delivery and payment models with a strong foundation on which to build these programs and achieve better care and better outcomes while reducing costs.

CONSIDER THIS   Nursing interest groups have seized the public's frustration with rising health care costs and promoted policies that emphasized the cost-effectiveness of advanced practice nurses (stream one—conditions, plus stream two—ideas/policies). President Obama has supported this idea and included advanced practice nurses (APNs) in his health care reform legislation (stream three—political change in values).

## Analyzing Policy Making and Professional Nursing

A more traditional approach to analyzing policy making uses a systems-based model that considers policy making in sequential stages. It is much like the nursing process: assess, plan, implement, evaluate, and assess again. In a policy system, a problem is identified and put on a policy agenda; then a policy is developed, adopted, implemented, evaluated, and extended, modified, or terminated; and the cycle begins again (Hanley & Falk, 2007). The challenge of using a traditional systems model approach is that it fails to consider that the elected government's policy agenda rarely, if ever, reflects a consensus.

For example, in the last two election cycles, the country has become more and more divided on a partisan and thus philosophical basis of how best to govern or what the government's role is on health policy as witnessed by the recent debates surrounding the Affordable Care Act 2010 (Nickitas, 2011c). Critics argue that the systems analysis of policy development leaves out the influence of interest groups, whether they are nursing organizations or health insurance companies. A case in point is using the nursing process for diabetic teaching of an adolescent without taking into consideration that the patient might not follow the diet because his or her peer group is eating fast food every day after school.

In contrast, policy development, adoption and implementation, and politics are inextricably linked in Kingdon's model, and the political environment in which policy is formed is considered. Nursing can play a role in all three of Kingdon's policy streams that create windows of opportunity. Again, using the recently released IOM report, nurses are considered the agent who will transform the health care system, ensuring care is patient centered, effective, safe, and affordable. This vision calls upon the entire nursing community to embrace this report as a blueprint for action and requires each and every nurse to use evidence-based research and collaboration to improve health care. It also means working for and within a remodeled health care system that guarantees high-quality, patient-centered care.

CONSIDER THIS   According to the IOM's definition, patient-centered care is "providing care that is respectful of and responsive to individual patient preferences, needs, and values and ensuring that patient values guide all clinical decisions" (IOM, 2011, p. 6).

It is up to the nursing profession and consumer groups to raise public awareness about the quality of care or lack of access to care. Professional nursing organizations and consumers collectively can develop ideas and propose policies to solve problems of health care access, health and safety, or quality of care. Nursing professional organizations and interest groups like AARP can lobby and engage in political action to influence policy.

In all of these examples, nursing is acting as an interest group. The unique thing about nursing as an interest group is that when nurse's advocate for nurses and nursing, patients and the public gets better care. Political action is a key part of interest group action. Interest groups do more than support or oppose policies; they help to elect the policy makers by engaging in grassroots campaign activity and raising money for campaigns.

### DISCUSSION POINT

Nursing has the potential to hold a significant leadership position in policy and politics. At the national level, the profession is represented by the ANA, the National League for Nursing (NLN), National Students Nurses Association, and many specialty organizations. What opportunities are available at the local, state, and national level for you to assume a leadership position?

## Policy Making and Politics: The Key to Involvement

Nursing's involvement in policy making and politics must rise to the level of engagement. If nurses truly want to influence health care and improve quality, access, and value they must engage the political process. For changes in health care reform to be fully realized, it will require nurses to envision themselves as leaders in the process and find others who will share and support their goals. Political engagement can be viewed along a continuum that extends from no engagement in politics to that of extreme activism. Individuals choose when and how much political engagement along the continuum they want throughout their lives in response to intrinsic and external motivators, time and energy resources, and situational opportunities and needs.

For many nurses, timing is everything in the continuum of political engagement from *nurse as citizen to nurse as activist*, and finally, to *nurse as politician* Mason et al. (2012). The classic description about the various levels of political activism comes from the perspective of an individual choice and emerges from the historical work of Kalisch and Kalisch (1982). They have described individual political participation along the continuum ranging from *spectator activities*, *transitional activities*, to *gladiatorial activities* (p. 316). Political engagement has often been described as people *who make things happen*, *people who watch what's happening*, and *people who wonder what's happened*. For example, nurses *who wonder what's happening vote* occasionally or not at all; they are not involved in improving the workplace or their community. Nurses *who watch things happen* are spectators; they expose themselves to political stimuli, they are members of their union, they vote, sometimes they wear buttons or put bumper stickers on cars, and they participate in community activities that are important to them such as parent–teacher organizations or nonprofit agencies for the homeless, veterans, or disabled.

---

CONSIDER THIS   Political engagement is when individuals make things happen. From where you sit right now, identify three activities that you can make happen in school, in the community, and at home that can make a difference.

---

## A Toolkit for Political Advocacy

Nurses *who make things happen* fall into three categories: professionals, leaders, and political change agents. Professional nurses vote in every election and stay informed regarding issues affecting the health care system. They participate in their union or speak out about working conditions and quality of care. They participate in their professional organization, know who their local, state, and federal elected officials are, and communicate with them regarding issues of concern. ANA President, Karen Daley (2011b), suggests there are a variety of ways that nurses can get involved and make a difference, including the following:

1. Don't let policy happen "to you"–get involved in the policy committees at work and through state associations.

2. Use your voice, experience, and expertise to help design and implement care environments and models. No one knows what patients want and need better than nurses do.

3. Participate in workforce planning surveys and data-collection opportunities. Nurses must measure the value of what they do.

4. Stays informed about and participate in the activities of a professional association. A few hours of voluntary time can make a big difference; remember there is strength in numbers.

5. Embrace and act on the power of nursing expertise and wisdom.

## Nursing Political Action Committees

The year 1974 brought new election laws allowing for contributions by Political Action Committees (PACs). The laws limited the amount an individual could contribute to a campaign and allowed groups to contribute up to US$5,000 per election. Contributions from nurses giving small amounts individually could not compare with what physicians gave; however, together, they could contribute to a PAC and give US$5,000. The Nurses Coalition for Action in Politics (N-CAP; the precursor of the ANA-PAC) was created by the ANA to establish political power through the endorsement of candidates and political contributions. The slogan "1 in 44" was worn on buttons when nurses visited their legislators to point out that 1 in 44 registered women voters was an RN.

When President Gerald Ford vetoed the Nurse Training Act of 1974 and attempted to eliminate the scholarship and student loan programs for nursing, the ANA lobbied Congress, which passed legislation extending the Nurse Training Act, which included, for the first time, funding for advanced practice nursing. President Ford vetoed the bill, and the ANA mounted a nationwide lobbying effort. Congress overrode the veto with many more than the two-thirds votes required (Kalisch & Kalisch, 1982). Again, a convergence of Kingdon's streams can be identified: a problem of not enough nurses and a powerful political interest group of nurses!

The proliferation of nursing specialty organizations and unions all claiming to represent "nursing" sometimes jeopardizes nursing's effectiveness because different nursing organizations bring different messages to elected officials. Elected officials tend to listen to the people who help elect them, so whichever nursing organizations are most active in political campaigns through contributions and through grassroots activity (usually only important in an official's first few elections because of the power of incumbency) are the organizations that will be heard.

It is essential for nurses to be involved in all organizations that represent nurses, especially those with PACs, because "money talks." Contributing to candidates that promote nursing's agenda to improve the quality of health care is important. It is unfortunate that campaigns are expensive, but it costs money to buy television ad time and to mail literature to people's homes.

Professional nurses must make things happen or they will find themselves not only wondering what happened but also complaining about it. Nurse are active members of nursing organizations that are political; they are active members of a political party and attend political meetings, forums, and rallies; they help register people to vote; they contribute and raise money for causes and campaigns through political action committees (PACs). The ANA PAC has grown over the years through contributions of members. The PAC considers the voting records of incumbent candidates for reelection and the relationships with the state constituent member of the ANA for candidates running for open seats. Keeping track of voting records is important, and PAC contributions are essential for successful reelection campaigns of friends of nursing. Song (2011) states,

> ANA does not use dues dollars to support candidates. Rather, ANA-PAC raises money through the voluntary donations from member nurses across the country. These nurses understand the importance of having a seat at the table when Congress is discussing nursing issues, such as appropriate staffing, home health, and safe patient handling. ANA-PAC donates to candidates who work to implement healthy public policy for our profession. (p. 15)

---

### DISCUSSION POINT

Do all RNs benefit from the contributions and work of the members of the ANA who make monetary contributions to the ANA PAC and help to elect "nurse-friendly" members of Congress?

---

## Understanding Political Parties and Their Politics

Nurses naturally work to affect policy in the workplace but often fail to realize that the work they do and the environment in which it is done are controlled by the government. So nurses must be involved beyond the private sector if they are to bring about change. To do so require nurses to examine their values and pick a political party that reflects their views and become involved.

From a health perspective, the primary difference between the two major parties in the United States is that Democrats typically favor "public" systems with taxpayers funding access to health services with a guaranteed benefit package and price controls. Criticism of this philosophy is that price regulation will stifle innovation and quality and that those taxpayers should not have to pay for the ills of others.

Republicans tend to favor a market strategy in which consumers will make choices based on cost and quality within private systems and that with consumers making market choices, competition will keep prices down. The major criticisms of this strategy are that education and health do not behave like traditional market systems and that market mechanisms in health care yield an advantage to the more affluent and healthier people, as well as for providers, suppliers, and insurers. In this system, the financial burden for the sick, disabled, and uninsured is left to the public (government) sector. The public risk pool—or the group of people being cared for by the public sector—is more costly than if the risk were spread among the entire population.

The Tea Party Movement (TPM) is an American populist political movement that is generally recognized as conservative and libertarian and has sponsored protests and supported political candidates since 2009 (Halloran, 2010). It endorses reduced government spending, opposition to taxation in varying degrees, reduction of the national debt and federal budget deficit, and adherence to an originalist interpretation of the U.S. Constitution (Barstow, 2010; Berman, 2010; Wallsten & Yadron, 2010).

The reality is that nurses are not born Republicans, Democrats, or Tea Party followers. Party affiliation is often a reflection of core personal values. It is important, then, to have nurses as leaders from all political parties.

---

### DISCUSSION POINT

Do your beliefs about health care align more closely with traditional Democratic, Republican, or Tea Party values?

---

## Nursing Moving Beyond the Bedside

The message throughout this chapter has been that nurses need to move beyond the bedside to the board room or at least be represented at tables of influence. These tables must increasingly involve issues around both politics and public policy. To become engaged in civic participation, will mean that nurses will have to balance the care of patients with the concerns of health care policy. Nurse must engage and move to new spheres of influence. A good way for most nurses to increase their influence is through involvement with a professional organization that is politically active. Find an organization that speaks to your professional and core values. Then investigate the organization's legislative and policy agenda, learn what legislations impacts nurses or nursing. There are several places where information about federal legislation can be located.

> CONSIDER THIS   Thomas website (http://thomas.loc.gov)
> - monitored by the Library of Congress
> - wealth of information available about the legislative process, including searches on bill status, public laws, House and Senate roll call votes, current activity in Congress
>
> Senate (www.senate.gov) and House (www.house.gov) websites
> - information about individual senators and representatives, committees, schedules, and search for legislation
> - members of Congress can be contacted directly from each of these sites
>
> ANA Government Affairs website (http://www.nursingworld.org/MainMenuCategories/Policy-Advocacy)
> - contains legislation that has been identified as important to nurses and information about how nurses can contact their legislators to express concern and voice their opinion
>
> National League for Nursing (NLN) website, the National League for Nursing's Public Policy Action Center (http://capwiz.com/nln/home)
> - provides information about legislation affecting nursing and allows searches for elected officials using zip codes

To become better informed about current issues affecting nursing and health care, consult additional websites of professional organizations. Other ways for nurses to learn about and increase their influence in politics and health care policy are shown in Box 23.3. These include becoming involved in electing candidates nurses want to win. This requires that nurses be knowledgeable regarding the candidates and their values. It is

politically smart for nurses to pick candidates that have a good chance of winning and who share nursing's values. The nurse who works for a losing candidate risks alienating the winner. In races in which the candidate is an incumbent and is in a district in which she is likely to be reelected, the candidate still needs help. Specific activities that might be undertaken to support such a candidate include telephone banking, precinct walking, fundraising, writing letters to the editor, and supporting the candidate in public forums, including other organizations in which one participates.

> CONSIDER THIS   Working together, speaking with one strong voice, nurses are a powerful political force.

Actions that nurses can take to increase their influence in the policy setting are also shown in Box 23.3. Again, becoming involved in a professional nursing

---

**BOX 23.3   ACTIONS NURSES CAN TAKE TO INCREASE THEIR INFLUENCE IN POLITICS AND POLICY**

**To Influence Politics**

- Be knowledgeable and get involved in campaigns (the earlier the better).
- Assist candidates in winning the endorsement of key organizations that you may be involved in, such as nursing organizations, parent–teacher organizations, and neighborhood organizations.

**To Influence Policy**

- Be a member of a nursing organization that influences policy at the local, state, and federal levels.
- Be informed. Subscribe to electronic listservs of elected officials that you agree with and compare the records of your officials.
- Get to know your elected officials.
- Write lobbying letters.
- Write letters to the editor.
- Participate in coalitions of organizations.

organization and being informed head the list. Nurses must also know the legislator who represents them. District office staff usually handles constituent case work dealing with local, state, or federal agencies. For example, if someone has a problem with the post office or is a veteran and cannot get benefits, they can seek help from their congressional representative's district office. The district chief of staff is often the only "policy person" in the district. The office in the Capitol deals with legislation and policy issues. Staff members are key in getting access to a legislator, so the politically astute nurse is polite and respectful in dealing with these individuals.

Finally, nurses who want to increase their influence in policy should write their legislative representatives regarding health care issues (Box 23.4). Letters should arrive before any proposed legislation is heard in committee because key decisions on proposed legislation are made in committee. Bills that have a financial impact are heard in a policy committee and a financial committee. Some bills are assigned to two or more committees. This is often a tactic used to defeat the bill before it comes to the floor. If your legislator is not on the committee, write to the Committee Chair at the committee office address. If you write to legislators who do not represent you

---

## BOX 23.4 SAMPLE LOBBYING LETTER

[1]Lillian Wald, RN, BSN
Henry Street
New York, New York 00251

[2]The Honorable Harry Nemo
Member, U.S. House of Representatives
House Office Building
Washington DC, 20015

[3]RE: SUPPORT for HR 1435

[4]Dear Representative Nemo,

[5]I am a registered nurse, and I have worked in the area of home health care for over 5 years. In the past 2 years, more and more of the elderly patients I care for have had to be readmitted to the hospital shortly after being discharged from the hospital because they are not taking their prescribed medications.
As you know, H.R. 1435 would provide a guaranteed, affordable prescription drug benefit within the Medicare program. Currently, despite many drug coverage programs for seniors, many remain unaffordable.
[6]It will save costly hospitalizations to provide needed prescription drugs at affordable costs to seniors. Please support H.R. 1435 and please advise me of your current position on this bill.
Sincerely,

[7]Lillian Wald, RN, BSN

### LEGEND

1. Include your address.
2. Use the proper form of address (most elected and appointed officials are addressed as "the Honorable").
3. State what the letter is regarding.
4. Use the office title in the salutation.
5. State your credentials and experience/belief/position.
6. Urge support/opposition, and *ask* for a response with the official's position.
7. Sign letter.

(Please be sure when signing your name, include RN after your name.)

(you do not reside in their district), however, they are unlikely to respond to your communications because you are not one of their constituents. It is a good idea to send a copy of the letter with a brief cover letter to your legislator urging his or her support when the bill comes to the floor (if bills pass out of committee, they go to the "floor" or the entire house of the legislature). If your legislator supports your position on legislation, *send a thank you note!* Thank you notes tell legislators that you are watching what they are doing. Nurses must understand the reality that global health care issues permeate our communities as well as our governmental agencies and health policies (Salmon & Guisigner, 2007, p. 998).

Finally, nurse political change agents are nurses who use their nursing expertise to lobby elected and appointed officials on issues of concern to the profession; write letters to the editor of professional journals and newspapers (see Box 23.5 for an example of a Letter to the Editor, which was sent to the editor of the *New York Times* and published). The work of health and public policy cannot be done in isolation. Nurses must build and participate in coalitions, encourage the participation of other nurses, and mentor future leaders. Most important, nurses must use their political muscle to enact and implement policies that enhance access, affordable quality health care, including nursing care; seek appointments or assist other nurses and friends of nursing in securing appointments to governing boards in the public and private sectors; be active members of political parties; query candidates about their positions on health care and assist with fundraising for candidates that support nurses and nursing; seek elected and/or appointed office and continue to identify themselves as an RN; work on staffs of elected/appointed officials; and extend their policy influence beyond the health system to the community and the globe.

## Nursing Leaders as Policy Pioneers

Nursing has a long history of involvement in politics and policy development. From its historic foundation to its essential core, nursing is political (Warner, 2003, p. 135). There are numerous nursing leaders who served as pioneers in public policy formation in the early to mid-1900s. Only a few are presented here, as is the area of policy they were most noted for. Yet their stories are similar; all of them shared passion, courage, and perseverance. In addition, they all shared a commitment to collective strength. These same attributes are recognized in nursing policy activists today.

---

**BOX 23.5 LETTER TO THE EDITOR**

### LETTERS

#### WHEN DOCTORS HUMILIATE NURSES

Published: May 14, 2011

Today, hospitals pride themselves on providing patient-centered care by a multidisciplinary team, a hallmark of their quality. When one team member bullies another, patient care suffers. As a nurse, I would not want my family member or my nursing student in a hospital where physicians demean and insult their nurse colleagues, thus hampering their ability to care.

A culture and a climate of respect and dignity not only win the day but also ensure patient safety and quality care. It's time physicians learned that nurses are on their team, poised to manage complex critical decisions and care for their patients. Please no bullying—It hurts.

Donna M. Nickitas

Old Greenwich, Conn., May 8, 2011

The writer is a nursing professor at Hunter College, Hunter-Bellevue School of Nursing.

## Lavinia Dock: Organizing Nurses for Social Awareness

At the 1904 ANA convention, Lavinia Dock, a founder of the ANA and the first to donate money to establish the *American Journal of Nursing* that same year, stated that it was essential that nurses exercise social awareness. As a result, delegates to the ANA convention that year considered social (policy) issues of the time, including child labor, women's suffrage, and sex education.

## Lillian Wald: Public Health and Child Welfare

Lillian Wald, one of the founders of the ANA, exemplified involvement in social change, community leadership, and politics. She was born to a family of Jewish scholars and rabbis. She graduated from nursing school and entered Women's Medical College in New York to become a doctor. During her first year of medical school, she volunteered to teach hygiene to immigrant women in a school on Henry Street in New York City.

She quit medical school, and, in 1893, she and a classmate, Mary Brewster, moved to the Lower East Side neighborhood to provide nursing care in the community (American Association for the History of Nursing [AAHN], 2004). A friend and philanthropist, Jacob Schiff, and Solomon Loeb agreed to fund Wald and Brewster's purchase of a house on Henry Street. This house became the Henry Street Settlement and is considered the founding place for public health nursing. Neighbors came to the house for help with their health, housing, employment, and educational needs.

Wald was also concerned about the living conditions of the neighborhood and the lack of safe places for children to play. She helped found the Outdoor Recreation League, which worked to gain attention for the need for public parks and raised funds for what would become the first municipal playground in New York City.

Fortunately, Wald's concern for children at the time was shared by many wealthy charity leaders. During the 1890s, close to 250 new orphanages were incorporated. Vast numbers of children were working in factories. Wald believed that the government needed to protect children and that child labor should be abolished. In 1904, she participated in a meeting with President Theodore Roosevelt lobbying for the creation of a national Children's Bureau. However, the powerful industrialist lobby made up of the wealthy factory owners who used child labor was successful in tabling the legislation through their lobbying and political support of legislators (Jewish Women's Archive, n.d.).

However, as an example of Kingdon's first stream (the conditions that are defined as problems sometimes come to the attention of policy makers through personal experiences), one of President Roosevelt's close friends was James West, who was an orphan. West joined Wald and others in 1909 to host a national Conference on Children that drew more than 200 leaders from all over the country. The publicity created a public sentiment largely among women of all classes that child welfare must be put on the national policy agenda.

Kingdon's third stream—politics—resulted in the creation of the Children's Bureau in 1912 (Krain, n.d.). Wald was appointed to New York's Immigration Commission in 1908 by Governor Charles Evans Hughes after he visited the Settlement House. Wald's efforts resulted in a report that called for improved living and working standards for workers and their families. The report led to the formation of a State Bureau of Industries in New York. Kingdon's three streams again appear to hold: conditions—of immigrant workers; idea/policy—need for government regulation; and politics—Wald's relationship with the governor.

By 1909, Wald convinced the Metropolitan Life Insurance Company that protecting the health of employees was good for business, and they funded nurses from the Henry Street Settlement to care for sick employees of companies they insured. The Henry Street Visiting Nurses Society began with 10 nurses in 1893. By 1916, it had 250 nurses and was serving more than 1,300 patients a day in their homes. Wald convinced the New York Board of Education to hire a nurse in 1902 and so began school nursing in the United States. She also lobbied successfully to change divorce laws so that abandoned spouses could sue for alimony, and she assisted the Women's Trade Union League in protecting women from "sweatshop working conditions" (National Association for Home Care and Hospice [NAHC], 2008, para. 6).

In 1912, Wald founded the National Organization for Public Health Nursing. She was also part of the peace movement against World War I and for that was cited as an "undesirable" citizen. In spite of this, she served as chairperson of the Committee on Community Nursing of the American Red Cross and worked with the International Red Cross in the campaign to fight the flu epidemic of 1918 (Jewish Women's Archive, n.d.). Wald was also active in the suffrage movement and believed women should have the right to vote and to be involved in politics.

Wald was active in nursing at the local, national, and international levels. At her insistence, Columbia University appointed the first professor of nursing at a U.S.

college or university. She was among the founders of the International Council of Nurses in 1899. Wald's nursing leadership also demonstrated that policy and politics are linked and that nurses must be active beyond their immediate workplace and also in the community, in business, and in government.

### Margaret Sanger: Birth Control

Among the many nurses whose training included a rotation through the Henry Street Settlement was Margaret Sanger. Sanger witnessed maternal and infant mortality resulting from uncontrolled fertility in the neighborhoods of the Lower East Side of New York City. She cared for women suffering from self-induced abortions and was motivated to make birth control available to women. In 1912, she began writing a column on sex education titled "What Every Girl Should Know," but it was soon censored (Steinem, 2004).

In 1914, Sanger was indited for disseminating contraceptive information. She jumped bail and fled to England. She returned to the United States and continued to promote access to birth control throughout her life. She opened a clinic in New York with her sister Ethel Byrne and was jailed, only being released after a hunger strike. She smuggled contraceptive diaphragms from Europe, and she founded the National Committee on Federal Legislation for Birth Control and the American Birth Control League, which became the Planned Parenthood Federation of America.

In 1965, after years of effort, the Supreme Court decision *Griswold v. Connecticut* made birth control legal for married couples. Sanger died shortly thereafter (Sanger, n.d.). Here again, Kingdon's streams took some time to come together: first conditions had to be compelling—maternal and infant mortality caused by lack of spacing pregnancies and poverty. Then the political stream converged with the women's movement and women demanding that they be able to control their pregnancies. Finally, policy change occurred with the legalization of birth control.

### Martha Minerva Franklin: Segregation and Discrimination

Martha Minerva Franklin was another pioneering public policy nurse in the early 20th century. She founded the National Association of Colored Graduate Nurses (NACGN) in 1908 with the fundraising assistance of Lillian Wald and Lavinia Dock, who mailed letters to more than 1,000 nurses (ANA Hall of Fame: Martha Minerva Franklin, n.d.). The NACGN was formed because many states barred Black nurses from membership in state nurses associations. Segregation and discrimination kept nursing education and hospitals separate.

The NACGN was instrumental, however, in political lobbying efforts to integrate Black nurses into the armed services during World War II. In 1951, the NACGN merged with the ANA (Flanagan, 1976). Today, the National Black Nurses Association exists as one of more than 70 national nursing organizations, some organized around clinical issues, some relating to ethnicity, and some relating to religious beliefs.

## Nurses and Social Change

Historically, nursing leaders have participated in many efforts to bring about social change. The efforts of nurse leaders in the suffrage movement have already been discussed. Nurse leaders in the early 20th century were also integrally involved in passing socially focused legislation that outlawed child labor and provided protection for women abandoned by their husbands.

Nursing was also at the forefront of and lent integrity to the civil rights movement. As a result of the civil rights movement, poll taxes and literacy tests were made illegal. In addition, politicians elected with the aid of newly enfranchised Blacks passed laws to eliminate discrimination based on race. Nursing was one of the first professions to eliminate segregation. However, educational opportunities remain out of reach for many students of color, and nursing's responsibility to ensure that the face of the profession reflects the faces of those entrusted to its care still requires much work.

Nursing did not formally participate in the "peace movement" against the Vietnam War, but some nursing leaders participated in the women's movement that emerged around that time. Nursing and teaching were professions almost exclusively made up of women, and employment ads at the time were separated for men and women.

In 1974, the ANA set up a special account to help pass the Equal Rights Amendment to the Constitution. The ANA joined a national boycott and moved its convention to a state that had ratified the Amendment. The Amendment failed ratification by a sufficient number of states. The women's movement continued, and nursing and teaching were often used as examples of professions requiring a significant amount of knowledge and skill for which compensation fell far below male-dominated jobs requiring the same levels of knowledge and skill, or "comparable worth." Nursing also became involved in the effort to establish comparable worth in employment settings during the 1970s. During this time, women were often paid less for the same work that men did. Many states passed "comparable worth laws" during the 1970s, supported by state nurses associations. During the 1980s and beyond, nurses at various places around the country went on strike to achieve wages of comparable worth. Nursing's involvement in the women's movement as its own interest group working in coalition with other women's interest groups strengthened that movement.

## TWENTY-FIRST-CENTURY NURSING LEADERS: POLICY AND POLITICS
### Mary Wakefield and the Nation's Health

Mary Wakefield, PhD, RN, was named administrator of the Health Resources and Services Administration (HRSA) by President Barack Obama on February 20, 2009. HRSA is an agency of the U.S. Department of Health and Human Services. HRSA seeks to close health care gaps for people who are uninsured, isolated, or medically vulnerable. The agency uses its US$9.6 billion annual budget (FY 2011) to expand access to quality health care in partnership with health care providers and health professions training programs. Wakefield joined HRSA from the University of North Dakota (UND), where she was Associate Dean for Rural health at the School of Medicine and Health Sciences. Wakefield has brought her expertise and wisdom from state politics and Capitol Hill to her post at HRSA.

In the 1990s, Wakefield served as chief-of-staff to two North Dakota senators: Kent Conrad (D) and Quentin Burdick (D). She also has served as director of the Center for Health Policy, Research and Ethics at George Mason University in Fairfax, Virginia, and worked on site as a consultant to the World Health Organization's Global Programme on AIDS in Geneva, Switzerland. Her extensive board experience and health care knowledge lead to an elected position to the IOM. She served on the IOM committee that produced the landmark reports *To Err Is Human* and *Crossing the Quality Chasm*. She also cochaired the IOM committee that produced the report *Health Professions Education* and chaired the committee that produced the report *Quality Through Collaboration: Health Care in Rural America*.

In addition, she has served on the Medicare Payment Advisory Commission as chair of the National Advisory Council for the Agency for Healthcare Research and Quality, as a member of President Clinton's Advisory Commission on Consumer Protection and Quality in the Health Care Industry, and as a member of the National Advisory Committee to HRSA's Office of Rural Health Policy. Wakefield's years of political acumen and commitment to nursing have been recognized by the President and her peers. As a nurse and appointed federal executive leader, Wakefield cares and seeks to protect the public's health while ensuring there are sufficient health professionals to care for the nation's citizens.

### Lorreta Ford—First Pediatric Nurse Practitioner Model

Loretta C. Ford, Dean and Professor Emerita, School of Nursing, University of Rochester, is an internationally known nursing leader. She has devoted her professional life and career to practice, education, research, consultation and influencing health services, community health, and military nursing. Her studies on the nurse's expanded scope of practice in public health nursing led to the creation of the first pediatric nurse practitioner model of advanced practice at the University of Colorado Medical Center.

Ford is a visionary leader who saw the need to meld nursing education, practice, and research. She provided administrative leadership for a unification model in nursing at the University of Rochester Medical Center in the position of Dean of the School of Nursing and the Director of Nursing in the University's Strong Memorial Hospital. She has authored more than one hundred publications on the history of the nurse practitioner, unification of practice, education, and research, and issues in advanced nursing practice and health care. Currently, she consults and lectures on the historical development of the nurse practitioner and on issues in advanced nursing practice and health care policy.

### Gaye Douglas and Nurse Managed Center

Gaye Douglas, APRN-BC, was featured in an article titled "Three Nurses Take the Lead on Change" in the *American Nurse*, January/February 2011 issue. She opened a nurse managed center after receiving her graduate degree. While working as a school nurse in a small, South Carolina community in a district with about 1,600 students in three schools and maintaining a clinical practice working weekends in the emergency room of a hospital, she worked two jobs to make ends meet. It was while working in the emergency room that she notice that some of the students that she saw during the school week for certain ailments, such as strep throat, that required a primary care visit were coming to the emergency room for that care (Trossman, 2011).

To solve the dilemma between providing primary care and emergency room care to her students,

Douglas decided to apply for a Duke Endowment Grant to become a family nurse practitioner. She went back to school while working both jobs and keeping up with her life as a single parent. Her commitment to her school work and vision for primary services led to the creation 4 years ago of the Campus Health Center, which is located on the high school campus of Florence County School District Five and is open to the public. She provides much needed primary care services to people of all ages who come from her county, as well as a neighboring county. The center staff consists of herself, an RN, and a billing clerk.

The nurse managed health center sees an average of about 15 patients a day, with some seasonal variations. To comply with state regulations regarding NPs' rural practice, Douglas has a formal collaboration agreement with a physician who must come to the health center once in every 2 weeks. She also must contact him to write prescriptions for schedule II narcotics, which sometimes affects how quickly she can meet patients' needs. Although Douglas has a good working relationship with him—she used to work with him in the ED—and consults him or physician specialists when the need arises, she would like to see South Carolina's law change to allow NPs to practice independently. Douglas like many APRNs understands that with the full implementation of the Affordable Care Act, an additional 3 million or more people becoming insured and need access to care. "There is no way the delivery system will meet the demand nor are there a sufficient number of physicians to provide primary care," said Douglas, who has been an NP for 6 years. "Also many don't want to work in rural communities." Just considering the communities that surround Florence County, Douglas said, "There still is so much that needs to be done" (Trossman, 2011).

At this point in time, Douglas is writing two new grants. One is focusing on getting funding to extend the health center's hours during the week and on weekends to increase access to care. The other is opening a health center in Williamsburg County, one of the poorest counties in the state with a population of 38,000 and one physician under 70 years of age (Trossman, 2011).

## HEALTH INSURANCE: THEN AND NOW

The fights for National health insurance and efforts to increase access to health care have been a steady and recurrent theme throughout nursing's long historical, political, and policy agenda. Indeed, nursing leaders such as Lillian Wald, Lavinia Dock, and Annie W. Goodrich supported the first unsuccessful platform for national health care proposed by Theodore Roosevelt in 1912. In fact, some critics labeled Goodrich and Wald socialists for their efforts.

The next proposal for national health care came during President Franklin Roosevelt's administration. It was made by Frances Perkins, the first woman to serve in the cabinet as secretary of labor. Perkins headed up a committee on economic security during the Great Depression that recommended both income security (Social Security) and health security. The American Medical Association (AMA), however, opposed national health care insurance and mounted a successful grassroots campaign to discredit a government-sponsored and -regulated health care system.

Roosevelt abandoned the linkage of health insurance to the social security provisions because he did not want to jeopardize the New Deal programs, which included Social Security, but he did promise to consider it in his next term. However, Roosevelt died in 1945 and was succeeded by Harry Truman. When Truman ran for his first full term as president, he promoted a prepaid medical insurance plan financed by increasing the Social Security tax. Again, the AMA opposed these efforts and likened national health coverage to totalitarianism in Nazi Germany. The ANA, the National League for Nursing (NLN), and the National Organization for Public Health Nursing, however, supported Truman's proposals (Kalisch & Kalisch, 1982).

In 1948, Truman won his first full term as President on a platform promoting universal health coverage—a comprehensive benefit package including prescription drugs, dental coverage, and nursing home care. However, just before the 1950 congressional election, the AMA again waged a successful campaign by assessing each of their members US$25 to fund a program designed to "educate" physicians and the public throughout the country about the dangers of socialized medicine and worked against candidates for Congress who supported Truman's plan. The AMA spent more than US$4.3 million dollars to defeat this health reform, and there were not enough members elected to Congress in 1950 who supported Truman's plan.

National health insurance was an idea that lost its attraction in the 1950s, despite the fact that families were losing their life savings and being forced into poverty by costly hospitalizations while science and technology were promising to save lives (Families USA, 1993). Again from Kingdon's perspective, this occurred because only one of the three criteria was met: conditions—because of the rising costs of medical care, the idea/policy had significant support; however, the politics—the opposition from powerful interest groups, the AMA, and organized labor who used health coverage as a tool to recruit members—made it impossible to pass national health reform (Families USA). This is an example of grassroots political activity by a group of health professionals (the AMA) directly in the electoral (political) process.

Efforts to create national health insurance did not die. In 1974, the ANA continued its support of national health insurance and adopted a resolution supporting national health insurance with the intent to increase nursing's participation in the policy debate. The resolution stated that a national health insurance program should be implemented that would "guarantee coverage for all people for the full range of comprehensive health services" and that nursing care should "be a benefit of the national health insurance program." The resolution also said that data systems necessary for effective management of the national insurance program should be in place to "protect the rights and privacy of individuals" and that nurses should be designated "as health providers in all pending or proposed legislation on national health insurance" (Flanagan, 1976, pp. 670–671). This was an example of the nursing profession's foresight: to cover all people, to protect privacy, and to include nurses as essential providers. Indeed, the legislative agenda of the ANA included all of these principles in subsequent health care legislation.

In 1978, the first Black president of the ANA, Barbara Nichols, was asked to testify on behalf of Senator Edward Kennedy's Health Care for All Americans Act. Television coverage of major issues meant that the organizations selected to testify had to have the trust of the public, and nursing was held in high regard. Nichols not only advocated for access to comprehensive health services for all but also specifically mentioned mental health services and nursing care in all settings. She insisted that we needed a health system and not a medical system. The AMA opposed the measure. It failed by only a few votes.

The ANA has remained active in advocating for access to quality, affordable health care. The ANA and the NLN drafted *Nursing's Agenda for Health Care Reform*

public health nurses providing primary care screening in community-based settings. More than 70 nursing specialty organizations signed onto the agenda so that nursing could speak with one voice about health care reform.

President Bill Clinton was elected in 1992 with the support of the ANA, and he promised to reform the health care system and to include nursing as part of the solution. Nurse leaders were a part of the task force that developed the Health Security Act. This legislative proposal was complex and was opposed by the insurance industry, the pharmaceutical industry, and the AMA.

In 1994, these powerful and well-financed interest groups successfully worked to defeat any member of Congress who supported reform. The proposal was completed and introduced after the 1994 elections, and enough members of Congress who supported it had lost that, like President Truman, President Clinton lost the majority he needed in Congress to pass health care reform. This including advocating for greater access for individuals in racial and ethnic minority groups and in lower social-class positions who have higher morbidity and mortality rates from virtually every disease (Syme, 2008).

On March 23, 2010, President Obama signed H.R. 3590, the Patient Protection and Affordable Care Act (PPACA). A week later, on March 30, 2010, the House and Senate both approved a package of fixes, H.R. 4872, the Health Care and Education Reconciliation Act of 2010. In reviewing the table of contents of the 974-page act, there are 10 major titles, and under each title, there are many subtitles, articles, and sections. Many of the health care reform activities over the next decade target new consumer protections, improving quality and controlling costs, increasing access to affordable care, and holding insurance companies accountable. Nurses have a role in ensuring better outcomes at lower costs. However, costs and coverage are only half the equation. "Nurses still have a responsibility to advocate for health care as a basic human right and for access to an affordable package of essential health services" (Nickitas, 2011c, p. 57).

The ANA has advocated for securing meaningful health care for all Americans for decades. Since the passage of the Affordable Care Act, ANA has and will continue to focus its efforts on the regulatory process to ensure that law is implemented as it was intended.

---

CONSIDER THIS   The ANA was selected to testify at key hearings on national health insurance, amplifying nursing's voice on television to households throughout the country in advocating for comprehensive health coverage, including nursing care in all settings for all Americans.

---

(ANA, 2001), which emphasized the cost-effectiveness of using the appropriate provider in the appropriate place at the appropriate level of care. An example of this tenet was

---

### DISCUSSION POINT

What can you do to help ensure nurses are able to use all of their knowledge, skills, and experience to better help patients?

## CONCLUSIONS

What would Lillian Wald do about health care coverage for children and access to health care? What would Minerva Franklin do about racial health inequalities? What would Florence Nightingale do to elevate nursing in the policy debates? Not since 2001, when the ANA called together all the nursing specialty organizations in a Call to the Profession to begin a dialogue on collaboration and to develop Nursing's Agenda for the Future, has progress been made on speaking with one voice in the policy arena. The ANA argued that it is essential that nursing speak with one voice (ANA, 2003), but how does nursing come together to do so?

So the question for today is "What should nursing say?" At a time when the country is deeply divided along party lines, nurses must voice their concerns and speak for the clients they serve. Nurses are stakeholders in what happens in health care (access, insurance coverage, cost, research), in the workplace (quality, staffing levels, safety, scope of practice, autonomy, working conditions), in the economy (unemployment's effect on mental and physical health and access to care, funding for Medicare and Medicaid), in international trade issues (foreign nurse licensure, importation of less expensive prescription drugs), and in the environment (preventing illness caused by pollution). That is, nurses are directly affected by the outcome of countless policies that are enacted or regulated.

There are many levels of political involvement and many spheres in which nurses can be influential, both public and private. Nurses can influence policies in the workplace (both public and private) and the community (both public and private). They can also influence policy within professional organizations (private) and within the government (Mason et al., 2002). The bottom line is that they must accept a responsibility to be involved in some way.

Pierce (2004) perhaps said it best:

> For the nursing profession to flex its collective political muscle and get involved with the redesign of the nation's health care system, we have to use our leadership to get the professional organizations to think and act collaboratively and to deliver a clear and strategic message to lawmakers.
>
> As nurses, as voters, and as constituents, we must be a part of the solution. Our elected officials truly want to know what nurses think and it is our obligation as professionals and as citizens to let them know. Our patients and the American public trusts nurses and are counting on us to advocate on their behalf. (p. 115)

Per capita, the United States has the most expensive health care system in the world, yet it ranks next to last on five dimensions of a high-performance health system: quality, access, efficiency, equity, and healthy lives (Davis et al., 2007). Nurses must be involved in policy debates to ensure that health care reform addresses cost, quality, and access simultaneously and preserves the notion that health care is a right and not a privilege.

## ACKNOWLEDGMENT

I would like to thank Catherine Dodd for her knowledge and contributions on ways nurses can become political advocates for themselves and for their patients. Her work was instrumental in building the structure for this chapter.

## FOR ADDITIONAL DISCUSSION

1. Are nongovernmental and governmental politics more alike than not? If not, how do they differ? If so, how are they alike?

2. Why do you believe nursing was the first profession to eliminate segregation?

3. What are the most significant nursing issues being debated in the policy arena?

4. With such limited membership in the ANA, will nurses ever have a political power base that is representative of the size of their voting block?

*continued*

5. Why are so many nurses reluctant to become active in the political arena? Do they lack the skills to do so? The confidence? Do nurses perceive a lack of congruity between professional behavior and politics?

6. With the AMA typically being far better represented than the ANA in legislative lobbying, is nursing's risk of being dominated by medicine greater than ever?

7. How well informed are most legislators about contemporary health care and professional nursing issues?

8. What do you believe will be the next major policy issue affecting nursing to be debated in the political arena?

## REFERENCES

American Association for the History of Nursing. (2004). *Gravesites of prominent nurses: Lillian D. Wald*. Retrieved from http://www.aahn.org/gravesites/wald.html

American Nurses Association. (2001). *Nursing's agenda for health care reform*. Washington, DC: Author.

American Nurses Association. (2003). *Nursing's agenda for the future*. Washington, DC: Author.

ANA Hall of Fame: Martha Minerva Franklin. (n.d.). Retrieved from http://www.nursingworld.org/FunctionalMenuCategories/AboutANA/WhereWeComeFrom_1/HallofFame/19761982/franmm5536.aspx

American Nurses Association. (2010). *Nursing's social policy statement*. Washington, DC: Author.

Aries, N. (2011). To engage or not engage: Choices confronting nurses and other health professionals. In D. Nickitas, D. Middaugh, & N. Aries (Eds.), *Policy and politics for nurses and other health professionals* (pp. 3–24). Sudbury, MA: Jones and Bartlett.

Barstow, D. (2010, February 16). Tea Party lights fuse for rebellion on right. *New York Times*, A1.

Berman, R. (2010, July 5). Gallup: Tea Party's top concerns are debt, size of government. *The Hill*. Retrieved from http://www.thehill.com.

Block, L. E. (2008). Health policy: What it is and how it works. In C. Harrington & C. L. Estes (Eds.), *Health policy: Crisis and reform in the U.S. health care delivery system* (pp. 4–14). Sudbury, MA: Jones & Bartlett.

Crigger, N. J. (2008). Nursing ethics in an era of globalization. *Advances in Nursing Science, 24*(2), 1–18.

Daley, K. (2011a). From your ANA president: Nurses lead the way. *American Nurse Today, 6*(5), 18.

Daley, K. (2011b). Lessons in leadership. *American Nurse, 43*(3), 3.

Davis, K., Schoen, C., Schoenbaum, S. C., Doty, M. M., Holmgren, A. L., Kriss, J. L., & Shea, K. K. (2007). *Mirror, mirror on the wall: An international update on the comparative performance of American health care*. Retrieved from http://www.commonwealthfund.org/publications/publications_show.htm?doc_id=482678

Dodd, C. (2008). Play to win: Know the rules. In C. Harrington & C. Estes (Eds.), *Health policy: Crisis and reform in the U.S. health care delivery system* (pp. 15–26). Sudbury, MA: Jones & Bartlett.

Families USA. (1993). *a.s.a.p.* Washington, DC: Author.

Flanagan, L. (1976). *One strong voice*. Kansas City, MO: American Nurses Association.

Ferris, G., Davidson, S., & Perrew, P. (2005). *Political skill at work-impact on work effectiveness*. Mountain View, CA: Davies-Black.

Freeman, J. (2008). *We will be heard: Women's struggles for political power in the United States*. New York, NY: Rowman & Littlefield.

Fry, S. (1983). The social responsibilities of nursing. *Nursing Economics, 1*, 61–72.

Gallop Poll. (2011). *Public rates nursing as most honest & ethical profession*. Retrieved from http://www.gallup.com/poll/9823/public-rates-nursing-most-honest-ethical-profession.aspx

Hall-Long, B. (2009). Nursing and public policy: A tool for excellence in education, practice, and research. *Nursing Outlook, 57*(2), 78–83.

Halloran, L. (2010, February 5). What's behind the new populism? *NPR*. Retrieved from http://www.npr.org/templates/story/story.php?storyId=123137382

Hanley, B., & Falk, N. L. (2007). Policy development and analysis: Understanding the process. In: D. J. Mason, J. K. Leavitt, & M. W. Chaffee (Eds.), *Policy and politics in nursing and health care* (5th ed., pp. 75–93). St. Louis, MO: Saunders/Elsevier.

Institute of Medicine. (2011). *The future of nursing: Leading change, advancing health*. Washington, DC: National Academy of Sciences.

International Council of Nurses. (2006). *Code of ethics.* Retrieved from http://www.icn.ch/images/stories/documents/about/icncode_english.pdf

Jewish Women's Archive. (n.d.). *Exhibit: Women of valor. Lillian Wald.* Retrieved from http://jwa.org/exhibits/wov/wald/lwbio.html

Johnson & Johnson's Campaign for Nursing's Future. (2011). Retrieved from http://campaignfornursing.com/

Kalisch, B., & Kalisch, P. (1982). *Politics of nursing.* Philadelphia, PA: Lippincott Williams & Wilkins.

Kelly, M. A., Connor, A., Kun, K. E., & Salmon, M. E. (2008). Social responsibility: Conceptualization and embodiment in a school of nursing. *International Journal of Nursing Education Scholarship, 5*(1), Article 28.

Krain, J. B. (n.d.). *Lillian Wald.* Retrieved from http://www.jewishmag.co.il/51mag/wald/lillianwald.htm

Kraft, M., & Furlong, S. (2010). *Public policy-politics, analysis, and alternatives* (3rd ed.). Washington, DC: CQ Press.

Leavitt, J. (2009). Leaders in health policy: A critical role for nursing. *Nursing Outlook, 57*(2), 73–77.

Lillie-Blanton, M., & Hoffman, C. (2005). The role of health insurance coverage in reducing racial/ethnic disparities in health care. *Health Affairs, 24*(2), 398–408.

Lowi, T., & Ginsberg, B. (1998). *American Government* (5th ed.). New York, NY: Norton.

Mason, D. J., Leavitt, J. K., & Chaffee, M. W. (Eds.). (2002). *Policy and politics in nursing and health care* (4th ed.). Philadelphia, PA: Saunders.

Mason, D. J., Leavitt, J. K., & Chaffee, M. W. (Eds.). (2012). *Policy and politics in nursing and health care* (6th ed.). St. Louis, MO: Saunders/Elsevier.

Milstead, J. (2011). *Health policy and politics: A nurses guide.* (4th ed.). Sudbury, MA: Jones and Bartlett.

National Association for Home Care and Hospice. (2008). *Why the U.S. should celebrate the birthday of Lillian Wald on March 10.* Retrieved from https://www.ncsbn.org/2403.htm

National Council of the State Boards of Nursing. (2011). *NCSBN embarks on an innovative multi-site transition to practice study to examine the effects of nurse transition to practice programs on patient outcomes.* Retrieved from https://www.ncsbn.org/2403.htm

National Council of the State Boards of Nursing. (2009). *Mission and Values.* Retrieved from www.ncsbn.org

Naylor, M. D., Brooten, D., Jones, R., Lavizzo-Mourey, R., Jacobsen, B. S., Mezey, M.,…Schawartz, J. S. (1999). Comprehensive discharge planning and home follow-up of hospitalized elders: A random controlled trail. *Journal of the American Medical Association, 28*(7), 613–602.

Naylor, M. D., Brooten, D., Campbell, R., Jacobsen, B. S., Maislin, G., McCauley, K. M., & Schawartz, J. S. (2004). Transitional care of older adults hospitalized with heart failure: A random clinical trail. *Journal of the American Geriatrics Society, 52*(5), 675–684.

Nickitas, D. (2011a). Defining nursing's expanded role in health care: An interview with Donna Shalala. *Nursing Economics, 29*(1), 23.

Nickitas, D. (2011b). In D. Nickitas, D. Middaugh, N. Aries (Eds.) *Policy and Politics for nurses and other health professionals* (pp. 95). Sudbury, MA: Jones and Bartlett.

Nickitas, D. (2011c). Cost and coverage in turbulent times. *Nursing Economics, 29*(2), 57–58.

Nickitas, D. (2011d). Nurses. In D. Nickitas, D. Middaugh, & N. Aries (Eds.), *Policy and politics for nurses and other health professionals* (pp. 75–102). Sudbury, MA: Jones and Bartlett.

Online Dictionary of Social Sciences. (n.d.). *Politics.* Retrieved September 18, 2008, from http://bitbucket.icaap.org/dict.pl

Pierce, K. M. (2004). Insights and reflections of a congressional nurse detailee. *Policy, Politics & Nursing Practice, 5*(2), 113–115.

Roberston, R., & Middaugh, D. (2011). Conclusions: A policy toolkit for healthcare providers and activists. In D. Nickitas, D. Middaugh, & N. Aries (Eds.). *Policy and politics for nurses and other health professionals* (pp. 327–352). Sudbury, MA: Jones and Bartlett.

Rushefsky, M. (2008). *Public policy in the United States: At the dawn of the 21st century* (4th ed.). Armonk, NY: M. E. Sharpe.

Sabatier, P. A. (Ed.). (1999). *Theories of the policy process.* Boulder, CO: Westview.

Salmon, M., & Guisinger, V. (2007). Global migration of nurses: Managing a scarce resource. In D. J. Mason, J. K. Leavitt, & M. W. Chaffee (Eds.), *Policy and politics in nursing and health care* (5th ed., pp. 982–991). St. Louis, MO: Saunders/Elsevier.

Sanger, M. (n.d.). *Encyclopedia Britannica profiles: 300 women who changed the world.* Retrieved from http://search.eb.com/women/article-9065508

Song, A. (2011). Defining ANA-PAC's role in the political process. *American Nurse, 43*(3), 15.

Steinem, G. (2004). *Margaret Sanger.* Retrieved from http://www.time.com/time/time100/leaders/profile/sanger3.html

Syme, S. L. (2008). Reducing racial and social-class inequalities in health: The need for a new approach. *Health Affairs, 27*(24), 459.

Tossman, S. (2011). Three nurses take the lead on change. *American Nurse, 43*(1), 14–15.

Wallsten, P., & Yadron, D. (2010, September 29). Tea-party movement gathers strength. *Wall Street Journal*. Retrieved from http://online.wsj.com

Watson, J. (2008). Social justice and human caring: A model of caring science as a hopeful paradigm for moral justice and humanity. *Creative Nursing, 14*(2), 54–61.

Warner, J. R. (2003). A phenomenological approach to political competence: Stories of nurse activists. *Policy, Politics & Nursing Practice, 4*(2), 135–143.

## BIBLIOGRAPHY

Adams, J. M., Chisari, G., Ditomassi, M., & Erickson, J. I. (2011). Understanding and influencing policy: An imperative to the contemporary nurse leader. *Voice of Nursing Leadership, 9*(4), 4–7.

Benton, D. (2012, January 31). Advocating globally to shape policy and strengthen nursing influence. *Online Journal of Issues in Nursing, 17*(1), Manuscript 5. Retrieved from http://www.nursingworld.org

Califano, J. (2009). *Bending the curve requires health care reform, not just sick reform: A history lesson.* Retrieved from http://www.kaiserhealthnews.org/Columns/2009/August/081009Califano.aspx

Center on Budget and Policy Priorities. (2010). *Policy basics: Introduction to the federal budget process.* Retrieved from http://www.cbpp.org/files/3-7-03bud.pdf

Jacobi, J., Watson, S., & Restuccia, R. (2011). *Implementing health care reform at the state level: Access and care for the vulnerable populations.* Retrieved from http://www.aslme.org/media/downloadable/files/links/1/5/15.Jacobi.pdf

Maryland, M., & Gonzalez, R. (2012). Patient advocacy in the community and legislative arenas. *Online Journal of Issues in Nursing, 17*(1), Manuscript 2. doi:10.3912/OJIN.VOL17No01Mar02

Matthews, J. (2012, January 31). Role of professional organizations in advocating for the nursing profession. *Online Journal of Issues in Nursing, 17*(1), Manuscript 3. Retrieved from http://www.nursing.org

Orszag, P. (2011). How health reform can save or sink America: The case for reform and fiscal sustainability. *Foreign Affairs, 90*(4), 42–56.

Sanford, K. (2012). Overview and summary: Nurse advocates: Past, present, and future. *Online Journal of Issues in Nursing, 17*(1). doi:10.3912/OJIO.Vol17No01MarOS

Selanders, L., & Crane, P. (2012). The voice of Florence Nightingale on advocacy. *Online Journal of Issues in Nursing, 17*(1), Manuscript 1. doi:10.3912/OJIN.VolNo01Mar1

Shamian, J., & Shamian-Ellen, M. (2011). Shaping health policy: The role of nursing research-three frameworks and their application to policy development. In A. S. Hinshaw & P. A. Grady (Eds.), *Shaping health policy through nursing research* (pp. 35–51). New York, NY: Springer.

The Henry J. Kaiser Family Foundation. (2011). *The uninsured and the difference health insurance makes.* Retrieved from www.kff.org/uninsured/upload/1420-13.pdf

Tomajan, K. (2012). Advocating for nurses and nursing. *Journal of Issues in Nursing, 17*(1), Manuscript 4. doi:10.3912/OJIN.Vol17No01Mar04

Watson, J. (2008). Social justice and human caring: A model of caring science as a hopeful paradigm for moral justice and humanity. *Caring Nursing, 14*(2), 54–61.

# Chapter **24**

# Nursing's Professional Associations

Marjorie Beyers

## ADDITIONAL RESOURCES

Visit thePoint for additional helpful resources
- eBook
- Journal Articles
- WebLinks

## CHAPTER OUTLINE

## LEARNING OBJECTIVES

*The learner will be able to:*

1. Examine how early professional nursing associations such as the American Nurses Association, the National League for Nursing, the International Council of Nurses, and Sigma Theta Tau International have affected the development of nursing as a profession.

2. Describe the organizational structure of a typical professional association.

3. Explore the multiple professional associations that exist in nursing and assess them for similarity and differences in functions.

4. Describe various types of membership in professional associations, including *full, associate, affiliate, honorary, organizational, retired,* and *liaison.*

5. Explore the challenges faced by professional associations, including sustaining membership, ensuring financial resources, ensuring current information, collaborating with colleagues from other professions, and responding to the need for membership diversity.

6. Identify common sources of non-dues revenue for professional associations.

7. Explore how professional associations can use technology to interact with members and their various publics.

*continued*

8. Explore the role professional associations can assume in shaping the future culture of professional nursing.

9. Question the future viability of associations and explore how professional associations may influence the future of nursing.

10. Debate whether professional nursing associations are the appropriate venue for sustaining the profession of nursing in the future.

11. Complete a self-evaluation regarding professional association involvement and reflect on whether greater involvement is desired.

Nursing's professional associations are a vital part of the profession. In this chapter, the evolution of professional associations over time and how they affect every nurse's practice are discussed. Professional associations are discussed in relation to how they work and how they may influence the profession's future.

The *Encyclopedia of Associations* lists more than 300 national nursing associations (Harper, 2011) representing registered nurses (RNs). Nurse aides and Licensed Practical Nurses also have their associations. Nursing and Healthcare Directories can be found at http://www.nursefriendly.com/associations

> **CONSIDER THIS**  Do you know nurses or other persons who belong to their professional association? Why do they join? Do you, as a student nurse, belong to the National Student Nurses Association? What do associations offer to you?

Some of the nursing associations are international, and others have international counterparts. The American Nurses Association (ANA) is the only national association recognized by the International Council of nurses, representing all nurses in the United States. Some nursing associations represent the function of the members, such as education, administration, or clinical practice. Still others are named to represent a cultural or ethnic background, such as the National Alaska Native American Indian Nurses Association or the Black Nurses Association.

The formation of associations and ongoing work reflect economic and political trends, changing values, and turbulence in organizations and institutions, the use of technology in both health care and in communications, and unique forces such as those related to the gender, age, and employment opportunities of nurses. Nurses in the past shaped nursing and today nurses are

a significant force in shaping the future of the profession. Members have a vital role in this work.

> ## DISCUSSION POINT
>
> Why are there so many nursing associations? Is the large number of nursing associations a value or a hindrance to the profession?

Associations are typically founded to further the work of the group they represent and individuals are drawn to the association by a common cause. An important role of professional associations is to protect the public interest, as well as to protect the interests of the members. The Internal Revenue Service (IRS, 2012) officially defines an association as a group of persons banded together for a specific purpose. Wikipedia also describes associations and provides a definition (Wikipeida, n.d.). Technically, professional associations must have a written document that shows their creation. Each state, however, has its own definition of associations. Most association are nonprofit. The IRS web site contains information about the tax status of associations (see charitable and non profit organizations) (IRS, 2012).

Associations generally have a mission, philosophy, vision, and strategic plan. Many nursing associations advance the profession by adopting a code of ethics, developing and updating the scope of practice, standards of behavior and practice, and definitions of competency important to protect the public. To serve their members, associations must remain viable to members and to the public that uses and supports their work. The common cause that brings members together to form and sustain an association must also be valued by the public served by the members. Each association has a valued history, and many have unique traditions. Membership and certification are used to recognize individuals who meet the criteria for being an active, competent member of the association.

Associations provide services and resources for nurses in the particular area of practice represented. Members and, sometimes, nonmembers have access to these services and resources, including education, conventions, annual meetings, communications, careers, mentoring, leadership development, and opportunities to become involved in shaping the association, the practice, and the profession. Some associations have research agendas. Another function of associations is to advocate for the practice of nursing with the public, government, and within health care. Major categories of professional association services are shown in Box 24.1. Leadership development is fostered for volunteer leaders through positions as elected offices or by participation in projects, committees, or other initiatives designed to sustain the association and to further the work of nurses.

## THE PUBLIC AND PROFESSIONAL ASSOCIATIONS

Professional associations serve members with a common bond and are formed, in part, to enhance the professional status of members. The public depends on associations as a way to reach members, to learn about practice, or to become informed about matters within

---

**BOX 24.1 MAJOR CATEGORIES OF PROFESSIONAL ASSOCIATION SERVICES**

**Professional development,** including opportunities for networking; publications such as newsletters, journals, and multimedia materials; careers and educational programs; conferences and conventions; information and resources such as tools and issue papers; and credentialing and socialization

**Advancing the profession** through activities, including research, standards of practice, designations, and productivity, and a code of ethics for the profession

**Policy and advocacy,** including government relationships, liaisons with related and influential groups, legislative advocacy to provide the resources and support for professional practice, and the appropriate environment for practice

---

the association's expertise. The mutual interdependency of professional associations and the public is grounded in trust. The professional association, through the collective work of its members, is expected to define and promote standards of behavior and practice.

---

CONSIDER THIS  Given that the public expects the association to be informed about practice, why do some nurses choose to become members of their professional association, whereas others do not seek membership?

---

## Disseminators of Information

As a source of information about standards of practice and qualifications of persons engaged in the practice, associations are viewed as credible sources of information about services needed by the public. They advocate for the public served, identifying and resolving issues surrounding practice, which can be raised by members, leaders, or the public. Effective associations serve members and protect the public safety and welfare by establishing, revising, or updating relevant standards, laws, rules and regulations. Practices that are harmful or no longer useful are changed or eliminated. Increasingly associations cooperate with other groups in these actions. Associations support or conduct research and participate in programs to advance the knowledge of the profession and to produce evidence used in professional decision making.

## Advocacy, Integrity, and Competency

Nurses, as members, have expectations of their professional nursing associations. It can be speculated that the large number of nursing associations is related to diversity within nursing education and practice. Associations advocate for their members. Some view this advocacy role as protecting the "property rights" of members to practice their profession. A counterview is that associations enhance the ability of members to fulfill their professional role with integrity. New associations reflect the needs of a group of nurses who value the potential to identify issues and resolve problems affecting their practice, to promote professional development, and to provide services useful to members. Joining a professional nursing association enables nurses both to provide input and to use the services that the association provides to enhance their ability to practice with integrity and competency. Associations serve as forums for communication with consumers, business, industry, and government on matters affecting nursing and nursing practice. Professional nursing associations are an integral part of the culture of nursing.

---

### DISCUSSION POINT

Could one nursing association represent all the diverse interests of nurses, or is having focused multiple nursing associations more effective to promote the profession and to protect the public?

---

### DISCUSSION POINT

What is the rationale for the professional association's continuing existence?

---

## THE GROWTH OF PROFESSIONAL ASSOCIATIONS

Nursing associations, like other types of professional associations, evolved over hundreds of years. Their history reflects the natural tendency of people to join together for a common purpose, the development of commerce and industry, and the political and societal realities of achieving public recognition and prestige. The impetus for the development of many professional associations of all types was and continues to be public safety and welfare. The growth of professional associations reflects the work of dedicated and energetic leaders who participated in founding and sustaining these associations over time, responding to changes in society, the economic and political environment and the often chaotic progress toward recognition of a given profession by society.

---

CONSIDER THIS  The professions of law, medicine, and the clergy were among the first to have professional associations, followed over time by a multitude of other groups.

---

Professional associations began to take shape during the Industrial Revolution, which was characterized by the emergence of trade associations, guilds, and professional associations. These associations were a vehicle used to deal with changes in society. Essentially, these groups provided for recognition; people were concerned about the quality of the goods and services they consumed, and "professionals" were seeking public recognition for their work. Professional associations recognized and met both of these needs.

## THE FORMATION AND WORK OF NURSING'S EARLY PROFESSIONAL ASSOCIATIONS

Associations have been integral to world cultures and societies, as evidenced by lore, historical texts, historical novels, and family legend. In the late 18th and 19th centuries, associations flourished and generally served the interests of the elite—the landowners, wealthy merchants, and other influential people. A wealth of information on "secret societies" and private clubs illustrates how people with common interests and affluence joined together to set their agendas. The growing number of scholars, trade groups, and individuals with common economic interests used associations to advance their work. Nursing associations have their roots in this movement, which was closely tied to the emancipation of women. Nursing leaders, driven by a common cause, clear direction for action, and passion for achieving the goals used associations to advance the profession for the benefit of the public and of nurses (Fenwick, 1901). Among the early associations that currently exist in new iterations are the National League for Nursing (NLN), the ANA, the International Council of Nurses, and Sigma Theta Tau International, Honor Society of Nursing (STTI).

### National League for Nursing

The NLN began as the Society of Superintendents of Training Schools for Nurses, formed in 1893. Renamed the National League for Nursing Education in 1912, a new association, the National League for Nursing, was formed in 1952 as a result of the reorganization of nursing's major professional associations (Henderson & Nite, 1978, p. 73; Spaulding & Notter, 1965, p. 335). Box 24.2 provides information about the NLN.

### American Nurses Association

The ANA began with a convening of alumnae groups in the 1880s. These alumnae groups adopted the constitution and bylaws for the organization, the Nurses

## BOX 24.2 MEMBERSHIP STRUCTURE OF THE NATIONAL LEAGUE FOR NURSING

The National League for Nursing was formed in 1893 as the American Society of Superintendents of Training Schools for Nursing, for the purpose of establishing and maintaining a universal standard of training.

- Named the National League for Nursing Education in 1912
- Renamed the National League for Nursing in 1952
- Established the National League for Nursing Accrediting Commission in 1997

**Mission**

The National League for Nursing promotes excellence in nursing education to build a strong and diverse nursing workforce to advance the nation's health.

The National League for Nursing implements its mission guided by four dynamic and integrated core values that permeate the organization and are reflected in its work:

- *Caring:* promoting health, healing, and hope in response to the human condition
- *Integrity:* respecting the dignity and moral wholeness of every person without conditions or limitation
- *Diversity:* affirming the uniqueness of and differences among persons, ideas, values, and ethnicities
- *Excellence:* creating and implementing transformative strategies with daring ingenuity

**Global/Diversity Initiatives**

With the new international realities of migration dissolving borders between countries, advanced communication technology, global health care needs, and a worldwide nursing shortage, preparing an ethnically and racially diverse workforce of faculty, researchers, and scholars to mentor future nurses and nurse educators is a critical priority.

**Membership**

Membership is open to all individuals, education agencies, health organizations, and other agencies committed to advancing excellence in nursing education. Constituent leagues, state level associations are affiliated with the National League for Nursing.

*Source:* National League for Nursing. (2012). *Homepage.* Retrieved October, 2012, from http://nln.org/

---

Associated Alumnae of the United States and Canada, in 1897. In 1911, the association was renamed the ANA. The ANA began its collective bargaining activities in the 1940s. Box 24.3 provides information about the ANA.

## Sigma Theta Tau International

STTI is an example of an association that was founded by six students at Indiana University who would probably be awed by the way the association has grown to represent nurses worldwide as presented in Box 24.4.

## International Council of Nurses

The early development of the ANA and the NLN was influenced by the women's movement at the end of the 19th and beginning of the 20th century. The June 1899 meeting of the International Congress of Women, held in London, was particularly notable for nurses. At this meeting, nurses from around the world founded the International Council of Nurses (ICN) to foster development of nurses throughout the world. The ANA is both a charter member and constituent member of the ICN.

## BOX 24.3   MEMBERSHIP STRUCTURE OF THE AMERICAN NURSES ASSOCIATION

The ANA is the only full-service professional organization representing RNs in the United States. The ANA advances the nursing profession by fostering high standards of nursing practice, promoting the rights of nurses in the workplace, projecting a positive and realistic view of nursing, and by lobbying the Congress and regulatory agencies on health care issues affecting nursing and the public.

**MEMBERS**

**INDIVIDUAL MEMBERS**

• ANA and state membership (formerly full membership)

• ANA-only membership (formerly direct membership)

• E-membership web-only virtual membership (formerly associate membership)

**CONSTITUENT MEMBERS**

There are 54 constituent nurses associations, which include the 50 states, the District of Columbia, Guam, the Virgin Islands, and the Federal Nurses Association.

**ORGANIZATIONAL AFFILIATES (A LISTING OF THESE ORGANIZATIONS CAN BE FOUND ON THE nursingworld.org WEBSITE)**

**SUBSIDIARIES**

• American Nurses Credentialing Center

• American Nurses Foundation

• American Academy of Nursing

*Source:* American Nurses Association. (2012). *Homepage.* Retrieved November 20, 2011, from http://nursingworld.org/; *The American Nurse, the Official Publication of the American Nurses Association,* September/October 2011 *43*(5).

## SHAPING THE NURSING PROFESSION

Nurse leaders in the United States, led by the National Associated Alumnae of the United States and Canada and the Society of Superintendents of Training Schools for Nurses, created the template for nursing's development in the United States. The three main prongs for development of the profession were uniform education, standards of practice, and regulation of the profession. Working with ICN members, nurses in the United States worked to achieve a legal basis for nursing in every country throughout the world. Nursing was not alone in this effort. Many other professional groups were also seeking licensure in the United States and the District of Columbia. From 1903 to 1923, these groups worked to achieve passage of a Nurse Practice Act in all of the states in the United States.

CONSIDER THIS   How does the early work to establish professional competence and licensure in the early 20th century affect your practice today?

Nursing and nurses continue to benefit from this work to establish nurse practice acts, mandatory licensure, the development of standards for nursing education and practice, and the promulgation of nursing's *Code of Ethics.*

## BOX 24.4    MEMBERSHIP STRUCTURE OF STTI

Established in 1922 by six students from the Indiana University Training School for Nurses in Indianapolis, Indiana, the honor society's charter members were Mary Tolle Wright, Edith Moore Copeland, Marie Hippensteel Lingernan, Dorothy Garrious Adams, Elizabeth Russell Belford, Elizabeth McWilliams Miller, and Ethel Palmer Clarke, advisor.

The STTI Foundation of Nursing was created in 1993. Its purpose is active fundraising and conscientious stewardship to promote honor society programs and initiatives.

### Organizational Mission

The mission of the STTI is to support the learning, knowledge, and professional development of nurses committed to making a difference in health worldwide.

### Society Vision

The vision of the STTI is to create a global community of nurses who lead in using knowledge, scholarship, service, and learning to improve the health of the world's people.

### Membership

Baccalaureate and graduate student nurses who have demonstrated excellence in scholarship and nurse leaders who demonstrate exceptional achievements in nursing are invited to become members.

### Nursing Knowledge International

Founded in 2002, Nursing Knowledge International is a not-for-profit, 501(c)3 subsidiary of STTI, which provides evidence-based knowledge solutions, offering free and fee-based content developed by organizations viewed as leaders around the world.

### Mission

The mission of Nursing Knowledge International is to help nurses help others. This is accomplished by providing products and services that serve the global community of nurses in its pursuit of health care knowledge, career advancement, research and continued development of the nursing profession. Nursing Knowledge International assists the nursing profession to improve the health and education of patients and the communities in which nurses practice, lead, teach, and conduct research.

*Source:* Sigma Theta Tau International, Honor Society of Nursing. (2011). *Homepage.* Retrieved November 20, 2011, from http://www.nursingsociety.org/default.aspx

In addition to the ANA and the NLN, several other nursing associations were formed by the 1940s. Nurse leaders, cognizant of the role of associations to serve nurses, commissioned Raymond Rich Associates to study what nurses needed from their professional associations. Changes in society and in health care delivery were considered. The *Rich Report* recommendations led to reorganization of the professional nursing associations formed between 1892 and 1949 to create larger associations with more assets and capability to advance the profession. Each association took on a mission that complimented the whole

(Henderson & Nite, 1978; "Raymond Rich Associates Report," 1946).

### DISCUSSION POINT

Imagine a world without any professional nursing associations. In this world, how are standards of education and practice, regulation of the practice, and advancement of nursing knowledge achieved?

## DEVELOPMENT OF SPECIALTY NURSING PROFESSIONAL ASSOCIATIONS

During the 20th century, a number of specialty associations were formed. The American Association of Industrial Nurses originating about 1915 is one of the oldest specialty nursing professional associations. Among the associations formed in the 1950s were the American Association of Nurse Anesthetists, established in 1952; the Association of Operating Room Nurses, formed in 1957; the American College of Nurse Midwifery, formed in 1955; the National Association for Practical Nurse Education and Service (NAPNES), established in 1941;

the National Federation of Licensed Practical Nurses, formed in 1949; and both the Catholic and Lutheran Nursing Groups (Spaulding & Notter, 1965). Box 24.5 illustrates landmark events that have affected the present.

## Nursing Professional Associations in the Last 50 Years of the 20th Century

Lacking definitive research, it can be speculated that factors leading to the proliferation of nursing associations were the development of specialization in health care following World War II, the growing number of nurses, and the expansion of specialty practice in hospitals and

---

### BOX 24.5    EVOLUTION OF NURSING PROFESSIONAL ASSOCIATIONS

- **1893:** American Society of Superintendents of Training Schools for Nurses was chartered.

- **1897:** Nurses Associated Alumnae of the United States and Canada—previously the Nurses Associated Alumnae Association and forerunner to the American Nurses Association (ANA)—was chartered.

- **1899:** International Council of Nurses was chartered.

- **1900:** *The American Journal of Nursing* was founded: renamed the *American Nurse Today*. Continues to be the official ANA journal now published by HealthCom Media.

- **1908:** National Association of Colored Graduate Nurses was founded (became part of the ANA in 1951, making the ANA one of the first national associations to declare membership open to all ethnic groups).

- **1911:** The ANA was formed from the Nurses Associated Alumnae of the United States and Canada.

- **1912:** The National League for Nursing Education was formed from Society of Superintendents of Training Schools for Nurses and functions of other associations.

- **1915:** The American Association of Industrial Nurses was originated, which is one of the oldest specialty nursing professional associations.

- **1922:** Sigma Theta Tau was founded.

- **1952:** The American Association of Nurse Anesthetists was established.

- **1955:** American Nurses Foundation was established. American College of Nurse Midwifery was established.

- **1957:** The Association of Operating Room Nurses was established.

*Source:* Websites for the representative associations; Spaulding, E. K., & Notter, L. (1965). *Professional nursing.* Philadelphia, PA: Lippincott.

*Note:* These associations continue to be viable today although most have been renamed and/or reorganized or reformed.

diversity in nursing practice. By the second half of the 20th century, nurses formed associations as an accepted way for all types of professional-, business-, and industry-related groups to gain recognition and acceptance of their work by the public. In nursing, diversity sometimes refers to the increasingly different opportunities to practice or to be employed. This latter diversity is considered by some to be a reason for so many specialty associations.

Some nurses were and continue to be concerned about how to bring the many nursing associations together to strengthen nursing and to unify the voice of nursing. Virginia Henderson observed the "proliferation of organizations is so marked that only through some federation of organizations could unity be achieved" (Henderson & Nite, 1978, p. 73).

---

### DISCUSSION POINT

How important are relationships among professional associations within health care to the work of nurses in health care?

---

## THE VITAL ROLE OF MEMBERS

Nurses join professional associations because it conveys professional status and a willingness to uphold the standards of the profession. The professional association provides benefits that are valued in today's culture of quality and patient safety. The benefits include certification, formal and continuing education, and participation in community or professional activities. Résumés often include a section for "professional development" or "professional accomplishments." Health care consumers now have technological resources to check professional credentials and performance or reputation when seeking services. Membership may serve as a seal of approval or as a mark of professionalism.

Nurses who want to participate in their professional associations have many opportunities for leadership development within associations as members of task forces that accomplish much of the work of associations and as members of committees and groups that work to carry out the mission of the association. In addition, they can serve as experts who inform the association about trends in practice, changes in competencies, and other aspects of the practice role. Members have great influence in the direction associations set for their work.

To be an effective member, one must know about the association, understand the issues and concerns the association faces, keep informed about new events and happenings, participate in association programs and projects, and contribute to the association through volunteer activities.

The first step is the decision to join an association. A self-evaluation regarding professional association involvement is given in Box 24.6. Once a decision is made to join an association, members must then decide their level of involvement in the selected association. Opportunities include participating in meetings, conventions, and educational programs or using products and services. Nurses wanting more involvement may participate in projects or programs. Some nurses seek appointment to committees or a leadership role, and a few serve as officers, committee chairs, spokespersons, or other type of action. Ensuring trust between the association and members also requires that associations identify, select, and elect leaders capable of visioning the future and leading the association.

Associations increasingly use the cyberspace vehicles to engage members in activities important to member

---

### BOX 24.6 SELF-EVALUATION: PROFESSIONAL ASSOCIATION INVOLVEMENT

- Do you belong to one or more professional associations in nursing or in other areas?

- Do you participate in activities or use services of professional nursing associations? Do you ever visit the websites? Do you use the Internet to learn more about nursing or related topics? Do you use the social media components of professional nursing associations?

- Do you subscribe to e-news provided by professional associations or by groups with similar interests?

- Do you attend meetings, conventions, or educational programs?

- Do you behave as a loyal member by being informed regarding issues?

- Do you share your opinions and concerns with leaders?

recruitment and retention, such as participating in surveys for member input, selecting leaders, and interactive activities such as blogging, sharing information, and networking. Recruitment and retention of members is guided by member input. Most associations routinely survey members to learn why they joined the association, what motivates their continued membership, what type of programs and services they need to support and advance their practice, and whether their expectations of the association are being met. Such surveys inform association leaders in the process of strategic planning. Being informed about the survey results helps associations respond to member needs and values. Many associations now reach out to former members to learn why they discontinued their membership and what factors would influence their return to full membership in the association.

Members seek value from professional associations and have a role to ensure that the association has the capability to produce that value. Typically nursing professional associations are voluntary, not-for-profit organizations formed to advance the profession. The key relationships of these associations are between and among members and between the association and external groups such as other nursing associations, related health care associations, and the public. The following section presents key aspects of associations important to volunteer members who are active in associations.

## THE ORGANIZATION OF AN ASSOCIATION

Associations are legal entities. The organizational structure of associations embodies volunteer leadership and, depending on the size and resources, paid staff to manage the association's business. The size of the association influences the mix of staff and volunteer involvement. Larger associations typically have more staff structure than smaller associations. Together, volunteer leaders and staff manage the business of the association, work with members to identify issues, develop positions and insights about the issues for public discussion, conduct meetings, engage members in forming and adopting resolutions that affect practice, plan and provide programs and services, and are accountable to the members.

> CONSIDER THIS   Member involvement is critical to maintaining relevant agendas for associations. Has anyone you know become involved in associations?

Associations continually work to sustain sufficient numbers of members to represent their interests and influence within the profession and in the public arena. Monitoring membership numbers, trends in membership, and member demographics are essential. Websites, social media, and other vehicles are used to communicate with members to provide current information and resources. Some sites are interactive and provide opportunities for give-and-take about the profession and proposed or needed changes. Maintaining interaction with members is more complex for associations with chapters or other forms of local or regional divisions that may be separate but related associations. In this situation, the interaction has two focal points—the local association and the member.

Most associations establish membership requirements in keeping with their mission to define eligibility and types of membership rights and responsibilities. Traditional types of membership categories may include *full, associate, affiliate, honorary, organizational, retired,* and *liaison.* Generally, full members have access to all programs and services and can vote. Associate members and affiliates might have access to selected programs and services at member cost. Honorary members are selected and recognized for their contributions to the association and to the profession. Liaison members might have access to information but often have limited member privileges. Some associations have dual membership for local and national branches. Some have organizational members with missions tied into the core functions of the association. Membership categories evolve over time and are usually tied to the association's needs and to the association's public agenda to foster working partnerships with companies and related businesses with mutual concerns and interests. Boxes 24.4 to 24.6 identify types of membership for three professional nursing associations.

> CONSIDER THIS   Associations achieve power that is more than the sum of members, but they depend on collective action of members and respected leaders to gain recognition and influence.

Because most associations are not-for-profit organizations and are eligible for tax-exempt status, they must carefully separate the not-for-profit activities from revenue or for-profit ventures. Associations do pay tax on their for-profit ventures. There are different types of tax-exempt codes that determine what the association may or may not do, such as accepting grants and becoming involved in political campaigns, to retain its tax-exempt status. Associations may create separate organizations such as foundations for these purposes. Leaders must keep abreast of changes in tax codes to keep associations up to date.

The Internal Revenue Service provides information about criteria for each of the different types of tax-exempt status (Internal Revenue Service, 2012). Generally, nursing professional associations have 501(c)(3) status, which includes religious, charitable, educational, scientific, and literary associations or those with selected social missions. Labor organizations engaged in educational activities to improve conditions of work and to improve products and efficiency have the 501(c)(5) designation. Tax-exempt status generally prohibits involvement in political action and campaigning, but allows associations to engage in lobbying or advocacy related to their exempt purposes (Internal Revenue Service, 2012). Many states also have requirements for registration by associations to maintain their tax-exempt status. Not-for-profit organizations and associations are increasingly scrutinized. Because criteria for associations are periodically revised, it is important to follow changes, which can be found at the IRS website.

Bylaws establish the governance structure, including board membership, committees and meetings, and staff accountabilities. Governance responsibilities are set forth in by-laws and sometimes in job descriptions. Board members are stewards of the association, and their functions typically include oversight of performance, including audits, decision making regarding membership eligibility, dues structure, policy, strategic direction, budget approval, and board development. Accountability of the board for keeping the association's bylaws up to date, ensuring financial stability with appropriate investment plans and budgets, and developing and implementing the strategic plan for the work of the association is shared with the staff.

The mission and goals of the association affect member eligibility. Nursing associations range from the most exclusive membership to the most inclusive membership. STTI and the American Academy of Nursing are examples of exclusive honor societies or associations that limit membership to RNs selected through an established process. Some nursing associations limit membership to RNs with credentials in a specialty field of practice. Others like state nurses associations limit membership to RNs. Increasingly, some associations are broadening their membership to include professionals with a common interest. Some associations deal with internal conflict of interest by forming subsidiaries or sections dedicated to a specific purpose.

Members of the association are responsible to be informed about the association's activities and to participate in keeping the association up to date. Nursing associations, like other organizations, are dynamic and influenced by internal and external forces. Over time, many associations undergo structural changes, renaming, or reorganization to keep up to date. For example, by 2000, the ANA had restructured the organization in response to member perceptions about internal conflict within the ANA. To retrieve the most recent information about ANA, please visit the ANA website now accessible online as ANA.org. Also can access ANA by using Nursingworld.org.

Like many businesses, nursing associations may also merge with others, form alliances with associations and groups with similar purposes, or change their mission and focus. As nurses fill positions in related health care fields, they often join associations relevant to the new field and may develop new arrangements to bridge nursing and the expertise in the related field. As practice changes, some associations are either finding new partners for collaboration or expanding membership eligibility to practitioners in other fields. Nurses may also be engaged in health care organizations their employers belong to, joining in innovations and best practices as members of the health care teams. Members may choose to belong to multidisciplinary associations as part of their employment and to belong to their selected nursing associations as part of their professional identity.

---

**DISCUSSION POINT**

Will the majority of professional health-related associations begin to merge and partner in significant ways in the next 20 years? If so, what is the potential effect on the nursing profession?

# CHALLENGES FOR CONTEMPORARY PROFESSIONAL ASSOCIATIONS IN NURSING

Key among the future challenges nursing professional associations face are sustaining and increasing membership, financing association programs and services, keeping information current, and changing practices to adapt to or shape nursing in a complex global environment. Perhaps the greatest challenge is preparing for an unknown future.

## Membership

Membership is a particular challenge in a world increasingly dominated by cyberspace. A pertinent question for associations is "how does an association use technology to ensure the continued valuing of membership in the professional association?" Many of the services formerly provided exclusively by associations are now available to nurses through the Internet, which may be perceived as competition for nursing associations. Entrepreneurs have found the critical mass of nurses and employers of nurses to be customers for their web-based products and services. Nurses can access newsletters and other publications, informational materials, chat rooms, message boards, and other venues to interact with colleagues. Some of these resources are short lived, whereas others tend to have longer life spans. Given all of the resources available in today's world, why do nurses need professional associations? Do professional nursing associations provide a way for nurses to engage in use of social media for blogging and interaction about matters important to nurses who have much in common in their practice?

> ### DISCUSSION POINT
>
> With all of the available resources for information and interaction, why do nurses need or why should they value professional associations?

Another membership challenge for associations is finding ways to meet the needs of diverse members. Associations must work to understand the motivation of people from various worksites and from various generations of nurses. Similarities between early nursing leaders and emerging leaders revolve around advancing the profession and therefore the members' practice. McKee and McKee (2008) considered passion to be the foundation for effective action in associations. Both early and present nursing leaders have passion and focus to accomplish the association's mission and share the importance of a sound strategic plan based on a vision of the future to make this vision real to members and to the public.

> **CONSIDER THIS** Conventional wisdom derived from previous studies indicates that there are "joiners" and "nonjoiners," but the reality is that the majority of RNs are not dues-paying members of one or more professional associations. There are more than 3 million nurses, yet membership in nursing professional associations ranges from 5,000 to almost 200,000.

Associations need members. The association's credibility and influence are related to the numbers and representation of its members. Does the association actually represent the field? Most associations work to attract eligible members through membership campaigns, aggressive marketing, and member-to-member interactions. Some associations strive to increase membership by changing eligibility requirements, taking care to gain member input and support for the changes. Many associations are broadening their eligibility requirements to attract more members. Associations need members to serve members and to be influential in practice and effective in public relations. The integrity of associations is threatened when membership numbers decline.

Some experts argue that professional associations have declining membership because they tend to be traditional, bureaucratic organizations that are preoccupied with sustaining the status quo, which tends to limit the capability to relate to changing member needs. The American Society of Association Executives (ASAE) serves leaders of member associations. Among the services provided are studies of the future, publications, association assessment and recommendations, and current information about matters related to association viability and management. Association 990, for example, provides all types of associations with benchmarking data (http://www.asaecenter.org/). Some doomsday predictors see the end of the association. The ASAE, however, envisions viable associations as essential to professional life and urges associations to develop realistic plans for a new future. In addition to futures studies and visioning materials, the association provides web-based information about how to meet future challenges (ASAE, 2012).

In a changing world, one expects increasing diversity from all sources—ethnic, gender, age, geographic location, type of function or specialty, and others. Each nursing association is challenged to relate its programs and services to a diverse membership. Many members value the traditions and rituals of their associations and enjoy the heritage and past practices of the association. Other members may seek the new and different and be drawn to nontraditional programs, services, and events. Most people in all age groups tend to seek community, colleagues, and support as well as ways to balance personal and professional life, using different modes of interaction.

## Finance

Financing the association is a long-standing concern. Dues are a base of financing. The number of members often affects an association's capability to partner with others or to benefit from support from others. Because member dues are a frequent issue, many professional nursing associations keep dues stable and charge for programs and services which are useful to the practice and which can be paid for by members or by others. Some associations have begun to partner in sharing services and products. Many seek vendors to participate in or support new programs and services, including web-based programs and interactive venues. It can be expected that associations will continue to develop sources of revenue, often finding unlikely partners with businesses that provide services or with industries, groups, or coalitions that may share a common interest in health care or a specific issue.

Sources of financing for associations include investments, fees for publications, services, (often with lower rates for members), major events such as conventions and educational programs. Advertising fees for careers, jobs, and promotions on websites and in journals and participation of vendors in meetings and conventions are another source of revenue. Development of foundations and solicitation of funding for member services is yet another approach, as is embarking on earned revenue ventures. The technology required in the current environment is often a major expenditure for associations but an essential one if the association is to be successful now and in the future. Seeking creative ways to finance these essential changes requires creativity and innovation.

Continued association effectiveness requires that members and leaders explore and pursue sources of funding and projects carefully. Decisions should be based on the mission, vision, values, strategic goals, and focused purpose of any activity. Retaining trust of members and the public is essential, especially in a turbulent environment. This trust is the core of any membership organization and is critical to effective advocacy and legislation. Valued as one of the most important services that associations provide for members and nonmembers, advocacy and legislation do not produce revenues. Maintaining a balance between emphasis on revenue-producing activities and essential advocacy is yet another challenge for associations.

### DISCUSSION POINT

What business approaches would be most effective for professional nursing associations to ensure continuation of essential services and to develop useful innovations?

## Communication: The Short Life Cycle of Information

Associations have historically been valued for their thoughtful and reliable communications on important matters requiring expertise, peer review, and testing for reliability. This professional communication is threatened by two sources. One is the increasingly short life cycle of knowledge, which may tax the association's capability to maintain up-to-date information. Another is the increasing accessibility to knowledge on the Internet. People have multiple sources for information. They also have high expectations for rapid communication, immediate feedback, prompt resolution of problems and issues, and customization of information.

Websites, online directories, chat rooms, message boards, social media, links, webinars, and other Internet venues and online resources are now used to facilitate member interaction online. Some associations use the web as well as print media to share proceedings of meetings and conventions. Methods used to disseminate information influence the way knowledge is produced and packaged. To incorporate technology in their work, associations often require large capital expenditures for research and development, costly production and staff training, outsourcing, or the addition of more staff.

Many associations continue to offer choices for print or web-based communications.

In an era of instant messaging, on-the-spot global reporting, and unfettered transmittal of information, associations are challenged to keep up with ever-changing communication strategies. Technology is a tool. It might change communication modes, but it does not change the importance of involving members to provide input and review and to ensure reliability in issue papers, educational materials, and increasingly evidence-based practice. Generating new knowledge and managing instant transmission of knowledge are important for associations to retain their position as expert sources of knowledge.

Members will seek the most convenient, reliable source of information. As members increasingly have access to communications from many sources, it is possible that some nurses may find these new sources to be just as or more effective than their association and may drop their membership. Those who have successfully used a search engine to rapidly and independently obtain reliable information on a multitude of topics may also be open to finding new networks with immediate entry that do not entail paying dues or attending to the requirements of professional associations for membership.

### DISCUSSION POINT

How will associations looking to the future balance traditional and evolving practices to meet members with diverse priorities, ways of accomplishing work and values? Do traditional rules of order, procedures, and protocol have a place in the association of today and the future?

## Changes in Nursing Practice

Nursing practice is changing. Many nurses now participate in multidisciplinary care teams. Their practice colleagues are more diverse. Their practice issues now extend beyond the nursing component of care, and they value networking with team members from a variety of disciplines. Chat rooms and new types of affinity groups and even new associations are forming around issues and topics of common concern that go beyond a given profession. The American Association of Critical Care

Nurses recognized this phenomenon and expanded their membership beyond nurses. also offers membership to health organizations with a nursing component.

### CONSIDER THIS    Associations of the future are challenged to respond to the complex issues of multidisciplinary practice and issues surrounding the new environment for practice.

This challenge involves concurrently supporting the domain of nursing practice and interprofessional interchange in a straightforward manner. Multidisciplinary groups now work together to deal with issues and resolve problems they experience with regard to today's integrated management and clinical systems, regulation, and legislation and concern for quality. They are joining in research. Will focus on multidisciplinary teams lead to merging of professional associations so that new, multidisciplinary associations are developed? Nursing's professional associations are challenged to deal directly with the new reality of partnerships, alliances, membership eligibility, and services as evidence-based practice and collaboration prevail. Some nurses prefer nurse-designated associations and others prefer associations that focus on the reality of their practice. Some nurses join multiple associations.

As society and nursing practice change, so do nurses' preferences for networking. Networking through meetings and conferences continues to be a mainstay of associations. Meeting colleagues, listening to respected leaders, and exchanging business cards are networking devices related to educational programs, conventions, and association gatherings. Either as follow-up or independently, the Internet allows nurses to exchange ideas and meet colleagues at any time through a computer, without travel expenses. Some associations, anticipating that networking practices change the way people communicate, are now incorporating interactive Internet communication and Internet resources in their member services. Will members continue to value the association for personal contacts, or will they be drawn to the increasing number of websites for this interaction and communication? Will members want to come to meetings, when they can review the proceedings online? Will they want informal groups and small convening's along with Internet access?

Association literature suggests that associations must become more flexible and more integrated to accommodate anticipated changes in member preferences. In the new environment, distinction among official meetings, conferences, and journals (all traditional marks of an effective association) is often blurred by instant communication and rapid exchange of information. Associations find that they have less control over communication and intellectual knowledge in the cyberspace environment.

To remain viable, associations must focus on understanding member needs, on balancing traditional attitudes and practices with contemporary ways of managing and interacting, and on prioritizing the use of resources. As society changes and as nursing roles change and expand, member needs will change. Balancing current programs and services with emerging expectations involves establishing a new way of approaching the business of associations. Some associations are enlisting participation of members with particular expertise to create the vision and plan for the future. Others are reaching out to other associations to share learning and to fill in gaps. Many associations have already begun to refocus services, becoming brokers for communication, mentoring, and professional dialogue.

The new demands on nursing's professional associations are beginning to change the perspective of what constitutes a "competitor." Previously, competitors have been other nursing and practice-related associations. Competitors, instead of having name recognition and elegant structure, may be flexible, open to experimenting with new approaches, and focused on member loyalty to services rather than to associations. Members and association leaders are now challenged to remain focused on their mission, their membership, and their services to make wise decisions about how to use and shape their resources for now and the future.

---

### DISCUSSION POINT

What should professional nursing associations do now to better understand networking, the motivation to network, and methods for effective networking? What steps should professional nursing associations take to keep pace with changing networking needs of members?

---

## Diversity

As the population becomes increasingly diverse, associations are challenged to ensure that their membership is representative of the cultural diversity of members. Representation of current and potential members is a strategic imperative. Definitions of diversity include age, gender, ethnicity, race, physical ability, religion, socioeconomic status, and geographic distribution.

Outreach to potential members to increase the association's member diversity may appear on the surface to be a simple task, but often it is complex. Staff and volunteer leadership, member involvement, programs, and services often need to be changed or adapted to reflect the diversity of the membership. For some associations, movement toward greater diversity is a giant step, whereas for others it is a natural evolution. Some of the strategies commonly used by professional associations to increase diversity are shown in Box 24.7.

---

### BOX 24.7   STRATEGIES FOR ACHIEVING DIVERSITY IN PROFESSIONAL ASSOCIATIONS

- Governing boards' commitment to diversity demonstrated in behaviors
- Allocation of funds to support activities to increase diversity
- Policy statements encompassing the vision and goals for diversity
- Goals and objectives for achieving diversity in the association's strategic plan
- Materials and tools to promote diversity among members
- Staff selection and staff development to promote diversity
- Management practices to promote involvement of diverse staff in all activities
- Outreach to diverse groups to gain support and mentors for diversity
- Evaluation and measurement of objectives to increase diversity

---

## THE ASSOCIATION FOR THE FUTURE

A hallmark of associations is the pattern used to elect officers, develop agendas, study problems and issues, obtain member responses to findings and recommendations, and transmit the information to members and to the public. How will associations in the future play a role in leading change as cultures, societal, economic, and political structures and mores evolve? Clearly, technology, the increasing complexity of issues, innovation, and societal changes are forces that currently and futuristically affect professional associations. Associations now and will continue to be challenged to be relevant to changing member needs. Those associations that remain understandable to members and dedicated to meeting members' needs will find ways to implement innovations while upholding their values. The relevant associations will be the ones that are most likely to survive in the face of generational gaps and changing values.

## Reinvention for Relevance

To remain relevant, it is predicted that many associations will recreate themselves to be viable organizations in a rapidly changing world. These recreated associations will be characterized by the ability to identify and resolve issues with a short life cycle and to change from a structured control and command pattern to become flexible organizations capable of meeting demands in a changing world. The culture and work of the association may change dramatically to reflect emerging cultures of work and of the profession, as well as changes in organizations (Principled Innovation, 2011). Most associations now participate in some form of social media to interact with and to draw members. Immediate access to information that can be shaped by people outside and inside the association is valued.

## Culture of the Future

Associations are part of nursing's culture, which is shaped through relationships, shared traits, and common purpose to achieve unity. Associations that build trust and communication among members are capable of defining ways to move the agenda, achieve support toward change, and have the potential to influence. Building on the legacy of early leaders, nursing associations have the capability to influence the cultures in which nurses function. Great strides have been made to achieve recognition of nursing as a profession and of nurses as professionals. The first half of the 20th century focused on solidifying the profession in society. The second half of the 20th century focused on expanding nursing capability to provide patient care. Which association or group of associations will step forward to identify the focus and lead the journey of the 21st century?

It is difficult to imagine a future so different from the present experience. However, change is inevitable, and forecasting the direction of change is difficult. Collaboration among nursing's professional associations to develop an awareness of forces that affect future nursing practice and the profession is well underway. The ANA continues to work with some nursing associations. In addition, many nursing associations participate in Nursing Organizations Alliance (NOA, 2011). Any nursing organization or structural component of a multidisciplinary organization may join The Alliance: NOA. The Alliance: NOA has developed its own bylaws and maintains autonomy of participating associations.

The ANA is the inclusive association with membership open to RNs in the United States, with constituent member associations (CMAs) in each state. As the U.S. member of the ICN, ANA is generally considered the representative of the nation's nurses in matters affecting the profession. ANA has the public recognition essential to shape the future. Other nursing associations, concerned with the future, also have a major role in exploring avenues to continue to shape the profession as the social and economic environment changes.

## Public Involvement

Because nursing is integral to society, the public must be involved in shaping nursing's future. Creating an agenda to inform the public and to gain support for the future is critical to advancing the profession. Nursing's influence relies on the support of every nurse and on the capability for effective communication between nursing and the public. Each nursing association has its circle of influence within health care and in the public arenas. The Internet is proving to be an effective way to communicate with many audiences and may be an important link in nursing's communication with the public, but it must be managed. As an experiment, put "nursing" in a search engine and analyze the results. The number of results is overwhelming.

---

### DISCUSSION POINT

What would an integrated professional nursing association look like? What resources would be needed to create a new association that could attract members and sustain member loyalty? Would it be beneficial for nursing to engage in a current type of Rich Study?

Associations of the future can be expected to evolve from changes in practice. In nursing, these associations would find ways to support nurses in maintaining their strong professional identity and their understanding and commitment to the profession while also supporting their capability to practice in integrated management and clinical patient care services. This association would grow from one that formerly concentrated on nursing to concentrate on building teamwork, bridging territorial domains, and recognizing issues and challenges of integrated systems.

> ### DISCUSSION POINT
>
> How can professional nursing associations develop services and programs for members that continue to support the nursing identity while also supporting participation in integrated systems?

Recreating professional associations can be considered undertaking a journey to the future. This journey begins with creating and sharing a vision of the future that is then continuously reinterpreted to evolving realities as change takes place. Once a vision is in place, other steps fall into place more naturally but not always easily.

## New Initiatives

Types of initiatives associations will undertake on this journey include evaluation of the complexity of nursing practice, needs of nurses, the environment for practice, and nursing roles in health care. Involvement of key stakeholders to grapple with key issues, make recommendations, and deliberate on action plans is important to the success. Preparing nurses and others for potential changes paves the way for action, especially when changes involve experimentation and some risk taking. Intentional outcomes should center on serving members within the constraints of the available resources through increasingly flexible and adaptable associations.

The journey to the future must be fueled by communication among members and between the association and the public. Understanding the nature and intent of change facilitates participation and support. Keeping in touch with members and the public provides both information and input about difficult decisions or radical change. If nurses examined their needs for nursing associations of the future, would they recommend radical change?

## Unification: A Radical Change?

An example of a radical change is creating a manageable unifying body that engenders cooperation of all nursing associations to identify issues for the profession as a whole and developing an action plan involving all. The proliferation of nursing associations in the 20th century might be viewed as strength or as a weakness. Each association must focus on its own mission and its role in shaping the nursing profession of the future. To create a unifying body of nursing associations, nursing must transcend some of the current and past issues. Even though the ANA is changing, nurses continue to seek and develop alternatives.

> ### DISCUSSION POINT
>
> Would it make any difference to you personally and professionally if the multitude of professional nursing associations did not exist?

Many association experts predict that radical change in professional associations is inevitable. Members of nursing's professional associations will look for evidence of performance outcomes, the effectiveness of political and legislative advocacy, member services, and collaboration to advance the profession and patient care. Demonstrating value is a key to future success of any association. This value is demonstrated by the design of future plans and initiatives, enhanced capability to meet new demands, and elegant communication on issues, change, and outcomes.

> ### DISCUSSION POINT
>
> What steps should professional nursing associations take now to develop new approaches to become associations that provide evidence-based performance reports to demonstrate value to members?

## Research Needed

Nursing would be well served by establishing a research agenda to investigate how, in the future, nurses can and should shape the future of the profession. Some starting points for developing research questions follow:

- What populations are served by nursing associations?
- To what extent are the purposes of the associations the same or different?
- What are the benefits of associations to nurses, to the profession, and to the public?
- What sustains associations over time?
- How are associations affected by societal, economic, and political forces?
- What factors influence changes such as merging or disbanding associations?
- What are the future needs of nurses in relation to developing their competency and practice standards?
- How should the profession structure itself to meet member needs?
- What role should associations have to advance the future of the profession?

To shape the future of nursing associations, there is a need to establish an evidence base for nursing associations. Associations are shaped and sustained by societal, political, and economic forces. Nursing associations are influenced by these forces and particularly by changes in health care, where change is now the norm. Research is needed to understand how these forces will affect the nursing profession and nursing associations. At issue is designing the most appropriate venue to advance nursing, to protect the public, to sustain the public recognition for the practice of nursing, and to sustain the profession. Strategies for continuing to advance the profession of nursing, whether led by associations or others, take time to formulate and longer to implement. Research is needed to inform these strategies.

---

### DISCUSSION POINT

Are professional nursing associations the appropriate venue for sustaining the profession of nursing in the future?

---

### CONCLUSIONS

Associations are integral to the cultures of work and society as we know them today. Associations serve members by engaging them in leadership initiatives and providing member services such as education and credentialing, initiatives to advance the profession, and advocacy for the profession and the health needs of the public. Legislative advocacy and policy development entail strong ties with influential persons and groups. Association work is informed by interaction with members and the public and by research. Support is facilitated by public relations to transmit information to members.

Nursing leaders are challenged by future demands and current resources. In previous millenniums, nurses with vision and passion were defining professionalism for nurses and designing strategies to achieve public recognition for nursing practice, to protect public safety and welfare, and to improve health. How will nurses, in this millennium examine their work to develop nursing, to evaluate the relevance of current definitions and strategies, and to reflect on what the nursing's profession needs in the future?

---

### FOR ADDITIONAL DISCUSSION

1. Do most RNs relate more directly to their workplace than to professional nursing associations on matters pertaining to the advancement of the nursing profession and protection of the public?

2. Some people join one or more professional associations, whereas others do not. What motivates RNs to become active in a professional association?

**3.** Should nurses, through professional associations, take responsibility for defining standards of practice and behavior? Regulation in the public domain is considered minimal. Is there a need to go beyond the public regulations?

**4.** What measures would be effective to engage every RN in activities that protect the public welfare and ensure quality nursing care in the policy and legislative arenas? Can this effort be accomplished without professional nursing associations?

**5.** What alternatives are there to professional nursing associations to provide professional nurses with opportunities to network, socialize, and grow in their profession outside the workplace

**6.** If you were to establish a professional nursing association today, what would you state as the mission and strategic direction for that association?

**7.** What research is imperative to better understand the role of professional nursing associations designed to meet member needs in the future? Who should conduct this research, and how should the findings be used?

**8.** How can nurses keep the profession alive? How can they capitalize on their resources to examine the nursing profession of the future from a global perspective to develop approaches and strategies to sustain nursing in the future? Can professional nursing associations play a part in this activity?

**9.** How can professional nursing associations become flexible and responsive to changing member values and needs and to new ways of providing members with information and resources to support their work?

**10.** Do nursing associations meet the current needs for ensuring quality of care such as through credentialing, production of information on evidence-based practice, and initiatives to advocate for the public?

**11.** Do all nurses benefit from the work of nursing associations in their practice? What are the consequences of a few nurses joining associations that produce work that benefits all nurses?

## REFERENCES

American Nurses Association. (2012). *Nursing World.* Retrieved July 12, 2012, from http://www.nursingworld.org/FunctionalMenuCategories/AboutANA/WhoWeAre/CMA

ASAE, the Center for Association Leadership. (2012). Retrieved October, 2012, from http://www.asaecenter.org

Fenwick, E. G. (1901). *The organization and registration of nurses.* Proceedings at the 3rd Quinquennia Meeting of the International Council of Nurses, Buffalo, NY.

Harper, K. A. (Ed.). (2011). *Supplement: National Organizations of the U.S.* (Encyclopedia of Associations, Vol. 3, 46th ed.). Farmington Hills, MI: Gale Cengage Learning.

Henderson, V., & Nite, G. (1978). *Principles and practice of nursing* (6th ed.). New York, NY: Macmillan.

Internal Revenue Service. (2012). *Facts about operating as an exempt organization.* Retrieved July 12, 2012, from http://www.irs.gov

McKee, J., & McKee, T. (2008). *The new breed, understanding and equipping the 21st century volunteer.* Loveland, CO: Group.

National League for Nursing. (2011). *Homepage.* Retrieved July 12, 2012, from www.nln.org/

Nursing and healthcare directories on: The nurse friendly nursing associations, organizations–National, state, local.

Nursing World. Retrieved October, 2012, from http://www.nursingworld.org

Principled Innovation. (2011). *Imagine a more vibrant future.* Retrieved November 22, 2011, from http://www.principledinnovation.com/

Raymond Rich Associates report on the structure of organized nursing. (1946). *American Journal of Nursing, 46*(10), 648–661.

Sigma Theta Tau International, Honor Society of Nursing. (2011). *Homepage*. Retrieved July 12, 2012, from http://www.nursingsociety.org/default.aspx

Spaulding, E. K., & Notter, L. (1965). *Professional nursing*. Philadelphia, PA: Lippincott.

Nursing Organizations Alliance. (2012). *Home page*. Retrieved October 1, 2012, from http://www.nursing-alliance.org/

Wikipedia. (n.d.). *Professional body*. Retrieved October, 2012, from http://en.wikipedia.org/wiki/Professional_Associations

## BIBLIOGRAPHY

Anderson, T. L. (2011). The foundational documents of professional nursing. *Nebraska Nurse, 44*(2), 9–10.

Byrne, M., Schroeter, K., & Mower, J. (2010). Perioperative specialty certification: The CNOR as evidence for magnet excellence. *AORN Journal, 91*(5), 618–622.

Eldredge, J. D., Morley, S. K., Hendrix, I. C., Carr, R. D., & Bengtson, J. (2012). Library and informatics skills competencies statements from major health professional associations. *Medical Reference Services Quarterly, 31*(1), 34–44.

Evaluation and implementation of clinical practice guidelines: A guidance document from the American professional wound care association. (2010). *Advance Skin Wound Care, 23*(4) 161–168.

Hill, K. S. (2011). Nursing leadership in professional organizations. *Journal of Nursing Administration, 41*(4), 153–155.

Hobbs, J. L. (2009). Defining nursing practice: The ANA social policy statement 1980–1983. *Advances in Nursing Science, 32*(1), 3–18.

Lukes, E., & Moore, P. V. (2010). The professional association and practice excellence. *AAOHN Journal, 58*(2), 47–49.

23rd annual survey of state boards of nursing and selected national professional certifying boards/associations. (2012). *Journal of Continuing Education in Nursing, 43*(1), 4–11.

Matthews, J. H. (2012). Role of professional organizations in advocating for the nursing profession. *Online Journal of Issues in Nursing, 17*(1), 3.

Macdonald, J. A., Edwards, N., Davies, B., Marck, P., & Guernsey, J. R. (2012). Priority setting and policy advocacy by nursing associations: A scoping review and implications using a socio-ecological whole systems lens. *Health Policy, 107*(1), 31–43.

McKenzie, H. (2010). Rekindle your passion for the nursing profession and home healthcare and hospice specialty. *Homehealthcare Nurse, 28*(2), 122–123.

Oncology Nursing Society, Association of Oncology Social Work, and National Association of Social Workers. (2010). Oncology Nursing Society, Association of Oncology Social Work, and National Association of Social Workers joint position on the role of oncology nursing and oncology social work in patient navigation. *Oncology Nursing Forum, 37*(3), 251–252.

Perlis, C., & Shannon, N. (2012). Role of professional organizations in setting and enforcing ethical norms. *Clinical Dermatology, 30*(2), 156–159.

Pierce, L. L. (2011). Invest in the future: Become a volunteer in your professional nursing organization. *Rehabilitation Nursing: The Official Journal of the Association of Rehabilitation Nurses, 36*(5), 191–195.

Resha, C. (2009). School nurse competencies. How can they assist to ensure high-quality care in the school setting? *NASN School Nurse, 24*(6), 240–241.

Sawin, K. J., Lewin, L. C., Niederhauser V. P., Brady, M. A., Jones, D., Butz, A.,…Trent, C. A. (2012). A survey of NAPNAP members' clinical and professional research priorities. *Journal of Pediatric Health Care: Official Publication of National Association of Pediatric Nurse Associates & Practitioners, 26*(1), 5–15.

Shekleton, M. E., Preston, J. C., & Good, L. E. (2010). Growing leaders in a professional membership organization. *Journal of Nursing Management, 18*(6), 662–668.

Sportsman, S., Wieck, K. L., Yoder-Wise, P. S., Light, K. M., & Jordan, C. (2010). Creating tomorrow's leaders today: The emerging nurse leaders program of the Texas nurses association. *Journal of Continuing Education in Nursing, 41*(6), 259–266.

Vioral, A. N. (2011). Filling the gaps: Immersing student nurses in specialty nursing and professional associations. *Journal of Continuing Education in Nursing, 42*(9), 415–420.

Walston, S. L., & Khaliq, A. A. (2012). Factors affecting the value of professional association affiliation. *Health Care Management Review, 37*(2), 122–131.

Your guide to certification. What you need to know to pursue professional recognition. (2011). *American Journal of Nursing, 111*(Suppl. 1), 22–34.

Yoder-Wise, P. S. (2010). The future of nursing begins now. *Journal of Continuing Education in Nursing, 41*(12), 533.

*Note*: Page numbers followed by *f*, *t* and *b* indicate figures, tables and boxes, respectively.